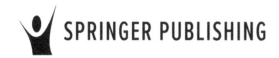 SPRINGER PUBLISHING

MW01097539

GET THE MOST FROM YOUR BOOK
Access your included eBook and educator resources today!

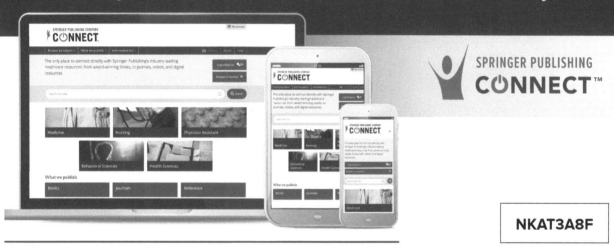

SPRINGER PUBLISHING
CONNECT™

NKAT3A8F

eBook Access

Your print purchase of *Textbook of Adult-Gerontology Primary Care Nursing* includes **online access via Springer Publishing Connect**™ to increase accessibility, portability, and searchability.

Insert the code at https://connect.springerpub.com/content/book/978-0-8261-8414-6 today!

Educator Resource Access

Let us do some of the heavy lifting to create an engaging classroom experience with a variety of educator resources included in your textbooks SUCH AS:

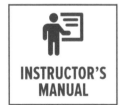
INSTRUCTOR'S MANUAL

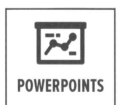
POWERPOINTS

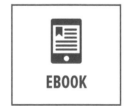
EBOOK

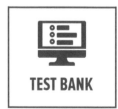
TEST BANK

Visit **https://connect.springerpub.com/** and look for the **"Show Supplementary"** button on your **book homepage** to see what is available to you! First time using Springer Publishing Connect?

Email **textbook@springerpub.com** to create an account and start unlocking valuable resources.

Textbook of Adult-Gerontology Primary Care Nursing

Debra J. Hain, PhD, APRN, AGPCNP-BC, FAAN, FAANP, FNKF, is a tenured professor, Interim DNP Director, MSN Co-Coordinator: AGNP Concentration at Florida Atlantic University (FAU), Christine E. Lynn College of Nursing (CEL), and a nurse practitioner (NP) seeing patients with or at risk of chronic kidney disease (CKD) at a free clinic serving a low-resource, uninsured community and at FAU, CEL Community Health Center, and HANDS of St. Lucie County. Dr. Hain retired from Cleveland Clinic Florida, Department of Nephrology, in 2019 after 25 years of service. She has more than 35 years of experience as a nurse and 20 years of that as an NP. Most of her expertise is in nephrology and the care of older adults. More recently, she has focused on palliative care for those with noncancer life-limiting illness after working as a hospice NP for many years. Dr. Hain received an associate degree in Nursing from Gateway Technical College in Kenosha Wisconsin; a Bachelor of Arts in Management and Communication from Concordia University in Mequon; Bachelor of Nursing from Florida International University; MSN Gerontological Nurse Practitioner/Clinical Nurse Specialist, Doctor of Nursing Science, Doctor of Philosophy, and post–master's certificate in Adult NP from FAU, CEL. Dr. Hain has received numerous awards including the Helen Feigenbaum Award for the Promotion of Excellence in Nephrology Nursing, Nephrology Nurse Researcher Award, and Nephrology Nurse Competence in Aging Award, all from the American Nephrology Nurses Association (ANNA). Other awards include Excellence in Research from the Gerontological Advanced Practice Nurse Association, the Tim Poole Memorial Award for Outstanding Nephrology Advanced Practitioner from the National Kidney Foundation, and the DAISY Faculty Award and Scholar of the Year, both from FAU. In addition, Dr. Hain was awarded Ronald and Elizabeth Blake Distinguished Professor from 2016 to 2020. Her research interests are developing strategies aimed at improving the health of adults with CKD and diabetes, structural racism in rural Black communities, palliative care in those with CKD, and reducing hospitalizations in residents of nursing homes. Currently, Dr, Hain is collaborating on research and educational projects with nursing faculty at Thammasat University and RBAC University in Thailand. She has published numerous manuscripts and is often invited to present at national and international conferences and educational events on the care of adults with CKD and, more recently, palliative care. Dr. Hain mainly teaches DNP courses and serves as an advisor for AGNP course curriculum. Dr. Hain has been the advisor for more than 30 DNP clinical projects, as well as several PhD students' comprehensive examinations and dissertation committees. She continues to be active in the ANNA, the American Society of Nephrology, and the American Nurse Practitioners. Dr. Hain is a Fellow in the American Academy of Nursing, the American Association of Nurse Practitioners, and the National Kidney Foundation.

Deb Bakerjian, PhD, APRN, FAAN, FAANP, FGSA, is a clinical professor at the Betty Irene Moore School of Nursing at the University of California (UC), Davis. Her education and research interests focus on patient safety, quality improvement, interprofessional team-based care, geriatrics, and expanding the workforce in rural and underserved areas. Over the past decade, she has taught geriatrics, patient safety, quality improvement, master's seminars, and leadership at UC Davis. Prior to coming to academia, she was a head nurse in ICUs for several years before becoming a nurse practitioner (NP). In 1998, she started an NP-owned practice for NPs to provide care to nursing home residents, one of the first such practices in California. Dr. Bakerjian earned a Doctor of Philosophy in Nursing in 2006 and a Master of Science in Nursing in 1992, both from UC San Francisco School of Nursing, and a Family Nurse Practitioner certificate from UC Davis in 1989. She received her ADN degree from Evergreen Valley College and a baccalaureate in Health Services Administration. Her doctoral study, "Utilization of Nurse Practitioners in Nursing Homes: A Comparison with Physicians," received the Distinguished Dissertation Award from UC San Francisco. She was a Pat Archbold Predoctoral Scholar and a Claire M. Fagin Postdoctoral Fellow at UCSF where she was also an assistant adjunct professor. She was also a Gordon & Betty Moore Postdoctoral Fellow at UC Davis in 2009 before becoming an assistant professor. Dr. Bakerjian has received a variety of awards over the years; most recently, she received the Dean's Award for Inclusion Excellence in 2016 from UC Davis Health, the Distinguished Educator in Gerontological Nursing in 2019 from the National Hartford Center for Gerontological Nursing Excellence in recognition for her teaching, and the Dean's Award for Research Excellence in 2021 from the Betty Irene Moore School of Nursing. Currently, Dr. Bakerjian is the co–editor in chief for the AHRQ Patient Safety Network (PSNet/WebM&M) and the co–principal investigator for CalQualityCare, a nursing home quality comparison website. She is also the director of four HRSA funded grants: SPLICE, Advanced NP PRACTICE-NP Residency Program, PA PROMISE, and PHN ENTRUST, all of which are focused on workforce development. She is also working on the DNP course development and a Graduate Academic Certificate on Quality and Safety. Dr. Bakerjian is active in several state and national organizations associated with older adults, quality improvement, and patient safety. Most recently, she has written extensively about the impact of poor staffing and COVID-19 in nursing homes. She is a Fellow in the American Academy of Nursing, the American Association of Nurse Practitioners, and the Gerontological Society of America.

Textbook of Adult-Gerontology Primary Care Nursing

Evidence-Based Patient Care for Adolescents to Older Adults

Debra J. Hain, PhD, APRN, AGPCNP-BC, FAAN, FAANP, FNKF
Professor (tenured) Director DNP Program, Graduate Co-Coordinator AGNP Concentration
NP Volunteer at FAU Community Health Center
Florida Atlantic University, Christine E. Lynn College of Nursing
AGNP for Mobile Medical Associates
Stuart, Florida

Deb Bakerjian, PhD, APRN, FAAN, FAANP, FGSA
Clinical Professor
Director, Advanced NP PRACTICE - NP Residency Program
Co-Editor-in-Chief, AHRQ Patient Safety Network (PSNet)
Betty Irene Moore School of Nursing, University of California, Davis
Sacramento, California

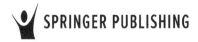 SPRINGER PUBLISHING

Springer Publishing Company, LLC
11 West 42nd Street, New York, NY 10036
www.springerpub.com
connect.springerpub.com/

Acquisitions Editor: Elizabeth Nieginski
Compositor: Amnet

ISBN: 978-0-8261-8413-9
ebook ISBN: 978-0-8261-8414-6
DOI: 10.1891/9780826184146

SUPPLEMENTS:
Instructor Materials:

Qualified instructors may request supplements by emailing textbook@springerpub.com

Instructor's Manual: 978-0-8261-6327-1
PowerPoints: 978-0-8261-8415-3
Test Bank: 978-0-8261-8416-0 (available via Respondus)
Image Bank: 978-0-8261-6327-1

22 23 24 25 / 5 4 3 2 1

The author and the publisher of this Work have made every effort to use sources believed to be reliable to provide information that is accurate and compatible with the standards generally accepted at the time of publication. Because medical science is continually advancing, our knowledge base continues to expand. Therefore, as new information becomes available, changes in procedures become necessary. We recommend that the reader always consult current research and specific institutional policies before performing any clinical procedure or delivering any medication. The author and publisher shall not be liable for any special, consequential, or exemplary damages resulting, in whole or in part, from the readers' use of, or reliance on, the information contained in this book. The publisher has no responsibility for the persistence or accuracy of URLs for external or third-party Internet websites referred to in this publication and does not guarantee that any content on such websites is, or will remain, accurate or appropriate.

Library of Congress Cataloging-in-Publication Data

Names: Hain, Debra J., editor. | Bakerjian, Deb, editor.
Title: Textbook of adult-gerontology primary care nursing : evidence-based
  care for patients across the lifespan / edited by Debra J. Hain and Deb
  Bakerjian.
Description: New York, NY : Springer Publishing Company, [2023] | Includes
  bibliographical references and index.
Identifiers: LCCN 2021047110 (print) | LCCN 2021047111 (ebook) | ISBN
  9780826184139 (paperback) | ISBN 9780826184146 (ebook)
Subjects: MESH: Primary Care Nursing | Geriatric Nursing |
  Aging—physiology | Evidence-Based Nursing
Classification: LCC RC954 (print) | LCC RC954 (ebook) | NLM WY 101 | DDC
  618.97/0231—dc23
LC record available at https://lccn.loc.gov/2021047110
LC ebook record available at https://lccn.loc.gov/2021047111

Contact sales@springerpub.com to receive discount rates on bulk purchases.

Publisher's Note: **New and used products purchased from third-party sellers are not guaranteed for quality, authenticity, or access to any included digital components.**

Printed in the United States of America.

For years I have been an adult-gerontology nurse practitioner who has been blessed by having many influential people in my life. I would like to first thank my mentors Dr. Theresa Touhy, Patricia Liehr, and Ruth Tappen. They have mentored me as I became and continued to grow as a scholar and educator. I want to thank Cleveland Clinic Florida, Department of Nephrology for all the opportunities to learn and gain experience as an expert in the care of adults with CKD. In addition, I want to thank my students and graduates of FAU CEL who inspire me every day. I owe much of my success to my family, my mother, father, stepmother Jody, sisters, and niece Stephanie. Most important are my children, Chris, Jeremy, Eric, Ashley, and Donald; their spouses, Kelly, Asuka, and Kevin; and my wonderful grandchildren, Abbey (her spouse, Elijah), Emily, Molly, Mackenzie, and Kevin Jr., who give me the energy to make a difference.

Debra J. Hain

I dedicate this book to my loving and consistently supportive husband, Stephen; he is my partner and my rock and is always willing to read my material and provide feedback. I also dedicate this to my four adult children, Jeff, Melanie, Patrick, and Matthew, who have supported me through my prolonged educational journey, my years of practice and on-call time, and now in my academic career. They have been steadfast in their enthusiasm as I pursued my dreams of making a difference in the lives of my patients, students, and colleagues throughout my 27 years as a nurse practitioner and 45 years as a registered nurse. I want to particularly thank Drs. Charlene Harrington and Jeanie Kayser-Jones for mentoring me as a doctoral student; they modeled academic nursing, research, and teaching at its best and I continue to work hard to live up to their standards. I also dedicate this book to my exceptional colleagues, staff, and students at the Betty Irene Moore School of Nursing at UC Davis who inspire me to keep improving.

Deb Bakerjian

Contents

Contributors

Vilija Abrute, MSN, APRN, ACNP-BC
Advanced Practice Provider
Department of Neurological Surgery
University of California Davis Health
Sacramento, California

Joshua Anderson, MS, PA-C
Physician Assistant Leadership and Learning Academy
(PALLA) Fellow, 2020–2021 Cohort
University of Maryland, Baltimore
Baltimore, Maryland

Demetra E. Antimisiaris, PharmD, BCGP, FASCP
Associate Professor
Assistant Dean, Continuing Medical Education
Director, Frazier Polypharmacy Program
University of Louisville
Schools of Medicine and Public Health
Louisville, Kentucky

Berit Bagley, RN, MSN, CDCES, BC-ADM
Diabetes Nurse Specialist
UC Davis Medical Center
Sacramento, California

Deb Bakerjian, PhD, APRN, FAAN, FAANP, FGSA
Clinical Professor
Director, Advanced NP PRACTICE -
NP Residency Program
Co-Editor-in-Chief, AHRQ Patient
Safety Network (PSNet)
Betty Irene Moore School of Nursing
University of California, Davis
Sacramento, California

Elise Buser, BSc
Junior Specialist
Department of Medical Microbiology and Immunology
School of Medicine
University of California, Davis
Davis, California

Deborah Chapa, PhD, ACNP-BC, FAANP, ACHPN
Program Director DNP
Associate Professor
Marshall University
School of Nursing
Huntington, West Virginia

Maureen Craig, DNP candidate, RN, CNS, CNN, APHN-BC
Clinical Nurse Specialist, Wellness Ambassador,
Mindfulness and Yoga Teacher
University of California Davis Health
Sacramento, California

Timothy W. Cutler, PharmD, DPLA
Assistant Chief of Pharmacy, Ambulatory Clinical
Services
Clinical Professor of Pharmacy, UCSF School of
Pharmacy
University of California Davis Health
Sacramento, California

Jennifer J. Edwards, MS, RN, CHSE
Assistant Clinical Professor
Betty Irene Moore School of Nursing
University of California, Davis
Sacramento, California

Damian Eker, DNP, APRN, GNP
Adjunct Professor
Florida Atlantic University School of Nursing
Boca Raton, Florida

Diane Esposito, PhD, APRN, PMHCNS-BC
Associate Professor, Lead Faculty PMHNP Track
PBA School of Nursing, DNP Program
Palm Beach Atlantic University
West Palm Beach, Florida

Rhonda Goodman, PhD, APRN, FNP-BC, AHN-BC, FAANP, FAAN
Family Nurse Practitioner
Associate Professor of Nursing (Retired)
Christine E. Lynn College of Nursing
Florida Atlantic University
Boca Raton, Florida

Debra J. Hain, PhD, ARPN, AGPCNP-BC, FAAN, FAANP, FNKF
Professor (tenured) Director DNP Program, Graduate
Co-Coordinator AGNP Concentration
NP Volunteer at FAU Community Health Center
Florida Atlantic University, Christine E. Lynn College of Nursing
AGNP for Mobile Medical Associates
Stuart, Florida

Nicole Hansen, MSN, RN, NEA-BC
Manager
Health Management & Education
University of California Davis Health
Sacramento, California

Nancy Harris, DNP, APRN
Assistant Professor
Christine E. Lynn College of Nursing
Florida Atlantic University
Boca Raton, Florida

Kathi Voege Harvey, DNP, FNP, APRN, NHDP
Adjunct Faculty
Christine E. Lynn College of Nursing
Florida Atlantic University
Boca Raton, Florida

Shelly L. Henderson, PhD
Clinical Psychologist and Associate Professor
Director of Behavioral Health, Family & Community Medicine
UC Davis School of Medicine
Sacramento, California

Tracian Kelly Hershorin, DNP, APRN, FNP-BC, PMHNP-BC
Assistant Professor and FNP Coordinator
Christine E. Lynn College of Nursing
Florida Atlantic University
Boca Raton, Florida

Gerald Kayingo, PhD, MBA, PA-C, DFAAPA
Assistant Dean, Executive Director and Professor
Physician Assistant Leadership and Learning Academy
Graduate School, University of Maryland
Baltimore, Maryland

Vasco Deon Kidd, DHSc, MPH, MS, PA-C
Associate Clinical Professor, Dept. of Orthopedic Surgery
Director of Advanced Practice Providers Program
University of California, Irvine (UCI Health)
Orange, California

Beth M. King, PhD, APRN, PMHNP-BC
Associate Professor
Christine E. Lynn College of Nursing
Florida Atlantic University
Boca Raton, Florida

Holly Kirkland-Kyhn, PhD, FNP, GNP, CWCN, FAANP
Director of Wound Care
UC Davis Medical Center
Sacramento, California

Kathleen Klein, MSW, CCM
Social Work Case Manager
Ambulatory Case Management
University of California Davis Health
Sacramento, California

Paul MacDowell, Pharm D, BCPS
Medication Safety Officer
University of California Davis Health
Sacramento, California

Natalie Murphy, PhD, APRN, FNP-BC
Director, School of Nursing
Associate Professor
Murphy Deming College of Health Sciences
Mary Baldwin University
Staunton, Virginia

Noelle Nelson, PharmD, MSPH, BCACP
Clinical Pharmacist, Ambulatory Care
UC Davis Health, Department of Pharmacy Services
Sacramento, California

Amy A. Nichols, EdD, RN, CNS, CHSE, ANEF
Associate Dean for Academics and Clinical Professor
Betty Irene Moore School of Nursing
University of California, Davis
Sacramento, California

Andrea Quinonez, PhD, MSN, RN, PHN
Quality Improvement Healthcare Specialist
Health Management and Education
University of California Davis Health
Sacramento, California

Humberto Reinoso, PhD, FNP-BC, ENP-BC
Assistant Professor and Nurse Practitioner Coordinator
Georgia Baptist College of Nursing
Mercer University
Atlanta, Georgia

Dianne Sandy, MD, FACP
Nephrologist
Cleveland Clinic Florida, Department of Hypertension
and Nephrology
Weston, Florida

Sumathi Sankaran-Walters, MBBS, PhD
Associate Adjunct Professor
Dept of Medical Microbiology and Immunology
UC Davis School of Medicine
Betty Irene Moore School of Nursing
University of California, Davis
Sacramento, California

Kathryn Sexson, PhD, APRN, FNP-BC
Program Director – Family Nurse Practitioner Program
Associate Director for Education – Family Caregiving
Institute
Assistant Clinical Professor
Betty Irene Moore School of Nursing
University of California, Davis
Sacramento, California

Sima Sitaula, DNP, APRN, FNP-C, BC-ADM
Nurse Practitioner Endocrinology, Diabetes &
Metabolism.
UC Davis Medical Center
Sacramento, California

Cynthia A. Skillsky, BSN, RN
Manager
Ambulatory Case Management
University of California Davis Health
Sacramento, California

Hannah Spero, MSN, APRN, NP-C
Nurse Practitioner, Departments of Emergency Medicine
and Geriatrics, UC Davis Health
Assistant Clinical Professor
Betty Irene Moore School of Nursing
University of California, Davis
Sacramento, California

Cathy M. St. Pierre, PhD, APRN, FNP-BC, FAANP
Associate Chief Nurse – Research
VA Bedford Healthcare System
Bedford, Massachusetts

Shannan Takhar, PharmD, BCACP
Ambulatory Care Clinical Pharmacist
University of California Davis Health
Sacramento, California

**Charity L. Tan, MSN, ACNP-BC, CDCES,
BC-ADM**
Acute Care Nurse Practitioner
Inpatient Glycemic Team
Division of Endocrinology, Diabetes and Metabolism
UC Davis Medical Center
Sacramento, California

Ashley Trask, PharmD
Clinical Supervisor, Medication Policy & Safety
University of California Davis Health
Sacramento, California

John R. Van Auker, PA-C, MSMT
Physician Assistant Family Practice
Sutter Medical Group
Auburn, California

**Laura L. Van Auker, DNP, APRN, FNP-BC, MSN,
SN-C**
Assistant Clinical Professor Health Sciences
Betty Irene Moore School of Nursing
University of California, Davis
Sacramento, California

**Justin M. Waryold, DNP, RN, ANP-C, ACNP-BC,
GS-C, CNE, FAANP**
Assistant Professor and Assistant Dean for Nursing
Education
SUNY Upstate Medical University
College of Nursing
Syracuse, New York

**Gordon H. Worley, MSN, RN, FNP-C,
ENP-C, FAWM**
Assistant Clinical Professor
Betty Irene Moore School of Nursing
University of California, Davis
Nurse Practitioner
Disaster Medical Assistance Team California-11
National Disaster Medical System, U.S. Department of
Health and Human Services
Sacramento, California

Foreword

The National Academy of Medicine *Future of Nursing 2020–2030*[1] issued a clarion call for nurses to act now to "improve the health and well-being of the nation." The ever-shrinking access to primary care, inequities in care delivery, increasing physician shortages, an aging population with complex healthcare needs, high degrees of comorbidity complicated by sociodemographic factors, and increasing numbers of persons with serious mental illness all demand that nurses be prepared and mobilized to support individuals' positive engagement with healthcare systems. For over five decades nurse practitioners have responded to challenges in healthcare by leading and collaborating with other disciplines to close the healthcare gap. They have provided primary healthcare, care coordination, health education, and advocacy, which have yielded positive health outcomes and patient/family experiences of care.

Their practice, whether at the point of care with patients and families, teaching students, conducting research, advancing policy, or leading healthcare systems, has earned nurse practitioners the respect and trust of the public. Adult-gerontology nurse practitioners (AGNPs), including the editors and contributing authors of this textbook, have been among those leaders and continue to be at the forefront of needed change in primary care across settings.

The continued trust of the public is contingent upon the competence and compassion of AGNPs. A critical way to ensure competency is to be informed of what constitutes best practice. *Textbook of Adult-Gerontology Primary Care Nursing: Evidence-Based Patient Care for Adolescents to Older Adults* was written for this purpose. Each of the 28 chapters is written by experts in the field, who bring years of experience working in primary care, and together offer a robust compendium to guide AGNP practice. I am particularly impressed by the depth and breadth of this body of work. The highly respected authors provide up-to-date information that supports not only clinical efficacy but also person-centered care, operational effectiveness, professional development, and leadership.

In my own experience, I have been challenged to find ways to work with administrators and staff to integrate best practices into the daily operations of the care setting. I was thrilled to see the content that focuses on quality improvement, patient safety, interprofessional collaboration, care coordination, and other content that supports the role of the AGNP as clinical leaders and change agents. Too often, we assume that the skills associated with these role functions come easily and/or do not need to be explicated and nurtured. The authors in this text give these topics the attention that they deserve, with clear, insightful guidance and, importantly, the evidence base. The chapters that address roles (including during disasters!), settings of care, billing, and medication use address salient issues that will help the fledgling AGNP to hit the ground running and the seasoned AGNP to keep current.

The clinical content is presented efficiently. The experts share the latest research and guidelines for clinical practice in adolescents and older adults, and for common health conditions. They also bring the content to life using actual case studies that skillfully illustrate best practice. A wide audience, including students, faculty, and AGNP clinicians, will find this text instructive, practical, and engaging.

AGNPs have an enormous responsibility when providing care to patients and families in this rapidly changing healthcare environment with its increasing regulatory requirements, variable staffing levels, and unpredictable reimbursement. AGNPs also have an amazing opportunity to positively change the daily experiences and health of those we serve. I believe that *Textbook of Adult-Gerontology Primary Care Nursing: Evidence-Based Patient Care for Adolescents to Older Adults* will help us meet those responsibilities and capitalize on our opportunities, with a well-deserved place in the libraries of many, many AGNPs across the country, as an authoritative source and reliable companion.

Marie Boltz, PhD, GNP-BC, FGSA, FAAN
Elouise Ross Eberly and
Robert Eberly Endowed Professor
Toss and Carol Nese College of Nursing
Penn State University

REFERENCE

1. Wakefield MK, Williams DR, Le Menestrel S, Flaubert JL, eds. *National Academy of Medicine; National Academies of Sciences, Engineering, and Medicine; Committee on the Future of Nursing 2020–2030.*

Preface

This much-needed AGNP-specific textbook provides comprehensive, evidence-based practice approaches to both common and complex health issues AGNPs may face in primary care. The editors' foresight in developing a textbook that emphasizes holistic, person-, and family-centered care for managing adolescent to older adult patients made this textbook a reality. Many of the chapters are written by practicing clinicians; their expertise is an essential contribution that integrates the best available evidence with a current clinical practice application and a focus on high-quality, cost-efficient, person/family-centered, safe care.

An innovative feature of this textbook is the way it is organized with five distinct sections that incorporate the entirety of the AGNP role to include fundamental concepts of AGNP practice, AGNP practice in various primary care practice settings, special health conditions for adolescents and older adults, practice-wide systems management, and disease-specific conditions. For example, unique to this textbook are chapters that focus on important practice issues, such as those in Part II illustrating the AGNP role in different primary care settings, and in Part IV, preparing the AGNP for practice in which the student will learn about billing, coding, and documentation. Many providers anticipate an AGNP to have the basic skills of billing when they are hired, so this chapter prepares the AGNP to have basic information that can be made more specific to their practice. Also unique is the focus on patient safety and quality improvement, starting not only with a chapter dedicated to these topics but also with these skills applied in the chapters on common health conditions.

As mentioned, the book is organized into five parts as outlined next, encompassing all of the aspects of AGNP care the editors thought were essential for students to know.

Part I: Fundamental Concepts in Adult-Gerontology Nurse Practitioner (AGNP) Care contains fundamental concepts such as healthy aging, person-centered care,

patient safety and quality improvement, interprofessional teams/team-based care, care coordination, and promoting wellness in AGNPs. One chapter emphasizes that it is essential that AGNPs care for themselves so that they can provide the best care possible to adolescents and older adults.

Part II: Providing Adult-Gerontology Nursing Care is focused on the AGNP role across healthcare settings, concepts in palliative and end-of-life care, and the role of AGNPs in disasters. So often we are called on to assist in disasters or we need to prepare our patients and families to be safe during a disaster. The inclusion of AGNPs' role in disasters is an important and unique aspect of this textbook.

Part III: Population Health examines the explicit health issues for older adults and adolescents that are exclusive to those two populations and essential to their care.

Part IV: Preparation for Practice provides a unique view of ensuring that AGNPs are ready for practice and the practice environment. The chapters include guidance on performing comprehensive screening and physical examinations, comprehensive medication review, and billing, coding, and documentation that prepares AGNPs to care for patients in the practice environment.

Part V: Common Health Conditions includes chapters that focus on common health conditions the AGNP may encounter in primary care no matter the setting. Each chapter provides an overview of anatomy and physiology, pathophysiology, common presentation of illness, diagnostic approach, evidence-based interventions, and patient education. Safety and clinical pearls are also included as well as one or more case studies to facilitate application to practice.

Debra J. Hain
Deb Bakerjian

Acknowledgments

We are grateful for the professional guidance of our Springer Team in facilitating the compilation of this textbook. We could not have done this without the expert guidance of Elizabeth Nieginski who brought the two of us together, Hannah Hicks who supported us through each editorial step, and Taylor Ball who provided input on the content development.

We also want to acknowledge the expert faculty and practicing clinicians who have contributed to the content of the textbook as well as the administrative staff who supported the coordination of meetings and communication. As with so many things, it takes a village!

Debra J. Hain
Deb Bakerjian

I am so grateful for Dr. Deb Bakerjian, my co-editor, for her expertise and dedication to providing AGNP and other NP students with evidence-based content to enhance their education and prepare for practice. Without her this book would have never become a reality. I would like to acknowledge all the authors in this textbook for their hard work and commitment to follow this through to publication.

Debra J. Hain

I want to acknowledge my family, friends, and many colleagues for their support in this endeavor that lasted well over a year. I invited many professional colleagues to contribute to the content in this textbook; not even one turned me down. In fact, they responded with enthusiasm, pouring their hearts and souls into the chapters. I am forever grateful for their expertise and willingness to make this the excellent textbook it has become. I also sincerely want to thank my co-editor, Dr. Debra J. Hain, for welcoming me into the fold somewhat late in the process to work on this textbook. She graciously embraced me and allowed me to feel an equal partner! We made quite a team!

Deb Bakerjian

PART I

Fundamental Concepts in Adult-Gerontology Nurse Practitioner (AGNP) Care

CHAPTER 1

Healthy Aging Across the Continuum

Debra J. Hain and Deb Bakerjian

LEARNING OBJECTIVES

At the conclusion of this chapter, the learner will be able to:

➤ Define healthy aging.
➤ Discuss life-span development.
➤ Present evidence-based health promotion strategies.
➤ Discuss the importance of Healthy People 2030 in guiding health promotion.
➤ Describe the health issues informal caregivers may experience.

INTRODUCTION

Healthy aging is defined by the World Health Organization (WHO) as "the process of developing and maintaining the functional ability that enables well-being in older age."[1] It requires that individuals adopt a set of behaviors and life habits that will help them engage in healthy behaviors that support well-being as they age. These behaviors start at adolescence and continue throughout the life span. Many factors can impact healthy aging, from the individual's genetics to the environment to the social determinants of health. Ultimately, the goal is to maintain optimal physical and mental function and a sense of well-being throughout life. This chapter reviews a brief epidemiology of aging, life-span development theories, health promotion, and Healthy People 2030 goals to provide the adult-gerontology nurse practitioner (AGNP) with a strong grasp of healthy aging from which they can provide person-centered care and assist their patients in optimizing health and well-being. In addition, it is essential to consider the important role informal caregivers have and the health conditions they may experience.

HEALTHY AGING

Healthy aging can be simply defined as embracing a set of behaviors and habits that promote health and well-being across the life continuum.[1] Healthy aging encompasses the goal of living a long and healthy life, free from serious disease, and maintaining optimal function.

Healthy aging can be impacted by a constellation of issues including the environment and exposure to health risks from air pollution and unsafe water, social determinants of health, and access to educational opportunities, safe work environments, and lifelong preventative healthcare.

The National Institute on Aging emphasizes a healthy diet[2] and physical activity[3] as two important actions that people must take to optimize health. Other actions include staying on top of health screening and maintenance such as immunizations and cancer screenings as well as managing risk factors for diseases. Healthy aging really starts when a person is of the age to begin to be accountable for their own lifestyle; for most people, that is somewhere during their adolescent years. Healthy aging is an active and ongoing process. It requires individuals to be cognizant of their health and take early steps to maintain health by developing healthy eating habits and integrating regular exercise into their daily and weekly routines.

Noncommunicable disease resulting in death affects about 41 million people each year.[4] The leading causes of death are heart disease, cancer, and diabetes. Many older adults have one or more of these chronic diseases that may have an insidious onset and are often identified during a primary care health screening. In younger adults, it is important to identify signs of pending chronic disease and intervene early to prevent future health problems.[5] Having chronic health conditions at a younger age is not related to the normal aging process but more often is related to unhealthy behaviors, although, in some situations, there is a genetic association. Major risk factors for chronic disease are smoking, a lack of exercise, and poor nutrition; active participation in healthy behaviors can reduce the risk of stroke, cardiovascular disease, and type 2 diabetes mellitus by 80%.[4] Prevention and healthy promotion strategies are important for healthy aging even in the presence of chronic disease.

Nutrition

The prevalence of obesity is increasing globally and is typically caused by a combination of an unhealthy diet and a lack of exercise. As people live longer there will be more older adults who are obese.[6] Healthy nutrition starts at a young age, and habits often are established in adolescent years. Despite this, at any time in a person's life, they can develop poor dietary habits or choose to change from an unhealthy diet to a healthier one. Physical inactivity also contributes to obesity and can be impacted by injuries or chronic diseases such as osteoarthritis, preventing older adults from being active. As stated earlier, healthy aging includes living healthy active years; however, the presence of one or more chronic diseases can also influence older adults' nutritional status as well as their physical function. Obesity is common in the United States, which ranks 12th in the world for obesity. In 2017 to 2018, the prevalence of obesity was 42.4% in the United States.[7] Even though an older adult is obese, they may still be frail, which we associate more often with malnutrition and weight loss.[8] Obesity in the older adult population is thought to contribute to the age-related decline in physical function, along with the many associated chronic diseases the obese older adults may also have.

Nutritional frailty describes a state that is often seen in vulnerable older adults. This is a state in which the person has unintentional weight loss, a loss of muscle mass and strength, and an essential loss of physiologic reserves, which increases the risk of frailty and disability. Frailty is a medical syndrome that involves vulnerability to stress or acute illness that results in negative outcomes from a new or coexisting illness. Frailty is further discussed in Chapter 10.

Adequate nutrition is essential for adolescents who experience rapid physiological, sexual, neurological, and behavioral growth. Poor nutrition can lead to delayed and stunted growth, impaired organ remodeling, and iron-deficiency anemia.[9] The growing concerns regarding childhood obesity and the impact on immediate and long-term health status warrant attention in primary care. There are many reasons for inadequate nutrition in people of all ages. One reason is related to food insecurity, which appears to be more prevalent during this pandemic.[10]

Food Insecurity

The AGNP should pay attention to risk factors for frailty and the physical, psychological, and social reasons why an individual may be experiencing food insecurity. *Food insecurity*, as defined by the U.S. Department of Agriculture (USDA), is when access to adequate

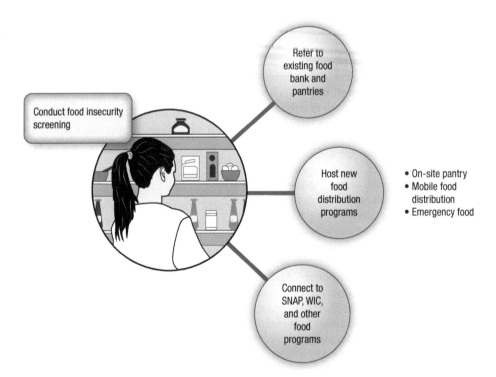

Figure 1.1: Identifying food insecurity and possible interventions

SNAP, Supplemental Nutrition Assistance Program; WIC, Special Supplemental Nutrition Program for Women, Infants, and Children.

Source: Data from Hunger + Health. Addressing food insecurity in health care settings. n.d. https://hungerandhealth .feedingamerica.org/explore-our-work/community-health-care-partnerships/addressing-food-insecurity-in-health-care -settings

food is limited by a lack of money or other resources. This is a pervasive problem in the United States, with Black Americans disproportionately affected compared to non-Hispanic Whites. In 2019, 89.5% of U.S. households were food secure, and the remaining 10.5% were insecure at least some time during the year. About 4.1% (5.3 million households) had very low food insecurity. There were about 13.6% of households with children that were experiencing food insecurity.[11] The first step in addressing food insecurity in primary care is identifying those who are at risk and assessing the situation (see Figure 1.1). Patients and their families can be referred to local food banks and can apply for assistance through the Supplemental Nutrition Assistance Program (SNAP) or other long-term nutrition supports.[12] Collaborating with a social worker or other social service organizations can be beneficial.

Malnutrition includes undernutrition, inadequate vitamins and minerals, overweight, and obesity, which can lead to chronic disease (e.g., diabetes) or be related to complications associated with chronic disease or acute illness.[13] When individuals experience undernutrition, they can have wasting (low weight for height), stunting (low height for weight), or be underweight (low weight for age). Micronutrient-related malnutrition occurs when there is a deficiency in a micronutrient (e.g., iodine, vitamin A, and iron are the most common deficiencies worldwide). Obesity, or being overweight, occurs when there is an imbalance between the energy consumed and the energy expended. Often this is the result of consuming too much food (high in sugars and fats) and not engaging in enough physical activity. People can be obese and still be malnourished due to micronutrient insufficiency.

Physical Activity

Physical activity is essential to promote healthy aging. The prevalence of global physical inactivity among all ages is high. Video gaming and e-sports have grown in popularity among adolescents and adults. Emerging evidence has demonstrated the negative impact on psychological, behavioral, and physical health indicators. Screen time (e.g., video gaming, watching TV, interacting on social media) can negatively impact health outcomes, such as difficulty falling asleep and staying asleep, altering circadian rhythm (if exposed to screen light before going to bed), and increasing risks for hypertension, diabetes, and being overweight or obese.[14] It is well known that regular exercise can help adolescents improve cardiorespiratory fitness, increase bone and muscle strength, control weight, and reduce symptoms of anxiety and depression. Physical activity in adolescents is linked to a reduction in heart disease, cancer, type 2 diabetes, hypertension, osteoporosis, and obesity as they age.[16] The problem is some adolescents have too much screen time and therefore are less likely to engage in the appropriate amount of physical activity. Monitoring screen time and encouraging physical activity are essential.

The WHO recommends that adolescents have at least an accumulation of 60 minutes of moderate-to-vigorous intensity physical activity daily.[15] Fewer than one-quarter (24%) of children aged 6 to 17 years participated in at least 60 minutes of physical activity each day. In 2017, only 26.1% of high school students participated in at least 60 minutes per day of physical activity each week, and only about half attended physical education classes in an average week (29.9% attended physical education on a daily basis).[15] Therefore, it is essential that AGNPs assess for screen time and physical activity and make recommendations for physical activity that include a balance between these two.

Physical activity, which is essential to healthy aging in older adults, can prevent health problems and promote health in those living with chronic disease(s).[7] The benefits are particularly relevant to older adults living with chronic medical conditions, such as osteoarthritis or cardiovascular disease.[17] Some physical activity is better than none, so try to get your patients moving even if it is only for short periods of activity (e.g., walk in the house or outside, or ride a stationary bicycle). It is important to discuss physical safety with exercises and how to prevent falls or other injuries. The more sedentary a person is, the higher the risk of deleterious health outcomes. Discussing with older adults the importance of avoiding inactivity and at the minimum engaging in 2 hours 30 minutes (150 minutes) of moderate-intensity aerobic activity (e.g., brisk walking) plus muscle strength activity for at least 2 days a week is important to their health.[17] Mutually establishing realistic goals can help the person develop a plan to achieve short- and long-term goals and revise as necessary.

EPIDEMIOLOGY OF AN AGING SOCIETY

The 2019 Census data indicated that there were 328,239,523 people in the United States; of these, 22.3% were younger than age 18 and 16.5% were older than age 65. For the first time in U.S. history, by 2034, the number of older adults is expected to outnumber children (see Figure 1.2). This demographic shift is new for the United States but not for some other countries such as Japan, which has the world's oldest population. Fewer births and longer life expectancy have led to this predicated change. Baby boomers (born between 1946 and 1964) will leave a substantial imprint on the population; by 2030, all boomers will be 65 years or older. In 2019, the population 65 and older was about 54.1 million (30 million women and 24.1 million men).[18] By 2060, about one in four Americans will be 65 years and older, the population 85 and older will triple, and there will be about

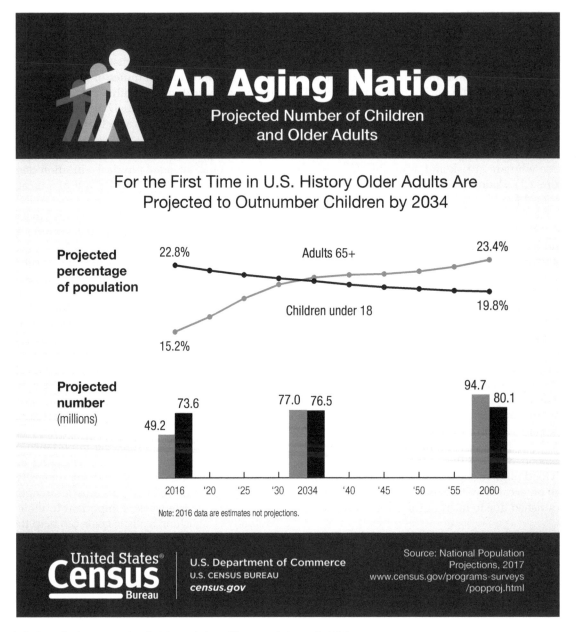

Figure 1.2: Population growth of older adults will exceed that of children

a half million centenarians. There will be an increase in demand for healthcare, in-home caregiving, and assisted living facilities.[19]

Most older adults live in a community; in 2019, 61% lived with a spouse or partner and 27% lived alone. In 2019, the median household income of older adults was $27,398, and about 4.9 million older adults lived below the poverty level, with 2.6 million being "near poor." Many adults 65 and older are still in the labor force (working or actively seeking employment).[18]

Racially and Ethnically Diverse Populations

Racially and ethnically diverse populations have increased from 7.8 million in 2009 (20% of older Americans) to 12.9% in 2019 (24% of older adults). This population is expected to increase to 27.7 million in 2040 (34% of older adult population). Between 2019 and 2040, the White (non-Hispanic) population will increase by 29% compared to 115% for other racial and ethnic populations; Hispanic older adults will increase by 161%, African Americans by 80%, American Indian and Alaska Natives by 67%, and Asian Americans by 102%.[18] As we witness an aging racial and ethnic population, it is critical that AGNPs are prepared to care and advocate for this diverse group of people across the life span.

Global Aging

There is a global aging population, which will present medical and social challenges worldwide. Although the WHO has proposed concrete action items to reach the objectives of the Decade of Healthy Aging (2021–2030), some low- to middle-resource countries will have financial difficulty engaging in efforts such as training and aligning healthcare systems to meet the needs of older people.[20] The Decade[21] is based on the Madrid International Plan of Action on Ageing (MIPAA)[22] and was developed by the United Nations and the WHO Global Strategy and Action Plan on Aging and Health.[23] There are more than a billion adults 60 years and older, and many don't have access to resources that promote healthy aging. There is a need to focus on population health that may influence individuals throughout the world as we attempt to implement strategies that foster healthy aging. As we witness an aging population, it is important to take a person-centered approach to care to assure the needs and preferences of adults and older adults are considered in the plan of care. There is a need for age-friendly communities and public health policies that address the diversity of health and functional states of older adults. Integrating actions at the macro level (legislation, funding), meso level (age-friendly communities), and micro clinical level that sustain quality, cost-effective care for all is needed.[20]

Globally, protein-energy malnutrition is among the top 10 reasons for death in adolescents. In 2016, iron-deficiency anemia was the second-leading cause of death and disability in adolescents.[13] Iron and folic acid supplements should be considered in this population. Globally, in 2016, undernourishment was highly prevalent in developing countries, with one in six adolescents (10–19 years) being overweight and many also being undernourished. The number of adolescents who are overweight or obese is increasing in low-, middle-, and high-income countries.

LIFE-SPAN DEVELOPMENT

Life-span development is known as the scientific study of ways in which people (infants, children, adolescents, adults, older adults) change and remain the same from the time of conception to death. The belief is that we change as we age, and life experiences have an impact on who we are and how we relate with others.[24] The terms "life-span development" and "life-course perspective" appear to be similar; however, there are unique differences.

A life-course approach highlights a time-based and social perspective, looking across an individual's or a population's life experiences and across generations to understand current patterns of health and disease. It recognizes that both past and present experiences are shaped by the wider social, economic, and cultural context and attempts to recognize the biological, behavioral, and psychosocial processes that function across an individual's or population's life span.[25]

Theories of Life-Span Development

Bates identified underlying principles of life-span development: [26,27]

- Development is lifelong, and change occurs across the life span.
- Humans change in many ways; there may be gains along with losses.
- People change across three general domains; change in one domain can lead to the next milestone (e.g., adolescent to adult):
  - Physical: includes changes in height and weight, sensory capabilities, neurologic system, and the risk for acute illness and/or chronic disease
  - Cognitive: intelligence, wisdom, perception, problem-solving, memory, and language
  - Psychosocial: emotion, self-perception, and interpersonal relationships with family, peers, and friends

Physical, cognitive, and personality development are characterized by plasticity, which provides an explanation for why we see natural changes in these areas. Plasticity can be defined as the idea of flexibility in developmental outcomes.

- Development occurs in many contexts:
  - Normative age-graded influences: People in a specific age group share similar experiences and developmental changes.
  - Normative history-graded influences: People born in the same time period go through life experiencing similar things.
  - Nonnormative life influences: We have unique experiences that make us who we are, which influences our development (Table 1.1).

It is important to note that life span is not the same as life expectancy. Life expectancy is the predicted number of years yet to be lived by a person of a particular age group.[28] A life-course perspective is the typical life span that describes regular periods, such as infancy, adolescence, adulthood, and older adult. "In medical and psychological research, it has long been recognized that certain conditions are influenced by one's stage in the life course."[28]

Other developmental theories focus on biological age, which is how quickly your body ages related to physical activity, sleep, unhealthy behaviors (e.g., smoking, excessive alcohol intake), mental stress, and genetics.

Table 1.1: Descriptions of Groupings of Generations

Generation	Born
Silent Generation	1928-1945
Baby Boomers	1946-1964
Generation X	1965-1980
Millennials	1981-1996
Generation Z	1997-Present

Source: Pew Research Center.

Table 1.2: Erikson's Psychological Development

Age Range	Psychological Stage	Health
12–18 years	Identity vs. Role Confusion	Develops sense of self and establishes relationships with other
19–40 years	Intimacy vs. Isolation	Ability to give and receive love and make long-term commitments
40–65 years	Generativity vs. Stagnation	Develops interest in guiding the development of the next generation
65 years to death	Ego Integrity vs. Despair	Acceptance of how one has lived

Psychological aging is the capacity to adapt compared to others of the same age. Social aging involves the expectations of society based on social norms of the culture. Chronological aging does not completely capture a person's age, so it is important not to determine treatment approaches based solely on age. Some older adults may be more physically and psychologically capable to engage in healthy behaviors than others who are the same age or younger.[24]

Age periods of development include prenatal, infancy, and toddlerhood (birth–toddlerhood); early childhood (2–6 years); middle and late childhood (6 years until the onset of puberty); adolescence (puberty–18 years); emerging adulthood (18–25 years); early adulthood (25 to 40–45 years); middle adulthood (40–45 to 65 years); and later adulthood (65 years and older).[24]

Erikson's psychological theory of development stages is well known and often provides a foundation for understanding development (Table 1.2). His theory is based on social expectations of a culture. Even though there are eight stages for this chapter, only those from 12 years to death will be presented.

Adolescence and Adulthood

Adolescence is a period of rapid physical, emotional, and psychological change. During this developmental stage, the person is experiencing puberty, which involves a growth spurt and sexual maturation. Adolescents are discovering their identity, thinking of new possibilities and abstract concepts of love, fear, and freedom.[24] It is during this stage they have a sense of invincibility, and peers are important in their lives.

Emerging adulthood is a transitional time between adolescence and entering adulthood. It is important that AGNPs caring for individuals living with a childhood illness and entering adulthood recognize that for years, the individual was most likely seeing a pediatric specialist. This transition from pediatric care to an adult primary care provider can be challenging because they will have to establish a new relationship. Identifying challenges a person may face during this transition is essential. At this stage, they are preparing to be independent from their parents and may be going to college or seeking employment. This is also a time the person may experiment with substances and alcohol.

Adulthood and Aging

During early adulthood, individuals begin to develop intimate relations and may get married and start a family. Young adults are mainly concerned with work and financial stability. Middle adulthood is when aging becomes apparent, and people are usually at the peak of their work and relationships with a significant other (i.e., spouse, life partner).

Late adulthood can be considered in two categories, young-old (65–84 years) and oldest-old (85 years and older). The major difference is that the young-old are usually healthy, active, productive, and live independently. Yet, even in the young-old, most people have one or more chronic diseases.[24]

HEALTH PROMOTION

Health promotion and disease prevention occur when people are empowered to increase control over their health. They cover a wide range of social and environmental interventions designed to benefit and protect the health of individuals while improving quality of life and well-being. The focus is on the root cause of disease and not just on treatment and cure. Social determinants are the economic, social, cultural, and political conditions in which people are born, grow, and live that affect their health status. Social determinants of health influence a person's ability to engage and can negatively influence behaviors that promote health and reduce the risk of disease. Social determinants of health are discussed later in this chapter in the Healthy People 2030 section.

Modifiable behaviors include smoking, excessive alcohol use, sedentary lifestyle, and poor nutrition, as previously mentioned.[29] Promoting health in those living with and without chronic health conditions is important. Viewing health promotion from a wellness lens embraces the "functional, physical, environmental, intellectual, psychological, spiritual, social, and biological dimensions of the human experience within the context of culture."[30] This textbook is based on a holistic approach of care provided by nurse practitioners (NPs) for adolescents, adults, and older adults with and without chronic health conditions in primary care.

Promoting Health in Adolescents

AGNPs should consider creative strategies to encourage adolescents to engage in healthy behaviors that promote health and prevent disease. The WHO and UNESCO have launched an initiative called "Making Every School a Health-Promoting School." Globally, over 90% of children who are of primary school age and more than 80% who are of lower secondary school age are enrolled in school, where they spend at least a third of their time. Partnering with schools to develop and implement health promotion programs may be an effective way to achieve the goal of promoting health in this population.[13] Mobile technology has grown since the introduction of smartphones. The use of smartphones and apps is high among adolescents. The findings of a qualitative study indicated that some adolescents use apps to manage disease, achieve a desired fitness goal, or improve health behaviors.[31] However, other participants reported that one barrier to using health promotion apps was the lack of knowledge about the apps. Others disclosed that health management was a low priority in relation to other social media or playing games. Several participants were concerned about social stigma from their peers when using health promotion apps.[31] Facilitators to using the apps were an interface and multimedia content that was considered "cool," being able to customize to goal setting, personal data tracking and tailored messaging, and intrinsic motivation.[31] Social influence (e.g., celebrity endorsement of health behavior activities) plays a major role in changing adolescent behavior, so keeping this in mind when engaging in discussions about health promotion with adolescents can be helpful.

Promoting Health in Adults

Health promotion and disease prevention in adults involves smoking cessation, healthy eating, physical activity, assuring alcohol intake is minimal, promoting lifestyle change, and disease management when appropriate. In addition, promoting women's reproductive health, men's health, and the use of clinical preventative services is important. Adults should have at least 7 hours of sleep

each night, but about one-third of adults report less sleep. Inadequate sleep increases the risk for chronic disease (type 2 diabetes mellitus, heart disease, obesity, depression) and can lead to motor vehicle accidents.[7]

Just like adolescents, most adults have smartphones with apps that can be used for health promotion messaging. However, Berry and colleagues[32] sought to determine if health promotion messaging was specifically targeted toward young adults and if the messaging motivated them to engage in health behaviors. The study participants ($n = 19$) didn't think the health messaging was tailored to them, so it didn't impact their participation in healthy behaviors. Therefore, it is important to collaborate with your patient to find the best app for them that will encourage healthy behaviors. Recognizing health promotion includes targeting interventions that reduce or alleviate stress in adults. Examples of preventative interventions that can help are mindfulness mediation, physical activity, yoga, and tai chi.

Promoting Health in Older Adults

Health promotion strategies for older adults are aimed at maintaining and increasing functional capacity, maintaining and improving self-care, and improving social connection through enhancing social networks with family and community members. As previously mentioned, it is important to prevent disease and promote health by considering physical, psychological/emotional, and spiritual domains. As people age, they experience losses (e.g., death of loved one or friend), which may impact their overall relationships and lead to loneliness and social isolation. Loneliness and social isolation in older adults can lead to serious health problems, including dementia (about 50% increased risk).

Loneliness is the subjective feeling of being alone regardless of how much social contact the person has; social isolation is objective and is the lack of social connection, or infrequent contact with others.[7] About one-third of adults 45 and older feel lonely, and nearly a quarter of adults 65 and older are socially isolated.[33] Social isolation is a public health problem linked to negative health outcomes such as depression and anxiety.[34,35] Other risks of social isolation are cardiovascular disease, hypertension, and obesity. Primary care providers play a vital role in identifying those at risk or experiencing loneliness and, in some circumstances, may be one of the few face-to-face encounters they have.[7] Social connection depends on the extent of the following:

- A connection to others or the existence of relationships and their roles
- A sense of connection that results from actual or perceived support
- A sense of connection to others based on positive and negative qualities[33]

Taking a person-centered approach to address loneliness and social isolation is important because not everyone who lives alone is lonely or has social isolation. The paucity of research addressing social connection supports the need for robust research studies examining the effect of interventions on loneliness and social isolation in both urban and rural communities. Rural communities often have challenges with distance to family or friends' homes, businesses, and primary care or other healthcare providers, thus increasing the risk of loneliness and social isolation.[33] Individuals that self-identify as gay/lesbian or bisexual tend to have more loneliness compared to their heterosexual peers.

Reducing loneliness and social isolation can be accomplished through indirect and direct methods. Direct interventions include having volunteers making face-to-face visits with a focus on socially connecting. Indirect could be encouraging the person to join other community-based groups. There are community-basedsenior centers that can help increase an older adult's social network and encourage social connection through various interactive programs (e.g., music therapy, current events, art therapy, exercise programs, tai chi). Social isolation increased during the pandemic, which has led to increased use of mobile technology. People using video chat apps (e.g., FaceTime and Skype) felt a connection to their family and other loved ones. In some nursing home facilities, residents have access to Skype, which enables medical visits with their healthcare providers and virtual visits with family members.[36] Older adults can be taught how to use these apps to reduce the risk of social isolation by improving social connections.

Participating in regular physical activity is extremely beneficial for older adults. For decades, the public has been aware of the cardiovascular benefits of physical activity, but other benefits patients may not be aware of are improved physical and cognitive function, reduced osteoarthritic pain, and overall well-being. In those with mild cognitive impairment, physical activity (primarily aerobic exercise) may potentially decrease the risk for dementia.[37]

HEALTHY PEOPLE 2030

Healthy People 2030 is the fifth in the series of Healthy People initiatives that started in 1979 with the first target goal in 1990 and has been revised and updated every decade. Each of the published initiatives focuses on enhancing the health of the population and sets measurable targets for that decade. The vision of the Healthy People Initiative is "a society in which all people can achieve their full potential for health and well-being across the lifespan."[37] The Foundational Principles listed in the text that follows are designed to help guide decisions about Healthy People 2030:[38]

- The health and well-being of all people and communities are essential to a thriving, equitable society.

- Promoting health and well-being and preventing disease are linked efforts that encompass physical, mental, and social health dimensions.

- Investing to achieve the full potential for health and well-being for all provides valuable benefits to society.

- Achieving health and well-being requires eliminating health disparities, achieving health equity, and attaining health literacy.

- Healthy physical, social, and economic environments strengthen the potential to achieve health and well-being.

- Promoting and achieving health and well-being nationwide is a shared responsibility that is distributed across the national, state, tribal, and community levels, including the public, private, and not-for-profit sectors.

- Working to attain the full potential for health and well-being of the population is a component of decision-making and policy formulation across all sectors.

Key overarching goals are for people to attain healthy, thriving lives that are free of preventable diseases, disabilities, injuries, and premature death and to eliminate health disparities and achieve health equity and health literacy of the population. A comprehensive action plan provides for national goals and measurable objectives, collects and makes available accurate data, provides relevant tools, and shares progress through biennial reporting.

A diverse group of people worked on the objectives for Healthy People 2030 for several years, ultimately developing 355 core objectives (about a third of the Healthy People 2020 objectives), which they hoped would focus on the most important health priorities. In general, the objectives revolve around common acute and chronic health conditions (e.g., diabetes, cancer, pain, chronic kidney disease, mental health, obesity, healthcare-associated infections, respiratory diseases, oral conditions), healthy behaviors (e.g., physical activity, drug and alcohol use, injury prevention, preventive care, violence prevention, tobacco use), populations (e.g., adolescents, adults, older adults, LGBT, people with disabilities, workforce), settings and systems (e.g., community, schools, workplace, hospitals and emergency services, public health and healthcare), and social determinants of health (e.g., economic stability, access to education and healthcare, neighborhoods and the built environment, social and communities).

The Leading Health Indicators (LHIs) are a subset of high-priority objectives; the following are LHIs that impact all ages:

- using the oral healthcare system
- reducing consumption of added sugars in the diet
- reducing drug overdose deaths and those due to homicides
- decreasing exposure to unhealthy air

- reducing food insecurity and hunger
- increasing the numbers of people who receive flu vaccines annually
- ensuring people know their HIV status
- reducing suicides

Key LHIs for adolescents include reducing major depressive episodes if they are receiving treatment, decreasing the use of tobacco products, and reducing obesity. LHIs for adults and older adults include improving physical activity and strength, improving colorectal cancer screening, controlling blood pressure in adults with hypertension, reducing maternal deaths, decreasing new cases of diabetes, reducing cigarette smoking and binge drinking, and increasing employment.

Health literacy was specifically considered in the Healthy People 2030 plan and has six associated objectives.

1. Increase the proportion of adults whose healthcare provider checked their understanding.

2. Decrease the proportion of adults who report poor communication with their healthcare provider.

3. Increase the proportion of adults whose healthcare providers involved them in decisions as much as they wanted.

4. Increase proportion of people who say their online medical record is easy to understand.

5. Increase the proportion of adults with limited English proficiency who say their providers explain things clearly.

6. Increase the health literacy of the population.

AGNP Integration of Healthy People 2030 Into Practice

The Healthy People 2030 site lists all 355 goals through links; readers can click on the links to read the specific objective of interest (https://health.gov/healthypeople/objectives-and-data/browse-objectives). The site also has many evidence-based resources that are available for the various conditions, including systematic reviews and other research on the various topics and goals (https://health.gov/healthypeople/tools-action/browse-evidence-based-resources/evidence-based-resources). The goals and resources are readily available for AGNPs to access to use as guidelines, particularly for preventive services and health promotion for all age groups.

For example, from the adolescent's health goals, the first general goal is to increase the proportion of adolescents who have had a preventative health examination in the past 12 months from 78.7% to 82.6%.[39] This goal is in the scope of practice of AGNPs and should be integrated into annual physicals and well-child checks as well as school and sports physicals. These types of

regular screening are the perfect times to assess an adolescent's progress, assess for risk, and redefine goals/focus for the coming year. These visits provide an opportunity to assess how well things are going physically and psychologically for the adolescents in the practice. The examinations should be comprehensive and include an assessment of objective parameters, such as physical growth and development, vital signs, and height and weight measurements, with documented percentage as well as body mass index (BMI), along with indications of substance abuse and sexual activity. These also provide the opportunity for early intervention if growth delays, obesity, malnutrition, and at-risk behaviors are detected. In addition, it is important to assess the mental health status of each adolescent who may be at risk for depression, suicidal ideation, or sexual promiscuity. Each visit provides an opportunity for appropriate and timely health education, including anticipatory guidance for both adolescents and their parents/caretakers. The current 2030 goals/objectives for adolescents are outlined in Table 1.3.

Similarly, the goals/objectives for older adults are outlined on the website and are easily accessible (https://health.gov/healthypeople/objectives-and-data/browse-objectives/older-adults). There are 17 baseline and 3 developmental objectives. Some examples of objectives are shown in Table 1.4.

Table 1.3: Top Five General Goals for Adolescents in Healthy People 2030

AH-1: Increase the proportion of adolescents who received a preventive healthcare visit in the past year from 78.7% to 82.6%.
AH-2: Increase the proportion of adolescents who speak privately with a physician or other healthcare provider during a preventive medical visit from 38.4% to 43.3%.
AH-3: Increase the proportion of children living with at least one parent employed year-round, full-time from 77.9% to 85.1%.
AH-4: Increase the proportion of high school completers who were enrolled in college the October immediately after completing high school from 69.1% to 73.7%.
AH-5: Increase the proportion of elementary, middle, and high schools that have official school policies and engage in practices that promote a healthy and safe physical school environment.

Source: Office of Disease Prevention and Health Promotion. Goal: Improve the health and well-being of adolescents. n.d. https://health.gov/healthypeople/objectives-and-data/browse-objectives/adolescents

Table 1.4: Examples of Goals/Objectives for Older Adults in Healthy People 2030

OA-01: Increase the proportion of older adults with reduced physical or cognitive function who engage in light, moderate, or vigorous leisure-time physical activities from 41.3% to 51%.
OA-05: Reduce the rate of hospital admissions for diabetes among older adults from 293.3 admissions per 100,000 adults older than 65 years to 264 admissions per 100,000.
DIA-01: Increase the proportion of older adults with diagnosed Alzheimer's disease and other dementias, or their caregivers, who are aware of the diagnosis from 59.7% to 65.1%.
OA-05: Reduce the rate of hospital admissions for urinary tract infections among older adults from 551.3 admissions for UTI per 100,000 age older than 65 years to 496.2 admissions for UTI per 100,000.
IVP-08: Reduce fall-related deaths among older adults from 64.4 deaths per 100,000 age older than 65 years to 63.4 deaths per 100,000.
OH-06: Reduce the proportion of adults aged 45 years and over with moderate and severe periodontitis from 44.5% to 39.3%.
O-D01: Increase the proportion of older adults (aged 65 years and older) screened for osteoporosis (developmental objective; no baseline data available yet).

Source: Office of Disease Prevention and Health Promotion. Goal: Improve health and well-being for older adults. n.d. https://health.gov/healthypeople/objectives-and-data/browse-objectives/older-adults

There are many different goals/objectives that are appropriate for older adults, particularly within the disease conditions that are not in the population section that are worth exploring to evaluate which ones to target in your practice. Some of these goals might be appropriate for a practice-wide quality improvement project if there are a lot of old adults in the practice.

INFORMAL CAREGIVERS AND HEALTH

Informal family caregivers are a primary source of support for the older adult population and are unpaid in most cases. In 2019, the AARP Public Policy Institute and National Alliance for Caregiving published an updated report, *Caregiving in the United States*, revealing that 41.8 million (16.8%) caregivers provided support to an adult age 50 or older; this was up from 34.2 million or 14.3% in 2015.[40] More caregivers (24%) reported that they provided care to two or more people in this latest report compared with

2015. It is suggested that the increased prevalence is due to the growing older adult population and shortages of community-based long-term services and support workers. AARP estimates the economic value of informal caregivers at $470 billion annually.[41]

Informal caregiving has been prevalent for decades; however, with the rapid growth of the older adult population living longer with more chronic diseases, this issue has become more widespread, with one in six Americans functioning as caregivers for older adults in 2020.[41] Adding to the prevalence is those aged 85 and older are the fastest growing segment of the population, an age when older adults are more likely to suffer from dementia, more serious chronic diseases, and frailty. In 2026, the first baby boomers will turn 80 years old, so this problem is not going away any time soon. At the same time, the American nuclear family is shrinking, often with both adults in families more likely to be working full-time and, therefore, less available for caregiving.

Caregivers of older adults are often older themselves; 56% are older than age 50, and 20% are older than age 65. Most caregivers (89%) are relatives and female (63%), and increasing numbers (24%) are providing care to two or more people, a 7% increase since 2015.[40] These caregivers are primarily providing care to one or more parents who are in their 80s and 90s. Because older adults are living longer with chronic diseases, caregivers are providing prolonged care to this population, sometimes for multiple years. Some caregivers in the older adult age range are providing care to a spouse or partner, and many of the caregivers also have declining health.

Caregivers are also a very diverse group, and cultural perspectives vary widely across the groups. In general, ethnic minorities tend to provide more care to their recipients when compared with White caregivers and suffer worse physical health.[42] However, Asian American and Hispanic caregivers had more depression than White caregivers in one study.[43] Studies have shown that the LGBTQ+ population are more likely to live alone than others who are not LGBTQ+ and, therefore, may have less caregiver support; they generally face more poverty as well.[44,45]

The Work of Caregivers

Older adults suffer from a variety of conditions from moderate to severe cognitive impairment to serious complex chronic diseases, and it falls to family and close friends to provide assistance when these adults can no longer care for themselves safely. And although there is a segment of the older population who remain healthy as they age, there are also large numbers who have complex chronic diseases, such as heart failure, diabetes, kidney failure, arthritis, and mental health disorders, and growing numbers have some type of cognitive impairment and dementia. This group of individuals requires additional supportive care to remain in their home environment and manage their health conditions.

Caregivers provide different types of support, such as assistance with housecleaning, preparing food, running errands, and activities of daily living (toileting, bathing, dressing, eating), as well as more complex healthcare tasks, including medication management, dressing, feeding tube changes, and administering injections. Additionally, caregivers assist in communication and coordination with medical providers and medical appointments. According to the AARP report, caregivers are providing care to people with greater comorbidities, 45% report that their care recipient has two or more chronic conditions, and almost 40% report providing care in high-intensity situations that may involve nursing-level care. As care recipients age, they are increasingly likely to have memory problems, with almost half of those age 85 or older reporting memory problems.[46] Depending on the type of support provided, this may be a significant commitment; 70% reported providing between 1 and 20 hours of care weekly, and 20% reported providing 41 or more hours weekly, making it very difficult to provide care to the older adult, provide care to their own family, and ensure their own health.

The Impact of Caregiving on Families

Caregiving can have both positive and negative effects on caregivers. There have been a few studies that have reported positive effects of caregiving; one qualitative study used a strengths-based perspective and found that family caregivers are able to discover personal strengths, view caregiving as a chance to give back, and grow closer to the care recipient.[47] Some cultures, including Asian and Hispanic cultures,[48,49] tend to have a more positive view of caregiving; however, some Latino caregivers experienced high levels of distress. Roth et al.[50] reported that African American and Hispanic caregivers were more likely to experience positive aspects of caregiving when compared with White caregivers. They reported a more positive attitude toward life, enabling them to appreciate life more fully.

Studies of caregivers have also found significant negative effects of caregiving, particularly on the health of the caregivers.[51] Role strain was noted by family caregivers who worked full-time, and some had more depressive symptoms in one study.[52] Caregiving for older adults with dementia has been associated with depression, anxiety, and mood disorders.[53] There can also be a significant financial impact on caregivers in terms of lost wages, reduced savings, diminished retirement, and higher healthcare costs.[54]

AGNPs must recognize the significant challenges that family caregivers face and work with families and caregivers to provide support and guidance as needed. In particular, AGNPs should watch for signs and symptoms of stress and anxiety in caregivers who accompany older adult patients to clinic appointments and allow opportunities for communication and discussion with the caregiver. If the caregiver is also a patient, set aside a specific appointment time to address these issues with the caregiver.

CONCLUSION

The concept of healthy aging is an ongoing process that applies to all age groups from adolescents to older adults. AGNPs must understand the epidemiology of healthy aging and the main contributors that prevent populations from achieving optimal physical and mental function and a sense of well-being. In particular, AGNPs should use person-centered approaches to health promotion and disease prevention in their practices and be familiar with the Healthy People 2030 goals to support their patients. A clear understanding of unhealthy behaviors and risk factors that contribute to chronic diseases must be part of the AGNPs armamentarium. And for those patients who have significant chronic diseases and/or frailty, it is essential to consider the important role informal caregivers play and the impact that caregiving has on their lives.

REFERENCES

References for this chapter are online and available at https://connect.springerpub.com/content/book/978-0-8261-8414-6/part/part01/toc-part/ch1.

CHAPTER 2

Toward Person-Centered Care

Shelly L. Henderson

LEARNING OBJECTIVES

At the conclusion of this chapter, the learner will be able to:

➤ Define "person-centered care."

➤ Define "motivational interviewing."

➤ Identify the spirit, principles, and core skills of motivational interviewing.

➤ Employ behavior-change techniques to assist older adults in reaching their identified lifestyle goals.

INTRODUCTION

Person-centered care (PCC) is focused and organized around the health needs and expectations of people and communities rather than on diseases. PCC involves respecting the values, needs, and preferences of people and families and applying the best evidence toward a shared goal of optimal health and quality of life. The PCC approach is particularly important in the care of older adults who may have multiple chronic diseases. Motivational interviewing (MI), as a person-centered counseling style, is one way of translating PCC into practice.

This chapter defines PCC and provides an overview of MI. The spirit, principles, and core skills of MI are reviewed. The goal is to provide adult-gerontology nurse practitioner (AGNP) students with communication tools that translate PCC into practice. While PCC is applicable to all populations, this chapter will focus on older adults. Examples of MI with older adults are provided.

IMPORTANCE OF PERSON-CENTERED CARE

PCC is empowering. By playing an active role in their care, patients take control of the decisions that affect their health. The PCC approach is considered fundamental to helping people live well with a chronic condition.[1] The World Health Organization has underlined the need to move toward comprehensive, PCC, considering it a central approach to improving the quality and efficacy of care of older people.[2] PCC supports autonomy and is respectful of each person's values, appraisals, and choices in daily life. Translating PCC into practice can help healthcare professionals understand each person's challenges and what they consider appropriate ways to overcome them.

Definition of Person-Centered Care

PCC extends the concept of patient-centered care to individuals, families, communities, and society. Whereas patient-centered care is commonly understood as focusing on the individual seeking care—the patient—PCC encompasses these clinical encounters and includes attention to the health of people in their families and communities.

The American Geriatrics Society defines PCC as an approach in which "individuals' values and preferences are elicited and, once expressed, guide all aspects of their health care, supporting their realistic health and life goals."[3] PCC is pursued through a dynamic relationship among individuals, others who are important to them, and all relevant providers. The PCC approach focuses on the improvement of care by reinforcing the importance of considering the preferences, needs, and personal identities of older adults and their families. Patients often lose their independence when they enter care, which puts their dignity at risk. PCC enables older adults to maintain that dignity by respecting their wishes and treating them with compassion and empathy. PCC involves respecting the values, needs, and preferences of older adults and applying the best evidence toward a shared goal of optimal health and quality of life.

MOTIVATIONAL INTERVIEWING AS AN APPROACH TO PERSON-CENTERED CARE

MI is an approach to counseling that aims to strengthen a person's motivation and commitment to behavior change by helping them resolve their ambivalence about the change.[4] MI fosters a partnership between clinicians and patients, allowing the clinician to demonstrate empathy, build rapport with the patient, learn about the patient's world, and help the patient achieve change.

MI was developed in the early 1980s by psychologist William Miller. Miller's experience working with individuals with alcohol problems convinced him that motivation to change was a frequent obstacle to reducing problem drinking. Miller described a way of talking with people to evoke and strengthen their motivation.[5] Since then, the principles of MI have matured, and it has become an evidence-based practice used worldwide as an approach to resolving an individual's ambivalence about changing behavior.

Although there are few randomized controlled trials of MI in older adults, most published studies indicate that MI is effective for influencing change in health behaviors including weight loss, medication management,[6] and increased walking to improve function in patients with peripheral vascular disease.[7] MI is a cost-efficient treatment and can be used in primary care and geriatric settings.

MI may be particularly useful for older patients because they often have multiple and interacting medical problems with treatment regimens that involve multiple medications, medication side effects, and changes in activity—all of which can be difficult to cope with unless patients are motivated to make changes in their daily lives.

Furthermore, older patients may be coping with other issues, such as grief over losses, physical illness, or disability. These complicating factors can impede behavior change and mistakenly be perceived as "resistance" or "noncompliance." Using MI to elicit the older adult's values and perceptions of barriers to change is an evidence-based approach to PCC.

MI has been used to address a number of behavior problems associated with lifestyle choices among older adults. In the area of diet, exercise, and weight control, MI has been found to produce significant changes among older adults including short-term weight loss, increased frequency and duration of physical activity, decreased health distress, decreased sodium intake, improved glucose control, decreased blood pressure, and improved adherence to weight control programs.[8] Regarding smoking cessation, all but one study found MI to be effective at increasing smoking cessation rates.[9]

Further areas in geriatrics where MI can be helpful include the following:

- Using a walker
- Moving into assisted living
- Stopping driving
- Decreasing drinking
- Talking with family members or inviting family members to engage in a different way
- End-of-life discussions

MI is a person-centered approach to navigate the delicate conversations that healthcare providers are charged with facilitating for their older patients.

Definition of Motivational Interviewing

Miller and Rollnick[4] describe MI as a "directive, patient-centered counseling style for enhancing intrinsic motivation to change by exploring and resolving ambivalence." MI is more than the use of a set of techniques or strategies. It is characterized by a particular "spirit" or clinical "way of being" that is the context or interpersonal relationship within which the techniques are employed. That is, the effectiveness of MI depends on the fundamental aspect of how the provider relates to the patient.[10]

Spirit of Motivational Interviewing

The spirit of MI is based on three key elements: collaboration between the provider and the patient, evoking or drawing out the patient's ideas about change, and emphasizing the autonomy of the patient.

Collaboration (versus confrontation) is a partnership between the provider and the patient, grounded in the point of view and experiences of the patient. This contrasts with the traditional biomedical model where the provider is the expert and the patient is passive. Traditionally, healthcare providers often specialize in one body system. While specialization has brought tremendous advancements in treatments for various acute and chronic diseases, it often comes at the expense of the patient's own expertise. The PCC approach acknowledges that patients are "specialists" in their own lives. Only patients know what their goals and values are. Collaboration assumes a whole-person approach that takes into consideration those goals and values that drive behavior change. It builds rapport and facilitates trust in the helping relationship, which can be challenging in a more hierarchical relationship where the provider is the "expert." This does not mean that the provider automatically agrees with the patient about the nature of the problem or the changes that may be most appropriate. Although the provider and patient may see things differently, the therapeutic process is focused on mutual understanding, not the provider being right or the patient dictating treatment.

Using MI, the provider draws out the individual's own thoughts and ideas rather than imposing their opinion. This tends to increase the patient's motivation as a commitment to change and is most powerful and sustainable when it comes from the patient. Lasting change occurs when the patient discovers their own reasons and determination to change. The provider's job is to "draw out" the person's own motivations and skills for change, not to tell them what to do or why they should do it, no matter how scientifically valid or clinically convincing the provider's reasons may be.

The final element is based on the bioethical principle of autonomy. Unlike the traditional biomedical model that emphasizes the clinician as an authority figure, MI recognizes that the true power for change rests within the patient. Ultimately, the patient is responsible to make a behavioral change that improves their health and pain management. This empowers the patient and increases their sense of responsibility to take action in their health-care. Providers reinforce that there is no single "right way" to change and that there are multiple ways that change can occur. In addition to deciding whether they will make a change, patients are encouraged to take the lead in developing a "menu of options" as to how to achieve the desired change.

Principles of Motivational Interviewing

There are four principles that guide the practice of MI: (a) express empathy, (b) support self-efficacy, (c) roll with resistance, and (d) develop discrepancy (Table 2.1). Empathy involves seeing the world through the patient's eyes, thinking about things as the patient thinks about them, and feeling things as the patient feels them to share in the patient's experiences. This approach provides the basis for patients to be heard and understood, and in turn, patients are more likely to honestly share their experiences in depth.

For example, a patient tells his provider, "I need to be strong for my wife. She can't know how much pain I'm in." The provider mentally places herself in the patient's life and states the following:

- "You're worried about your wife and you don't want to be a burden."
- "You feel like you need to push through the pain."

In the preceding scenario, the provider communicates to the patient the core emotion that another would feel if they "put themselves in the patient's shoes." Ultimately, the patient feels emotionally heard. This opens the door to the initial stages of building mutual trust.

Regarding self-efficacy, MI promotes a strengths-based approach. This means that patients have within themselves the capabilities to change successfully. A patient's belief that change is possible (i.e., self-efficacy) is needed to instill hope about making those difficult changes. Patients often have previously tried and been unable to achieve or maintain the desired change, creating doubt about their ability to succeed. In MI, providers support self-efficacy by focusing on previous successes and highlighting skills and strengths that the patient already has. For example, the provider may state the following to promote self-efficacy:

- "You were successful in coming here today and voicing what's important to you in your health."
- "You have managed many hardships in your life."
- "Managing pain takes time and energy just like you dedicated time and energy in the past when you stopped your alcohol use."
- "You value living independently. Let's keep this value in mind as we discuss your pain management."

These simple statements of affirmation serve to bolster the patient's confidence and direct the conversation toward existing strengths within the patient. Recognizing these strengths and prior successes lays the groundwork for future change.

Table 2.1: Motivational Interviewing Principles

MI Principle	Rationale	Skills/Tools	As Compared to ...
Express empathy	• Demonstrate acceptance and understanding of patient ambivalence	• Reflective listening • Open-ended questions • Summary	• Providing data and statistics to convince patient of need for change
Support self-efficacy	• Build patient's confidence in their ability to change	• Affirmations • Reflect change talk • Identify patient's strengths	• Getting too far ahead of patient (misalignment with stage of change) • Focusing on what's going wrong rather than patient's attempts to change
Roll with resistance	• Refrain from confronting or arguing about patient's behavior • Use as opportunity to learn about patient's experience	• Reflective listening • Open-ended questions	• Engaging in power struggle • Arguing with patients about why they should change • Giving ultimatums
Develop discrepancy	• Evoke/illuminate discrepancy between patient behavior and patient's beliefs/values	• Use decisional balance • Use change rulers • Reflective listening • Open-ended questions • Summary	• Arguing for healthy behavior based on provider's values • Pointing out inconsistencies in patient behavior

MI, motivational interviewing.

Rolling with resistance means slowing down and reflecting back the patient's concerns. From an MI perspective, resistance in treatment occurs when the patient experiences a conflict between their view of the "problem" or the "solution" and that of the clinician or when the patient experiences their freedom or autonomy being impinged on. These experiences are often based on the patient's ambivalence about change, which is a normal part of the change process. In MI, providers avoid eliciting resistance by not confronting the patient. When resistance occurs, the provider recognizes the need to slow down, de-escalate the interaction, and "roll with resistance." For example, a provider may recommend physical therapy for low back pain. Well-intentioned, and even evidence-based, recommendations are sometimes met with a "yes, but" response from patients: "Yes, I've tried that, but it doesn't seem to help." Rather than seeing this response as a lack of adherence, the MI approach suggests that this is an opportunity to understand barriers to treatment. A simple reflection, "You're worried that another round of physical therapy won't help," serves to disarm the patient and can be followed with an open-ended request, "Tell me about your experience with physical therapy." This can elicit important points about the patient's expectations and use of a recommended treatment.

Actions and statements that demonstrate resistance remain unchallenged, especially early in the treatment relationship. The MI value on having the patient define the problem and develop their own solutions leaves little for the patient to resist. A frequently used metaphor is "dancing" rather than "wrestling" with the patient. In exploring patient concerns, healthcare providers invite patients to examine new points of view and are careful not to impose their own ways of thinking. A key concept is that providers avoid the "righting reflex," a tendency born from concern, to ensure that the patient understands and agrees with the need to change and to solve the problem for the patient. The following is an example of rolling with resistance.

After a fall at home, a patient presents to their primary care provider (PCP). The PCP recognizes that polypharmacy may be contributing to dizziness or sedation and would like to reduce or change the medication regimen.

- **Patient:** "I need my medication! I've been taking these pills for years. I don't think I'll be able to get out of bed without them."
- **Provider:** "It's stressful to even think about making a change to your medication. You worry that you won't be able to get out of bed." (*Reflection*)
- **Patient:** "Yes! And I'm always hearing 'use it or lose it.' If I don't stay active, I'm worried I'll go downhill fast."

This empathetic and reflective response builds rapport and trust between the patient and provider, allowing for further conversation. If resistance continues, the provider may respond, "I see that staying active is important to you. Can I have your permission to return to medications at a later time? I really want for us to spend a good amount of time thinking about medication options that are right for you, in line with your goals of staying active, and that I feel comfortable with."

Motivation for change occurs when people perceive a mismatch between where they are and where they want to be.[11] Providers practicing MI work to develop this by helping patients examine the discrepancies between their current behavior and their values and future goals. When patients recognize that their current behaviors place them in conflict with their values or interfere with accomplishing self-identified goals, they are more likely to experience increased motivation to make important life changes. It is important that the provider using MI does not use strategies to develop discrepancy at the expense of the other principles (such as empathy and self-efficacy). The provider aims to gradually help patients become aware of how current behaviors may lead them away from, rather than toward, their important goals. For example, providers may highlight the discrepancy by stating the following:

- For the patient who is ambivalent about taking antidepressants: "You mentioned that your goal is to get up in the morning and feed the birds. How do your current problems with your mood get in the way of that plan?"
- For the patient who is ambivalent about physical therapy: "Your goal is to wean off pain pills. How does physical therapy fit in with that goal?"
- For the patient who is ambivalent about dietary changes for weight loss: "You want to lose weight as a way to manage your back pain. How does your soda intake fit in with that goal?"

The responses to these questions provide information about the patient's knowledge of the "problem" and how they perceive solutions. Gathering this information is in line with the PCC approach and is essential to developing a treatment plan that "fits" the older adult.

The practice of MI involves the skillful use of certain techniques for bringing to life the "MI spirit," demonstrating the MI principles, and guiding the process toward eliciting change talk and commitment for change. Change talk involves statements or nonverbal communications indicating the patient may be considering the possibility of change. We will return to change talk and go through specific examples in an upcoming section of this chapter.

SKILLS OF MOTIVATIONAL INTERVIEWING

Often called micro-counseling skills, open-ended questions, affirming, reflective listening, and summarizing (OARS)[12] is a brief way to remember the basic approach used in MI: OARS are core provider behaviors employed to move the process forward by establishing a therapeutic alliance and eliciting discussion about change.

Open-Ended Questions

Open-ended questions are not easily answered with a yes/no or short answer. Open-ended questions invite elaboration and thinking more deeply about an issue. Although closed questions have their place and are at times valuable (e.g., when collecting specific information in an assessment), open-ended questions create forward momentum used to help the patient explore the reasons for and possibility of change. For example, the provider suspects their patient is drinking alcohol for sleep. The provider may ask the following open-ended questions to better learn about the patient's experience of drinking alcohol:

- "What role does alcohol play in your life?"
- "How does alcohol impact your relationships or activities you enjoy?"
- "What are the things you would do in your life if alcohol were not in the picture?"

These open-ended questions allow for an honest and open discussion without judgment. Asking questions in this way creates space for patients to express ambivalence.

Affirmations

Affirmations are statements that recognize patient strengths. They assist in building rapport and in helping the patient see themselves in a different, more positive light. To be effective they must be congruent and genuine. Using affirmations can help patients feel that change is possible even when previous efforts have been unsuccessful. Affirmations often involve reframing behaviors or concerns as evidence of positive qualities. Affirmations are a key element in facilitating the MI principle of supporting self-efficacy. For instance, a provider may state the following:

- "I appreciate you being honest with me about sharing your medication with your spouse."
- "I want to thank you for your openness and trust in me to talk about the sadness you are experiencing."
- "You showed courage and strength when you stopped smoking in the past. I can see your courage and strength now, too, as we work together to help you cut back on alcohol."

- "You're working hard to get your strength back after your surgery."
- "It took a lot of effort for you to get your appointment today. I can tell how important your health is to you."

These simple statements serve to bolster the patient's confidence in their ability to make a change. Affirmations are a testament to the basic tenets of MI—that all people are capable of change and are motivated to be their best selves.

Reflections

Reflections (also called reflective listening) are perhaps the most crucial skill in MI. They have two primary purposes. The first is to bring to life the principle of expressing empathy. By careful listening and reflecting responses, the patient comes to feel that the provider understands the issues from their perspective. Beyond this, strategic use of reflective listening is a core intervention toward guiding the patient toward change, supporting the goal-directed aspect of MI. In this use of reflections, the provider guides the patient toward resolving ambivalence by highlighting the negative aspects of the status quo and the positives of making change.

There are several levels of reflection ranging from simple to more complex. Different types of reflections are skillfully used as patients demonstrate different levels of readiness for change. An amplified reflection, for example, is more helpful when the patient seems resistant. Reflecting what the patient has said in an exaggerated or amplified way encourages the patient to argue less and can elicit the other side of the patient's ambivalence. For example, a patient with mild cognitive impairment may say: "I'm here because my daughter made me come here." The provider could respond with an amplified reflection (in an empathetic and matter-of-fact tone): "That's the only reason why you're here." The double-sided reflection is more appropriate when the patient offers statements indicative of ambivalence: "I know this cough is because I've smoked for so long, but I can't imagine quitting cigarettes now." To which the provider might respond, "On one hand, it's scary to think about quitting, but on the other, you're concerned about how smoking affects your health." Reflections serve to validate the patient's experience while also guiding the conversation toward resolving ambivalence about change.

Summaries

Summaries are a special type of reflection where the provider recaps what has occurred in all or part of a healthcare visit. Summaries communicate interest and understanding and call attention to important elements of the discussion. They may be used to shift attention or direction and prepare the patient to "move on." Summaries can highlight both sides of a patient's ambivalence about change and promote the development of discrepancy by strategically selecting what information should be included and what can be minimized or excluded. Finally, summaries give patients the sense that they have been heard and offer an opportunity for the patient to correct any misunderstandings.

CHANGE TALK

"Change talk" is defined as statements by the patient revealing consideration of, motivation for, or commitment to change. In MI, the provider seeks to guide the patient to expressions of change talk as the pathway to change.[13] Research indicates a clear correlation between patient statements about change and outcomes. This means that the more someone talks about change, the more likely they are to change. Different types of change talk can be described using the mnemonic DARN-CAT:[14]

- ■ **D**esire (I want to change.)
- ■ **A**bility (I can change.)
- ■ **R**eason (It's important to change.)
- ■ **N**eed (I should change.)
- ■ **C**ommitment (I will make changes.)
- ■ **A**ctivation (I am ready, prepared, willing to change.)
- ■ **T**aking Steps (I am taking specific actions to change.)

Commitment, activation, and taking steps are examples of implementing change talk and are the most predictive of a positive outcome.

Strategies for Evoking Change Talk

There are specific therapeutic strategies that are likely to elicit and support change talk in MI. The following is a list of 10 tools that can be used in any given patient encounter:[12]

1. **Ask Evocative Questions:** Ask an open-ended question, the answer to which is likely to be change talk.

2. **Explore Decisional Balance:** Ask for the pros and cons of both changing and staying the same.

3. **Good Things/Not-So-Good Things:** Ask about the positives and negatives of the target behavior.

4. **Ask for Elaboration/Examples:** When a change talk theme emerges, ask for more details: "In what ways?" "Tell me more?" "What does that look like?" "When was the last time that happened?"

5. **Look Back:** Ask about a time before the target behavior emerged. How were things better, different?

6. **Look Forward:** Ask what may happen if things continue as they are (status quo). Try the miracle question: If you were 100% successful in making the changes you want, what would be different? How would you like your life to be in the time you have?

7. **Query Extremes:** What are the worst things that might happen if you don't make this change? What are the best things that might happen if you do make this change?

8. **Use Change Rulers:** Ask: "On a scale from 1 to 10, how important is it to you to change [the specific target behavior], where 1 is *not at all important* and a 10 is *extremely important*? Follow up by asking: "And why are you at ___ and not ___ [a lower number than stated]?" "What might happen that could move you from ___ to [a higher number]?" Alternatively, you could also ask "How confident are you that you could make the change if you decided to do it?"

9. **Explore Goals and Values:** Ask what the person's guiding values are. What do they want in life? Ask how the continuation of target behavior fits in with the person's goals or values. Does it help realize an important goal or value or interfere with it, or is it irrelevant?

10. **Come Alongside:** Explicitly side with the negative (status quo) side of ambivalence. "Perhaps _____ is so important to you that you won't give it up, no matter what the cost."

STAGES OF CHANGE

Assessing readiness to change is a critical aspect of MI. Motivation, which is considered a state, not a trait, is not static and thus can change rapidly from day to day. If providers know where patients are in terms of their readiness to change, they will be better prepared to recognize and deal with a patient's motivation to change. The Stages of Change model[15] shows that, for most people, a change in behavior occurs gradually, with the patient moving from being uninterested, unaware, or unwilling to make a change (precontemplation) to considering a change (contemplation) to deciding and preparing to make a change (preparation). Genuine, determined action is then taken (action), and, over time, attempts to maintain the new behavior occur (maintenance). Relapses are almost inevitable and become part of the process of working toward lifelong change.

A simple and quick way to assess the stage of change is to use a Readiness to Change Ruler.[12] This scaling strategy conceptualizes readiness or motivation to change along a continuum and asks patients to give voice to how ready they are to change using a ruler with a 10-point scale, where 1 = definitely not ready to change and 10 = definitely ready to change. Depending on where the patient is, the subsequent conversation may take different directions. The central dilemma for most people confronting health behavior change is ambivalence. Ambivalence is a state of having simultaneous, conflicting feelings toward both a current behavior and a new behavior. Ambivalence is most prominent during the contemplative stage.

When using MI with older adults, it is essential to focus on one behavior at a time. Once the provider and patient have agreed on an agenda for the visit and the patient has identified a behavior of concern, the provider can use a three-step process to frame the conversation. Elicit–Provide–Elicit is a simple approach congruent with MI. The steps are as follows: (a) Determine what the patient already knows, (b) reflect what they know and add information to help them understand more fully, and (c) ask what they want to know more about. For example, after determining that a patient is ambivalent about using a walker, the provider may elicit from the patient,

- "Tell me, what are your concerns about using a walker?"
- "What do you think would be the benefits of using a walker?"
- "What would you be most interested in knowing about using a walker?"

After listening to the patient's perspective and understanding, the clinician asks for permission before offering advice. This increases the likelihood that the patient will not be resistant to the suggestions offered. The clinician expresses empathy and provides information:

- "I hear that you're afraid of losing muscle mass and becoming frail. I'm aware of some strategies we can use to mitigate this. Would you like to hear about some of these?"
- "I wonder what you will think about this. . . . See which of these you think might apply to you. . . ."

Finally, the provider follows with open-ended questions to check in with the patient and elicit their feedback:

- "What else would you like to know?"
- "What do you think is the next step for you?"
- "What do you think about that?"
- "What does all of this mean to you?"

CONCLUSION

The MI approach is consistent with the values of PCC and is one way to implement PCC into practice. PCC is an antidote to a fragmented healthcare system that dissects patients into body parts. In such a system, the disease model of healthcare dominates, and the very strengths that can support better health outcomes are minimized or overlooked. Communication errors lead to a lack of trust and undermine the patient–provider relationship. For older adults, this can mean deadly medication errors, delays in care, and a sense of abandonment.

MI is an evidence-based approach to health behavior change. Core clinical strategies include reflective listening and using open-ended questions to elicit the person's values and priorities in order to support inherent motivation for change. MI encourages individuals to work through their ambivalence about behavior change and to explore discrepancies between their current behavior and broader life goals and values. MI is a person-centered way of communicating with older patients that respects the autonomy and the rich lived experience that every elder embodies.

CASE STUDY
PATIENT IN REHABILITATION AFTER A STROKE

Mrs. Santiago is a 78-year-old woman who was admitted to a skilled nursing facility for rehabilitation following a stroke.

Physical Examination

AGNP Provider: Hi Mrs. Santiago, my name is Laura, I'm an AGNP in the practice. I wanted to follow up with you about how your rehab is going here. How did the swim class go? *[open-ended question]*

Patient: I went once. The instructor was very nice, but I felt self-conscious. And the water was cold.

AGNP Provider: That must have taken a lot of courage to try it at all. *[affirmation]*
What were you hoping to achieve by going to the swim class? *[open-ended question]*

Patient: Well, the doctor told me it helps with balance. My balance has to get better. But I still feel pretty wobbly.

AGNP Provider: You were hoping it would help, but you're not seeing the results yet. *[reflection]*

Patient: Right.

AGNP Provider: What is your overall goal? What are you working toward? *[open-ended questions]*

Patient: Going home. I just want to get home to my life.

AGNP Provider: What is important to you about getting home? *[open-ended question]*

Patient: I'm a very independent person. I like to cook for myself, and I want to work in my garden.

AGNP Provider: So you want to get home to your life, your independence. *[reflection]* What do you need to do to achieve that goal? *[open-ended question]*

Patient: They told me I need to be able to walk down the hall and back with the walker.

(cont.)

AGNP Provider: Do you agree that's what you need to do to get home? *[closed-ended question]*

Patient: (With some hesitation) Yes, I don't want to fall. I've had friends that have had that happen. I guess I agree.

AGNP Provider: And tell me how your other physical therapy is going. *[open-ended question]*

Patient: Oh, it's better. It still hurts, but I'm getting better.

AGNP Provider: So, it sounds like you can see you're making progress in physical therapy and you're hoping swim class will help you with the balance. *[summary]*

And so, do you want to go back to swim class? *[closed-ended question]*

Patient: (With some hesitation) Yes, my friend loves it. I just wish I wasn't so self-conscious.

AGNP Provider: It's important that you know that you're the one who gets to make the decision about whether swim class works for you. *[support autonomy]*

Patient: Well, I don't know after one time. I guess I can't tell after just one time.

AGNP Provider: So, you haven't seen the results you want yet, but because we have recommended it could help with balance and your friend does it, it sounds like you'd like to give it another chance. *[double sided reflection]*

What has to happen for you to get there again?

Patient: I'd have to make arrangements, and I'd have to get over feeling self-conscious.

AGNP Provider: I think we can help you make arrangements. Feeling self-conscious is not uncommon, but you're right, it's something you'll have to decide how to handle. How confident are you on a scale of 1 to 10, with 1 being *not at all confident* and 10 being *the most confident* that you can learn to feel less self-conscious? *[self-efficacy scale]*

Patient: I guess I'm a 5. I know I can, but it is really hard when I look in the mirror.

AGNP Provider: What would help you to feel more confident?

Patient: I think if I go at the same time my friend is there I won't care as much. Or maybe if I get a new swimsuit.

AGNP Provider: Are there any other barriers to getting to swim class?

Patient: Not that I can think of right now.

AGNP Provider: You can see that you're making progress with physical therapy, and you're hopeful that swim class will give you that extra push toward regaining your balance. If we can help make arrangements and you can coordinate with your friend, you're willing to give it another chance. *[summary]*

REFERENCES

References for this chapter are online and available at https://connect.springerpub.com/content/book/978-0-8261-8414-6/part/part01/toc-part/ch2.

CHAPTER 3

Integrating Patient Safety and Quality Improvement into Practice

Deb Bakerjian and Amy A. Nichols

LEARNING OBJECTIVES

At the conclusion of this chapter, the learner will be able to:

➤ Demonstrate an understanding of patient safety and quality improvement principles.

➤ Compare and contrast the patient safety and quality improvement competencies.

➤ Apply patient safety and quality improvement principles in practice.

INTRODUCTION

Knowledge and skills in patient safety and quality improvement principles and processes are vital for all healthcare professions students during their educational journey to ensure that the healthcare workforce is well prepared to provide high-quality and safe care. Adult-gerontology nurse practitioners (AGNPs), along with other primary care nurse practitioners, play an important role in leading patient safety and quality improvement efforts in the primary care environment, particularly pertaining to the care of older adults. Therefore, it is critical that they understand the overarching principles and specific processes and metrics to identify medical errors and quality problems to prevent harm to patients. Additionally, knowledge of key agencies, such as the Agency for Healthcare Research and Quality (AHRQ), that are involved in quality and safety will assist in their ability to tap into evidence-based resources and toolkits will help them provide optimal care in their practices. It is incumbent that AGNP programs ensure that they have the knowledge, skills, and abilities to ensure high-quality, safe care.

Background and Significance

Many Americans believe that the U.S. healthcare system is the best in the world and expect that they will always receive the highest quality and safest care. In 2019, the United States spent almost $11,000 per capita on healthcare (Figure 3.1); Switzerland was second at $7,730, and the mean expenditure for comparable countries was about $5,700.[1]

Although the United States spends the highest amount of money on healthcare of any nation in the world (17.1% of the gross domestic product [GDP]), unfortunately U.S. health outcomes are not the best in the world. The World Health Organization (WHO) ranked the U.S. healthcare system 37th in the world in 2019, a similar ranking to where they have been for the last few decades.[2] In 2019, the United States was ranked 40th in the world for life expectancy at birth, 78.5 years, compared with Japan, which was first at 84.3 years. Similarly, the United States ranked 33rd for infant mortality according to the Organisation for Economic Co-operation and Development in 2019.[3] Figure 3.2 shows the overall health rankings of westernized nations based on the Institute of Medicine (IOM; now the National Academy of Medicine [NAM]) quality domains first identified in *Crossing the Quality Chasm*.

Given the high cost of care and the lower quality outcomes, one must ask, Where is the value? Value equals the quality of care divided by the cost of care. These rankings provide strong incentives for the United States to improve the quality and safety and increase the value of healthcare. AGNPs can impact quality and safety through their individual efforts and collectively by collaborating with other members of the interprofessional team to ensure that the overall organization embraces quality and safety practices.

Defining Patient Safety and Quality Improvement

There are several definitions of patient safety in the literature; however, for the purposes of this chapter, the definition from the AHRQ[3] will be used, which is "avoiding harm to patients from care that is intended to help them."[4] Preventing harm to patients is a fundamental tenet in patient safety with multiple components to consider depending on the role of the healthcare worker and the situation with the patient. Harm in patient safety is typically related to the care provided or not provided to the patient. For example, patients might be harmed when there is a diagnostic error and care is either not provided or the wrong care is provided.

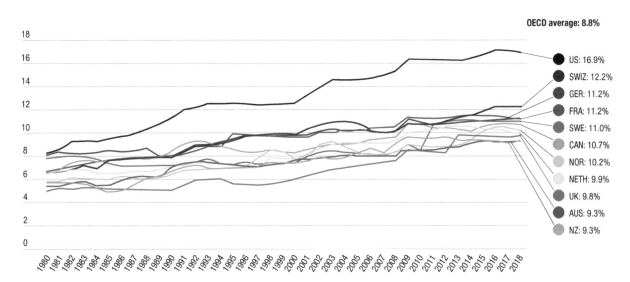

Figure 3.1: U.S. spending compared with other westernized nations

Source: Tikkanen M, Abrams MK. U.S. health care from a global perspective, 2019: higher spending, worse outcomes? Published January 30, 2020. https://www.commonwealthfund.org/publications/issue-briefs/2020/jan/us-health-care-global -perspective-2019

Country rankings

	AUS	CAN	FRA	GER	NETH	NZ	NOR	SWE	SWIZ	UK	US
Overall ranking (2013)	4	10	9	5	5	7	7	3	2	1	11
Quality care	2	9	8	7	5	4	11	10	3	1	5
Effective care	4	7	9	6	5	2	11	10	8	1	3
Safe care	3	10	2	6	7	9	11	5	4	1	7
Coordinated care	4	8	9	10	5	2	7	11	3	1	6
Patient-centered care	5	8	10	7	3	6	11	9	2	1	4
Access	8	9	11	2	4	7	6	4	2	1	9
Cost-related problem	9	5	10	4	8	6	3	1	7	1	11
Timeliness of care	6	11	10	4	2	7	8	9	1	3	5
Efficiency	4	10	8	9	7	3	4	2	6	1	11
Equity	5	9	7	4	8	10	6	1	2	2	11
Healthy lives	4	8	1	7	5	9	6	2	3	10	11
Health expenditures/Capita, 2011**	$3,800	$4,522	$4,118	$4,495	$5,099	$3,182	$5,669	$3,925	$5,643	$3,405	$8,508

Legend: Top 2* / Middle / Bottom 2*

Figure 3.2: Overall health rankings of westernized countries based on quality domains

Source: The Commonwealth Fund. US health system ranks last among eleven countries on measures of access, equity, quality, efficiency, and healthy lives. Press release. Published June 16, 2014. https://www.commonwealthfund.org/press -release/2014/us-health-system-ranks-last-among-eleven-countries-measures-access-equity

"Quality of care" can be defined very simply as doing the right things in the right way, which requires healthcare providers to perform at the highest level using the best available evidence in an effective and efficient manner. The AHRQ[4] definition of "quality improvement" is "the framework we use to systematically improve the ways care is delivered to patients."[5] Although the concepts of patient safety and quality of care have been around for centuries, these topics were brought to the forefront when the IOM (whose name changed in 2020 to the National Academy of Medicine or NAM) Committee on Quality of Health Care in America published two landmark reports early in the 21st century.

Two Landmark Reports

To Err Is Human: Building a Safer Health System revealed stunning findings that as many as 98,000 people die annually from avoidable causes in healthcare.[6] At that time, this report revealed that medical errors were responsible for more deaths than several other significant and more well-known causes of death, such as motor vehicle accidents, breast cancer, and AIDS. Furthermore, the authors reported that the national cost of preventable medical errors (adverse events) that cause injury was between $17 and $29 billion annually. The study unquestionably broke the silence that had existed for decades about medical mistakes, which was attributed to provider concerns about the fear of liability. It also emphasized that healthcare providers are human and that humans make mistakes, normalizing this phenomenon by highlighting several systems-level causes of medical errors and identifying several barriers to reporting these adverse events. One of the most important messages from this report is that Americans need to reframe how they think about adverse events caused by human error. Instead of blaming individuals, focus should be placed on analyzing the error and the system of care and putting systems-level measures in place to prevent errors.

High-quality care begins with ensuring safe care and adverse events or medical errors provide the motivation for quality improvement (QI). Therefore, it makes sense that 2 years after *To Err Is Human* was published, the NAM committee followed with a second landmark study, *Crossing the Quality Chasm: A New Health System for the 21st Century.*[7] This report focused on the failures of the U.S. healthcare system and what was needed to bring about improvements. To quote the committee that worked on this report, "Quality problems are everywhere, affecting many patients. Between the health care we have and the care we could have lies not just a gap but a chasm." The report called for urgent changes to close the gap in quality of care in the United States and set performance expectations, rules to guide patient–clinician relationships, an organizing framework for making improvements, and steps to promote evidence-based practice and strengthen clinical information systems. The organizing framework is particularly helpful in thinking

about an approach to quality. The original quality dimensions included safety, timeliness, effectiveness, efficiency, patient centeredness, and equity. In 2010, the Committee revised the framework for the National Healthcare Quality Reports (NHQR) and National Healthcare Disparities Report (NHDR). The revised framework saw equity and value as crosscutting dimensions across all other components and settings of quality care.

The Triple Aim

The Triple Aim is a framework initially developed by the Institute for Healthcare Improvement (IHI) that focuses on optimizing the performance of health systems of all types. The framework covers three domains:

- Improving the health of populations
- Improving the patients and family experiences and outcomes of care
- Reducing healthcare per capita costs[8]

This overarching framework provides a useful guide for improving population health at a lower cost and without sacrificing the positive experience of patients and families. According to Don Berwick, a former administrator of the Centers for Medicare and Medicaid Services (CMS) and former president and CEO of IHI, organizations are responsible for partnering with individuals and families and redesigning primary care, population health management, financial management, and macro-system integration. AGNPs participate by using the IHI framework as a lens for approaching their practice, using the best available evidence to provide care, embracing a person-centered approach, and implementing effective and efficient processes of care.

As practices began to embrace the Triple Aim, there was increasing evidence of the negative impact on healthcare providers. In response to reports of dissatisfaction and burnout in the healthcare workforce and the ensuant challenges, such as workforce turnover and increases in medical errors, Bodenheimer and Sinsky posited a growing gap between society's expectations of the primary care workforce and the ability for primary care providers to overcome the barriers in achieving the Triple Aim.[9] They proposed that healthcare organizations must address the increasing burnout of the workforce and suggested the need for a fourth aim, creating the Quadruple Aim, which adds the aim of improving clinicians' experience of healthcare. Causes are that burnout is similar for physicians and nurses, starting with long work hours, a high-stress environment, extensive time on bureaucratic tasks instead of patient care, the amount of time documenting care in electronic health records, and a lack of autonomy.[10] Shah et al.[11] conducted a study of a sample of 50,273 nurses who represented a population of 3,957,661 nurses. In the total weighted sample of nurses who left their job, 9.5% reported burnout as the cause, and of those considering leaving their job, 43.3% reported burnout as the cause.[11] These numbers are significantly higher than in a 2007 study that reported only 17% citing burnout as a reason for leaving their job.[12] Subsequently, there have been numerous efforts on the part of workforce stakeholders, including employers and workforce agencies such as the Healthcare Resources and Services Administration, to identify ways to reduce burnout.[13,14]

Advanced Practice Quality and Safety Competencies

The American Association of Colleges of Nursing (AACN) led a national effort designed to enhance the ability of nurse faculty to effectively develop quality and safety competencies among graduates of their programs. The AACN hosted a series of regional Quality and Safety Education for Nurses (QSEN) Faculty Development Institutes in 2010 and 2011; the program gave nurse faculty key training and information to improve their curricula. QSEN was developed to inspire healthcare professionals to put quality and safety as a core value to guide their work either in practice or within a school of nursing

curriculum. There are six major QSEN competencies developed for prelicensure and graduate nursing programs: patient-centered care, teamwork and collaboration, evidence-based practice (EBP), QI, safety, and informatics.[15] In addition, competency requirements are defined and agreed on by the National Organization of Nurse Practitioner Faculties (NONPF). The NONPF created the first set of competencies in 1990; the most recent updates were incorporated in 2012. These core competencies apply to all nurse practitioners, regardless of their medical specialty or patient population focus. Nurse practitioner core competencies were created by experts in clinical practice and education. The task force behind the 2012 update included various nurse practitioner organizations and certification boards, and it created subgroups of experts for each population focus. NONPF has defined nine broad areas of core competence: scientific foundations, leadership, quality, practice inquiry, technology and information literacy, policy, health delivery system, ethics, and independent practice. Table 3.1 describes the knowledge, skills, and attitudes for the QSEN and the NONPF.

Table 3.1: Graduate Competencies for Patient Safety (QSEN) and Quality (NONPF)

QSEN Graduate Competencies: Safety		
Knowledge	Skills	Attitudes
Analyze factors that create a culture of safety and a "just culture."	Use existing resources to design and implement improvements in practice (e.g., National Patient Safety Goals). Use evidence and research-based strategies to promote a "just culture."	Commit to being a safety mentor and role model. Accept the cognitive and physical limits of human performance. Value a systems approach to improving patient care instead of blaming individuals.
Identify best practices that promote patient, community, and provider safety in the practice setting.	Integrate strategies and safety practices to reduce risk of harm to patients, self, others (e.g., risk evaluation and mitigation [REM] strategy).	Value the process of risk reduction in health systems.
Analyze human factors safety design principles as well as commonly used unsafe practices (e.g., work-arounds, risky behavior, and hazardous abbreviations).	Demonstrate leadership skills in creating a culture where safe design principles are developed and implemented. Engage in systems focus when errors or near misses occur. Promote systems that reduce reliance on memory.	Appreciate the role of systems problems as a context for errors. Accept the limitations of humans.
Identify effective strategies to promote a high-reliability organization.	Create high-reliability organizations based on human factors research. Report errors and support members of the healthcare team to be forthcoming about errors and near misses.	Commit to working to achieve a high-reliability organization. Value the contribution of standardization and reliability to safety.

(continued)

Table 3.1: Graduate Competencies for Patient Safety (QSEN) and Quality (NONPF) (*continued*)

	Anticipate/prevent systems failures/hazards.	Value open and honest communication with patients and families about errors and hazards. Encourage reporting of errors as a foundational element to improve quality and systems.
Describe evidence-based practices in responding to errors and good catches.	Use evidence-based best practices to create policies to respond to errors and "good catches."	Value the use of organizational error and reporting systems.
Identify processes used to analyze cause and error and allocation of responsibility and accountability (e.g., root cause analysis and failure mode effects analysis).	Design and implement microsystem changes in response to identified hazards and errors.	Commit to the identification of errors and hazards. Commit to individual accountability for errors.
Summarize methods to identify and prevent verbal, physical, and psychological harm to patients and staff.	Encourage a positive practice environment of high trust and high respect. Develop culture in which a hostile work environment is not tolerated. Use best practices and legal requirements to report and prevent harm.	Value a work and patient care culture where dignity and respect are fostered inclusive of prevention of assaults and loss of dignity for patients, staff, and aggressors.
Analyze the potential and actual impact of national patient safety resources, initiatives, and regulations on systems and practice.	Use national patient safety resources to design and implement improvements in practice.	Value the relationship between national patient safety campaigns and implementation of system and practice improvements.

NONPF NP Core Competencies: Quality

Quality Competencies	NP Core Competencies	Content to Support Competencies
	Use the best available evidence to continuously improve the quality of clinical practice. Evaluate the relationship among access, cost, quality, and safety and their influence on healthcare.	QSEN principles and content
	Evaluate how organizational structure, care processes, financing, marketing, and policy decisions impact the quality of healthcare. Apply skills in peer review to promote a culture of excellence. Anticipate variations in practice and be proactive in implementing interventions to ensure quality.	Evaluate outcomes of care such as quality improvement projects with an evaluation component. Have a reflective practice. Participate in a culture of safety. Evaluate cost-benefit analysis. Participate in peer-review process. Collaborate in team processes and practices. Use skills for leading change for quality clinical practice.

NONPF, National Organization of Nurse Practitioner; QSEN, Quality Safety Education in Nursing
Source: QSEN Institute. Graduate QSEN competencies: safety. n.d. https://qsen.org/competencies/graduate-ksas; Thomas A, Crabtree M, Delaney K, et al. *Nurse Practitioner Core Competencies Content*. National Organization of Nurse Practitioner Faculties; 2017:5. https://cdn.ymaws.com/www.nonpf.org/resource/resmgr/competencies/2017_NPCoreComps_with_Curric.pdf

Quality and Safety Agencies

To Err Is Human and *Crossing the Quality Chasm* were groundbreaking reports that set the foundation for the patient safety and quality movements that followed in the next two decades.[3,15] Most of the recommendations in these reports resulted in actionable change. For example, Congress established the Agency for Health Care Policy and Research in 1989 as the lead federal agency responsible for improving the safety and quality of the U.S. healthcare system. In 1999, about the time of *To Err Is Human* was published, it was renamed the AHRQ. Since that time, the AHRQ has been a leader in improving systems of care in America. Its website (www.ahrq.gov) has a myriad of helpful information, research, programs, and toolkits available for clinicians.

Patient Safety and Quality Organizations and Accrediting Agencies

There are several other important organizations that focus on patient safety, quality, and QI. These are listed in Table 3.2. The table provides the name of the agency and its main purpose.

There are also several organizations that establish national standards and accreditation processes for healthcare organizations in the United States. Healthcare facilities voluntarily sign up with the organizations of their choice to go through the accreditation process, which is required by most payers such as Medicare, Medicaid, and private insurers. Table 3.3 lists the main organizations that accredit healthcare organizations.

Implications for AGNPs

It is important that AGNPs understand the various national and state agencies and organizations that may impact the healthcare work environment by establishing quality standards of care and ensuring safe patient care. AGNPs will have opportunities to interact with these agencies in a variety of ways. For example, the AGNP may be asked to lead the QI efforts at their organization; therefore, understanding what metrics are being tracked nationally and how their organization compares with others in their state and in the United States will be important. The AGNP may be part of the accreditation team that helps to review the organizational standards and prepare for accreditation visits. In those roles, it will also be critical to understand what the accreditation standards are as they pertain to quality and safety and how the healthcare team provides care.

Table 3.2: U.S. Quality and Safety Agencies

Agency	Organization	Purpose/Work
National Quality Forum www.qualityforum.org/About_NQF	Not-for-profit, nonpartisan, membership-based	Leads U.S. healthcare providers to come to consensus on measurable healthcare goals; goals considered best, evidence-based approach to improving care
AHRQ–Patient Safety Organization www.ahrq.gov	Can be government, industry, professional, or consumer organizations	Collects and analyzes voluntarily reported data to help establish national benchmarks and goals to improve quality
Quality Improvement Organizations (QIOs) www.cms.gov/Medicare/Quality-Initiatives-Patient-Assessment-Instruments/QualityImprovementOrgs	Not-for-profit	These organizations have health quality experts and work with guidance from CMS to support healthcare facilities such as hospitals and nursing homes to improve quality. They also respond to consumer appeals on behalf of CMS.
Centers for Disease Control and Prevention www.cdc.gov	Government	
CMS Compare Website www.medicare.gov/care-compare/?providerType=Hospital&redirect=true	Government	Website allows consumers to select and compare hospitals, nursing homes, home health agencies, hospice, inpatient rehabilitation, long-term care hospitals, doctors and clinicians, and dialysis centers
Institute for Healthcare Improvement www.ihi.org	Not-for-profit	Provides education and tools for quality improvement and patient safety

CMS, Centers for Medicare & Medicaid Services.

Table 3.3: Accrediting Bodies for U.S. Healthcare Organizations

The Joint Commission (TJC) www.jointcommission.org	Not-for-profit	Sets healthcare standards and accredits thousands of hospitals and other healthcare facilities. It also sets National Patient Safety Goals that are updated annually and collect quality and safety data from its evaluation processes.
National Committee for Quality Assurance (NCQA) www.ncqa.org	Not-for-profit	This organization has programs that provide accreditation and monitoring of health facilities and organizations through multiple programs: Patient-Centered Medical Home (PCMH) Recognition program is how PCMH practices are evaluated and recognized; Health Plan Accreditation sets standards, surveys, and collects performance data from health plans. The NCQA also accredits other healthcare organizations, particularly ambulatory healthcare offices. Healthcare Effectiveness Data and Information Set (HEDIS) are the measures NCQA uses to compare facilities.
American Medical Accreditation Program (AMAP)		Offers accreditation to physician practices based on 12 core standards based on domains of education, licensure, ethics, and practice. AMAP is an offshoot of the American Medical Association (AMA).
Utilization Review Accreditation Commission (URAC) www.urac.org		Accredits health plans, pharmacies, mental health organizations, disease management, dental networks, call centers, case management, and multiple other programs. Focuses on a quality improvement approach.
Accreditation Association for Ambulatory Health Care (AAAHC) www.aaahc.org		Only accredits ambulatory healthcare organizations including ambulatory surgery, endoscopy, student health, retail clinics, and medical and dental practices
Commission on Accreditation of Rehabilitation Facilities (CARF) www.carf.org		Accredits disability, addiction, substance abuse, and home and community services organizations based on quality of care and demonstrating value

APPROACH TO PATIENT SAFETY AND QUALITY IMPROVEMENT

In general, all healthcare organizations and individual healthcare providers have a goal of providing high-quality and safe care. Federal and state governments have a role in ensuring that the public is provided safe care and establish minimum standards of care derived to achieve those quality standards. Accrediting agencies evaluate the different healthcare organizations and certify that they meet these standards; when organizations fail accreditation, it puts them at risk of losing their contracts with commercial insurers and the federal government. This system of national standards and oversight through accreditation is what helps achieve the best quality of care possible in the United States.

Despite these efforts, medical errors and adverse events occur in large numbers each year, and the U.S. healthcare rankings are poor in many of the areas that impact Americans' overall health. Advanced practice providers must work with the rest of the healthcare team to improve healthcare in the United States by integrating patient safety principles into their practice and implementing QI processes.

Donabedian's Conceptual Framework

An excellent way to approach patient safety and quality improvement is by understanding the Donabedian Conceptual Framework (Figure 3.3). Avedis Donabedian was a physician who was commonly known as the Father of Quality. Dr. Donabedian studied medical quality for many years and was the first physician to explore quality assessment and the monitoring of medical quality. He created a "quality framework," which he proposed was a useful way to think about healthcare quality. His framework involved identifying characteristics of healthcare and categorizing them as structures (the conditions under which care is provided), processes (the activities that constitute healthcare), or outcomes (changes attributable

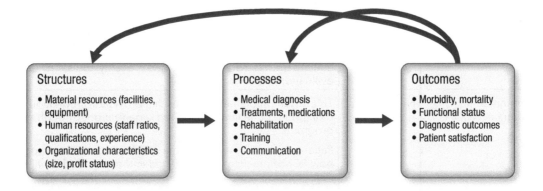

Figure 3.3: Sample Donabedian's structures, processes, outcomes (SPO) framework

to healthcare). Donabedian posited that good structures would lead to good processes and ultimately to good patient outcomes. Donabedian's initial model was criticized as being too linear, but later work recognized the existence of the feedback loop that outcomes would affect structures and processes.

UNDERSTANDING ERRORS AND ADVERSE EVENTS

One of the first steps to improve safety in healthcare settings is to understand the epidemiology and connection of safety events and to appropriately classify events. Medical errors are events that lead to a negative outcome or have the potential for a negative outcome.[16] An "adverse event" is defined as an unintended injury or complication due to management or medical care that affects the patient. A "near miss" is a medical error that is identified and caught before it reaches or harms the patient. Classifying and identifying errors, adverse events, and near misses allow healthcare systems to analyze events, track trends, and make improvements to prevent future errors. Ambulatory care-related errors and adverse events differ from those related to hospital-based care. Events in outpatient settings are classified as related to diagnosis, treatment, medication prescriptions, and surgery.[17] Diagnostic-related errors in the process of care are more problematic in outpatient settings, and a variety of factors contribute to their occurrence.

PATIENT SAFETY ESSENTIALS

There are several important patient safety concepts that AGNPs must be familiar with to prevent medical errors and adverse events and avoid causing harm to patients. The next several sections describe the most important of these patient safety concepts. Students should familiarize themselves with the concepts and be able to apply them within the practice environment.

Reducing Harm

A patient in the care of a healthcare provider, whether inpatient or outpatient, should not be harmed due to medical errors. Although not all errors can be prevented, the healthcare team should put special focus on those errors that harm patients. For example, an AGNP may inadvertently order a comprehensive metabolic panel by error when the intent was to order a basic metabolic panel. In almost all cases, this error would not cause harm to the patient. There may be a greater cost associated with the more expensive test, but that can be mitigated by the provider. Common medical errors that AGNPs may make that can also cause the patient harm include diagnostic errors (misdiagnosis or delayed diagnosis), medication errors, delayed diagnostic tests or other treatments, and failure to act on diagnostic test results. Other patient safety issues include overtreatment (e.g., unnecessary surgeries or procedures, unnecessary medications, or other treatments) and undertreatment (e.g., failure to prescribe a medication or provide a treatment).

There is a subset of medical errors called "never events." TJC refers to these as "sentinel events"; hospitals are asked to voluntarily submit sentinel events to TJC, which requires that the hospital perform a root cause analysis (RCA) for each sentinel event. These are medical errors that cause substantial harm or death to a patient. Examples include wrong site surgery, wrong surgery, inpatient suicide, retained foreign objects, mismatched blood transfusion, severe (stage 3 or 4) pressure injuries, or preventable product or device errors.[18]

AGNPs should be able to recognize serious medical errors and work with the healthcare team in their organization to put appropriate systems in place to prevent errors from occurring. Despite efforts at prevention, sometimes errors do happen. In that case, it is important to determine why the error happened. One of the main ways that a patient safety or QI team determines why an error occurred is through the RCA process.

Root Cause Analysis

TJC defines RCA as "a process for identifying the factors that underlie variation in performance, including the occurrence or possible occurrence of a sentinel event."[19] The purpose of an RCA should be focused on systems and processes rather than on individual performance, and the product of this analysis is an action plan that identifies strategies to reduce the risk of similar events occurring in the future. Action plans should address the responsibility for implementation and oversight, pilot testing (when appropriate), timelines, and measures of effectiveness of the plan. A typical RCA incorporates six steps (Figure 3.4):[20]

Step 1: Identify what happened. The team must try to describe what happened accurately and completely.

Step 2: Determine what should have happened. The team must determine what would have happened in ideal conditions.

Step 3: Determine causes ("Ask why five times"). This is where the team determines the factors that contributed to the event.

Step 4: Develop causal statements. A causal statement links the cause (identified in Step 3) to its effects and then back to the main event that prompted the RCA in the first place.

Step 5: Generate a list of recommended actions to prevent the recurrence of the event. Recommended actions are changes that the RCA team thinks will help prevent the error under review from occurring in the future.

Step 6: Write a summary and share it. This can be an opportunity to engage the key players to help drive the next steps in improvement.

Once the RCA is completed, it becomes part of the planning document. The root causes need to be prioritized and an action plan put in place. Which of the causes will the team act on first? Sometimes it makes sense to act on more than one cause. The RCA informs the intervention(s) the team will test to determine if they will prevent the problem from occurring in the future.

The Human Component of Patient Safety

A key component of any model of patient safety must consider the human factor or component of a system. Human factors is a body of knowledge about human abilities, human limitations, and other human characteristics relevant to design. Human factors engineering (HFE), also called ergonomics, is a discipline that conducts research regarding human psychological, social, physical, and biological characteristics and works to apply that information with respect to design, operation, or the use of products or systems that optimize human performance, health, safety, and/or habitability. Understanding human factors and the impact on their interplay on safety is very important for healthcare providers. The application of human factors methodology to help us better understand the issues and problems in clinical care and design meaningful solutions to improve the delivery of healthcare has become increasingly more common.[21] For example, for many years, it was possible to connect an intravenous line connector to other types of devices, such as a nasogastric tube, and vice versa. Because providers are often distracted in emergencies or other urgent situations in healthcare, errors happened when a tube feeding intended for a nasogastric tube was instead attached to an intravenous or central venous line. Humans get distracted and errors happen; to mitigate these kinds of errors, manufacturing can change the connectors so that IV fluid tubing can only connect to an IV line and the same for a tube feeding.

Human factors are an issue in many industries, not just healthcare. The airline and auto industries have

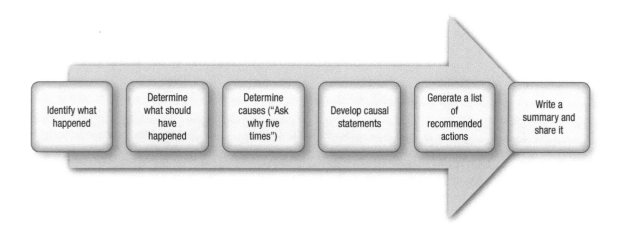

Figure 3.4: The IHI six steps of a root cause analysis

identified common human errors in their industries. The WHO published a report in 2009, *Human Factors in Patient Safety Review of Topics and Tools,* which describes the major human factors topics relevant to patient safety.[22] They developed an organizing framework with four main categories:

- Organizational/managerial
- Team
- Individual
- Work environment

Within these categories, there are 10 topics described: organizational culture, managerial leadership, communication, teamwork, team leadership, situation awareness, decision-making, stress, fatigue, and work environment. Each of these topic areas interacts throughout the four categories.

Human factors encompass human beings and how we interact with products, devices, procedures, workspaces, and the environment in our workplace. For example, our workspaces can be stressful and disruptive, cause distraction, and lead to fatigue. Human factors research involves studying human behaviors, applying the knowledge about human strengths and their limitations, and applying that information to designing better products and equipment and improving systems designs to ensure that humans can interact safely, efficiently, and effectively within their environment. This involves intensive examination of the healthcare environment, the products and machinery that clinicians work with, the culture of the organization, and the many activities performed to enhance performance and reduce error.

Several other organizations and agencies have created frameworks that are useful in understanding human factors in the work environment. Figure 3.5 shows the model developed by the Collaborative Healthcare Patient Safety Organization, a patient safety organization in 13 states, which is straightforward and easily understood. It shows the integration of humans, their work environment, and the human–machine interface, all of which are important in understanding human factors and HFE.

Understanding human factors is critical for healthcare providers to work toward a safer environment and to reduce medical errors and adverse events, thereby reducing patient harm.

The Swiss Cheese Model

The Swiss cheese model of accident causation is a model used in risk analysis and risk management, including aviation safety, engineering, healthcare, and emergency service organizations, and is the principle behind layered security, as used in computer security and defense in depth. It likens human systems to multiple slices of Swiss cheese, stacked side by side, in which the risk of a threat becoming a reality is mitigated by the differing layers and types of defenses that are "layered" behind each other. Therefore, in theory, lapses and weaknesses in one defense do not allow a risk to materialize because other defenses also exist to prevent a single point of failure. This model has gained widespread acceptance and is sometimes called the "cumulative act effect." In the Swiss cheese model, multiple failures in safeguards must happen for an error to reach a patient. When multiple systems are put in place to prevent an error, none of the individual failures is sufficient to cause harm; multiple failures must occur along the system safeguards. The model's name comes from the concept that each barrier to a bad outcome is like a

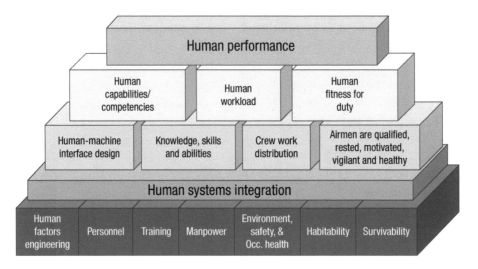

Figure 3.5: Human factors model of human performance and human systems integration

Source: Reproduced with permission from Pew RW. Some new perspectives for introducing human-systems integration into the system development process. *J Cogn Eng Decision Making.* 2008;2(3):165–180. doi:10.1518/155534308X377063

piece of Swiss cheese, with the holes in the cheese being analogous to potential errors, circumstances, or events. If enough of the holes line up in a series of slices of cheese, a bad outcome could occur (Figure 3.6).

There are different types of errors in the Swiss cheese model. Active errors are readily apparent and occur at the point of contact, typically between the healthcare provider and the patient (or the sharp end). An example might be an error in programming the intravenous pump so that the patient received the incorrect amount of fluid or dose of a medication. In contrast, latent errors are less obvious and typically upstream (or the blunt end); an example might be in the intravenous pump error that the hospital uses for many different types of pumps, each of which requires a different programming process, making it easy for a nurse to make an error.

Metrics

A valid, reliable, and usable system of metrics is essential to any patient safety program, including ambulatory care settings. Much of the early data focused on inpatient metrics, and ambulatory settings were not on the radar. Later, the focus on patient-centered care and framing care on a healthcare continuum shifted the evaluation of quality and safety to include outpatient care settings. Data related to patient safety can be used for a range of purposes, including selecting improvement initiatives, measuring the success of safety improvement efforts, and enhancing transparency by public reporting, organizational accreditation, and even contracting and reimbursement.[23] With the increase in patient safety data applications, the importance of the data has increased commensurately.

Several data elements should be contemplated in the context of patient safety metrics. First, are the data feasible to collect? Are the collected data reliable and valid? Do the data support their intended use? What is the rationale for using a given patient safety metric? It is the rationale for using a given patient safety metric that underlies the rationale for collecting it. The mere creation or use of patient safety measures does not ensure that they will be useful for improving safety and reducing harm. Even worse, invalid measures can lead to poor decision-making, whereas measures that do not lead to safety improvements can be viewed as lost opportunity costs.

There are many different agencies that measure the safety of healthcare. Some examples are TJC, the CMS, and the Leapfrog Group. In the past decade, it has become more common for these patient safety measures to

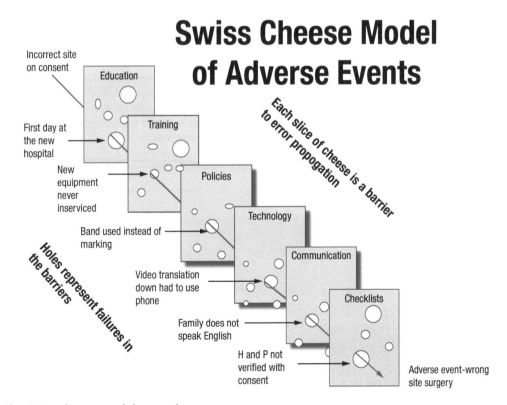

Figure 3.6: The Swiss cheese model example

Source: Stein JE, Heiss K. The Swiss cheese model of adverse event occurrence–closing the holes. *Semin Pediatr Surg.* 2015;24(6):278–282.

be publicly available on the internet. For example, CMS publishes data about many different types of organizations including hospital, nursing homes, dialysis centers, home health services, and others on their "compare" website (www.medicare.gov/care-compare). At this site, consumers can look up healthcare organizations in their geographic region to find out which are the safest and have the highest quality. Organizations and healthcare providers are rated on a 5-star system, with 5 stars being the best. Metrics for each of these categories vary, but examples for hospitals and nursing homes may include how many preventable falls happened in a given time (quarter or year) or the number of infections or serious complications that occurred. In fact, comparison data are becoming available about individual physicians and advanced practice providers on that same website. Data include whether the practice uses an electronic health record; whether it participates in quality metrics, such as ensuring that older adults have gotten a pneumonia vaccine; or whether it has followed recommended best practices to provide safe care.

Safety Culture–Just Culture

A safety culture environment is one in which members are accountable, respectful, and trustful toward each other; one in which errors or near misses can be reported free of shame and blame in an atmosphere of nonnegotiable mutual respect, and one in which all staff clearly know the difference between acceptable and unacceptable behaviors. "Just culture" is a notion related to systems thinking, which emphasizes that mistakes are generally a product of fault by organizational culture or the system rather than solely brought about by the person or persons directly involved. In a "just" culture, after an incident, the question asked is "What went wrong?" rather than "Who caused the problem, and who is to blame?" A just culture is not the same as a no-blame culture; it is a culture where individuals are accountable for their willful misconduct or gross negligence (see Figure 3.7).

A just culture helps create an environment in which individuals at all levels feel free to speak up when noticeable obvious errors are about to happen and to report errors to help the organization learn from mistakes. This contrasts with a "blame culture," which is much more punitive in nature, in which individual persons are fired, fined, or otherwise punished for making mistakes but the root causes leading to the error are not investigated and corrected. In a blame culture, mistakes may not be reported but rather hidden, leading ultimately to diminished organizational outcomes. In a system of just culture, discipline is linked to inappropriate behavior rather than harm. This allows for individual accountability and promotes a learning organizational culture.

In this system, honest human mistakes are seen as a learning opportunity for the organization and all its employees. Typically, the mistake is a systems or organizational error in which the individual who made the mistake is a part of this broken system. The individual who made the mistake may be offered additional training and coaching. However, willful misconduct may result in disciplinary action such as termination of employment, even if no harm was caused. As can be seen in Figure 3.7, there are three types of behaviors related to risk: human error, at-risk behavior, and reckless behavior. How the behavior is managed depends on the type of error. If it is human error, an inadvertent action, the goal is to console the person who made the error, offering additional training, modifying the systems that led to the error, or redesigning the process. At-risk behavior is a choice to increase risk when mistakenly believed to be justified and managed by coaching and incentivizing the right behaviors. And reckless behavior is a conscious disregard for obvious and known risk and should be managed through remedial actions.

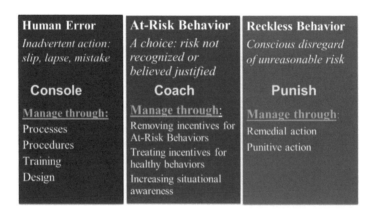

Figure 3.7: Accountability within a just culture

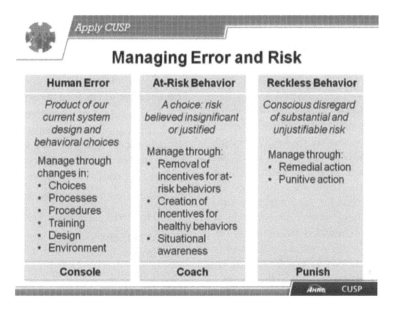

Figure 3.8: Managing error and risk

Source: Agency for Healthcare Research and Quality. Comprehensive Unit-based Safety Program: Apply CUSP module: Facilitator notes [Slide 7]. https://www.ahrq.gov/hai/cusp/modules/apply/ac-cusp.html

From the organizational culture perspective, punitive culture makes transparency impossible, yet a blame-free culture means no accountability. A just culture is designed to optimally support a culture of patient safety (Figure 3.8).[24] When healthcare workers exhibit reckless behavior, remedial actions must be put in place. However, the majority of medical errors and adverse events are simple human error, so modifying systems to prevent these errors is an appropriate action. This is called systems engineering, which is used to revise the system to prevent errors.

INTEGRATING PATIENT SAFETY IN PRACTICE

Key Aspects of Patient Safety in Primary Care

Multiple strategies are needed to prevent errors or mitigate harm in ambulatory settings. This includes cultivating a culture of patient safety, providing consistent leadership, making patient safety a top priority, having a strong commitment to improve quality of care, and instituting systems and mechanisms to ensure safety in ambulatory settings. Leadership in ambulatory settings with safety measures includes establishing a system for reporting adverse events, including near misses, and not forgetting to include disruptive behaviors. Confidential reporting systems should include a systematic analysis of reports

to discern root causes and factors contributing to events that inform changes for safer care. Should an error or an adverse event occur, the patient and/or family should be notified on what happened following a fact-gathering and situational investigation. Diagnostic errors in ambulatory practice are problematic. There are a variety of issues that stem from the process of care, including, but not limited to, the areas of history/physical evaluation of symptoms, ordering a diagnostic/lab test, interpreting tests, following up with providers, and referral management. Cognitive errors in clinical decision-making and diagnosis are challenging to address and resolve. Croskerry detailed more than 30 cognitive errors in diagnosis, including those associated with biases, failures in perception, and failures in solving problems using shortcuts.[25] Medication errors in ambulatory care that harm patients occur less frequently than diagnostic errors. Adverse drug events and medication safety are among the most studied topics in safety-related ambulatory research. Partnering with patients is at the cornerstone of patient-centered care as defined by the NAM (previously the Institute of Medicine). Increasing patient engagement helps to reduce the risk of adverse events and improve patient outcomes, satisfaction, and adherence to treatment. Research in patient-centered care found that achieving effective communication, partnership, and health promotion are critical to improving outcomes by improving the patient's experience and mitigating errors.[26]

CASE STUDY: PATIENT SAFETY

Angie Reed, AGNP, had just seen Ms. Martinez, a 60-year-old woman, for a well-woman check and discovered a breast mass. Angie ordered a diagnostic mammogram and an ultrasound. The radiologist report indicated there was dense breast tissue but ultimately interpreted the results as probably benign, which Angie reported to Ms. Martinez and asked her to return in 6 months. When the patient returned, the mass had increased in size. Angie was surprised by this and immediately referred her to a surgeon for a breast biopsy; however, there was a 2-month delay getting that appointment scheduled because the patient thought the surgeon's office would reach out to her to schedule the appointment. When Angie was informed about the issue, she reached out to the surgeon herself to arrange for an urgent appointment. Unfortunately, the biopsy showed invasive breast cancer that was found to have metastasized to her axillary nodes and her spine. Angie's collaborating physician, Dr. Alexander, berated her for not turning this case over to him, telling her that Ms. Martinez suffered due to her lack of judgment. Angie was devastated by what happened and, soon thereafter, quit her job and stopped practicing as an AGNP, returning to a nursing position.

1. What are the patient safety problems in this case?
2. What healthcare professionals were involved?
3. Was it appropriate for Dr. Alexander to have reacted in the way he did?
4. What are the implications of Angie leaving the profession?

QUALITY IMPROVEMENT ESSENTIALS

QI offers a structure and process that can be used to enhance the way care is delivered systematically, with an eye toward continually improving system performance and patient outcomes. QI is the natural follow-up to identifying medical errors and adverse events.

Quality Improvement Models

Three main QI approaches are currently used in healthcare—the IHI's Model for Improvement, Lean, and Six Sigma—although there have been several other approaches in the past. Key components of these models include

- emphasizing system improvements rather than blaming the individual for mistakes or shortfalls;
- including all team members involved in, or who have knowledge of, the issue at hand, with active solicitation of participation from frontline staff;

- having clear goals and transparent metrics and using data to identify issues and guide decisions; and
- using structured, iterative processes to support improvements over time.

The IHI Model for Improvement

The IHI model for improvement is the most widely used approach, as it is easily learned and applied without advanced training.[27] It also provides a foundation for Lean, Six Sigma, and Lean Six Sigma improvement cycles. This model asks three main questions:

1. What are we trying to accomplish?
2. How will we know that a change is an improvement?
3. What change can we make that will result in improvement?

Figure 3.9 shows the model for improvement and the Plan–Do–Study–Act (PDSA) process used to accomplish answering these questions. The model for improvement is founded on iteratively and incrementally changing clinical practice through a "trial and learning" approach, making small but progressive changes in rapid PDSA cycles.[28]

The Lean and Six Sigma Approaches

Lean and Six Sigma are two different approaches to quality improvement that can also be combined into Lean Six Sigma. Both approaches are used effectively in healthcare.

Lean

Lean arose from the automobile industry, primarily the Toyota Motor Corporation; these organizations embrace a culture that integrates production efficiency and product quality with an overall goal of eliminating waste and optimizing efficiency. "Kaizen," a Japanese word for "improvement," is a business philosophy that embraces continuous quality improvement with frequent, iterative small tests of change. The three pillars of Kaizen are housekeeping, elimination of waste, and standardization.

1. **Housekeeping:** The method of managing the work environment to be clean, orderly, and efficient is called *Gemba*. Staff conduct a Gemba Walk, in which they can look for wasteful activities; they observe, ask why, and show respect to the workers. In other words, participants can observe the care processes, ask why things are done that way, and take notes respectfully and without confrontation.

2. **Elimination of Waste:** *Muda* is the Japanese term for "waste." This refers to resources that are being used but are not adding value to the end product. Waste can be human or material resources or can focus on time, such as wait times in a healthcare office. The goal is to optimize efficiency without compromising quality.

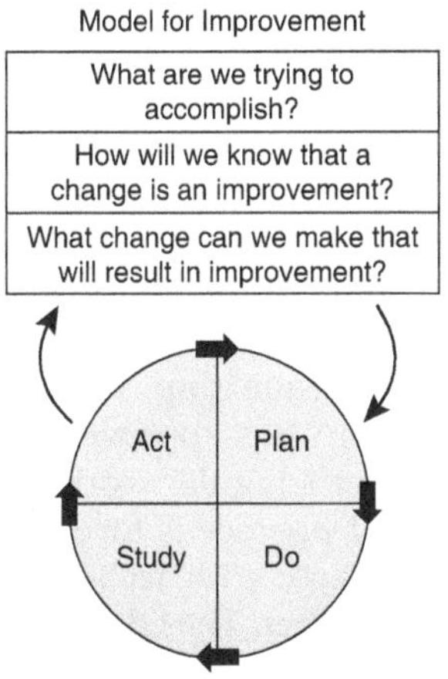

Model for Improvement

What are we trying to accomplish?

How will we know that a change is an improvement?

What change can we make that will result in improvement?

Act | Plan

Study | Do

Phases of a PDSA Cycle

Plan: Plan for the test. This includes stating the objective of the test, making predictions about what will happen, and developing a detailed plan for implementation, including data collection.

Do: Try out the test on a small scale. This could be as small as one provider trying out the change with one patient, one time. Results and any unexpected observations are documented. Data analysis begins.

Study: Time is dedicated to a more full data analysis and consideration of results. Data analysis is completed, results are compared to predictions set earlier, and any lessons learned are reviewed.

Act: Based on what was learned, refine next steps. Any needed modifications are identified, and plans fot the next cycle begin.

Figure 3.9: IHI model for improvement and phases of a Plan-Do-Study-Act cycle

PDSA, Plan-Do-Study-Act.

Source: Institute for Healthcare Improvement. How to improve. http://www.ihi.org/resources/Pages/HowtoImprove/ScienceofImprovementTestingChanges.aspx

3. **Standardization:** The process of developing standard for work is known as standardization and involves establishing preset specifications for each process with a goal of eliminating waste. Standardization means eliminating variation; when done well, it can lower costs and increase productivity due to stable workflows.

There are also five principles that are fundamental to Kaizen: Know your customers, let it flow, go to the Gemba, empower people, and be transparent. Lean defines value based on the customer's perspective. Lean, applied to healthcare, focuses on minimizing waste in all processes, procedures, and associated tasks in the organization.

Six Sigma

Six Sigma is a slightly different approach to quality improvement. It also focuses on reducing waste and eliminating defects or errors. It uses a process of DMAIC, which stands for define, measure, analyze, improve, and control. This is very similar to the PDSA process of the IHI model. Six Sigma uses data to drive change and places more emphasis on improving services and making them more effective.

Lean Six Sigma

Many healthcare organizations, particularly acute care hospitals, use Lean Six Sigma, which combines the principles and processes of Lean and Six Sigma. The combined goal is to use data to increase efficiency, eliminate waste, and reduce variation, thereby improving processes and patient outcomes in healthcare. Several organizations offer training in Lean Six Sigma methodologies for healthcare clinicians and staff.

THE QUALITY IMPROVEMENT PROCESS

QI is a team process that starts by identifying a problem, which often is associated with a patient safety adverse event or medical error. Problems can be identified through patient complaints, failure to meet targeted population metrics, or a problem that the provider or staff have identified. In hospitals or nursing homes, the problems could be identified from quality metrics or the outcome of an accreditation or survey visit. The target of the QI process can also be focused on improving efficiency or effectiveness or the patient experience of care. Using the quality dimensions or the Triple Aim as an overarching framework can help the QI team to identify issues that can be improved.

Initial team activities focus on establishing a project aim, determining measures, and selecting change strategies, which is guided by three fundamental questions: "What are we trying to accomplish?" "How will we know a change is an improvement?" and "What change can we make that will result in improvement?" Aims should be expressed in a SMART (specific, measurable, achievable, realistic, and time-bound) format; example aims might include:

- 90% of diabetic patients in the practice will get a HgbA1C drawn at least three times a year
  - meet an age-appropriate HgbA1C
  - sub-aims

- 80% of adult patients older than age 70 will undergo depression screening annually

Once project aims, measures, and change concepts are identified, the team moves into PDSA cycles to test the impact of implementing specific ideas for change, with the goal of rapidly putting readily accessible changes into action, learning which changes (or associated modifications) lead to improvement, and then scaling up or disseminating those positive changes for more widespread improvement effects through sequential PDSA cycles.[28] As a project starts, specific changes or a group of changes are implemented on a small scale. If changes show a positive response (as demonstrated by monitoring the determined measures), the tests are incrementally expanded to larger groups and settings if improvements continue to be noted.

For clinical practices interested in incorporating or improving care coordination, QI frameworks provide an accessible platform for introducing changes. While a brief overview is presented here, there are many resources available to learn more about QI methods, including training and strategies for implementation (see Table 3.4).

Identifying an Area or Areas for Improvement

QI is a process that starts by identifying a problem, which is often associated with a patient safety adverse event or medical error. Problems can be identified through patient complaints, failure to meet targeted population metrics, or a problem that a provider or staff has identified. In hospitals or nursing homes, the problems could be identified from quality metrics or the outcome of an accreditation visit or complaint investigation. The target of the QI project can also be focused on improving efficiency or effectiveness or the patient experience of care. Using the quality dimensions or the Triple Aim as an overarching framework can help the QI team to identify issues that can be improved. In many organizations, senior leadership develops the list of problems or assigns a committee specific problems.

Table 3.4: Quality Improvement Resources

Agency for Healthcare Research and Quality	www.ahrq.gov
American Medical Group Association	www.amga.org
American Society for Quality	www.asq.org
Institute for Clinical Systems Improvement	www.icsi.org
Institute for Healthcare Improvement	www.ihi.org
Lean Enterprise Institute	www.lean.org
Medical Practice Management Association	www.mgma.org
National Committee for Quality Assurance	www.ncqa.org

Put Together a Team

Forming the right team is an important step. In general, the team should have members who are knowledgeable about the specific problem, members who have expertise in QI, and someone from senior leadership who can facilitate approval of the process. Teams should meet regularly at a time that allows the most members to attend. Leadership should support the committee membership but approve time away from the committee member's regular work to participate in the QI activity. A best practice is for there to be a core group on the committee, with technical experts joining for a specific QI project. The QI team is accountable for their work, which means there should be meeting minutes and regular reporting of their progress to leadership.

Goal Setting

Once the team is formed and its members understand the problem to be improved, they should have aims or objectives for the project. Aims should be expressed in a SMART format:

- **Specific:** Is the information goal-focused and detailed enough to isolate the problem and identify an outcome? The aims should not be vague.
- **Measurable:** There must be a specified way to measure whether the project is successful. This is typically accomplished by observation, a survey, a checklist, or some other means for quantifying progress.
- **Achievable or Attainable:** While the goal should be challenging, it should also be reasonable for the organization to achieve. This is often referred to as a stretch goal.
- **Realistic or Relevant:** The goal should be important, practical, and aligned with the organization's mission, vision, and values.
- **Time-Bound:** This refers to having a target date for accomplishing the goal.

As an example, an aim might be that 90% of diabetic patients in the primary care practice who have visits in the next 90 days will have a HgbA1C drawn and discuss the results with their provider. It is specific to diabetic patients, measurable through drawing the HgbA1C labs, achievable as this is a best practice, relevant to diabetic patients' health, and time-bound within the next 90 days. Many times, the main aim of a QI project will have sub-aims. These are often interim process steps. For example, for the example aim, a sub-aim might be that the medical assistants will review the charts 1 week ahead of time to call the patients with diabetes who do not have a recent HgbA1C on record.

Understanding the Current Process and Root Cause Analysis

To be able to create an intervention, the team must understand what went wrong. This involves understanding the current way that specific process is accomplished and then determining what went wrong. This involves reviewing relevant policies and procedures as well as interviewing experts on the process in addition to team members who have that knowledge. For this step, the team wants to know what is expected of the staff based on existing policies and procedures. In addition, the team should conduct a literature search to ensure that existing policies and procedures are consistent with current best practices. The problem could be either that an error was made by a person or persons or that the policy and procedure are outdated. Sometimes it is helpful to create a process map or algorithm to represent the process, as it may be easier to identify where things went wrong in general.

The next step in this is to conduct an RCA. The RCA is a comprehensive team effort to understand the root causes of what went wrong. It is usually easy to determine interim or high-level causes of the error through the earlier step, but that is typically not the root or most important cause. Most of us understand that when we see a weed and just pull the visible part out of the ground, the weed will grow back because we did not remove the root. It is a similar issue in healthcare. If the QI team designs an intervention to solve an obvious cause but fails to address the root cause, the problem will return. Here is an example:

Joseph Lawson is an AGNP in a busy family practice and on the QI team. He informed the medical director that there had been a trend of patients with elevated international normalized ratios (INRs) and was concerned because of the potential for errors in prescribing the correct anticoagulant dose. The clinic uses a point-of-care (POC) INR test prior to prescribing warfarin. However, a few patients were found to have markedly different INR results from the reference lab that coincidentally had drawn blood within a few hours of the clinic test. Joseph, who leads the anticoagulant clinic, was assigned to determine the reasons for these errors but was given a very short timeline to get the improvement plan in place. Because time was limited, Joseph just made a list of potential problems and prioritized a lack of knowledge in performing the POC testing as the main cause. After talking with a few other providers, Joseph decided that better staff education was needed to resolve the problem. Staff education was developed, and 95% of the staff completed the training. Unfortunately, there continued to be problems with correct dosing. When the RCA was finally performed with the QI team, additional causes were identified, and although the POC testing was still identified as the main
problem, it was not because staff did not know how to conduct the test. Instead, it was discovered that clinicians were not considering patients who had abnormal hemoglobin levels, either too high or too low, which would cause results to be falsely high or low.

Develop an Intervention

Once the RCA is completed and the key problems are identified, an intervention or interventions can be developed. Typically, it is best to do small tests of change, which means there is a group of interventions consisting of incremental steps that will lead to the desired outcome.

Determine Measures

It is essential to develop a way to measure the outcome of the intervention. Examples include observing the activity, developing a survey, using a checklist, using diagnostic values, or doing chart abstraction. The QI team is responsible for developing the measure and determining how to display the outcomes. In most cases, the QI team uses a run chart that shows the results of the measurement over time; however, histograms, control charts, and other graphic representations of data can also be used.

Develop an Implementation Strategy

The previously discussed steps are part of the planning process. After the plan is completely developed, the team needs to develop an implementation strategy. It is best to have a strategy that allows for pilot-testing processes with a small group before rolling out the project through an entire organization. This allows the QI team to improve the processes along the way.

Implementing the Plan: The Plan-Do-Study-Act Cycle

Once project aims, measures, and change concepts are identified, the team moves into PDSA cycles to test the impact of implementing specific ideas for change, with the goal of rapidly putting readily accessible changes into action, learning which changes (or associated modifications) lead to improvement, and then scaling up or disseminating those positive changes for more widespread improvement effects through sequential PDSA cycles.[28] As a project starts, specific changes or a group of changes are implemented on a small scale. If changes show a positive response (as demonstrated by monitoring the determined measures), the tests are incrementally expanded to larger groups and settings if improvements continue to be noted.

For clinical practices interested in incorporating or improving care, QI frameworks provide an accessible platform for introducing changes. While a brief overview is presented here, there are many resources available to learn more about quality improvement methods, including training and strategies for implementation (see Table 3.5).

Metrics

QI processes must be measured so that the team can show that an improvement has or has not been achieved. To do this, the QI team must determine what they are going to use as a measurement and then obtain baseline measurements prior to starting the improvement process. Metrics can be anything that will help to show progress toward the goal. For example, if the team is trying to improve diabetes care, it might be counting the number of patients who have an HgbA1C ≥ 8.0 who receive quarterly HgbA1C labs. It may also entail counting the number of eye and foot examinations conducted on all patients with diabetes.

Once the improvement has been implemented, the team regularly remeasures (usually weekly) until the goal is achieved or until the team decides that the improvement plan is not working. The team has three actions to take:

- adopt the plan because the goals were met
- adapt the plan because parts of the plan worked, or some improvement was noted
- abandon the plan because no improvement was achieved.

Pilot Testing

Pilot testing involves implementing the plan with a small group. This might mean implementing the plan with a small percentage of patients, or it could be that the plan is implemented on one shift or with one practitioner.

The reason for pilot testing is that this will allow the team members to determine whether their plan works, and if not, they can make modifications and retest on the same small group until the plan works and makes headway toward the project goal. From there, the project can be expanded to additional units, practices, or practitioners until it has been implemented throughout the organization.

Sustainability is the biggest challenge that most organizations face. Typically, improvements are made in the first few months of a project but then will start to plateau. It is then that many organizations stop measuring and reinforcing the improvement, the patient safety or QI team disengages, and the staff stop focusing on that achievement. Over time, new staff come on board who don't know about the project, existing staff are no longer focusing on that work, and the improvements that were made begin to revert back. Sustainability requires that the organization maintain focus on the project and measure it for a prolonged period; this may be as long as several years. However, over time, the measurement can be less frequent unless the organization sees that the measures are backsliding, and then they can refocus on the project.

QI takes hard work in an organization, so finding ways to integrate new processes in the daily routine will help sustainability.[29] The best QI teams employ strong or at least intermediate actions to implement their improvement plan (see Table 3.5). Weak actions are easy to abandon along the way when healthcare workers get busy or stressed. Stronger actions have a greater impact on systems and are less prone to being inadvertently discontinued. In many cases, a combination of actions is needed, including creating a new policy, educating staff, devising a checklist, and making software enhancements, particularly if stronger actions are not feasible.

Table 3.5: Actions Taken to Implement Improvements in Quality Improvement

Stronger Actions	Intermediate Actions	Weaker Actions
• Change physical surroundings • Usability testing of devices prior to purchase • Simplify process & unnecessary steps • Standardization • Forcing functions	• Increase staffing/decrease workload • Software enhancements • Eliminate/reduce distractions • Checklist • Enhanced communication: read-back; documentation	• Double-checks • Warnings & labels • New procedure or policy • Training • Additional study or analysis

CASE STUDY (CONTINUED)

Review the patient safety case study involving Angie Reed, AGNP, from earlier in the chapter.

Prompted by Angie's abrupt departure, the quality and safety committee from this multipractitioner ambulatory care office investigated this case. As it turns out, there had been more than 40 patients who had delayed diagnostic tests in the office within the previous 3 months. The office had difficulty in maintaining trained staff in their office, which had doubled in size with almost 10 new providers during the previous 6 months. Many of the staff had been frustrated and complained to the leadership, but nothing had been done.

1. Assume that you are a member of this committee. What steps should be taken to address the issues in this case?
2. What kind of a plan needs to be put together? What would be the goals?
3. Who would participate in this activity?
4. How would you determine the causes of this problem?
5. What interventions should be initiated?
6. How would you measure progress?

CONCLUSION

AGNPs play an important role in leading patient safety and quality improvement in the primary care environment. The content in this chapter provides the fundamental knowledge needed to begin to integrate patient safety and quality improvement processes into their practice environments. AGNPs should utilize the knowledge, skills, and abilities and access the resources reviewed in this chapter to ensure they are practicing optimally and providing high-quality and safe care.

REFERENCES

References for this chapter are online and available at https://connect.springerpub.com/content/book/978-0-8261-8414-6/part/part01/toc-part/ch3.

CHAPTER 4

Interprofessional Collaboration and Team-Based Care

Deb Bakerjian and Jennifer J. Edwards

LEARNING OBJECTIVES

At the conclusion of this chapter, the learner will be able to:

➤ Demonstrate an understanding of the key themes in team-based care.

➤ Identify two to three methods for developing collaborative relationships with interprofessional staff.

➤ Differentiate between siloed and team-based care.

➤ Identify three ways in which the learner can encourage collaboration through their own practice.

INTRODUCTION

Adult-gerontology nurse practitioners (AGNPs) are important members of the interprofessional primary care team and are often asked to take a leadership role on teams. Thus, AGNPs must be familiar with the knowledge and skills necessary to model team-based care and be ready to lead high-quality teams to provide person-centered care. There are a variety of competencies that AGNPs must embrace and integrate into their practice related to team-based care. Several organizations have developed competencies that evolve from three landmark Institute of Medicine (IOM) reports: *To Err Is Human*,[1] *Crossing the Quality Chasm*,[2] and *Health Professions Education: A Bridge to Quality*;[3] all relate to team-based care.

Accrediting bodies from nursing, including the National Organization of Nurse Practitioner Faculties (NONPF) and the American Association of Colleges of Nursing (AACN), are requiring schools of nursing to provide education on interprofessional practice and team-based care. Furthermore, the Quality and Safety Education for Nurses (QSEN) Institute integrated team-based care into their patient safety and quality improvement competencies. In a follow-up, the Interprofessional Education Collaborative (IPEC), comprising accrediting bodies from multiple professions including medicine, nursing, pharmacy, and therapy, published core competencies for interprofessional education and practice that are essential to building the high-quality healthcare teams necessary to meet the needs of patients with complex, chronic conditions across the care continuum. This chapter illustrates the work of these experts across all health professions who contributed to the development of these important competencies and describes the AGNP's role in integrating the competencies into practice.

BACKGROUND

Over the past few decades, a significant shortage of primary care physicians has developed as a consequence of greater specialization in medicine, which impacts access to healthcare. This is evidenced by the 83 million Americans who live in a primary care health professional shortage area (HPSA). The shortage of primary care physicians is even more evident in rural areas, which make up 61% of primary care HPSAs in the United States, impacting the 23 million people living in those areas.[4] This shortage has led to new healthcare roles and an increased focus on efficient, effective team-based care.

Advances in technology and science have meant that people are living for decades with chronic health conditions that used to be fatal at younger ages (e.g., diabetes, certain cancers), creating more demand for care. These same advances have led to the increased specialization of healthcare roles as it has become more challenging to be a "jack of all trades." Increased specialization, along with shortages of primary care physicians, has spurred the development of new healthcare roles, including those of advanced practice nurses and physician assistants.[5]

Increasing patient demand, greater specialization in the healthcare profession workforce, and the need for more complex patient care have also forced a change in the delivery of healthcare, resulting in the need for the various professions and disciplines to work closely together. One could argue that healthcare professionals have a history of working closely together, with physicians and nurses providing care to patients since the 1800s. However, since those times in the 19th and early 20th centuries, society has continued to evolve and with it the healthcare needs of the U.S. population; consider how the population demographic and healthcare landscape has changed in the last 100 years. The U.S. population is aging and is more diverse; there have been extensive technological advances that have impacted the types of diagnostic and surgical procedures available, the types of medications that can be prescribed, and the ways in which healthcare providers communicate. In addition, shifting societal norms and the ease of access to information via the internet have also changed the dynamic between healthcare providers and patients. These changes have brought about a paradigm shift emphasizing person- and family-centered care, establishing new expectations for the way that healthcare providers interact with patients and families and resulting in new models of healthcare delivery. These new models of healthcare are becoming more team focused, which has been associated with improved outcomes. Therefore, it is essential that the AGNP student be exposed to the fundamentals of interprofessional, team-based care.

The Shift Toward Interprofessional Practice

In the 1990s, the IOM, now the National Academy of Medicine (NAM), initiated a multiphased effort to improve the quality of care in the United States. Between 1999 and 2003, the IOM released two landmark reports, *To Err Is Human* and *Crossing the Quality Chasm*, which highlighted significant gaps in healthcare quality and serious patient safety concerns in the U.S. healthcare system. The reports revealed shocking data that quantified the significant preventable harm caused by the healthcare system and the need for radical transformation to improve the quality of care (see Chapter 3).

Several strategies to address these challenges were laid out by the two committees, including the need for a sweeping redesign of the healthcare system to address the problem of preventable harm caused by medical errors in healthcare. An imperative that came from that work was to prepare the workforce, which included redesigning the way in which health professionals are trained. The committee focused on needed efforts to effectively implement workforce redesign. Their recommendations were targeted throughout healthcare and included all health professions with the goal of working in teams to provide coordinated patient care.

Health Education Reform

In response to the call for redesigning the workforce, the third phase of the IOM quality initiative was implemented, bringing more than 150 experts and thought leaders from a wide range of professions together to tackle the challenge of redesigning health professions education and training. It focused on the future healthcare system and the strategies and recommendations from the two previous reports. Its report, *Health Professions Education: A Bridge to Quality,* was released in 2003 and listed five

competencies central to the education of all health professions.[3] These were

1. provide patient-centered care.
2. apply quality improvement.
3. employ evidence-based practice.
4. utilize informatics.
5. work in interdisciplinary teams.

They named four key processes to achieve coordinated team-based care: communication, cooperation, coordination, and collaboration in teamwork. However, the report did not define the interprofessional competencies that would be necessary to address working in interdisciplinary teams. That work came some years later.

Team-Based Care and Health System Reform

Early efforts at team-based care focused on a multidisciplinary approach, in which efforts were made to involve various disciplines (e.g., geriatrics, cardiology, pulmonology) in the care of a patient. Although it was an important first step, there was little coordination between the specialties, and each discipline felt responsible only for those items within their clinical scope, maintaining professional silos.[6] Communication between disciplines was limited, and patients often received conflicting information from various specialists.[6]

As more research and reporting became available and as part of a rapidly changing healthcare landscape, there has been a move toward interdisciplinary teams, in which linked disciplines create a coordinated whole, and transdisciplinary teams, in which disciplines are integrated, allowing them to break through traditional boundaries.[7] Unlike multidisciplinary approaches, these interdisciplinary teams often work within the same office or setting and coordinate care between disciplines. A good example is the interdisciplinary team in a nursing home that typically includes a nurse, a pharmacist, and a therapist, among other professions. The group of clinicians works in the nursing home and provides care for or consults on the same group of patients. Thus, the interdisciplinary team communicates about shared patients and develops unified care plans. Patients are placed at the center of the care team, and shared-decision making is a focus.[6]

With even greater emphasis on teams that include different professions, the term "interprofessional" more commonly refers to various professions such as nursing, medicine, pharmacy, psychology, social work, and others working or learning together no matter the setting. Interprofessional collaboration is the effort of various professions to collaborate across the healthcare continuum. When education and training include various health professions schools it is called interprofessional education. This movement toward team-based care has forced changes in both education and clinical practice.

Healthcare reforms at both the education and practice levels have been influenced by a series of organizations that have developed competencies for interprofessional and team-based practice. Several of these are described in the following section.

COMPETENCIES

As the importance of interprofessional and collaborative practice has grown, competencies have been developed at both the student and professional levels. While not exhaustive, key interprofessional competencies are outlined next and are followed by a discussion on incorporating these competencies into the AGNP role.

Quality and Safety Education for Nurses

The QSEN competencies were developed based on the 2003 IOM competencies of patient-centered care, interdisciplinary team care, evidence-based practice, quality improvement, and informatics and were tailored to nursing. They were originally designed to guide curriculum development in prelicensure nursing programs to provide new nurses with the knowledge, skills, and attitudes required to improve the healthcare environment. Later, they were adapted to guide curriculum development for graduate-level programs, including graduating advanced practice nurses. There are six QSEN competencies that align with the five education competencies and add a competency to patient safety:

1. **Patient-Centered Care:** Recognize the patient or designee as the source of control and full partner in providing compassionate and coordinated care based on respect for patient's preferences, values, and needs.

2. **Teamwork and Collaboration:** Function effectively within nursing and interprofessional teams, fostering open communication, mutual respect, and shared decision-making to achieve quality patient care.

3. **Evidence-Based Practice:** Integrate best current evidence with clinical expertise and patient/family preferences and values for delivery of optimal healthcare.

4. **Quality Improvement:** Use data to monitor the outcomes of care processes and use improvement methods to design and test changes to continuously improve the quality and safety of healthcare systems.

5. **Safety:** Minimize the risk of harm to patients and providers through both system effectiveness and individual performance.

6. **Informatics:** Use information and technology to communicate, manage knowledge, mitigate error, and support decision-making.[8]

The teamwork and collaboration competency highlights the importance of knowledge of one's own role and communication style and the role and importance of other members of the team. Importantly, the competency also highlights having the necessary skills to negotiate with team members when roles overlap, which is common in advanced practice. This skill is incredibly important to maximize the effectiveness of a team. This QSEN competency also highlights the importance of communication skills and attitudes that recognize the importance of the unique attributes of each team member in the success of the team as well as the role of the patient and family as team members.

CASE STUDY
TEAM VACCINATION TASK DELEGATION CONSIDERATIONS

Dr. J., DNP, AGNP, works on a team that includes a medical assistant, a registered nurse, a physician, and a pharmacist. Everyone on the team can appropriately give a vaccination.

Case Study Question

How should the team decide which member completes that task?

National Organization of Nurse Practitioner Faculties and American Association of Colleges of Nursing Competencies

The NONPF and the AACN collaborated on the development of the adult-gerontology primary care competencies, developed by a multi-organizational task force, which are the entry-level competencies for AGNPs:[9]

1. Scientific foundations
2. Leadership
3. Quality
4. Practice inquiry
5. Technology and information literacy
6. Policy
7. Health delivery system
8. Ethics
9. Independent practice

While the NONPF competencies do not specifically list team-based collaborative practice as one of the nine competencies, the principles are woven throughout. For example, the leadership competency includes describing one's current and evolving role to both other healthcare providers and the public and providing leadership in facilitating coordination and planning in patient care. In fact, the competency updates imbedded a recommendation for leadership curriculum content to include teams and teamwork. The competency on practice inquiry describes interprofessional research. The health delivery system competency emphasizes seven interprofessional/team competencies that include three of the IPEC competencies. The independent practice competency highlights the importance of AGNPs in collaborating with and providing consultation as appropriate with other health professionals to achieve optimal care outcomes.

All AGNP students should familiarize themselves with these competencies, which can be found online at https://cdn.ymaws.com/www.nonpf.org/resource/resmgr/files/np_competencies_2.pdf. The AGNP primary care competencies start in the middle of the document. In reviewing the competencies, pay close attention to what differentiates the AGNP from the NP core competencies.

Interprofessional Education Collaborative Core Competencies

The IPEC came together to address the interprofessional competency challenges identified in the three IOM reports. This group was composed of experts from six national health profession accrediting bodies for nursing, osteopathic medicine, pharmacy, dentistry, allopathic medicine, and public health. Its vision was linked to the five IOM core competencies for health professions and reinforced that interprofessional collaborative practice was essential to high-quality, safe, accessible, and patient-centered care.

The 2011 Core Competencies of Interprofessional Practice report was the product of their work, which identified four overarching competency domains as essential for all health professions: (a) Values and Ethics, (b) Roles and Responsibilities (c) Interprofessional Communication, (d) Teams and Teamwork. The report included several implementation recommendations for each of these competency domains.[10] Throughout the next 5 years, the IPEC disseminated its work through its IPE PORTAL at the University of Iowa (https://interprofessional.uiowa.edu/article/ipe-portal-advances-interprofessional-collaborative-practice-education), with multiple team projects and the publishing of healthcare literature (Figure 4.1).

In 2016, the IPEC added nine additional institutional members, thereby expanding represented professions to include optometrists, social workers, physician assistants, podiatry, physical therapy, occupational therapists, psychologists, allied health professions, and veterinary medicine. With 15 accrediting organizations on board, the group updated the competency domains to integrate population health, enhance communication with fields

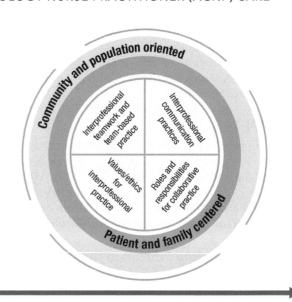

The learning continuum pre-licensure through practice trajectory

Figure 4.1: Interdisciplinary learning continuum and IPEC domains

Source: Courtesy of the Interprofessional Education Collaborative.

outside of health, place greater emphasis on health promotion and disease prevention, and respect the diversity of the team and the impact of unique cultures, values, roles, and expertise of all health professions.[11]

The four IPEC core competencies are:

1. **Values and Ethics:** Work with individuals of other professions to maintain a climate of mutual respect and shared values. This includes prioritizing the interests of patients and communities; respecting and embracing individual, team, and community diversity; and developing strong and trusting relationships with all parties. Ethical dilemmas, as well as all relationships, are managed with honesty and integrity.

2. **Roles and Responsibilities:** Use the knowledge of one's own role and those of other professions to appropriately assess and address the healthcare needs of patients and to promote and advance the health of populations. This includes understanding one's own limitations and strengths and ensuring each team member is working at the top of their scope of practice to optimize care. To do this effectively requires clear communication about each member's role and their responsibility in completing tasks, as well as developing interdependent relationships among professions with a shared focus on providing efficient, effective, equitable, timely, and safe care.

3. **Interprofessional Communication:** Communicate with patients, families, communities, and professionals in healthcare and other fields in a responsible

manner that supports a team approach to the promotion and maintenance of health and the prevention and treatment of disease. This includes organizing and communicating information, expressing one's knowledge and opinions, and recognizing one's own role in developing positive team culture. This competency also highlights the importance of listening actively, encouraging contributions from team members, and sharing constructive and timely feedback with others while receiving the same with respect.

4. **Teams and Teamwork:** Apply relationship-building values and the principles of team dynamics to perform effectively in different team roles to plan, deliver, and evaluate patient-/population-centered care and population health programs and policies

that are safe, timely, efficient, effective, and equitable. This includes applying leadership practices that build team effectiveness, engaging other health professionals, and integrating their knowledge and experience into care decisions that also respect a patient's values, priorities, and preferences. Members should perform effectively on teams and in team roles in a variety of settings.

Table 4.1 outlines the competencies and subcompetencies with a short explanation for each. AGNPs should acquaint themselves with these competencies and learn to integrate them into their practices when working with other professions. These competencies are not only for working with physicians and pharmacists but for all professions as well and should be applied in the office with medical assistants, lab technicians, and front-office staff.

Table 4.1: IPEC Core Competencies From the 2016 Revision

Roles/Responsibilities: Use the knowledge of one's own role and those of other professions to appropriately assess and address the healthcare needs of patients and to promote and advance the health of populations.	
Subcompetencies include the following:	
RR1.	Communicate one's roles and responsibilities clearly to patients, families, community members, and other professionals.
RR2.	Recognize one's limitations in skills, knowledge, and abilities.
RR3.	Engage diverse professionals who complement one's own professional expertise as well as associated resources to develop strategies to meet specific health and healthcare needs of patients and populations.
RR4.	Explain the roles and responsibilities of other providers and how the team works together to provide care, promote health, and prevent disease.
RR5.	Use the full scope of knowledge, skills, and abilities of professionals from health and other fields to provide care that is safe, timely, efficient, effective, and equitable.
RR6.	Communicate with team members to clarify each member's responsibility in executing components of a treatment plan or public health intervention.
RR7.	Forge interdependent relationships with other professions within and outside of the health system to improve care and advance learning.
RR8.	Engage in continuous professional and interprofessional development to enhance team performance and collaboration.
RR9.	Use unique and complementary abilities of all members of the team to optimize health and patient care.
RR10.	Describe how professionals in health and other fields can collaborate and integrate clinical care and public health interventions to optimize population health.
Interprofessional Communication: Communicate with patients, families, communities, and professionals in health and other fields in a responsive and responsible manner that supports a team approach to the promotion and maintenance of health and the prevention and treatment of disease.	
Subcompetencies include the following:	
CC1.	Choose effective communication tools and techniques, including information systems and communication technologies, to facilitate discussions and interactions that enhance team function.
CC2.	Communicate information with patients, families, community members, and health team members in a form that is understandable, avoiding discipline-specific terminology when possible.

(continued)

Table 4.1: IPEC Core Competencies From the 2016 Revision (*continued*)

CC3.	Express one's knowledge and opinions to team members involved in patient care and population health improvement with confidence, clarity, and respect, working to ensure common understanding of information, treatment, care decisions, and population health programs and policies.
CC4.	Listen actively, and encourage ideas and opinions of other team members.
CC5.	Give timely, sensitive, instructive feedback to others about their performance on the team, responding respectfully as a team member to feedback from others.
CC6.	Use respectful language appropriate for a given difficult situation, crucial conversation, or conflict.
CC7.	Recognize how one's uniqueness (experience level, expertise, culture, power, and hierarchy within the health team) contributes to effective communication, conflict resolution, and positive interprofessional working relationships.[33]
CC8.	Communicate the importance of teamwork in patient-centered care and population health programs and policies.

Values/Ethics for Interprofessional Practice: Work with individuals of other professions to maintain a climate of mutual respect and shared values. Subcompetencies include the following:	
VE1.	Place interests of patients and populations at center of interprofessional healthcare delivery and population health programs and policies, with the goal of promoting health and health equity across the life span.
VE2.	Respect the dignity and privacy of patients while maintaining confidentiality in the delivery of team-based care.
VE3.	Embrace the cultural diversity and individual differences that characterize patients, populations, and the health team.
VE4.	Respect the unique cultures, values, roles/responsibilities, and expertise of other health professions and the impact these factors can have on health outcomes.
VE5.	Work in cooperation with those who receive care, those who provide care, and others who contribute to or support the delivery of prevention and health services and programs.
VE6.	Develop a trusting relationship with patients, families, and other team members.[32]
VE7.	Demonstrate high standards of ethical conduct and quality of care in contributions to team-based care.
VE8.	Manage ethical dilemmas specific to interprofessional patient-/population-centered care situations.
VE9.	Act with honesty and integrity in relationships with patients, families, communities, and other team members.
VE10.	Maintain competence in one's own profession appropriate to scope of practice.
Teams and Teamwork: Apply relationship-building values and the principles of team dynamics to perform effectively in different team roles to plan, deliver, and evaluate patient/population-centered care and population health programs and policies that are safe, timely, efficient, effective, and equitable. Subcompetencies include the following:	
TT1.	Describe the process of team development and the roles and practices of effective teams.
TT2.	Develop consensus on the ethical principles to guide all aspects of teamwork.
TT3.	Engage health and other professionals in shared patient-centered and population-focused problem-solving.
TT4.	Integrate the knowledge and experience of health and other professions to inform health and care decisions while respecting patient and community values and priorities/preferences for care.
TT5.	Apply leadership practices that support collaborative practice and team effectiveness.
TT6.	Engage self and others to constructively manage disagreements about values, roles, goals, and actions that arise among health and other professionals and with patients, families, and community members.

TT7.	Share accountability with other professions, patients, and communities for outcomes relevant to prevention and healthcare.
TT8.	Reflect on individual and team performance for individual and team performance improvement.
TT9.	Use process improvement to increase effectiveness of interprofessional teamwork and team-based services, programs, and policies.
TT10.	Use available evidence to inform effective teamwork and team-based practices.
TT11.	Perform effectively on teams and in different team roles in a variety of settings.

IPEC, Interprofessional Education Collaborative.

Source: Interprofessional Education Collaborative. *Core Competencies for Interprofessional Collaborative Practice: 2016 Update.* https://ipec.memberclicks.net/assets/2016-Update.pdf

CASE STUDY
SUPPORTING SCOPE OF PRACTICE DISCUSSIONS

Dr. J, DNP, AGNP, has been at her current practice for a few months and has noticed the medical assistants do not give vaccinations, something known to be within their scope of practice. When asked, they report the policy of the clinic has always been for providers to give their own injections.

Case Study Question

Thinking about the four IPEC competencies, how might Dr. J address this with the clinic administration, fellow providers, and the medical assistants?

Box 4.1: Definitions

Interprofessional Team-Based Care: When healthcare organizations deliver care through specific small work groups that are recognized as having a mutual identity and shared responsibility and accountability for a patient or group of patients.

Interprofessional Education: "When students from two or more professions learn about, from and with each other to enable effective collaboration and improve health outcomes."[13]

Interprofessional Collaboration: "Collaborative practice happens when multiple health workers from different professional backgrounds work together with patients, families, caretakers, and communities to deliver the highest quality of care across settings."[13]

Summary

The competencies from the IPEC, the QSEN, the NONPF, and the AACN are worded and formatted differently, but they share common threads of collaboration, role definition, communication, shared values, and respect. Each emphasizes the importance of the team in providing evidence-based, patient-centered care and the need to include the patient and family as a central member of the team itself, with "family" defined broadly as being who the patient says they are as opposed to genetic or legal definitions (Box 4.1).

TEAM-BASED CARE

Team-based care has been recommended as a partial solution to poor quality and safety in healthcare by the three IOM reports described earlier in this chapter and multiple healthcare experts.[5,14] It is also highlighted throughout the professional competencies as described earlier.

Why Is Team-Based Care Important?

The impact of teamwork can be significant, and its lack has been identified as a contributing factor in sentinel events that have resulted in grave bodily harm and death of patients.[5] Team-based care is one of the 10 key building blocks of high-performing care as described by Bodenheimer et al.,[15] but it does come with challenges. In her book *Teaming: How Organizations Learn, Innovate, and Compete in the Knowledge Economy*, Edmondson asserts that thriving in today's economic climate will require a seismic shift in how we think about and use teamwork. Edmondson, who has been studying teamwork for two decades, says, "We've seen fewer stable, well-designed, well-composed teams, simply because of the nature of the work, which is more uncertain and dynamic than before."[16]

Team-based primary care models have been shown to have numerous benefits to both patients and healthcare professionals and have been suggested to build primary care capacity through the idea of "sharing the care."[17] A meta-analysis of team-based care interventions for patients with diabetes found improvements in blood glucose management, blood pressure, and total cholesterol when compared to usual care, as well as slight improvements in patient satisfaction and physical and mental health.[18] Among healthcare professionals, working in team-based environments was shown to contribute to reduced utilization of healthcare services by chronically ill patients[19] and to greater work satisfaction.[20]

What Makes a Good Team?

Several healthcare professionals have conducted research and developed conceptual models on this topic. Reeves et al.[5] synthesized teamwork literature and identified five shared elements across concepts. Team members (a) have a shared team identity; (b) have clear roles, tasks, and goals; (c) are interdependent; (d) have integration of work; and (e) have a sense of shared responsibility. These elements are consistent with the IPEC competencies and those introduced by Mitchell et al.[21] and are important concepts for AGNPs to embrace in their work:

1. Shared goals that reflect patient/family priorities, are well articulated, and are supported by all members.

2. Clear roles and expectations for each team member, allowing for efficient division of labor and maximizing team output.

3. Mutual trust in which reciprocity is the norm.

4. Effective communication that is prioritized and refined continuously. All team members feel comfortable communicating across all settings.

5. Measurable processes and outcomes in which the team obtains feedback on team functioning and goal achievement in a reliable and timely manner.

Factors impacting teamwork fall into categories of interprofessional (e.g., relationships between team members), organizational (e.g., working conditions or policies), and systemic (e.g., professional systems),[22] as well as the urgency of tasks to be completed.[5] Various models have been proposed for different types of teams. An in-depth discussion of these is beyond the scope of this chapter, but AGNPs should be alert to types of teams in various clinical settings.

Box 4.2: Activity

Think about one or two teams you have been a part of or observed closely. If possible, select one that worked on a specific, time-limited project (e.g., organizing a health fair) and another that was long-lasting (e.g., a primary care team). How were the teams different? What traits did they have in common? How did you feel being a part of each? Share your thoughts and discuss this with a colleague.

INTEGRATING TEAM-BASED CARE INTO PRACTICE

The following section focuses on tools AGNPs as healthcare providers can use to encourage and incorporate team-based care into their practice. Use the framework of the four IPEC competencies described earlier as a lens throughout this section.

Roles and Responsibilities

The roles and responsibilities competency speaks to the importance of understanding your own role and the roles of others on your team and enabling each person to work at the top of their scope and as part of an efficient team.

The AGNP Role

As a team member, it is important that each member can speak to their own scope of practice. The role of the AGNP is relatively new compared to that of a physician. AGNPs should be prepared to explain their scope succinctly to patients and colleagues who may not be familiar and to communicate how they would like to be addressed to patients. Forms of address can vary by clinical practice; some are less formal than others, so observe and check in with colleagues if you are unsure. If you have completed a doctoral degree, it is essential that you always introduce yourself as an AGNP so as not to confuse patients over the term "doctor." You may still use the term "doctor" in many cases, but it must go along with an explanation of your role as a nurse practitioner.

In primary care, the front office staff and medical assistant will most likely be in contact with the patient first. Confirm they know how to respond to questions about your role and how to introduce you to patients. This can have legal ramifications in some cases, so it is an important step.

CASE STUDY
CONSIDERATIONS AROUND INTRODUCTIONS AND ROLE CONFUSION

Dr. J, DNP, AGNP, recently graduated and started at a geriatric practice. She is the first AGNP to work at the practice, and many of her colleagues and patients are unaware of the scope of her role. She has found herself providing role education to many of her patients, taking up a significant amount of patient visit time. She suggests to the medical assistant that going forward she be introduced as Dr. J without explaining that she is an AGNP.

Case Study Questions

1. What are the legal, ethical, and team considerations?

2. What are alternative methods of addressing this challenge?

Write a 15-second explanation of your role. Practice your delivery with friends and family. How will it be different if you are speaking with another health professional versus a patient?

Role of Others

A key element of the roles and responsibilities competency and team-based care is recognizing the importance of what each profession brings to the team. Understanding the role and scope of each member of the healthcare team is necessary for the efficient, effective division of tasks among the team. Beyond the scope of licensure, professionals should be familiar with the expectations of the organization in which they work and the skills, comfort, and training of teammates. This is especially important when there is a supervisory relationship (e.g., medical assistant).

It is also vital that AGNPs articulate the roles of other members of the team to patients, focusing on the various professions' strengths and building patients' confidence in the team. This also helps patients understand who can help them with specific tasks, enhancing efficiency. When communicating about the role of others, ensure the accurate professional name is used. The term "nurse" is often used in primary care to describe both a medical assistant and a licensed vocational nurse, yet their scopes are different. It is confusing for patients when the incorrect or generic term is used, and it takes away from the professional identity of the team member.

It is important for AGNPs to consider professionals outside their organization and develop relationships with other healthcare and community resources. In addition to medical specialists, it is important to get to know the home health and private duty nursing companies in the area. Where possible, it is beneficial for AGNPs to make connections with these organizations and understand their communication pathways to ease referrals. It is also helpful to form relationships with local pharmacists if the practice does not employ a pharmacist, as they are an important resource. Broad professional relationships are an important aspect of effective team-based care.

List all the staff you interact with on a regular basis and practice explaining the role of each to a friend or family member. Ask them to listen for hierarchical or confusing language. Did you realize any gaps in your knowledge?

CASE STUDY
TEAM-BASED CARE POSTHOSPITALIZATION

Gino Romano, a 74-year-old man, and his wife come to see their primary care physician, Dr. J, DNP, AGNP, for a hospital follow-up visit. Gino recently had a stroke and was left with changes to his mobility. The hospital coordinated a home health registered nurse (RN), prothrombin time (PT), and occupational therapy (OT) upon discharge, but the Romanos declined the services. They feel Dr. J does a great job of managing their care, and they do not need anyone else.

Case Study Question

Thinking about the IPEC roles and responsibilities subcompetencies and the desired outcome for Gino poststroke, how could Dr. J respond?

Communication

Communication is multifaceted. Healthcare professionals communicate via multiple avenues, in written and verbal forms, using words as well as tone, expression, and body language. Poor communication between professionals has been shown to have a negative impact on patient safety.[10] Historical hierarchies can inhibit communication, whereas fast-paced environments further reduce opportunities to break down barriers and encourage collaboration.[23] An integrative review of the literature by Foronda et al.[24] identified the impact of profession-specific communication styles. Frustration may occur when nurses, trained with a holistic and descriptive focus, communicate with physicians who prioritize succinct, factual conversations. This can leave physicians feeling that nurses' communication is disorganized and sometimes irrelevant, while nurses feel unsure of the amount of detail to provide, how to offer a suggestion, and afraid of being incorrect or humiliated.[24] Formats like SBAR (situation–background–assessment–recommendation), which provide an agreed-on framework by both parties, have been promoted to address these challenges both between providers and between providers and caregivers.[25] Additionally, opportunities for professions to learn communication skills together such as with Agency for Healthcare Research and Quality's (AHRQ) TeamSTEPPS (an evidence-based collection of tools designed to improve communication and teamwork) or by participating in interprofessional simulation experiences have improved self-reported communication skills.[24]

AGNPs should work within their teams and organization to identify agreed-on formats and norms of communication and take advantage of opportunities to practice communication skills together through workshops or simulation experiences.

Values and Ethics

Values and ethics include both ethical conduct and developing a strong set of team values. Mitchell et al.[21] describe five personal values characterized by effective members of high-functioning teams. These are honesty, discipline, creativity, humility, and curiosity. Inherent in this section is placing patients at the center of healthcare delivery, promoting health equity, and respecting the dignity and privacy of individuals along with embracing the diversity of patients and populations. Healthcare teams must develop trusting relations and act with honesty and integrity, demonstrating highly ethical conduct. In placing the patient at the center of care, the healthcare team must recognize the inherent power differential between healthcare providers and patients and find ways to balance power to favor the patient. One way to accomplish this is to approach patients with cultural humility. The concept of cultural humility is described as "a lifelong commitment to self-evaluation and critique . . . and to developing mutually beneficial and non-paternalistic partnerships with communities."[26]

Implicit bias also ties into this competency, as it acknowledges the ways in which people make assumptions based on factors such as age, race, gender, sexuality, income level, or nationality. Health disparities among minority populations in the United States have been well documented as has the potential negative impact implicit bias can have on healthcare.[27] AGNPs must actively engage in the lifelong process of exploring their own implicit biases and be aware of implicit bias among team members. Team values of equity and respect should be established and reinforced.

Implicit bias may emerge when faced with ethical dilemmas in which the provider's own beliefs or values differ from that of the patient. It is important for healthcare professionals to recognize these situations and have a plan in place to ensure patients receive evidence-based, equitable treatment. In extreme cases, this may involve transferring care to another provider or involving an ethics board.

Teams and Teamwork

As discussed earlier in the chapter, strong teamwork is a key component of effective, efficient patient-centered care. Coordinated team-based care is particularly relevant for those working with older adults, such as AGNPs, where the insight of a diverse group of professionals is often needed in the management of chronic disease and long-term planning.[28] Team-based care in primary care practices has been shown to improve access to care and services.[29] Hierarchy, gradients of real or perceived power, can spark conflict between professions, negatively impacting team collaboration, decision-making, communication, and overall team performance.[30] Hierarchy can come from within the clinical team or more broadly from within the organization. Consider the role of administrators. They have a great deal of power to shape clinic practices yet are often further removed from the day-to-day actions of the team and may be less familiar with the role of advanced practice providers. In a mixed-methods study by Poghosyan et al.,[31] 60% of NPs surveyed reported an inequality in comparison with how physicians were treated by administrators, which may have been because the administrators did not understand their skill set or role. In those instances where administrators were familiar with the NP role and competencies, they were often strong advocates of NPs working at the top of their scope.

A concept that is gaining traction is that of interprofessional socialization, the process by which learners develop both a professional and an interprofessional identity, ideally leading to a sense of belonging both to one's profession and to a larger interprofessional community.[32] Within this, it is important for AGNPs to advocate for broad inclusion of everyone working within a practice, including those outside of a direct clinical role.

Patient and Family as Team Members

The importance of patient-centered care has come to the forefront in recent years. A key component of this is the inclusion of the patient and family as members of the healthcare team. Chapter 2 speaks to this topic, so it will not be addressed here, but when reviewing the IPEC competencies, consider how they apply to the patient in this context.

CASE STUDY
MANAGING CONFLICTING MEDICAL AND PERSONAL VALUES AS A PROVIDER

Dr. J, DNP, AGNP, is approached by the granddaughter of a patient who is suffering from terminal cancer. She would like Dr. J to discuss medically assisted death with her grandmother, as she knows she is in a great deal of pain. She shares that her grandfather is not comfortable with this idea, but she believes it is her grandmother's right to know her options. Dr. J does not support medically assisted death, and it is not something offered as part of the practice.

Case Study Questions

1. What are Dr. J's ethical and medical responsibilities to the patient?
2. How might Dr. J handle the differing family opinions and support the patient's right for self-determination?

CONCLUSION

AGNPs play an influential role in team-based care at both a team and organizational level. They must be familiar with, become skilled in, and integrate the IPEC competencies in their practice setting. Additionally, AGNPs should be familiar with the competencies required by U.S. nursing accrediting bodies, such as the AACN, and other nursing organizations that provide input into the education and training of AGNPs. Leading by example, AGNPs can develop and lead inclusive, interprofessional teams that deliver efficient, effective, and person-centered care. A clear understanding of their own role and the roles of other professions and the ability to articulate those roles makes AGNPs well positioned to influence organizational culture as well. Shared ethics and values, high-quality communication, and purposeful teamwork must also be part of the AGNP's knowledge and skills in the primary care practice environment.

REFERENCES

References for this chapter are online and available at https://connect.springerpub.com/content/book/978-0-8261-8414-6/part/part01/toc-part/ch4.

CHAPTER 5

Care Coordination

Andrea Quinonez, Kathleen Klein, Cynthia A. Skillsky, and Nicole Hansen

LEARNING OBJECTIVES

At the conclusion of this chapter, the learner will be able to:

➤ Describe common care coordination activities in primary care and outpatient settings.

➤ Compare the concepts of care coordination and care management.

➤ Construct a care plan.

➤ Differentiate care team member roles in care coordination efforts.

➤ Describe the impact of communication in care coordination and mechanisms to strengthen communication among teams.

➤ Identify how performance measurement and quality improvement efforts can be leveraged to introduce or improve care coordination approaches in clinical practice.

INTRODUCTION

Care coordination is an essential strategy to providing safe care transitions along the continuum of care. Collaboration among care teams located in multiple settings is integral to the process, including those in inpatient and outpatient settings, primary and specialty care, and other settings such as home health or skilled nursing facilities. Care coordination activities focus on creation of a seamless model of care across the care continuum. These activities involve contributions from multiple disciplines and care team members, require excellent communication among all care providers, and include the development of an effective goal-oriented care plan. The patient's needs and preferences are central to the interdisciplinary care team's approach throughout the process and are communicated in a clear and timely manner. This chapter provides an overview of key components of care coordination and considerations for practice, including methods of ongoing monitoring and evaluation of care coordination efforts.

CARE COORDINATION OVERVIEW

The Institute of Medicine (IOM) identifies care coordination as a key approach to improve efficacy, safety, and efficiency of the American healthcare system, which benefits all involved: patients, providers, and payers.[1,2] Care coordination strategies have been associated with reduced hospital admissions, lower 30-day readmission rates, reduced emergency department and provider visits, and a reduction in overall cost of care, as well as improved quality of chronic disease management, improved patient satisfaction, and better access to specialty care.[3 5,9]

While there is no consensus definition, the Agency for Healthcare Research and Quality (AHRQ) describes "care coordination" as "the deliberate organization of patient care activities between two or more participants (including the patient) involved in a patient's care to facilitate the appropriate delivery of health care services."[35] Organizing care involves the marshaling of personnel and other resources needed to carry out all required patient care activities and is often managed by the exchange of information among participants responsible for different aspects of care."[5] These activities are performed with the goal of meeting patients' needs and preferences, while also delivering high-quality, high-value healthcare.

Care coordination is founded on a person-centered approach and includes key aspects of care management, development of goal-oriented care plans, team-based care, information sharing, and ongoing performance measurement and quality improvement.[6–9,46] Successful care coordination involves multiple elements—access to multiple healthcare services and providers, as well as good communication and transitions between care team members, with priority given to the total healthcare needs of the patient and information provided to patients they can easily understand.[10] As these elements come together, the goal is to create a seamless model of care around the patient throughout their journey across the care continuum, in which "the patient's needs and preferences are known ahead of time and communicated at the right time to the right people."[1]

Indications for Care Coordination

Care coordination is an ongoing, fluid process that begins when a patient first engages with a provider. As care needs and systems with which to access care have become increasingly complex, the care team is in a constant process of coordinating patient care, all the while understanding the patient from both social and medical standpoints. Significant consideration should be given to the potential barriers experienced in coordinating care efforts of patients.

In the absence of a designated healthcare team member to address care coordination needs, the expectation is for the primary care provider (PCP) to coordinate all care needs and facilitate communications among specialties and throughout different levels of care.[11] Designating a person on the care team, be it the PCP or another team member, to assist with these responsibilities is necessary, as the process of tracking and coordinating care needs can be overwhelming, confusing, and difficult for patients with complex care needs to navigate.[12] This may include coordination of care provided by multiple specialties, ancillary care needs such as lab work and imaging, and maintaining appropriate follow-up for each. As navigation of health systems in general is complex and patients may receive care in multiple health systems, it follows that care needs can, and do, get dropped due to patients' lack of understanding and system barriers.

With the severe time limitations that exist for a PCP to provide comprehensive medical care while also effectively managing all the care coordination needs of a patient, it is important to leverage assistance where and when available. Larger health systems may have opportunities for nurses, medical assistants, or other support staff to assist with care coordination activities. Most commercial insurance companies offer support with care coordination activities as requested by the patient and/or PCP. Medicare also provides some limited monetary reimbursement for care coordination activities for medically complex patients; however, the responsibility falls onto the PCP office to manage these activities.[9,14,47] There are some community opportunities for case management and care coordination as well. For instance, in California, there are several case management and care coordination services available for medically complex, frail, and/or older adult persons receiving Medi-Cal (the California state Medicaid program), such as the Multipurpose Senior Services Program (MSSP; www.dhcs.ca.gov/services/medi-cal/Pages/MSSPMedi-CalWaiver.aspx).

In considering barriers to care coordination, one must examine potential system barriers as well as patient-level barriers. An initial intake exploring potential barriers might examine how seeing multiple providers in multiple locations may create difficulty for the patient and consider how receiving care in multiple health systems can impede flow of communication and patient understanding of the process. A review of social influencers of health (SIOHs; see Box 5.1) should also be performed to better understand an individual patient's current social stressors. This may include limited (or absence of)

Box 5.1: Social Influencers of Health

In recent years, there has been a shift to move away from the term "social determinants of health" to the more inclusive "social influencers of health." In swapping out "influencers" for "determinants," the healthcare community adopts the stance that a person's socioeconomic environment may influence the probability of health outcomes, rather than determining them. This allows room for the potentially positive effects of hope, resilience, and/or effective interventions.

Source: Simon G. *What's Wrong With the Term 'Social Determinants of Health'?* KP Washington Health Research Institute; 2017. https://medium.com/@KPWaResearch/whats-wrong-with-the-term-social-determinants-of-health-8e69684ec44213

---

transportation, food insecurity, housing insecurity, depression, or financial resource strain. Taking these factors into account while planning care and coordination needs can have positive results in patient adherence and health outcomes, as well as reduce healthcare spending.[15]

While barriers should be evaluated at intake, it is important to note that care coordination is an ongoing process. It requires regularly checking in with the patient and their support system to understand any changes to the patient's condition and/or social situation. This is especially pertinent during times that the patient moves across different levels of care, such as a hospital discharge to home, or handoff from primary to specialty care for managing a chronic disease. Transitions of care present particularly vulnerable times for patients, and effective care coordination throughout the transitions of care for medically complex patients has a positive impact in both patients' and caregivers' perceptions of care.[17] Patients often find that during times of transition, there are conflicting and/or confusing instructions regarding medications as well as after-care needs, requiring the assistance of their identified medical provider (usually the PCP) for clarity regarding follow-up needs.

Consistency in care coordination is especially important for patients with cognitive impairment, as cognitive issues pose unique challenges in patients' ability to follow complex directions, arrange for follow-up care, and maintain medication adherence. When a patient is seen longitudinally by the same set of providers, it is more likely that the nuances of potential cognitive impairment will be noticed and addressed.[18] Gaining an understanding of the home environment and support system available to a patient with cognitive impairment is paramount in the successful medical management of complex issues.

PATIENT AS THE CENTER IN CARE COORDINATION

Historically, medical care has been provided within a provider-driven context, but there has been a shift in recent years to move toward "patient-centered" or "person-centered" care in order to highlight consideration of a person's needs and preferences, beyond strictly clinical or medical concerns.[6] Person-centered care (PCC) "means that individuals' values and preferences are elicited, and once expressed, guide all aspects of their health care, supporting their realistic health and life goals. PCC is achieved through a dynamic relationship among individuals, others who are important to them, and all relevant providers. This collaboration informs decision making to the extent that the individual desires."[6] In this approach, the patient is a central determinant in their own healthcare decisions, and options are considered with their own values, preferences, and needs in mind.

PCC-driven communication has three core concepts. The first is to elicit information during your time with the patient to understand their perspective—problems, needs, feelings, expectations—so that a foundation is laid to guide further communication. Next is understanding the patient "within his or her unique psychosocial and cultural contexts."[19] The final core concept is having a shared understanding of the patient's values and goals of care that are centered around those values. In PCC, the patient/person, in consideration of their values and preferences, is empowered to "guide all aspects of their health care."[6] This will include developing a care plan, care plan revisions over time, and continual information sharing between patient/provider as well as provider/provider. According to the American Geriatrics Society Expert Panel (AGSEP),[6] common barriers include the following:

- Traditional approaches to clinical practice
- Physician workload
- Misaligned incentives
- Identifying appropriate indicators
- Provider concerns or risk and safety
- A lack of advance care planning
- A lack of payment structures that span healthcare and community-based organizations
- A lack of continuity in health records
- Communication

These common barriers should be taken into consideration by the medical team and addressed during attempts to initiate or adhere to PCC over longitudinal care.

Individual patients are the expert on their own situation, experiences, and overall care. As medical visits can be subject to strict time constraints, often leaving little room for understanding the breadth of social complexities for the patient, involving additional team members to build a relationship with the patient in order to learn about the complexities of that individual's needs can benefit both the patient and provider(s). According to Kogan et al.,[20] "PCC is increasingly recognized as central to health care" and recognizes "there is a great need for PCC approaches in outpatient care." Creating the space and environment that allows a provider to tap into the wealth of knowledge that individual patients have regarding their own needs coupled with recognizing the inherent barriers that exist within PCC will create the building blocks for developing PCC in an individual practice.

CASE STUDY
PERSON-CENTERED CARE

SL is a 70-year-old female who is calling her PCP's office up to five or more times per day demanding the PCP's attention to her social situations (needing food, inability to pick up medications, conflict with landlord). SL is referred by her PCP to case management for assistance with her home support, transportation, and specialty coordination needs (multiple "no-shows" for medical appointments).

MEDICAL HISTORY

Asthma, chronic obstructive pulmonary disease (COPD), cognitive impairment, vertigo, diabetes mellitus (DM), new diagnosis chronic kidney disease (CKD) stage IV, bipolar, cluster B personality disorder traits, mild cognitive impairment

SOCIAL HISTORY

Lives alone in an apartment (hoarding tendencies), relies on public transport/bus, experiences some challenges with ambulation, relies on local food banks and congregate meal sites for nutrition; low-income apartment building has been sold and all residents have been given 90-day notice to vacate, no social support system and estranged from family

CASE MANAGEMENT

- SL works with a social worker case manager (SWCM) to address her immediate housing needs, eventually moving to a local room and board where her meals are included in monthly rent.
- SWCM works with the patient on identifying barriers to medical adherence, connecting her with a local transport company to provide Medi-Cal–funded rides to all medical appointments.
- By building a relationship with SL, providing the space for her to express her concerns and frustrations, and addressing her complex social needs, she

is, over time, able to engage with providers and follow-through on recommendations.

- ■ SWCM notes likely limited understanding and adherence with medications and low medical literacy regarding chronic disease management. SWCM enlists the support of a pharmacist case manager for increasing medication adherence and RN case manager for disease management for diabetes, CKD IV, and COPD.

SL's health conditions are optimized through the work of the team based on an understanding of SL and her complex social situation, resulting in better health outcomes. She gains a stable housing situation including regular access to food, improved medication adherence due to home delivery and simplified packaging, attends all scheduled medical appointments, and is observed to have an improved relationship with her medical providers.

CARE MANAGEMENT AND CARE COORDINATION

For complex patients, care management comprises a key factor within care coordination efforts across the care spectrum. The overarching goal of care management is to provide appropriate interventions for patients within a given population to reduce health risks and decrease the cost of care.[21] This includes a team-based, patient-centered approach to assist patients and their support systems in managing their medical conditions more effectively. In this setting, care coordination activities are embedded in ongoing chronic condition management.

Of note, while one of the main activities of care management is to improve care coordination, not all care coordination must happen in the setting of care management. Care management may be provided on an "as needed" basis, as care management provides disease-specific support, whereby there are modifiable risk factors with a goal of achieving self-management by the patient.[21] Once self-management is achieved, care management generally supports or follows a patient with less intensity or frequency of contact, although that same patient may continue to require care coordination support by other team members for ongoing identification and support in navigating barriers.

Typically, care managers are nurses or social workers who work with patients and their PCP to provide education regarding medical conditions, utilizing motivational interviewing (MI) and small, manageable, incremental changes with the patient in achieving self-management of their medical condition(s). Care management recognizes that the patient is in charge of the process toward change, utilizing established disease-management protocols. Other activities involved in care management and

care coordination include identification of, and outreach to, high-risk populations, provision of services aligned to the needs of those populations, and addressing care gaps, with particular attention to communications, support during transitions of care, and provision of any additional social supports as needed (Table 5.1). Program

Table 5.1: Strategies and Activities in Care Coordination and Care Management

Strategy	Related Activities
Identification of populations with modifiable risks	• Registry review • Chart review • Outreach • Patient needs assessment

Align services and support with the needs of the population	• Self-management support
	  ○ Education/motivational interviewing
	• Care planning
	  ○ Includes goal setting
	• Facilitate completion of advance directives
	• Medication therapy management
	• Depression screening and follow-up
	• Previsit planning
	  ○ Flag screening or disease-specific testing needs
	  ○ Collect pertinent information ahead of time (i.e., hospital records or glucometer readings)
	  ○ Provide screening tools or questionnaires to patient
	  ○ Adjust appointment lengths as needed

Support in care transitions	• Follow-up after:
	  ○ ED or hospital discharge
	  ○ Specialist visits
	• Appointment scheduling
	• Medication reconciliation
	• Referral coordination

Preventive care	• Contact patients overdue for screenings (either preventive or disease-specific)

Patient-centered care	• Act as patient advocate
	• Provide health literacy interpretation
	• Provide emotional support
	  ○ Act as "sounding board"
	  ○ Recognize and validate patient experience

(continued)

Table 5.1: Strategies and Activities in Care Coordination and Care Management (*continued*)

Strategy	Related Activities

Resource support	• Connect patient with community resources, including housing, fuel, food, transportation
	• Cultivation of relationships with community organizations
	• Assistance in obtaining affordable care options
	  ○ Low-cost medications
	  ○ Insurance navigation
	• Arrange for durable medical equipment

Communication facilitation	• Establish communication methods between care settings (i.e., hospital discharge to community physicians, primary and specialty care, etc.)
	• Participation in huddles or other team meetings
	  ○ Develop agenda and/or case reviews for staff meetings
	  ○ Lead team discussion to plan individual patient care

Program measurement	• Data collection • Monitor process and outcomes data • Provide reports to funding agencies or other stakeholders • Engagement in quality improvement efforts

Source: Data from Farrell T, Tomoaia-Cotisel A, Scammon D, Day J, Day R, Magill M. *Care Management: Implications for Medical Practice, Health Policy, and Health Services Research.* AHRQ Publication No. 15-0018-EF. Agency for Healthcare Research and Quality; 2015. https://www.ahrq.gov/sites/default/files/publications/files/caremgmt-brief.pdf; O'Malley AS, Gourevitch R, Draper K, Bond A, Tirodkar MA. Overcoming challenges to teamwork in patient-centered medical homes: a qualitative study. *J Gen Intern Med.* 2015;30(2):183-192. doi:10.1007/s11606-014-3065-9; Friedman et al., 2016; Kianfar S, Carayon P, Schoofs Hundt A, Hoonakker P. Care coordination for chronically ill patients: identifying coordination activities and interdependencies. *Appl Ergon.* 2019;80:9-16. doi:10.1016/j.apergo.2019.05.002; Wagner EH, Flinter M, Hsu C, et al. Effective team-based care: observations from innovative practices. *BMC Fam Pract.* 2017;18:13. doi:10.1186/s12875-017-0590-8

data collection and outcomes monitoring are also activities embedded within care management and care coordination efforts.

Few forms of reimbursement by payers exist for care management activities.[21] Outside of a larger health system, care management services may be difficult to implement as it is a cost savings rather than a revenue-generating service. From the patient perspective, the ability to access multiple pieces of care in the same visit, such as office visits, labs, and imaging, and pharmacy (for medication changes/refills) is a cost-savings in taxing areas of their social needs as multiple visits to the same location can incur stress/burden on the caregiver, transportation complications (including money spent for each transport), and difficulty maintaining overall adherence with the plan of care. Care managers can assist with co-ordinating ancillary care needs with both the PCP and specialty providers to consolidate trips and lessen the burden on the patient/support system.

Complex medical issues and behavioral health struggles are often concurrent.[23] Care managers can address both medical concerns and specialty needs, as well as access to appropriate behavioral health professionals, to support all needs of the patient. Depending on the funding source, county of residence, and healthcare system, accessing the appropriate and relevant behavioral health resources can be quite complex, which is something that care managers can assist in navigating.

GOAL-ORIENTED CARE PLAN DEVELOPMENT

Care planning identifies a patient's current and long-standing needs, coordination gaps, and goals for care, as well as actions needed to achieve those goals.[5] This is performed as a collaborative effort among the patient, provider, and care team, in a person-centered manner in alignment with the patient's values. Once developed, the care plan becomes a working document for the care team to be able to share the mutually set goals and coordinate care based on those goals.[22] The key elements of a care plan include the following:

▪ Patient current state

▪ Collaborative development of goals and identification of concerns

▪ Actions and interventions

▪ Planning for transitions of care

▪ Ongoing review of goal progress and plan[24,25]

Rather than creating multiple discipline-specific care plans, it is most meaningful to work toward the development of one interprofessional shared care plan. The care plan should also highlight the process of care rather than a chronologically arranged list of tasks.[25] Once the care plan is collaboratively established and goals are agreed on, care teams must also have an effective system for coordinating care and sharing the information with all stakeholders responsible for meeting the goals, including identification of specific tasks and which team members are best suited to complete those tasks.[26] A discussion of patient and care team communication strategies and barriers follows later in this chapter.

Patient Current State

The current state section of a care plan can be described as "About Me."[25] It includes patient information, such as demographics and medical history, as well as an assessment of patient functioning. Additional information in this area includes care team members, along with their contact information, roles, and responsibilities, as well as community contacts and resources, or others involved in patient care. As with the rest of the care plan, this section should be reviewed and updated on a regular basis for all information to remain pertinent.

Collaborative Development of Goals and Identification of Concerns

Considered by many to be the central focus of a shared care plan, this area of a care plan includes patients' goals and concerns and considers patients' values, needs, and expectations, as well as goals recommended by the care team.[25] Working from a goal-based framework helps not only the care team but also the patient better understand what all team members are working toward, as well as identify what all involved, including the patient, can do to work toward those desired outcomes. Care team members provide support to patients while mutually setting goals and considering how those goals might be achieved by focusing on the patient's values, cultural influences, priorities, and personal interests. This is especially important in setting realistic, achievable goals, resulting in actionable, relevant care plans both from the patient and care team perspectives.

Enlisting the patient in the execution of their own care plan requires a shift in the mindset of both providers and patients alike. Providers move from a "telling" communication approach to one that is more inquisitive and inclusive to bring the patient's viewpoints and values into the formulation of the plan and its respective goals; a collaborative approach, including agenda setting, problem-solving, and teamwork, is recommended.[27] Providers may also need to offer patients additional education and support in order to help them achieve successful outcomes, as patients may not understand the purpose of the care plan or follow through on their own tasks.[22] In addition, not all patients may be interested or motivated to participate in care planning or to follow up on set

goals.[21] In this case, MI may be a helpful tool to meet the patient at their level of readiness for change; a brief discussion of this approach is presented later in this section.

A variety of goals may be included in the care plan, including health and well-being outcome goals, behavioral goals, or care or service goals.[26] As goals are driven from the patient perspective, each care plan and its respective goals will be unique to each person. Care team members work with patients in determining what they would like to work toward by first establishing trust and then learning about what is important to them. While some patients may be able to clearly express what end outcomes are most important to them (i.e., continuing to live in their home, be able to ambulate without a walker, etc.), others may not be as clear and tend to express their goals through stories or behavior. Tips in eliciting goals include adopting the stance of a learner by acknowledging the patient as the expert in their own care, understanding the patient's history and current circumstances, and encouraging the patient to talk about what matters to them.

While setting goals, cases do arise in which the patient's preferences and desires differ from the priorities of others involved in their care, such as the care team, family, or other caregivers. In those instances, the care team member should respect those preferences while also facilitating conversations with others involved in the patient's care.[26] If patient preferences or values are in contradiction with clinical recommendations, the care team member should also inform the patient about available options and potential consequences of choices. In this negotiation process, the desired end outcome is a shared goal with a plan to attain it.

CASE STUDY
ELICITING GOALS

BL is a 100-year-old female, living with her son, who is also her primary caregiver.

MEDICAL HISTORY

Bell's palsy, hypothyroidism, hypertension, hyperlipidemia, chronic respiratory failure, diaphragmatic hernia, dyspnea, interstitial lung disease, osteoporosis, compression fracture of vertebra, sarcoidosis, essential tremors, gout, low back pain radiating to leg bilaterally

SOCIAL HISTORY

BL is widowed and lives with her son, who is her primary caregiver. Her daughter lives in a neighboring town and assists with her care. BL is a retired teacher. BL is full assist for activities of daily living (ADLs), unable to ambulate, and uses a wheelchair.

The original referral was placed by the PCP after a recent office visit with BL, her son, and her daughter. BL presented with increasing shortness of breath (SOB), resulting in respiration rate into the 40s. The referral stated "patient has difficulty with appointments and leaving her home. Please provide resources for in home MD and lab draws." The referral requested the nurse case manager call the daughter, "as the son is currently caring for patient and is overwhelmed."

CASE MANAGEMENT

■ A call is placed to BL's daughter as requested. BL's daughter and son are having difficulty asking for hospice and find it easier when telling the story of BL's current state of health, how far she has declined in the last 30 days, and the difficulty watching her suffer. After further assessment and education, BL's daughter and son opt for hospice and request an urgent referral.

■ The nurse case manager requests an urgent referral from the PCP. The hospice nurse contacts the family within 24 hours. During the initial intake by the hospice nurse, BL's son declines the services.

■ After follow-up 24 hours later by the nurse case manager, and further education provided by the hospice nurse, the family decides to proceed with hospice. The family is referred to chaplain services as well as a licensed clinical social worker to assist with the transition of care to hospice.

What seems like a family in need of community resources for home laboratory draws is actually a family in need of help with making the very difficult decisions that come with caring for loved ones at the end of life.

After arriving at a mutually agreed-on goal, it should be documented clearly. While either the care team or patient's own words can be used, the goal should be documented in a SMART format: specific, measurable, attainable, relevant, and time-bound.[24-26] Using the SMART format not only supports a shared understanding of what is important to the patient but also specifies what mark the patient and care team are striving for, as well as how to know when that mark has been met. Once identified, the patient should review and give feedback on the SMART goal to ensure it accurately reflects their priorities and preferences in a manner that is realistic and achievable (Table 5.2).

Table 5.2: Writing a SMART Goal

S	Specific—statement, for example, who, what, where, and how.
M	Measurable—the goal must be able to be quantified and tracked over time.
A	Achievable—goals should cause the team to stretch but should be something that can be accomplished.
R	Relevant—the goal should be important to the patient and relevant to patient care.
T	Time-bound—this sets the length of time to achieve the goal in days, weeks, or months.

Throughout care planning and goal-setting conversations, MI can be a useful tool to assist patients in moving to a higher level of readiness for change and care participation. MI is described as a counseling approach that draws on a patient's own motivation and commitment to change in a setting of compassion, acceptance, and partnership.[28] Communications founded in MI techniques incorporate four processes:

■ **Engaging:** "The process of building and supporting a relationship where trust and respect go both ways"

■ **Focusing:** "The ongoing process of choosing and keeping a specific direction"

■ **Evoking:** "Bringing out another's strengths, knowledge, and ideas about the situation and themselves"

■ **Planning:** "Being with someone while they form specific actions to take"

These processes are used throughout patient interactions and are not necessarily linear; rather, different processes may be drawn on at different times. While moving through the four processes of MI, core communication skills are employed in conversations as abbreviated in the acronym OARS: asking open-ended questions, affirming, reflective listening, and summarizing.[29] Not every interaction will conclude with a plan. Rather, interactions take place within the context of a helping relationship with the long-term objective of change; ambivalence about change is also accepted as a natural part of the process. By using an approach of open exploration and empathetic reflection, the care team member aids the patient to recognize their own motivations for change, as well as identify and resolve sources of ambivalence.

While training is often needed to fully bring MI techniques into clinical interactions, MI strategies can be used by all care team members, and many tools can be readily incorporated into usual communications. As with any new skill set, MI communication techniques become

Table 5.3: Motivational Interviewing and Goal Setting Resources

Agency for Healthcare Research and Quality (AHRQ): Self Management Support	www.ahrq.gov
Centre for Collaboration Motivation & Innovation	www.centrecmi.ca
Guilford Press: Applications of Motivational Interviewing Series	www.guilford.com
Michigan Center for Clinical Systems Improvement	www.miccsi.org
Motivational Interviewing Network of Trainers (MINT)	www.motivational interviewing.org
Positive Psychology	www.positivepsychology .com
Psychology Tools	www.psychologytools.com

easier and more consistently employed with practice over time. While this introduction to MI is not extensive, it is intended to familiarize the reader with the MI approach. There are many good resources available to learn more about goal setting and MI, some of which are outlined in Table 5.3.

Actions and Interventions

Once SMART goals have been established, care team members work together with the patient to identify individual strategies and actions to move toward achieving those goals, including who is responsible for which actions or tasks.[25] To assist the patient in achieving any actions they are responsible for, care team members adopt a self-management support perspective. In this approach, the care team member helps the patient break down goals into smaller tasks by not only helping them identify what steps they will take but also how they will make those steps happen, as well as support problem-solving for any issues that may arise and identification of support in accomplishing those steps.[30] Further enlistment of support networks or other resources may be leveraged to assist in patient execution of the action plan; to this end, awareness of resources available to a patient, and ability to assist the patient in navigating those resources, for a variety of areas of concern is a crucial component of care management.

CASE STUDY
GOAL SETTING

RC is a 59-year-old female referred by her PCP to case management for assistance with access to psychiatry to address benzodiazepine use and ongoing prescription concerns.

MEDICAL HISTORY

Asthma, depression with anxiety, history of cerebrovascular accident (CVA) with left-side hemiparesis & associated contractures of the lower extremity (LE), hypertension (HTN), opioid-dependence, posttraumatic stress disorder (PTSD), history of physical and sexual abuse, history of domestic violence in marriage

SOCIAL HISTORY

Lives alone (divorced) in an apartment with her cat, wheelchair-dependent, relies on public transport/bus with wheelchair lift access; CVA at age 45 (related to untreated HTN) necessitated early retirement and reliance on disability

CASE MANAGEMENT

- Upon discussion with the patient and eliciting the patient-centered goals RC identifies accessing coordination of care for surgical clearance re: orthopedic procedure as her primary concern. RC has LE contracture and is having increased pain and difficulty with transfers due to this contracture.

- Working together with the PCP and RC reveals that the PCP will see RC to provide general surgical clearance once she is seen by psychiatry to address benzodiazepine use. RC is willing to access psychiatry consult arranged by the case manager with the understanding that the case manager will also assist with the steps needed for surgical clearance. The case manager arranges for a psychiatry consult; the patient attends the appointment and receives recommendations regarding ongoing benzodiazepine use.

- Regarding surgical clearance, RC will require pulmonology clearance and recent pulmonary function tests (PFTs) prior to PCP clearance. Due to RC's mobility, transportation, and financial challenges in accessing primary medical group facility for PFTs, the case manager is able to arrange for PFTs within an alternate medical system in close proximity to RC's home. With PFTs completed, pulmonology provides surgical clearance.

■ RC has an appointment set with the PCP. Psychiatry consult reviewed, and both agree to ongoing recommendations re: benzodiazepine use, and surgical clearance is provided.

By engaging RC in a patient-centered goal-setting environment, both provider and patient goals are able to be addressed and achieved in a manner that is satisfactory to all involved parties.

RC has her orthopedic procedure completed with a very satisfactory outcome.

Planning for Transitions of Care

Planning for how information will be communicated in transitions of care is another important part of the care planning process.[24] Transitions of care can be defined as "the movement of patients between health care practitioners, settings, and home as their condition and care needs change."[31] Any time the patient moves from one setting to another, such as from the hospital to a skilled nursing facility, from primary care to specialty providers, or even from the clinic to home, there is the potential for pertinent information to be lost, conflicting recommendations to be developed, or for multiple plans of care to arise. To avoid fragmentation, delays, and potential duplications in care, it is important that all members of the care team across the care continuum have access to and understand the coordinated care plan, and use the care plan as a base point for the care they provide as well. This section of a care plan also addresses pertinent information regarding the handoff process, including contact information, follow-up plans, and coordinating communications as a patient moves from one setting to the next (Box 5.2).[24]

Box 5.2: Components to Include Regarding Transitions of Care

■ Where the patient is going

■ How they are going to get there

■ When they are going

■ Contact for the individual(s) on the receiving end

■ Confirmation that the care plan has been shared with each of the health and/or community care providers

■ Confirmation that the patient's family has been notified about the transfer

■ Contact information for the individuals responsible for the creation of the care plan so that caregivers on the receiving end know whom to contact should they require additional information about the patient

■ A schedule of medical appointments or community care interactions that are to take place within the days following the transition

■ A reconciliation of medications being taken by the patient

■ A space for the care coordinator to describe the handoff or transfer of information that took place, including dates, times, contact persons, position, and contact information

■ Any follow-up plans or instructions for the caregivers or care coordinator at the originating facility (i.e., call to confirm the patient made it to their first appointment)

Adapted from Ontario Medical Association. *Key Elements to Include in a Coordinated Care Plan.* Published 2014. https://content.oma.org//wp-content/uploads/coordinatedcareplan_june2014-1.pdf

Ongoing Review of Goal Progress and Plan

The care plan should be revisited with the patient regularly not only to track patient progress and offer further support and encouragement as needed but also identify any need to modify the plan based on changes in the person's goals, as well as any changes in medical, functional, psychological, or social status.[6,25,26] Establishing a plan for revisiting goal progress also provides a timeline and a method of accountability for care team members and patients alike. Any barriers to goal attainment should also be assessed; these might include social barriers, such as financial concerns, or medical barriers, such as medication side effects.[26] In some circumstances, patients may not be able to identify or express what keeps them from achieving progress; for these scenarios, probing questions such as "What don't you like about . . ." and "What do you like about it?" may help elicit the underlying challenges a patient may be experiencing. Patient motivation comprises another key aspect of attaining and maintaining success in reaching goals; to this end, MI techniques as discussed earlier are also useful to support ongoing motivation for change.[26]

TEAM-BASED CARE

Teamwork and shared values help to break down walls and convert fragmented care into integrated care.[32] Health professionals working together as integrated teams draw on individual and collective skills and experience across disciplines, allowing each provider to practice at a higher level and provide better patient care.[33] Simply put, a well-coordinated team optimizes the experience and outcomes for a patient. Providers should take inventory of the availability and scope of resources for their patients as this could look different depending on the practice setting. Healthcare professionals who assist with care coordination activities, including care management, may not always be embedded within the provider setting; resources may be centralized at the organization or health plan.

AGNP Role in Care Coordination

Due to their advanced training, NPs are in a unique position to bridge gaps between teams across various disciplines and care settings. Care coordination in the AGNP role may include activities such as proactive surveillance for escalations in care and outreach to patients, with associated tasks such as assessment of needs in transitions of care, and review and revision of the multidisciplinary care plan as needed, as well as pulling in other care team members for follow-up on patient needs as identified.[34-36] Activities may be performed in an office or a home visit setting. Incorporation of the NP role may be especially helpful in at-risk populations with particularly complex needs.[34,36]

Registered Nurses

RNs assume a variety of case management roles in primary and specialty care settings. RNs typically assume these specialty roles after extensive experience in an acute care setting. In an ambulatory setting, the RN should be leveraged to closely follow medically complex patients who are at high risk for hospitalization. RN case managers may specialize in a clinical specialty, such as oncology or cardiology, while other nurse case managers perform complex case management for a broader patient population with multiple chronic conditions. RNs perform assessments of needs and report patient goals, document care planning, provide disease management through self-management education, monitor clinical results, facilitate transitions of care, and provide community resources. Lower acuity activities can be supported by licensed vocational nurses, medical assistants, or unlicensed staff. Examples of these activities include scheduling appointments, following up on referrals, sending appointment reminders, monitoring care gap reports, and escalating complex barriers to an appropriate team member.

Social Workers

Because of their training in mental health, systems navigation, and care coordination, social workers are particularly well poised to assess the complexity of patients' nonmedical issues and link patients with appropriate resources.[34] Transportation, housing, food assistance, mental health, and substance use all heavily influence

a patient's ability to self-manage care coordination and comply with treatment plans. Priority should be given to addressing social influencers of health to mitigate barriers to care and optimize health outcomes. An example of how social workers can be leveraged in care coordination can be found in Rush University Medical Center's Ambulatory Integration of the Medical and Social (AIMS) model (Box 5.3). In this model, the social worker assesses the needs of complex patients and then provides risk-focused care coordination guided by a standardized protocol.

Box 5.3: Ambulatory Integration of the Medical and Social (AIMS) Model

The AIMS social worker (SW) assists patients and/or their caregivers with biopsychosocial and functional issues impacting their medical care plan adherence or physical condition, moving through five steps in the process:

1. **Patient/Caregiver Engagement:** SW contacts the patient to explain the intervention and schedule the full assessment. Goals include developing rapport and trust, ensuring the patient understands the rationale for the intervention, and beginning to identify issues important to the patient.

2. **Assessment and Care Plan Development:** The SW performs a standardized comprehensive biopsychosocial assessment with a focus on strengths and barriers in multiple domains including finances, functional abilities, cognition, and mental health. Care plan goals are developed collaboratively with the patient using MI techniques in order to select up to three person-centered goals based on complexity, safety concerns, and the patient's ability to independently work on a goal.

3. **Telephonic or In-Person Case Management:** The SW regularly assesses progress on goals and supports or shifts the goal attainment plan as necessary. The SW and the patient problem-solve barriers to goal attainment using evidence-based MI and psychoeducation techniques.

4. **Goal Attainment:** The SW and patient summarize goal achievement and ensure community-based resources are in place to support the patient in the community. Resources and methods for additional goal attainment independent from an active AIMS intervention are discussed, and patients are encouraged to contact the SW should new challenges emerge.

5. **Ongoing Care:** If goals are not attained, the SW assists the patient in problem-solving barriers to goal attainment using MI techniques and

psychoeducation. If continued social work intervention regarding agreed-on goals is warranted, the SW and patient reevaluate the care plan and reengage in active case management.

Source: Rizzo VM, Rowe JM, Shier Kricke G, Krajci K, Golden R. AIMS: a care coordination model to improve patient health outcomes. Health Soc Work. 2016;41(3):191-195. doi:10.1093/hsw/hlw029; The AIMS Model. AIMS model. n.d. https://www.theaimsmodel.org/aims-2

Pharmacists

Pharmacists should be leveraged to support care coordination goals for patients to mitigate medication-related adverse events, readmissions, and preventable errors.[39] This is particularly true during periods of transitions from one level of care to another because inpatient or ED providers may not be fully informed of the patient's history; therefore, new or changed medication orders may not align with patients' home medications, lifestyle, or financial situation. During medication reconciliation, pharmacists review medications for indication, appropriateness, effectiveness, and safety and are verified with most recent orders to ensure accuracy. When medication reconciliation occurs in collaboration with a patient, an assessment can occur to determine a patient's unique burdens that impact adherence such as cost or pill burden, prior experiences or preferences, or other perceived barriers. Furthermore, a pharmacist can assess and reinforce a patient's health literacy regarding proper administration and self-care behaviors to improve adherence.[39]

CASE STUDY
TEAM-BASED CARE

MT is a 62-year-old female referred by her primary care physician (PCP) to case management for assistance with care coordination after multiple "no-shows" to appointments.

MEDICAL HISTORY

Traumatic brain injury (TBI), cognitive impairment, diabetes, splenomegaly, hyperlipidemia, hypertension, hypothyroidism, esophageal varices, peptic ulcer disease, hepatitis C, pancytopenia

SOCIAL HISTORY

Has a poor support network, lives alone in a single-story, one-bedroom apartment. MT is fully independent with ambulation. MT is unable to drive due to TBI. MT has limited/fixed income. MT has Medicare and Medicaid (known as "Medi-Cal" in California).

CASE MANAGEMENT

- A telephonic assessment by the RN case manager (RNCM) finds multiple barriers, home safety concerns, overdue annual screenings, and risk factors that require a team approach to her care coordination. The RNCM is concerned about safety issues at home due to cognitive impairment and isolation. An adult protective services (APS) report is filed with the county.
- The RNCM determines MT is eligible to have in-home assistance for her care, including assistance at home, with medication management, shopping, cleaning, and transportation to appointments through her Medicaid benefits. MT is unable to independently complete the paperwork; the RNCM collaborates with the APS social worker to complete the paperwork.
- The RNCM arranges for transportation with a Medicaid-approved provider at no cost to MT and establishes a process for the patient to utilize this transportation benefit moving forward.
- RNCM enlists the support of the RN diabetes educator to perform an in-person assessment and determine educational needs related to diabetes self-management. The RN diabetes educator determines MT has limited ability to accurately measure blood sugars and self-manage high/low values. MT is also unable to read/interpret numbers/charts/sliding scale without written instructions to remind her. A new strategy is developed which includes a continuous glucose monitor and regular administration times for insulin.
- The RNCM enlists the support of a pharmacist related to concerns of polypharmacy and insulin use.
- With the transportation barrier resolved, RNCM reschedules missed appointments with the endocrinologist, and external specialty providers in ophthalmology and podiatry.

The RNCM relies on multiple healthcare and community team members to support MT's complex care coordination needs. MT subsequently maintains scheduled appointments with her primary and specialty providers with the support of the RNCM and in-home support caregiver. MT adheres to regular appointments with the RN diabetes educator; her HgbA1c improves from 11.0 to 9.1 within a year of engagement.

INFORMATION SHARING AND COMMUNICATIONS

Patient-Care Team Communication

Clear, effective, and efficient communication is crucial to healthcare, and care coordination, in particular.[11] Communication streams involving the patient and members of the care team should aim to accomplish eliciting information from the patient perspective, an understanding of the patient within their own psychosocial and cultural contexts, and a shared understanding of the goals of care.[19] However, communication gaps exist between patients and providers, which can lead to adverse health outcomes.[40] The practice of teach-back can enhance the patient-provider relationship by ensuring a thorough understanding of the medical information discussed.[40]

The teach-back method incorporates confirmation of understanding, by requesting the patient explain back to the educator the information that was discussed, in an iterative manner focused on reaching a state of clear patient recall. Talevski et al.[40] describe this process:

> Teach-back involves asking patients to explain in their own words what a health provider has just told them. Any misunderstandings are then clarified by the health provider and understanding is checked again. This process continues until the patient can correctly recall the information that was given. (p. 2)

This process aims to reduce the barriers presented by the utilization of medical jargon by providers and to address potential communication gaps. Communication gaps can present a challenge in patient–provider communications. These gaps/barriers include awareness of differently abled patients (including sight impairment, hearing impairment, cognitive impairment, primary language, and differing literacy levels, to name a few). Using teach-back can help address barriers by eliciting input and understanding from the patient, engaging them in the healthcare process, and leading to reductions in readmission rate, complications, and medication errors.[41]

There are several avenues of patient–provider and provider–provider communication modalities:

- **Face-to-Face, In-Person, and Video Visits:** Facilitates direct communication
- **Telephone:** Facilitates direct communication; not widely used for provider–provider due to lack of reachability/limited availability by providers
- **Written:** Includes indirect communication and medical documentation of visits with the patient, as well as emails/secure electronic messaging. Electronic messaging allows for confirmation of material being accessed and ease of provider–provider communication streams. It is becoming more widely used for patient–provider communication.[9]

Strategies to improve communication between the care team and the patient also include providing visit summaries to patients after both inpatient and outpatient encounters, outreach after hospital discharge, and electronic health record (EHR) patient portals.[12] Another person-centered approach includes designating one lead or primary point of contact on the care team for the patient, thereby streamlining communication and continuity of care as the patient moves across care settings.[6] Other practices have limited point persons for patient communication to two or three team members or provide a card outlining key team member roles and contact information.[22]

Interdisciplinary Care Team Communication

Challenges in Care Team Communication

Common areas of breakdown in collaboration and communication between providers include challenges in information exchange, such as unclear care plans, or unavailability of notes in a timely manner; unclear roles and responsibilities between providers; and limited access to, or rapport with, other providers, limiting the ability to interact with each other for consults or other concerns.[11,42–44,48] When considering EHR use, similar issues have also been reported, such as limited access to the EHR, inadequate information available in the EHR (either due to unavailable, incomplete, or untimely documentation or test results), limited usefulness posed by structural limitations (i.e., inability to see or access referral orders, inability to run needed reports), and difficulties in using the EHR itself.[12,45,49] Team members involved in care coordination may also rely on multiple health information technology systems, further complicating how care is delivered and communicated. Incomplete information, time spent on workarounds, waiting for needed information, or repeat testing in the absence of access to current results ultimately leads to the potential for conflicting plans of care, inefficient delivery of care, and avoidable duplications in care. A lack of care team communication also leads to a negative experience of care provision, both from a patient and provider perspective, as well as increased patient concern that important aspects of care may be missed.[11,12,42,48]

Strategies to Strengthen Team Communication

Despite its challenges, EHR use is recommended to improve the availability of information across team members and across healthcare settings, offering a centralized and accessible location for data-driven teamwork. EHR functionalities beneficial to care coordination efforts include the availability of visit notes across care settings, the specification of care team member roles, and the support of practice-based registries.[41] The EHR can also be leveraged as a platform for team functioning, in which tasks can be assigned into team "buckets" or organized into lists. Effective use of EHRs has been reported positively from a patient perspective as well, as providers have access to medical history, treatment plan, and recent care information, including test results and current medications. However, as noted earlier, for health information technology to be used effectively, all members of the healthcare team must enter complete, clear, up-to-date information in a timely manner. Using structured templates in EHR communications and interoperability among various EHR systems have also been identified as areas for potential improvement opportunities.[11,12]

Communication establishing clear role definition is recommended to allow for team members to function in a streamlined manner based on established expectations.[22,39,48] One example of this is with the use of care coordination agreements, a set of documents outlining agreed-on processes, mechanisms, and criteria for referrals, as well as roles and responsibilities for providers comanaging the patient's care.[39,42] These agreements also outline timelines for reviewing these documents to make any needed improvements over time. Clear role definition is also recommended specific to the care coordination role in a team, to improve communication and trust among team members as well as with patients.[43] This might include designating one team member as the primary point of contact, whose role is to facilitate coordination across care settings and communicate the coordinated picture to the patient.[6]

Personal interactions are essential in building rapport, trust, and collaborative relationships among team members, both in terms of communications between primary care and specialty providers, as well as among clinic team members and other providers involved throughout the patient's care, such as those in ED, inpatient, and home care settings (Box 5.4).[9,40,48]

Box 5.4: Essential Personal Interactions

According to the National Committee for Quality Assurance, communication is essential to build trust, develop relationships, and coordinate care. Inherently, there are multiple processes involved:

1. Involve all the appropriate people.
2. Work together to create common goals.
3. Recognize each person's or organization's needs as well as strengths.
4. Find specific opportunities to collaborate.
5. Work to identify and remove potential barriers.
6. Create and implement a shared plan for communications that includes both regular communications and a way to address urgent issues.

Source: Data from The National Committee for Quality Assurance. Goals to care: how to keep the in "person-centered." https://www.ncqa.org/wp-content/uploads/2018/07/20180531_Report_Goals_to_Care_Spotlight_.pdf

Regular interdisciplinary team meetings offer an example of how care team members can build an interdependent dynamic while organizing and establishing priorities in individual patient care.[44] These meetings may include goal-focused collaboration, which incorporates all team members' perspectives as well as the patient's stated goals, as well as build rapport and relationships to support interprofessional problem-solving. These meetings also help the team in identifying opportunities to streamline care, including avoidance of duplicative care or overuse of services. Other opportunities to facilitate personal interactions include colocation of team members into team pods, daily clinic huddles incorporating standard processes to relay pertinent information to off-site team members, designating one person to whom team members can bring communication gaps forward, and seminars held by varying specialties for primary practices and vice versa.[19,40]

CARE COORDINATION PERFORMANCE MEASUREMENT AND QUALITY IMPROVEMENT

When implementing care coordination strategies in practice, it is important to monitor how well those efforts are working and to adjust as needed. Care coordination is not one-size-fits-all and may be implemented in different ways across varying healthcare organizations. A multilayered approach is likely most effective; using multiple strategies has also been associated with better overall hospital quality ratings as defined by the Centers for Medicare and Medicaid Services.[3]

Care Coordination Measures

As care coordination can be interpreted and implemented in a variety of ways, there are several approaches and measures for tracking these efforts. Potential types of measures that may be used include the following:

- Structural measures, such as the presence of an EHR system or care coordination agreement
- Process measures, such as frequency of communication with other clinicians or development and implementation of care plans
- Appropriateness, overuse, or efficiency measures, such as tracking duplicate services, such as imaging or labs, or provision of unnecessary services
- Outcome measures, such as rates of preventable hospital admissions or readmissions
- Patient experience measures, such as patient satisfaction surveys or care coordination reports[45]

In any evaluation efforts, exactly which types of measures and perspectives are incorporated may vary depending on the specific care coordination strategy to be examined, as well as what knowledge is deemed most important to make decisions about which aspects of the approach to maintain, improve, or remove as care coordination efforts continue to evolve. Incorporating multiple perspectives also produces more holistic insights into how a given strategy may be performing, aids incorporation of a person-centered approach, and provides the opportunity to give feedback to multiple stakeholders in the process.[6]

Taking a global approach, the AHRQ outlines care coordination mechanisms by domain, including effects and experiences from the patient, healthcare provider, and health system perspectives. The AHRQ's Care Coordination Measures Atlas is recommended as a useful starting point in performance measurement planning, including a detailed guide in how to choose measures, as well as a comprehensive measure index mapped to pertinent domains and perspectives (Box 5.5).[5]

Box 5.5: AHRQ Domains of Care Coordination Measurement
Coordination Activities
Establish accountability or negotiate responsibility
Communicate
Facilitate transitions
Assess needs and goals
Create a proactive plan of care
Monitor, follow up, and respond to change
Support self-management goals
Link to community resources
Align resources with patient and population needs
Broad Approaches
Teamwork focused on coordination
Healthcare home
Care management
Medication management
Health information technology-enabled coordination

Source: Adapted from McDonald KM, Schultz E, Albin L, et al. *Care Coordination Atlas Version 4.* AHRQ Publication No. 14-0037-EF. Agency for Healthcare Research and Quality; 2014. https://www.ahrq.gov/sites/default/files/publications/files/ccm_atlas.pdf

Continuous Quality Improvement Methods

Tracking care coordination measures provides insight into whether care coordination processes are working, or desired outcomes are being achieved, and prompts consideration of where improvements can be made. Quality improvement (QI) offers a framework that can be used to systematically enhance the way care is delivered, with an eye toward continually improving system performance and patient outcomes. For clinical practices interested in incorporating or improving care coordination, QI frameworks provide an accessible platform for introducing changes. There are many resources available to learn more about quality improvement methods, including training and strategies for implementation. Chapter 9 focuses on quality improvement; students should review that chapter for further information.

CONCLUSION

Effective care coordination is essential in a patient-centered care setting. The benefits of care coordination include improved health outcomes, reduction in hospital admissions and avoidable readmissions, improved patient experience, and cost savings. Engaging others on the healthcare team to assess and address a patient's clinical and social needs, developing and updating personalized care plans, and monitoring outcomes are necessary to ensure optimal patient care in a fragmented healthcare system.

REFERENCES

References for this chapter are online and available at https://connect.springerpub.com/content/book/978-0-8261-8414-6/part/part01/toc-part/ch5.

CHAPTER 6

Promoting Well-Being in AGNPs

Maureen Craig

LEARNING OBJECTIVES

At the conclusion of this chapter, the learner will be able to:

➤ Identify three contributors to burnout in healthcare providers and one or more actions an adult-gerontology nurse practitioner (AGNP) can implement to respond with resilience building behaviors.

➤ Differentiate the four foundations of well-being and one self-care behavior that supports each foundation.

INTRODUCTION

As a healthcare provider, promoting client well-being and client self-care is best accomplished when we understand the foundations of human health and personally live aligned with that understanding. As healthcare leaders, supporting provider well-being and a healthy work environment sets the stage to efficiently deliver quality patient care, improving our community's health, carrying out the Institute on Health Care Improvement's Triple Aim. Yet why is it important for nurse practitioners to care about personal well-being? Well-being is an important step toward preventing burnout.

The healthcare workforce has faced unprecedented strain with the pandemic, heightening the need to routinely assess one's well-being and institute self-care measures to mitigate burnout and improve resilience. Sleep, nutrition, movement, and social connection are key areas where healthcare providers can initiate self-care and commit to changes that positively evolve life experience. To make change last, healthcare professionals must know how to reform unhealthy habits. Humans are creatures of habit and deeply integrated with their physical and social environment. Understanding these connections is a critical component of achieving and maintaining well-being for the AGNP, helping make the better choice the easy choice!

BURNOUT AND RESILIENCE

Burnout Risk

The AGNP is tasked with managing and caring for a growing population of aging patients with ever-lengthening lists of chronic health conditions in a system with shrinking resources. In response to this growing burden and the strain of facing multiple roles, the advanced practice provider's risk for burnout can be as high or higher[1] than many other healthcare professionals.[2] The combination of high responsibility for the care of human physical and emotional well-being, limits on control of how that care is delivered, and continuing demands to produce more product (billable patient care) produces the triad that leads to burnout for many dedicated healthcare professionals. The informed AGNP does well to understand this risk and select and participate in a work design that mitigates this risk. However, much of how healthcare is delivered is determined by healthcare employers, insurance companies, and government agencies, demonstrating the importance of the advocacy role the proactive AGNP might inhabit.

Burnout is more common than not in the healthcare workforce. Survey data on burnout in 2013 and 2014 from 740 primary care clinicians (21% nurse practitioners [NPs]/physician's assistants [PAs]) was matched to employment roster data from 2016. The survey revealed, 53% of clinicians reported burnout, predicting clinician turnover.[3,4] Although data are lacking specifically for AGNPs, burnout is common, and rates are increasing in the healthcare workforce in contrast to the steady rates seen in the general U.S. working population. In a study conducted by the Mayo Clinic in partnership with the American Medical Association, researchers found that 54.4% of physicians reported at least one symptom of burnout in 2014 compared with 45.5% in 2011, a 9% increase in 3 years.[5] For the foreseeable future, the AGNP as a healthcare practitioner is likely to face uncertainty and stress from the changing healthcare needs of the population. From long-standing problems like cancer and heart disease to more recent surges in dementia and the COVID-19 pandemic, the challenges and unpredictable care demands of this population add to the stress and risk of burnout for the healthcare workforce.

What Is Burnout?

The *International Classification of Diseases-11* defines "burnout" as a syndrome conceptualized as resulting from chronic workplace stress that has not been successfully managed. It is characterized by three dimensions: (a) feelings of energy depletion or exhaustion; (b) increased mental distance from one's job, or feelings of negativism or cynicism related to one's job; and (c) a sense of ineffectiveness and a lack of accomplishment. Burnout refers specifically to phenomena in the occupational context and should not be applied to describe experiences in other areas of life.[6] The diagnosis of burnout is specific to the work or caregiver environment and is distinct from disorders related to adjustment, stress, anxiety, or mood. From a clinical perspective, burnout can be considered a type of adaptive disorder related to psychosocial work stressors and the existence of a persistent imbalance between demands and available resources for fulfilling them, expectations, and perceived results, as well as performed effort and obtained reinforcements. The pathology results from an accumulation of risk factors, whether they are personal, organizational, role-related, or other, and from the lack of protective factors and resistance to experienced stress.[7] The person experiencing burnout in addition to the triad of exhaustion, cynicism, and a sense of low productivity may experience any of the following symptoms or behaviors: headaches, gastrointestinal disturbances, sleep difficulties, cold and flu symptoms, overwhelm, depression, depersonalization, irritability, impatience, frustration with and social withdrawal from coworkers and patients, desire to not start or give up on work, an inability to concentrate, and/or the misuse of food, drugs, or alcohol to feel better or not to feel.[8]

Management of workplace stress leading to burnout is best addressed jointly by the healthcare provider and the healthcare organization/system. Focusing solely on the individual for intervention creates a "blame the victim" culture that is counterproductive in resolving work-related stress and burnout and results in rapid turnover of talented and dedicated healthcare providers. Forward-thinking organizations seeing the link between provider well-being and quality and safety of patient care are paying close attention to how to have the workplace environment support the healthcare provider human resource.

Costs of Burnout

The significant costs of burnout are borne by the individual AGNP, the healthcare employer, and the patient/family. The burnout experience combining job-related exhaustion, cynicism, and a reduced sense of efficacy is a disappointing state of reduced work satisfaction for the individual who has applied their efforts to finishing a long journey of education and training in a respected profession. The burnout experience at work often influences overall life satisfaction, reducing work happiness[9] and leading to an increased risk of alcohol abuse/dependence[10] and suicide.[11]

The healthcare organization also faces loss as burned-out providers have increases in sick leave,[12] increased job turnover,[3] and decreased work effort,[13] adding to healthcare provider shortages. Burnout also correlates with the delivery of lower quality of care, increased hospital-transmitted infections,[14,15] increased rates of medical errors,[16] higher standardized mortality ratios,[17] and reductions in patient satisfaction.[18]

The way to better patient care is through better provider care. Healthcare providers experiencing burnout will not be able to improve the quality of care; burnout in the workforce must be addressed first. Systemwide policy and practice that advocates for the healthcare provider's well-being can lead to the delivery of improved quality of care at a lower cost, with higher patient satisfaction, and would guide a globally improved experience in healthcare delivery, optimizing the experience for all.

What Is Resilience?

Merriam-Webster defines "resilience" as an ability to recover from or adjust easily to misfortune or change.[19] Resilience in the workplace can be explored in at least two different contexts. Resilience is a developed robustness that can take on the stressors as they arise (e.g., increases in workload, changes in workplace rules) with a degree of physical and emotional flexibility. Resilience is also the ability to respond to a larger scale difficulty or loss (e.g., medical error, unexpected loss of a patient, job loss) in a way that integrates the event into life experience and includes profound personal growth,[20] allowing the person to adapt, evolve, and move forward in their life experience, again able to access energy, positive emotions, and a sense of efficacy.

Correlating Factors in Burnout and Resilience

All individuals and organizations looking to improve the quality and safety of patient care and increase patient and provider satisfaction will want to be aware of and preventively address factors that correlate with burnout. These correlating factors are here categorized as role-related, organizational, and personal.

Role-Related Factors

The role of the AGNP was well discussed earlier and has areas of emphasis in clinical practice, research, education, consulting, and administrative/leadership. Consideration for which roles present the best alignment for the individual AGNP can aid the nurse practitioner in career planning with more time spent in the roles that support personal resilience and prevent and/or mitigate burnout.

Inherent components of the AGNP role that increase the risk for burnout include the strong emotional nature of the work,[21] the ethical challenges of considering the burden, and the benefits of life-sustaining therapies often leading to moral distress when the AGNP cannot act in accordance with individual beliefs due to organizational constraints.[22] The most significant job/role variable that has been linked with employee burnout is role stress. Role stress includes both role conflict (role demands that conflict with the employee's abilities, goals, values, or beliefs) and role ambiguity (employee does not have the necessary information to perform the role adequately).[8] Assessing and mitigating role stress is an area in which the healthcare employer can make a significant impact.

Organizational Factors

Leaders in professional organizations, healthcare systems, and learning institutions who are now aware of the strong links between burnout and the influence it has on patient safety and healthcare quality have a vested interest in promoting the wellness of those they employ, train, and represent.[23] Individuals may weather brief periods of challenge, but prolonged or repeated negative stress leads to healthcare provider burnout and reduced quality of patient care. The six main risk factors for work burnout are organizational factors: having an overwhelming workload, limited provider autonomy, unrewarding work, unfair work, work that conflicts with values, and a lack of community in the workplace.[24] Significant improvements in the quality of the organization's healthcare product can be achieved by addressing these workplace conditions that contribute to burnout.[25]

Workload

When an individual has workload needs beyond the resources to accomplish them, the situation quickly leads to burnout. In most healthcare settings, the workload is unpredictable and often heavy relative to the resources. Resources are both the human resource and the equipment, supplies, and personal protective equipment needed to accomplish the work needs safely and with a degree of ease and sustainability. Healthcare providers, as part of clinical and administrative leadership, must continuously assess workforce needs and use their knowledge and voice to quickly respond to the rise in workload with additional resources. Leadership must ensure the culture of the workplace supports each healthcare provider's time away from work to recover, time off during work for meals, and breaks with freedom from connectivity to the work (e.g., pagers and messaging apps).

Practices such as retaining and recruiting the workforce to accomplish the work at hand avoid healthcare provider burnout and the loss of valuable employees who are a good fit for the organization and the work. An environment where it is safe to speak up and there is good listening by leadership can be a supportive bridge through times when the workload to workforce ratio is elevated; however, timely action to increase the workforce is critical to prevent individual healthcare provider exhaustion, cynicism, emotional distancing, and a loss of work efficiency (e.g., increases in sick calls), which are all symptoms of burnout.

In addition, leadership must continuously assess what tool and equipment updates are of value in the effective delivery of the care and managing the workload. The electronic health record (EHR) is a tool that has some clinical merit (provider access to data); however, since its inception, it has become an oppressive documentation device[26] that has largely prioritized billing and administrative functions over care delivery and clinical decision-making. The EHR was incentivized by the 2009 Health Information Technology for Economic and Clinical Health Act. While intended to improve care quality and efficiency, the EHR has inadvertently burdened clinicians (documentation time, influences on provider–patient relationship, worsening quality of documentation) and is now considered a leading cause of their frustration and burnout.[27–29] Improvements in the EHR rely on human factors engineering, a science that considers the benefits and fallibility of human interaction with a system. The EHR documentation must be optimized, requiring less effort (e.g., reduced steps and clicks to accomplish a single task), allowing for more succinct notes with meaningful content pushed forward while preserving revenue generation. In-basket management would minimize autogenerated alerts and prioritize tasks and messages to appropriate team members, keeping them practicing at the top of their license and skill (correlated with provider satisfaction).[30] Clinicians are at twice the risk for burnout when their inboxes have an above-average number of EHR-generated messages.[28] Training, at the elbow, with real-time feedback after observation, provided at regular intervals, helps improve clinician efficiency and satisfaction with the EHR tool.

Provider Autonomy

Excessive bureaucracy and a lack of autonomy in the workplace are strongly linked with the development of burnout.[8] Individual healthcare providers often have limited control of healthcare organizational policy and decisions, call time, work hours, and a lack of control of patient adherence to prescribed treatment. A workplace culture that includes healthcare providers in decision-making processes at all levels, that allows individuals to lead on problem-solving efforts and maintain ownership of results (e.g., setting their own work performance goals), and that provides leadership support of provider decision-making at the lowest level possible, respecting professional autonomy and practice control, all leads to provider satisfaction, a sense of independence, and a reduced risk of burnout.[8,23,27]

Reward Management

Evolutionary psychology[31] notes that humans are constantly performing a cost/benefit analysis of every interaction. Taking this principle to the organizational level, the organization will thrive if rewards (i.e., benefits) are managed to minimize the cost-to-benefit ratio for all parties (i.e., patients, providers, staff, and leadership) involved in the interaction, creating win–win experiences. Healthcare providers look for work experiences with varying degrees of clinical predictability combined with opportunities for learning, growth, and reward for invested time and effort.

Rewards for the healthcare provider are both tangible (e.g., income) and intangible (e.g., the emotion and gained esteem of being valued for one's service by the patient/family, colleagues, and/or leadership).

Organizational leadership optimizes the work environment when verbalizing and modeling a clear vision of the organization's mission, evidenced in the details of defined work expectations and rewards. Bridgeman[23] notes an unclear mission with contrasts between what the leadership/organization says it values and how it is leads to moral distress. Values represent the ideals and motivators that draw an individual to the profession; if they are incongruous, dissatisfaction results. Ideally, organizational leaders speak and deliver a clear mission/vision, share goals with healthcare providers, and create a safe space for structured debates on big decisions. Effective leaders will keep roles and work clear, and document/communicate changes in expectations so when providers return to work, they can easily be updated. Healthcare providers experience increased work satisfaction and retention when they are aware of and have input into the measurable processes and outcomes that leadership uses to evaluate work performance, especially when qualitative measures are included. In addition, the possibility for individual learning, growth, recognition, and promotion (e.g., career ladders with clarity on promotion) increases the sense of fairness and work satisfaction for the healthcare provider.[8] Providers are at increased risk of burnout when the reward target keeps moving or is unreachable or when the reward is unevenly distributed or unfair relative to the workload.[32] Those who perceive their supervisors as fair and equitable are less likely to develop burnout symptoms, indicating that workplace fairness and equity influence the perceptions of effort–reward balance.[23]

Payment, income, and practice finances; concerns related to professional liability and regulation; and healthcare reform were all cited as concerns and factors potentially influencing healthcare quality and contributing to

professional dissatisfaction.[27] Notably, Medicare pays 85% of the physician fee schedule (PFS) rate when a service is billed under the NP's own national provider identifier (NPI) number, but Medicare pays 100% of the PFS rate when the same service provided by an NP is billed "incident to" a supervising physician, making independent practice (i.e., autonomy) at the top of license financially (i.e., reward) disadvantageous, a potentially specific factor in burnout for NP and PA providers.

Whereas the direct feedback between patients and providers during engagement can be a powerful source of satisfaction for both the patient and provider, some providers experience increased stress from patient satisfaction survey results.[27] The organization can support the successful patient/provider engagement with enough time and repeat exposure to allow these relationships to evolve and be experienced by the humans engaging in them. A schedule that is overbooked (too large a workload) squeezes out the positive experiences, keeping the provider in a sympathetic dominant state, seeing threats over opportunity.

Belonging to the Tribe (Team Building)

The most consequential organizational characteristic mitigating burnout is social support.[21] Healthcare organizations attenuate burnout and support resilience by structuring the work and provider interactions to build relationships with leadership, with the multidisciplinary team, and, most important, with those who can best empathize with the experience, that is, peers. Providers can be protected from isolation through practices of new-hire mentoring, buddy systems, career mentors, and especially teams. There are strong and independent associations between teamwork, clinician occupational well-being, and patient safety.[33]

DNP lead team-based care improves the quality of care delivered in many clinical environments (ICU, OR, ED to primary care clinics), and is associated with reduced costs and clinician well-being.[30] A study involving 327 providers found burnout was significantly associated with independently intervening or educating patients on lifestyle disease-specific self-care activities, without reliance on the multidisciplinary team (intervening on lifestyle, 95% CI = [0.39, 7.83], $p = 0.03$, while educating patients, 95% CI = [0.33, 7.32], $p = 0.03$).[34] This study supports reducing primary care provider burnout by redistributing some of the patient education to other healthcare professionals while maintaining team collaboration and communication.

High-performing teams have shared values and goals, strong team identity, defined and complementary roles, effective leadership, regular meetings, adequate staffing, shared physical space, effective communication, mutual trust and respect, constructive conflict resolution, task sharing and shifting, and practice observation and feedback focused on measurable processes and outcomes. Successful teams have the capacity to improve patient outcomes, the efficiency of care, and the satisfaction and well-being of healthcare clinicians. Team training is a means for investing in the continuous professional development of clinicians, keeping them engaged and practicing at the top of their licenses. Multidisciplinary team training can also break down the silo-ed approach to the undergraduate and graduate education of many clinicians.[35]

Humans are social beings and sensitive to reputation (e.g., belonging to the tribe) as this meant survival to our ancestors. Today with reputation being more available for the tribe to witness in social media, individuals face unprecedented social comparison triggering the fear of others' opinions, especially for those with more agreeable personality traits. Healthy teams can give individuals feedback to buffer unhelpful, underinformed outside opinion.

The nature of providing healthcare services includes adverse events (e.g., unexpected death of a patient, workplace violence, or medical error—the third-leading cause of death in the United States). These work-related events and other life stressors will be part of the healthcare provider experience and can be mitigated with peer support, preventing a second victim. Although stress reduction techniques and supervisor support are helpful, peer support is more effective to help a worker mitigate work-related stressors and prevent burnout.[8] Healthcare organizations can support team-based and/or organization-based peer support training and programs so practitioners are ready to effectively respond when difficulty arises. The support offered may include a text message, a phone call, a cup of coffee, a walk and talk, or a group debriefing, providing a listening understanding presence for all involved. Peer support can be activated by the provider themselves, or a colleague or manager, yet the interaction with the peer always remains confidential. Peer support is separate from adverse event investigation and quality improvement efforts of the organization yet is a profound contribution to patient care quality and safety and provider well-being.

Healthy Work Environment

Humans find work that allows deep focus engaging and cognitively rewarding. Work that is perceived as repetitive and/or chaotic without mental space for deep focus (frequent and/or meaningless alerts, distractions or interruptions, and prioritizing urgency over the importance of work) causes work quantity and quality to suffer and is a risk factor for burnout.[36] A healthy physical work environment that supports work that is largely predictable yet has some engaging novelty, supporting a sense of growth, provides the most sustainable experience for worker engagement and increases quality and quantity of work output while supporting worker well-being.

Modern work environments are often riddled with noise and frequent meaningless interruptions! When considering highly productive healthy work environments, organizations will create a variety of comfortable, quiet work spaces with good lighting and options for natural light (shown to promote calm, peaceful moods and reduce stress)[36] and support a culture that is flexible and allows employees to work where and when they want so employees can create their own ideal work conditions and help them get into the flow of their work.

Additional environmental factors that support the healthcare work and worker include a work culture that supports, trains in, and practices taking breaks and time off work and time off connectivity to work; and also provides wellness programs, peer-support training programs accessible to all workers, healthy whole plant food in the cafeteria and locations food is sold, mindfulness and exercise programs, gym memberships, and protected time to engage in these activities. Healthcare providers learn much of their work behavior patterns in school and residential training programs, suggesting educational and workplace settings must change the culture to expect engagement in self-care activities.[37]

Personal Factors

Some personal factors correlating with burnout are not changeable, yet awareness of them allows the individual to take actions to support themselves when they have the given risk factor. Healthcare providers are at increased risk of burnout when they are younger than 55 years of age (200% increased risk); female (30%–60% increased risk); have high caregiver responsibility in the family, for example, a child younger than 21 years of age (54% increased risk); or a spouse that is a nonphysician healthcare provider (23% increased risk).[38] When considering personality, it is not the work, but the person–environment fit that determines the perceived stress. Stress levels can vary widely even in identical situations based on the work demand and perceived control.[39]

The AGNP role may well attract individuals with the personality trait conscientiousness, that is, perfectionism,[40] which has a positive relationship with both deep work engagement (e.g., best patient outcomes) and yet also burnout.[41] The AGNP with a strong personality trait of sensitivity/emotional lability, that is, neuroticism, may empathize beautifully with patients and families and yet this trait correlates positively with burnout.[42] The AGNP where these personality traits dominate or the individual who has had more challenging life experiences benefits from more frequent and increased use of resilience behaviors, deliberately and systematically engaging self-care tools[79] to regulate negative emotion intensity.

Beneficial self-care practices include disconnecting from work, for example, no missed breaks; prioritizing relationships, especially those that provide empathetic listening;

taking care of the body with good nutrition (quality, quantity, timing, e.g., no skipped meals), sleep, hydration, and exercise; taking care of the mind with meditation, mindful self-compassion, yoga, and/or journaling; avoiding negative outlets such as numbing with food, alcohol, or other substances; keeping challenging experiences in perspective, accepting what you cannot change, learning from past experiences, maintaining hope, finding purpose, moving toward your goals, and looking for opportunities for self-discovery and growth.[20] Although personal factors are important to emphasize when optimizing the healthcare provider experience, organizational factors (e.g., workload, autonomy, and reward management) are the dominant driving force behind burnout and must not be ignored.

Burnout Recovery Plan

Burnout, with its triad of exhaustion, cynicism, and ineffectiveness, results in lower quality of experience for the provider and at the same time a lower quality of patient care and reduced patient safety. When examined, a meta-analysis of 82 studies of 210,669 healthcare providers showed a statistically significant negative relationship between burnout and quality, implying greater burnout among healthcare providers was associated with poorer quality healthcare and reduced safety for patients.[43] When patient safety and quality care are waning, moving from burnout to resilience in the provider workforce is critical and challenging. Organizational leaders can begin with lots of infusions of listening, mindfulness and compassion, and briefings and debriefings. Tailor the tools to the needs of the area and assess the workgroups one team at a time. Check in on their self-care; for example, provide a burnout assessment tool, make it easy to ask for help, pace work intensity in intervals (about 60–90 minutes) with mental and physical breaks, allow providers to develop deep focus, minimize multitasking to provide a sense of control and reward from work, ensure meals and meal breaks are taken, encourage providers to leave work on time with little to no paid or unpaid overtime, assess and prioritize sleep quality and quantity, include movement and opportunity for movement throughout the day, offer and promote sound nutrition throughout the organization, and encourage providers to create personalized wellness goals based on their perceived needs. When needs are identified, individuals can develop and implement a personal burnout recovery plan, for example, take time off, connect with friends and family, be active, connect with nature, continue learning, help others, take a mindfulness meditation training, and so on. Organizations can look at ways to restructure the work so there is an emotional payoff of autonomy (do not micromanage), mastery (novel skill building), and purpose (meaning in the work, recruit them to the vision of the mission). Wait to work on

quality and safety after the workforce is engaged and self-care is the norm. Improvements in provider self-care will lead to better patient care.

When particularly stressful events occur (e.g., violent patients, medical error, unexpected loss, moral distress, an extra heavy workload, vicarious trauma), organizations can encourage resilience by listening (e.g., group or individual debriefings) and promoting peer support, mental health, and wellness resources, encouraging time off to connect to the bigger picture. Adverse events are part of the human experience, and humans have evolved to be resilient and experience growth from and through these events.

WELL-BEING AND SELF-CARE

One concept in nursing that desperately needs revolution is that there is some virtue in sacrificing one's self. The fact that we, who provide our communities healthcare, are more often than not suffering from one or more symptoms of poor mental or physical health is a paradox that can be solved. As educators, researchers, and clinicians, we must be committed to changing the culture, insisting that assertive, radical, shameless well-being, and self-care are part of any health professional's training and personal journey. Healthcare professionals at every stage of our training and career can boldly commit to our well-being and self-care as part of our personal and professional journey.

The Wisdom of Living by Listening

Our bodies communicate with us through our feelings and emotions, not words. Raising our cognitive awareness of the body's feelings and emotions is a powerful guide in self-care. For example, the feeling of hunger, satiation, or overfullness can guide us to optimize the quantity and type of food consumed; the feeling of fatigue or energy can guide the needs for rest or activity; and the feeling of loneliness can be a signal to seek connection. Cognitively, we can suppress feelings and emotions, lowering their priority during times of work and focus, yet our needs remain. According to evolutionary psychology, emotions are best understood as regulatory mechanisms whose evolved function is to coordinate a variety of programs in the mind and body to ensure their harmonious coactivation in the service of solving an adaptive problem for the organism.[44]

Humans evolved to have emotions as a guidance system to help us pursue our goals. When we sense opportunity, we experience desire and then pleasure or disappointment once the opportunity materializes into a success or failure. When we sense threat, we experience fear and then pain or relief once the threat has become a loss or a narrow escape. Boredom and frustration help us know when to abandon less valuable pursuits. Emotions reveal less about success or failure; rather, they tell us whether we're making meaningful progress toward our goals.[32] Emotions carry millennia of evolved wisdom and taking time to listen and reflect on the causes of those feelings and emotions, rather than ignoring or suppressing them, can guide the individual toward opportunity or alert them when an endeavor is best set aside. Fortunately, as we get in touch with listening to our experience, the very activities that support our well-being can be innately pleasurable.

Habits Are Destiny

Knowledge is power, but habits are destiny! What we do day in and day out is our life. Habits are involuntary behaviors controlled by the subconscious mind. Studies by neurobiologists, cognitive psychologists, and others indicate that up to 95% of human behavior—how we think, what we say, and our overall actions—falls into the habit category.[45] Understanding how to build new habits or change existing habits using the habit loop is the first step; putting this knowledge into practice has the potential to evolve our lives.

Building new habits moves us through the four stages of competence to new behavior mastery:[46]

- **Unconscious Incompetence:** a level at which a person is unaware of how bad they are at a particular skill or how bad a particular behavior is for them. This is when a coach or mentor can be critical to raising personal awareness of behaviors.

- **Conscious Incompetence:** a level at which a person's awareness informs them that they are poor at a particular skill or are engaging in a habit that is not in alignment with their interests

- **Conscious Competence:** a level at which a person is using tremendous cognitive energy from the newer part of the brain (neocortex) to override old behaviors and practice new behaviors

- **Unconscious Competence:** a level at which a person uses little effort to perform the new behavior. If conscious competence continues, the brain becomes more efficient and moves the behavior from the slow, more cumbersome part of the conscious brain to the more reflexive and faster, older (reptilian and limbic) part of the brain, sometimes described as "in the flow."

People may not maintain conscous competence long enough to get to unconscious competence. Looking more closely at the habit loop provides insight into navigating this period.

The Habit Loop

The habit loop, seen in Figure 6.1, begins with a cue that brings on craving. This cue may be time of day, a particular person, location, preceding event, environment (e.g., food in the breakroom), or emotional state (e.g., uneasiness, anxiety). The craving is an emotion; the brain is anticipating reward and urges us toward the routine or behavior. The behavior is the action we do (e.g., eat a snack). Finally, the reward comes. The reward always includes an emotion (e.g., relief, reduced anxiety).[47]

Building a New Habit

How does the brain build new habits (e.g., which shoe you put on first, how you brush your teeth, how and when you eat) and how can we intentionally build habits that support our well-being? Begin by focusing on process, not outcome (e.g, taking a morning walk rather than losing weight). Once the new behavior is chosen, consider what might cue us to engage in that behavior (e.g., walking shoes next to my scale and alarm on my phone). Cues that are part of our existing routine work very well to add a behavior onto, so if we weigh each morning, having the walking shoes next to the scale would be an effective cue. If we engage in the behavior, the reward may be natural (e.g., feeling good from walking), yet we can increase the chance that the new habit will develop if we amp up the reward (pause after we have walked, throw our hands up in the air, and celebrate loudly for a moment or two congratulating ourselves on the behavior). The brain learns from these actions and emotions and with repetition builds a new habit that takes less and less effort to execute to get the reward.

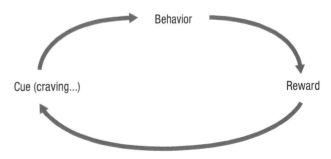

Figure 6.1: Habit loop

Evolving an Existing Habit

What about when we want to extinguish an existing habit that no longer serves us? The brain doesn't really extinguish habits; when it gets the cue, it wants the reward. However, it turns out we can evolve the existing habit as seen in Figure 6.2 by changing the behavior the brain associates with the reward. If the existing habit is a cue (seeing a cookie in the breakroom), behavior (eating the cookie), and reward (feeling relaxed), then you can interrupt the habit loop by stopping the cue (don't go to where the cookies are). Often, however, the cue is internal (an uneasy feeling, "I could use a break to relax with a cookie"). To evolve this existing habit of eating cookies when we have an uneasy feeling, we must substitute a new behavior (deep breaths, peaceful visualization) for the brain to associate with that cue and get to the reward (feeling relaxed). Some habits are much harder than others to evolve, so the first time you practice the new behavior the effort is high, and the reward may seem small relative to the reward of the old behavior. The reward may only last a moment or two, so you may need to repeat the new behavior (deep breaths) many times in a row to get an adequate reward. With many repetitions, the required effort declines and the reward grows as the brain learns from the practice. It is important to note that after the new behavior begins to take hold, there can be a surprising spike in craving for the old behavior here and there on the path to evolving the habit loop. When we stick with the new behavior these spikes diminish with time. If, however, we reengage in the old behavior we again reinforce the old pattern in the brain. To make the threshold for change lower, we can both support ourselves environmentally (don't use the breakroom with the cookies) and practice the new behavior (deep breaths), giving ourselves an increased chance for success. We never know what little change might be the

Reflection: Exploring My Habits and Motivations

Take a pause right now, finding a comfortable place to sit or even lie down. Let your hands be free of holding anything and resting. Begin by deepening the inhale and lengthening the exhale, letting your exhales be complete. Repeat this pattern for 5 to 10 breaths. Then inquire: What habits do I already have that support my well-being that I might reinforce or grow? What new habit might I want to build? What habit might I benefit from changing? What is my motivator for change, my "why" that makes me cry? Take a moment to journal on your "why" or on the habit loop you wish to build or change. Remember, this is a new path, so expect to bumble a bit; be generous with yourself as you explore and experiment with change in your life over days and weeks. Keep reflecting on what works and what might need to be edited to work. Analyze your experiences, especially failure, with kindness. Be willing to try again and again to find what works. Once you learn the technique of habit change it can be applied in countless ways to positively evolve your life experience.

tipping point to evolve our behavior. We keep exploring, expecting to bumble, and are willing to experiment, fail, and try again. The path is not straight to the new behavior. When we fail our expectations the brain may shout, "What the hell, I already failed my expectations! I might as well indulge fully in the old behavior." We want to be aware of this tendency and, when we have the slightest engagement in the old behavior, quickly physically move to a safe place where we can reflect and analyze the details that brought on the old behavior over the new behavior and what we might be able to do differently next time to continue moving toward our best life experience.

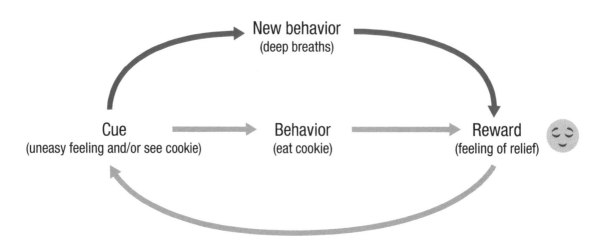

Figure 6.2: Evolving the habit loop

Motivation to Change

We will not embark on behavior change without motivation, sometimes referred to as the "why that makes you cry," to emphasize the importance of emotional intensity. Behavior is the result of motivation, ability, and prompts, that is, cues.[48] The stronger our emotions when exploring our "why," the more we know we are ready for personal change. One of the most effective time frames for behavior change is when we are acutely aware of a potential loss or fearing death (e.g., new medical diagnosis, experiencing pain or other concerning symptom, aware of another's pain or death, especially if the person is emotionally vulnerable). These opportunities can provide motivation for profound change.

Foundations of Well-Being

There are countless aspects to our well-being and here we will explore the four foundations: sleep, nutrition, movement, and connection. The framework's value is in its simplicity and the demonstrated interconnection between the foundations of well-being, as seen in Figure 6.3. When we improve self-care in one foundation, it usually leads to improvements in the other foundations, improving our overall well-being.

Sleep

Why do we sleep? When you are asleep, you cannot gather food, socialize, or mate; worse still, sleep leaves you

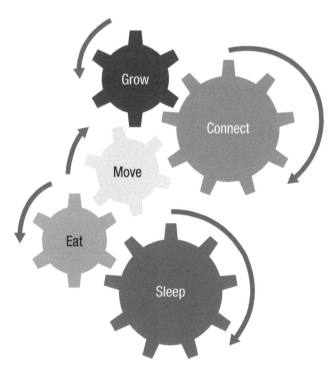

Figure 6.3: Interconnectedness of the foundations of well-being

vulnerable to predation. There was strong evolutionary pressure to prevent the emergence of sleep, yet sleep persisted in offering some survival advantage. Sleep is the most important foundation of well-being. The impairments caused by one night of bad sleep dwarf those caused by an equivalent absence of food or exercise. Sleep is the single most effective thing we can do to reset our brain and body health each day. Mentally sleep and dreaming prepare our brain to learn, make logical decisions, consolidate meaningful memories, and inspire creativity. Physically sleep restocks our immune system, fights malignancy, prevents infection and all manner of autoimmune disease, prevents metabolic disease, regulates appetite, helps control our body weight, maintains a flourishing microbiome, and prevents diabetes and unwanted weight gain; protects the cardiovascular system, lowering blood pressure and the risk of heart attacks and stroke; wards off dementia; makes us happier, less suspicious, less depressed, and less anxious; and even makes us look more attractive. There are more than 20 large-scale epidemiological studies that have tracked millions of people over many decades, all of which report the same relationship: the shorter your sleep, the shorter your life and the unhappier your life.[49]

So how much sleep is enough? Adults need 7 or more hours of sleep per night for the best health and well-being.[50] As our sleep efficiency declines quickly with age, we must prioritize at least an 8-hour sleep opportunity every night to get these benefits. Small, consistent sleep deprivation adds up; individuals who went 10 days with 6 hours of sleep a night (like many of us do) became as impaired in performance as those going without sleep for 24 hours straight; their lapses in concentration (missed responses) increased by more than 400%, yet they failed to recognize any degree of their own compromise.[49]

So how do we get more sleep? Sleep deprivation is the ability to generate sleep, yet we are not giving ourselves a full sleep opportunity. Giving our sleep the priority it deserves by offering ourselves a full 7 to 9 hour sleep opportunity will resolve this deficit. However, sometimes we find that when we do prioritize sleep, we are unable to generate a full 7 hours of sleep. We can pay attention to our sleep hygiene (see Table 6.1) by keeping a sleep journal to see what we can improve. If this situation persists for more than 3 months before adding in any sleep medication, we need a thorough assessment with a sleep expert.

Nutrition

How can we optimize the quality of our nutrition? Researchers have shown that a whole-food plant-predominate dietary pattern[51] may help prevent, treat, or reverse some of our leading causes of death, including heart disease, that is, our number one killer; type 2 diabetes; and high blood pressure. Plant-based-diet intervention

Table 6.1: Sleep Hygiene: Practices That Are Conducive to Sleeping Well on a Regular Basis

Sleep Hygiene Tips	
Include	*Avoid*
<ul><li>Keep a sleep journal.</li><li>Work with your provider to treat medical conditions, e.g., sleep disorders, sleep apnea, narcolepsy, restless leg, sleepwalking, reflux disease, pain, anxiety, depression.</li><li>Exercise daily.</li><li>Mental comfort prior to bed:<ul><li>Write tomorrow's to-do list and set it aside.</li><li>Meditate.</li><li>Expressive writing.</li><li>Keep a bedtime routine, for example, brush teeth, change, read, toilet, stretch, retire to bed.</li></ul></li><li>Physical comfort prior to bed:<ul><li>Empty bladder.</li><li>Stretch/massage.</li><li>Comfortable bed and pillow.</li></ul></li><li>Reduce noise in the sleep environment with earplugs or white/pink noise.</li><li>Light: Live with the circadian rhythm:<ul><li>Exposure to natural daylight at sunrise and sunset.</li><li>Dim all lighting 1 to 2 hours prior to bedtime.</li><li>Avoid or filter out the blue light from devices 1 to 2 hours prior to bedtime.</li><li>Keep sleep room pitch black. If some light is included for safety, red light is least disturbing.</li><li>Eat in the early part of the day avoiding the 3 hours prior to bedtime.</li><li>Keep a regular sleep window moving no more than 1 hour off the set sleep start time on all days of the week.</li></ul></li><li>Temperature:<ul><li>Warm bath or sauna followed with a rapid cool down; the fall in temperature promotes deeper sleep.</li><li>Keep room temperature lower than 68° F.</li><li>Keep the head cool.</li></ul></li><li>Use the bed only for sleep and sex.</li></ul>	<ul><li>Never take someone else's sleeping medication.</li><li>Never take over-the-counter sleeping aids without your provider's knowledge.</li><li>Avoid intense exercise 1 to 2 hours prior to bedtime as it elevates the core temperature.</li><li>Avoid participating in stimulating mental activities just prior to bedtime, e.g., intense movies, competitive games, important conversations with loved ones, or stressful emails.</li><li>Avoid lying in bed awake for more than 20 minutes; get up and do a quiet activity in another room until drowsy, then return to bed.</li><li>Avoid naps if you can. Otherwise, keep them to 20 minutes prior to 3 p.m.</li><li>Avoid heat-trapping pillow or bedding.</li><li>Don't sleep with pets; they disturb our sleep and we disturb theirs! Play with them prior to bedtime and tuck them into their beds.</li><li>Don't let a partner interfere with sleep; consider noise control for snoring or twin beds for tossing and turning or separate sleeping rooms.</li><li>Avoid alcohol as it significantly disrupts REM sleep.</li><li>Avoid eating 3 hours prior to bedtime and especially avoid large meals prior to bedtime as they signal the gastrointestinal system it is active time.</li><li>Avoid caffeine after noon due to its 6-hour half-life.</li><li>Avoid nicotine as it is a stimulant.</li><li>Avoid stimulating medications, for example, decongestants.</li><li>Avoid drinking lots of liquids right before bedtime.</li></ul>

groups have reported greater diet satisfaction than control groups, as well as improved digestion, increased energy, and better sleep, and significant improvement in their physical functioning, general health, vitality, and mental health. Studies have shown plant-based eating can improve not only body weight, blood sugar levels, and ability to control cholesterol but also emotional states, including depression, anxiety, fatigue, sense of well-being, and daily functioning.[52] For most of us, the countless dietary patterns commercially promoted and a plethora of hyperpalatable, highly processed foods that are widely available make eating to support our well-being more challenging than was the case for our ancestors. With the balance of scientific evidence suggesting that the healthiest way to eat is a vitamin B12-fortified diet of whole-plant foods, we should be sure to include in our daily diet, as depicted in Figure 6.4, not only an array of whole grains, beans, nuts, seeds, fruit, and as many vegetables as we can eat, but also specifically dark green leafy vegetables, berries, water, and white (or green) tea, giving special attention to ensure adequate B12, omega-3 fatty acids, vitamin D, calcium, iodine, iron, and selenium.[53] To learn more about this evidence-based eating pattern, visit https://nutritionfacts.org.

Knowing what we currently are eating (e.g., food journaling) and the direction we want to move our nutritional intake is valuable when we are looking to harness the incredible power of nutrition in supporting our well-being. Choosing to have the foods we want to eat (e.g., fruits, vegetables) in our environment increases the chance we will eat those foods, just as keeping our environment (e.g., kitchen, office, breakroom) free of foods we wish to avoid (e.g., processed food) increases the likelihood that we will not eat those foods. We begin with an awareness of what we are eating now and change one habit at a time, so over our lifetime, we continue to move toward the best evidence-based nutrition available.

As we improve food quality and avoid the hyperpalatable, processed foods with added salt, oil, and sugar,

eating when hungry and stopping when satiated rather than beyond becomes more common. The skill of intuitive eating, that is, listening to our hunger and eating to satiation, is a habit that requires practice. A key intuitive eating principle is discovering the pleasure of eating this way, figuring out what you really want to eat, paying close attention while eating, and savoring the food and eating experience.[54] When we are triggered to eat and notice we are not hungry, we can use the "evolving an existing habit" information earlier to build an alternative pathway, for example, deep breathing, to find emotional relief in the moment. With careful and kind attention, we can make time and space to care for the emotions that arise in daily life in ways that best meet those emotions, which usually do not involve food. As this is a new path, we expect to struggle a bit. Being kind and compassionate with ourselves as we explore and experiment over days and weeks cannot be overemphasized as harsh criticism leads to giving up. Self-compassionate people engage in healthier behaviors[55] like exercise,[56] eating well,[57] and drinking less.[58]

The time of day we eat and fast signals the circadian rhythm in our digestive system when to be active or recover, just like light activates the circadian rhythm for the sleep/wake cycle. These endogenous rhythms dampen with age and erratic eating patterns can disrupt the temporal coordination of metabolism and physiology, leading to chronic diseases that are characteristic of aging. However, sustaining a robust eating–fasting cycle, even without altering nutrition quality or quantity, can prevent or reverse these chronic diseases. Restricting our eating to 6 to 10 hours per day, especially in the light-filled early part of the day, demonstrated improved beta-cell responsiveness and insulin sensitivity, lowered 24-hour glucose levels, improved lipid metabolism, reduced appetite, increased weight loss, prevented unwanted weight gain, improved sleep quality and quantity, reduced blood pressure, reduced cardiovascular disease risk preventing age-related deterioration of cardiac performance, offered protection from breast cancer, reduced oxidative stress, increased autophagy, and provided additional human antiaging effects[59–64]

Movement/Activity

For most humans today, the physical activity levels required to gain food and shelter are significantly less than what our genes evolved under, one of the main reasons our activity levels have significantly declined. Increasing physical activity offers protection from our top killers, improves quality and quantity of life, and includes diverse benefits in modern life, for example, lowering the risk of heart disease, stroke, type 2 diabetes, high blood pressure, dementia, some cancer, complications of pregnancy, and symptoms of depression and anxiety, while improving sleep, cognition, memory, attention, bone

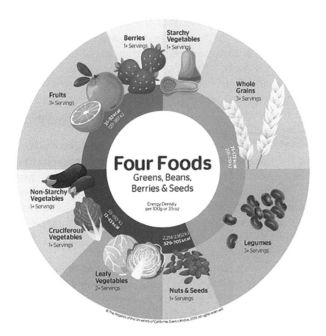

Figure 6.4: The whole-food plant-based plate.

Fill half the plate with fruit and nonstarchy vegetables and half the plate with starchy vegetables and legumes with some seeds and nuts for optimum balanced nutrition. Learn more at https://ucdintegrativemedicine.com.

Source: Reproduced with permission from the Regents of the University of California, Davis campus. 2019. All rights reserved

health, and an overall sense of well-being. Current Physical Activity Guidelines[65] state that adults should move more and sit less. Some physical activity is better than none. Adults who sit less and do any amount of moderate to vigorous physical activity gain some health benefits. For substantial health benefits, adults should do at least 150 minutes to 300 minutes a week of moderate-intensity or 75 minutes to 150 minutes a week of vigorous-intensity aerobic physical activity or an equivalent combination, spread throughout the week. Additional health benefits are gained by engaging in even more physical activity. Adults should also do muscle-strengthening activities that involve all major muscle groups on 2 or more days a week, as these activities provide additional health benefits. Although many do not exercise at these recommended levels, and thus lose the benefits described, those of us who do leverage social and personal factors to influence the amount and type of exercise chosen see the benefits. Social factors include self-presentation management, improving physical appearance, establishing images of being physically active in others' eyes, and social interaction with others;[66] we choose to exercise and move to present the best image of ourselves. Personal factors include self-satisfaction, improving health and physical fitness, and personal enjoyment;[66] we are likely to start and stay with exercise if we feel the joy and pride of strength and movement. Once physical activity patterns are established, habits do make the better choice the easier choice.[67]

Additional emerging evidence notes the deleterious effects of sedentary behavior, that is, too few breaks from sitting and notes future activity guidelines might indicate limits in continuous inactivity.[68,69] Environmental factors, for example, computer screen time, work against moving more. To optimize activity throughout all waking hours we must build personal habits and support a healthcare organizational and professional culture that endorses some movement of any intensity every hour of our waking day. To move more throughout our day, we can begin with an activity tracker looking both at our active and inactive time. Then reflect on what activity changes we want to make in our personal and professional life. We can walk and take the stairs to move between locations, make one-on-one meetings walking meetings, schedule all virtual or in-person classes or meetings for 50 minutes, share cultural wellness expectation of a 10-minute movement opportunity each hour, invest in a sit–stand desk and an under-desk elliptical stepper, walk and talk while taking a coffee break, walk while listening to our email read to us through an app or making phone calls, and place weights or exercise bands near the couch or chair to add in some muscle-strengthening activities during normally sedentary time. We can get creative and build movement habits throughout our day, enhancing how we feel all day long and improving our performance on both physical and cognitive tasks, not to mention how well we sleep during the 8-hour opportunity we take to rest at night.

Connection

Our social connections are the most consistent predictor of a happy and healthy life.[70] The Harvard Study of Adult Development,[71] one of the world's longest studies of adult life, looks closely at predictors of physical and mental health. Close relationships with happy and healthy people protect us from mental and physical decline and are better predictors of long and happy lives than social class, IQ, genes, money, or fame.[72] Our social networks, even out to the third degree (friends of friends of friends) significantly influence our chance of gaining weight,[73] smoking,[74] or being happy.[75] Our friends and acquaintances really are our future; we can examine our entire social network, direct its influence on our life, and make sure we are in the social environment that supports the health and happiness we want.[76]

We can begin by assessing our relationships with mates, trading partners, and friends and how they are influencing our own experience, then choosing the relationships we want to deepen or distance ourselves from. To strengthen relationships we value, we can give unconditional positive regard. We should not try to control anyone, because the truth is, we cannot; personality is relatively fixed. Instead, we can think of how to work with who they are, listen and validate the other person, and express gratitude for being who they are in our lives. We like people because of the way they make us feel. With intention, we can bring joy, entertainment, novelty, and laughter into our valued relationships. We can nurture our valued relationships by turning everyday moments into moments with more connection, pausing, and engaging, including eye contact.

Distancing from a relationship can be very challenging for those of us with highly agreeable personalities. When a relationship is unhelpful or imbalanced, we practice saying "no" to additional time and commitments. Releasing relationships that no longer serve us is easier when our time is firmly committed to relationships that do build the life we want.

Connection with others is the outward journey, whereas connecting with ourselves is the inward journey. Having routines, rhythms, and rituals that let us turn inward with reflection fosters our insight, complex learning, and growth.[77] We can engage in reflection through contemplative practices like mindful noting, open awareness or focused attention, meditation, self-compassion and gratitude practices, and expressive writing. Many universities, for example, the University of California, Berkeley, now offer training in person or online (Greater Good in Action website: ggia.berkeley.edu) to help support this area of human life.

Reflection: Listening to Pain as a Teacher

Take a pause right now, finding a comfortable place to sit or even lie down. Let your hands be free of holding anything and resting. Begin by deepening the inhale and lengthening the exhale, letting your exhales be complete. Repeat this pattern for 5 to 10 breaths. Then inquire, where am I experiencing the most pain and discomfort in my life? Pain and discomfort have wisdom informing us where change can increase our happiness and alignment with our best life experience. Use the breath to lean into the pain, knowing you may not even have awareness of what change to pursue. Take a moment to journal on whatever is coming up for you, where you might apply your energy to evolve your life in a positive direction, and what changes to your physical environment or social network might support your best life. Pause again and reflect: What is my motivation for this change? Dig deep here; knowing this source of power carries you through the big hurdles. Take a moment to write down what is coming up for you. Remember, change is rarely easy or a direct path, so expect the ups and downs to happen, practice kindness with difficult moments, and keep reflecting to learn what works and what is it time to let go of. You can turn to this reflection again and again as you explore progress, not perfection, in your journey toward well-being. Namaste.

We want to spend time looking at what we want to do with this human life (a gift from the universe), what matters to us, and what delivers meaning in our lives. When we connect our learning to these important areas, learning and retention are optimized and our life direction has a chance to align. Undoubtedly, there are also painful moments in reflection. Every human suffers, and sometimes there is nothing to be gained from the pain and all one can offer is kindness. However, often pain and discomfort have the wisdom to inform us where we need change. As we develop and use the tools of mindfulness and self-compassion, we can use this discerning wisdom to progress in our well-being and self-care.

Engaging in Self-Care

When we know better, we don't always do better. Participating in health promotion activities is influenced by intrinsic factors, including one's personal characteristics, perceived costs, and perceived benefits, and by extrinsic factors, including environmental, situational, and interpersonal influences, such as norms, social support, and role modeling.[78] When we don't have success motivating ourselves to do the health-promoting activities we know will benefit us, we might have more leverage on changing our behavior by placing ourselves in a physical and social environment that will tip us in the direction of positive change.

CONCLUSION

Healthcare providers are human and, more often than not, at one point or another, will experience one or more symptoms of burnout. The good news is that with careful assessment the forces leading to burnout can be identified and addressed. Healthcare providers can find the freedom to enjoy their life and work again and the organization and patients they serve will benefit as well. Why wait for stress to overwhelm? One can begin each day with a commitment to self-care. Take time to reflect on how one can honor the foundations of well-being in modern life: sleep, nutrition, movement, and connection. Set a clear aim and focus on one change at a time. When the inevitable missteps occur, turn a "bad day" into "good data" and begin again. This leads to living one's best life.

REFERENCES

References for this chapter are online and available at https://connect.springerpub.com/content/book/978-0-8261-8414-6/part/part01/toc-part/ch6

PART II

Providing Adult-Gerontology Nursing Care

CHAPTER 7

The AGNP Role and Settings of Care

Holly Kirkland-Kyhn and Deb Bakerjian

LEARNING OBJECTIVES

At the conclusion of this chapter, the learner will be able to:

➤ Analyze the roles of the adult-gerontology nurse practitioner (AGNP) in primary care.

➤ Critique the regulatory framework for AGNPs.

➤ Describe at least 10 types of settings of care where AGNPs work.

INTRODUCTION

The American Association of Nurse Practitioners (AANP) identifies nurse practitioners (NPs) as licensed independent practitioners who provide nursing and medical services to individuals, families, and groups according to their practice specialty and according to state and federal regulatory guidelines. NPs are an important part of the primary care workforce. As of May 2021, there are more than 325,000 licensed NPs in the United States.[1] Almost 70% are family NPs, with about 18% of all NP certifications comprising adult, adult-gerontology, and gerontology NPs.[1] AGNPs play a critical role in providing primary care to the aging population in a variety of traditional, innovative, and emerging healthcare settings.

History of Adult Geriatric Nurse Practitioners

Historically, adult nurse practitioners (ANPs) and geriatric nurse practitioners (GNPs) were separate roles requiring distinct educational preparation and separate certifications; however, in 2015, the roles were combined into the adult geriatric nurse practitioner (AGNP) through the APRN Consensus Model. Although GNPs were important contributors to the care of older adults in primary care, they represented less than 3% of all NPs, whereas ANPs were about 15% of NPs. The rationale for combining the roles was mainly to address the critical shortage of NPs who had special education and training focused on the care of older adults.[2]

The APRN Consensus Model came together through the work of several national advanced practice nursing professional organizations who worked collaboratively to author the APRN Consensus Model. The goal was to provide guidance for states to adopt uniformity in essential elements of licensure, accreditation, certification, and education (LACE) of APRN roles. The APRN Consensus Model identified six population foci of the APRN as (a) family across the life span, (b) adult-gerontology, (c) neonatal, (d) pediatrics, (e) women's health, and (f) psychiatric/mental health and defined four advanced practice roles: (a) NP, (b) clinical nurse specialist, (c) nurse anesthetist, and (d) nurse midwife (see Figure 7.1). They also established that the roles should be distinguished between acute care and primary care.[3] The AGNP role has subsequently evolved to meet the increasing demand of a growing aging population, particularly in providing coordinated chronic disease management[4] and emphasizing healthy aging.[5]

The continued growth of AGNPs as a profession has been driven by the growing need for a stronger primary care workforce, particularly to help with chronic disease management and preventative care of medically complex patients.[6] Stakeholders advocate that AGNPs are part of the solution for improving healthcare in our aging population as concerns materialize around physician shortages and rising demand for care in older adults.

LICENSURE, REGULATION, AND SCOPE OF PRACTICE

AGNPs must be licensed to practice by the state in which they provide care. To be licensed, AGNPs must graduate from an accredited AGNP program with either a master's or doctoral degree. Most states also require AGNP graduates to pass a national-level certification examination to obtain a license and practice in their respective states.[48]

National Certification

The AGNP certification process requires that individuals graduating from AGNP programs take a national certification examination to assess both the adult and the geriatric knowledge obtained during training.[7] There are two organizations that provide certification for AGNPs. The first one is the AANP Certification Board, which provides an Adult-Gerontology Primary Care Nurse Practitioner

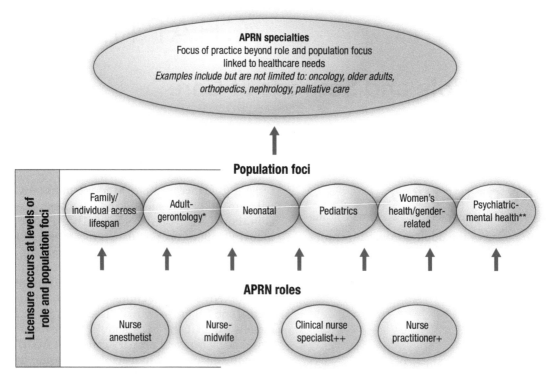

Figure 7.1: The APRN regulatory model.

Source: APRN Consensus Work Group, National Council of State Boards of Nursing APRN Advisory Committee. *Consensus Model for APRN Regulation: Licensure, Accreditation, Certification & Education.* Published July 7, 2008. https://www.ncsbn.org/Consensus_Model_for_APRN_Regulation_July_2008.pdf

Certification examination; passing the examination allows the AGNP to use AGNP-C to signify their national certification. More information can be found on the AANP Certification Board website at www.aanpcert.org/certs/agnp. The second certifying body is the American Nurses Credentialing Center, who offers the Adult-Gerontology Primary Care Nurse Practitioner Certification. AGNPs that pass this examination receive a credential that is good for 5 years. More information about the certification can be found at www.nursingworld.org/our-certifications/adult-gerontology-primary-care-nurse-practitioner. AGNPs who pass the ANCC certification can use the credential AGPCNP-BC.

There is also a separate certification examination specific to advanced practice geriatrics. This certification is through the Gerontological Advanced Practice Nurses Association and its Gerontology Nursing Certification Commission. This examination is open to all APRNs who meet their eligibility criteria, which is available on its website at www.gapna.org/certification. APRNs that pass this certification examination are signified as APRN Gerontological Specialist-Certified or GS-C.

Scope of Practice

Scope of practice is based on the graduate education within a defined patient population for the advance practice

NP role and is based on the LACE[3] of each NP. The APRN Consensus Model outlines that the services provided by APRNs are not defined or limited by the practice setting but by patient care needs.[48] Clarification of the scope of practice within the education, state regulatory board, and certification is essential to ensure the quality and safety of NP practice.[8]

Historically, the scope of practice has varied based on the setting of care and the state of practice, with some states allowing full practice authority and other states restricting practice in various ways. Recent policy and regulatory changes have been nationally driven to support full practice authority for NPs based on recommendations put forward by the 2010 Institute of Medicine report *The Future of Nursing: Leading Change, Advancing Health.*[9] Unfortunately, challenges exist in restrictive barriers to practice among many state boards and facility credentialing bodies, which contribute to NP role confusion, so not all states have full practice authority (FPA) for NPs. The AANP maintains a current map delineating states with full, reduced, or restricted practice available at www.aanp.org/advocacy/state/state-practice-environment.

The expansion of the NPs' scope of practice is important to meet new and ongoing national demands for healthcare since passing the Affordable Care Act (ACA) legislation that insures more Medicare and Medicaid beneficiaries. FPA has been shown to increase the number of NPs available to provide care and thereby increase utilization of their services.[10] States that have restricted FPA for NPs have less accessibility for healthcare in rural areas and for vulnerable populations that may be uninsured or underinsured.[10] Research and clinical expertise within the profession must inform FPA regulation in individual states without FPA for progress to occur. There are several different types of primary care NPs including family, pediatric, women's health, and AGNPs. What sets AGNPs apart in their primary care role is their unique focus on older adults and in ensuring care coordination. While they are trained to provide care for adolescents and adults, a large part of their education is dedicated to the older adults and working as part of a team of healthcare providers. Family NPs also receive some preparation in the care of older adults, but it is not as in depth as that for AGNPs.

AGNP ROLES

AGNPs may serve in a variety of roles in the care of older adults and practice in many different types of settings. The most obvious roles are as a clinician, but there are many other roles for AGNPs depending on their interests and goals. In general, AGNPs perform important roles in research, education, and practice. Once the AGNP is certified and licensed, it is important that they register for a National Provider Number (NPI) to ensure recognition of their role and opportunities to bill for patient services as a provider.[11] The NPI is a 10-digit number issued by the National Plan and Provider Enumeration System (NPPES) to all healthcare providers; see https://nppes.cms.hhs.gov/#. The NPI number is used for health insurance reimbursement and makes all providers' names, specialties, and practice addresses available to the public.

Research Role

In 2015, the NP research roundtable met and set priorities for NP research specifically in four areas: policy and regulation, workforce, education, and practice.[12] NPs must act as key leaders in areas of quality improvement and evidence-based practice to meet the Quadruple Aim goals to decrease cost, improve safety, and improve patient and provider/staff satisfaction for best measurable outcomes.[12] There are multiple opportunities for AGNPs to participate in research and education in addition to providing direct patient care in a clinical practice.

AGNPs often participate in applied research activities, such as when new clinical practice guidelines are announced. Implementing research into the practice environment is an important role for AGNPs. Another principal area is research in areas of AGNP practice, education, and patient outcomes. This type of research is essential to ensure that the public is aware of the high-quality care that AGNPs provide. Knowledge about the numbers of AGNPs and other types of NPs is important to identify gaps and to ensure a safe and sufficient number of NPs are available to meet rising patient numbers with complex medical needs.[5] Some AGNPs may not be familiar with undertaking research or in promoting their research through publication or other means of dissemination; however, these research-naïve NPs should be encouraged to seek out colleagues who are conducting research for support and leadership guidance if this is an area of interest.

Many professional nursing societies and NP associations are preparing priority research agendas. A consensus on research agendas can be performed at brainstorming round tables or with a Delphi method. Some research agendas are broad to allow for identifying priority areas that are important to the clinical population, while others are wide-ranging practice areas and patient populations. Many research agendas are published on society websites as research agendas for the next 5 to 10 years. Policy makers are calling for the identification of new and innovative models of care delivery to include variability in tasks and professional roles.[17] Tasks alone do not define a discipline; the nature of the discipline; is determined by the philosophical approach adopted.[49] NPs should take a more active role in partnering with healthcare institutions to lead the transformation of healthcare, define workforce composition, and guide health policy.[50] This NP–policy maker partnership, combined with supporting research and evidence, requires cooperation between NP organizations and a willingness to adapt policy as new evidence emerges.

NP researchers are well positioned to assess quality outcomes and lead outcome-driven interdisciplinary research to test emerging care delivery models designed to meet the Quadruple Aim.[16] Innovative care delivery models are currently being implemented to improve access to care, reduce waiting times for appointments, and reduce costs.[17] NPs are well positioned to lead the evaluation of innovative changes and modifications to healthcare based on clinical practice and evidence.

Educator Role

The education provided by the AGNP as a clinician is aimed at patients/caregivers, medical providers, administrators, and the community. Historically, providing patient education on lifestyle and behavior change was found to increase the burden and burnout of primary care physicians.[18] The burden of managing complex patients with chronic health conditions in a reduced resource setting further strains a system stretched by an aging chronically ill population. A recent study involving 327 providers found that engaging patients in lifestyle disease-specific self-care activities, without reliance on their interdisciplinary team, was significantly associated with burnout.[18] This study provides evidence to support that primary care physician burnout may be reduced by expanding the role of nurses and other healthcare professionals to assume and redistribute the tasks and education on behavior change while improving shared communication and collaboration (see Chapter 6). Physician–NP comanagement has also been found to alleviate individual provider workload and prevent burnout while increasing access and quality of care for patients.[17]

AGNPs as Academic Educators

AGNPs are essential to fulfill the role of educator in AGNP programs, but also may play an important role in family NP and other advanced practice programs because of their expanded knowledge of the care of older adults. AGNPs also play an important role in teaching interprofessional teams, in both the theory courses and the experiential learning that take place in simulation laboratories in health professions schools. Interprofessional education in academic centers provides a collaborative practice-ready workforce that provides comprehensive healthcare for best health outcomes—see Chapter 4. Specifically, the AGNP is an excellent team member to provide education for graduate nurses, PAs, and public health students to improve knowledge of chronic care management, health promotion, respectful communication, and teamwork skills.[19] AGNPs who are DNP-prepared are the primary educators in DNP AGNP programs.

Practice Role

There are two aspects of practice that AGNPs participate in, as a direct care clinical provider or as an administrative leader. Often, these two roles may be intertwined whereby the AGNP provides direct patient care part of the time and fulfills a leader or administrator role part-time.

Clinical Role

NPs go through an important role change from expert nurse to novice NP when they graduate and transition to the advanced practice NP role.[20] The NP role is dynamic in which the knowledge and skills are practiced, maintaining clinical expertise and competence. The AANP identifies NPs as licensed independent practitioners who practice in ambulatory, acute, and long-term care as a primary area of practice. These NPs provide nursing and medical services to individuals, families, and groups according to their practice specialty. The AACN recently completed work on the *Adult-Gerontology Acute Care and*

Primary Care NP Competencies, which address AGNP care based on the entire spectrum of adults, including adolescents to older adults.[50] Adult gerontology primary care nurse practitioners (AGPCNPs) provide primary care services in an outpatient setting or specialized support for health challenges, such as obesity, diabetes, dementia, and heart disease.

Primary care was the original setting for the NP role development, and as of 2015, 86% of NPs worked in primary care.[15] Specialty NPs have emerged to provide services for specific populations, settings, and within roles requiring expert clinical, administrative research or in education.[50] Acute care AGNPs play an important role in hospitals, often in the consultant role. The primary care role for the NP workforce is essential for the development of high-functioning teams that expand the supply of primary care providers and develop optimal team-based care. The NP is an effective team member in developing interprofessional teamwork.[17]

Appropriately trained AGNPs with a foundation in nursing science and advanced clinical practice can function in a substitutive or complementary role delivering effective integrated care across settings.[21] Most primary care NPs work in collaboration with physicians either in substitutive roles by filling the role while collaborating with a physician or in a comanagement or complementary role. In the substitutive role, the AGNP provides patient care typically to a different set of patients and substituting for the physician role, which requires a trusting relationship between the NP and the physician as there is less communication for these patients between the two providers. In a complementary role, the AGNP comanages that same set of patients, providing specific care (e.g., chronic disease management) or procedures that would have formerly been performed by physicians, such as additional primary care visits, follow-up visits, procedures, and expanded education for patients, caregivers, and family. The complementary role often adds services to individual patients, while the substitutive role may increase the number of patients in the practice, but those patients may not receive extra services. Many practices are a combination of both roles.

Depending on the practice environment, AGNPs may collaborate with various healthcare providers including physicians, registered nurses, licensed practical or vocational nurses, medical assistants, social workers, pharmacists, therapists, and others. This effort to collaborate comes naturally for AGNPs based on their experiences as registered nurses facilitating care coordination for patients. This also provides a strong foundation for AGNPs to work within an interprofessional team, which has been shown to improve the overall quality of care.[22]

One of the advantages that NPs bring to any practice environment is that they are registered nurses and can incorporate the roles, responsibilities, and functions of the registered nurse into the care that they provide to patients and their families. For example, an AGNP that goes out to visit an older adult patient in their home can assess their acute illness or chronic diseases, order treatments, write prescriptions, and provide comprehensive wound care as needed. In the nursing home, they can order pain medications for residents in pain and work directly with the nursing staff to develop a comprehensive care plan for pain management. The ability of AGNPs to integrate the role and their experiences as a registered nurse into their daily work greatly enhances the value of the care they provide.

Administrative or Leadership Role

Leadership is an important role for the AGNP in assessing the current needs for providing care in a variety of new environments. In 2020, healthcare providers were challenged with providing adequate healthcare services to an aging, more diverse, immigrant, climate-changed, pandemic-impacted population. This was a time of constant change and great uncertainty and, under emergency waivers, to reduce restrictions on NP scope of practice, NPs played important roles in leading teams in various healthcare settings, stepping up to manage ventilated patients with COVID-19 and lead vaccine clinics.[23] AGNPs have stepped up to lead chronic care teams to help manage the 25% of all Americans that have two or more chronic health conditions.[6] In this year of the nurse/year of the COVID-19 pandemic, AGNPs have been trusted to address the health impact of our changing world and its consequences, particularly to the older vulnerable population.

Another AGNP important role is leading quality improvement activities. AGNPs lead teams of staff to identify and implement practice change to improve efficiency and reduce cost; they work with the staff on team building, improving communication, and ensuring high-quality, safe care. They also examine patient outcomes, identify areas of improvement, and lead teams in implementing evidence-based practices to improve patient outcomes, particularly for chronic disease management and population health. Examples might be improving practice management of patients with diabetes and heart failure or enhancing staff skills to work with patients with cognitive impairment.[24] AGNPs initiate interprofessional collaboration and guide practice and policy to improve healthcare for the needs of this patient population.[25] AGNP practice promotes evidence-based, age-appropriate guidelines that correct disparities in screening while addressing the challenge of pervasive ageism among providers.[5] The leadership role for the NP workforce is essential for the development of high-functioning teams that expand the supply of primary care

providers and develop optimal team-based care.[26] The NP is an effective team leader in developing interprofessional teamwork[26] for quality and safety project development and education and operationalization of implementing change for best outcomes.

NURSE PRACTITIONER RESIDENCY PROGRAMS

NPs face a significant challenge when transitioning from the registered nurse role to an advanced practice role. NPs are key to addressing the future shortage of primary healthcare providers; however, successful role transition is imperative for new NPs to fully operate on a complex medical team. Many factors have been identified as central to a successful transition for the new NP, including supportive colleagues who understand the NP role, mentorship with an experienced NP or physician, continued NP didactic and clinical education, and collaboration with the care delivery team, with eventual greater autonomy and self-efficacy.[26] This evidence supports formal transition programs such as postgraduate residencies, which are expanding with varying curriculum to accommodate NP settings and roles. Residency programs for new NPs build confidence, clinical preparedness, and eventual autonomy for fulfilling the NP role. New mandates in some states (e.g., California) are requiring 3 years of postgraduate supervision by a physician to obtain full practice authority as an NP,[51] and an NP residency would partially fulfill this mandate.

In 2019, the Health Resources and Services Administration (HRSA) released a call for proposals for the Advanced Nursing Education Nurse Practitioner Residency Program, the first-ever federally funded NP residency program. The program funded thirty-six 12-month-long residency programs in 25 states across the United States to prepare new primary care NPs to practice in community-based settings. The grants were for 4 years, and the HRSA will likely evaluate whether to continue funding based on the outcomes. There are also several residency programs across the United States that are funded in other ways, such as through the reimbursement from visits or through donor support. AGNP graduates may want to consider a residency program as these programs provide a salary (mean was $69,301 annually) along with substantial educational support from preceptors and mentors.[28]

SETTINGS OF CARE

Currently, NPs are employed in several different practice settings ranging from ambulatory clinics, EDs, acute care hospitals, long-term care hospitals, skilled nursing homes, hospice and palliative care, and industry. The most common practice settings include hospital outpatient clinics (14.5%), private group practice (14%), private physician offices (8.5%), hospital inpatient clinics (8.1%), community health clinics and federally qualified health centers (6.5%), and emergency department/urgent care (4.7%).[1]

AGPCNPs primarily provide primary care services and work collaboratively with other healthcare professionals, but in some cases, they practice in a consulting model where most of their patients are referrals specifically for issues related to the patient's age and overall condition. The consulting model is most common in acute care hospitals, where AGNPs examine patients and make recommendations to physicians or advanced practice providers who are not geriatric certified in how to best manage the care of older adult patients.

Hospital Setting

Older adults make up a large proportion of a hospital's core business, with the hospitalization rate of adults older than age 65 three times the comparable rate for persons of all ages.[7] The AGNP in the hospital-based or acute care setting acts as part of an interdisciplinary team member and was initially adopted in response to limiting resident physician work hours.[29] AGNPs have been found to deliver equivalent or better care for high use, high-cost, chronically ill geriatric patients.[6] In addition, AGNPs had similar service utilization requests when compared to physicians, and patient satisfaction was positive.[21] Acute care NPs were found to spend more than 85% of inpatient hospital practice time delivering direct or indirect patient care activities,[25] while the remaining nonclinical activities for administrative, research, and education were less evident in the NP workweek.[25]

Ambulatory Care

Ambulatory care historically entailed traditional physician offices located in the community, often close to acute care hospitals. These office practices provided primary care services based on the specialty of the provider such as family practice or pediatrics. Over the past few decades, these single-provider offices have merged with the multiprovider office, which is now much more common. Additionally, to better meet the healthcare needs in rural and underserved communities, there has been a rise in community health centers (CHCs) and Federally Qualified Health Centers (FQHCs). CHCs and FQHCs are grant-funded through the federal government and provide a variety of services to communities that are health professional shortage areas (HPSAs). CHCs and FQHCs are known to employ NPs as key members of the care team. With the increased numbers of insured people and improved access to care brought about through the ACA, primary care offices have been challenged to meet the demand, and this is expected to get worse in the future.[30,31]

In response, the federal government and various foundations have funded demonstration projects to trial new ways to provide primary care services.

Many different innovative models of care have emerged in the past few decades. Many of these were in response to CMS Innovation Center grants and demonstration projects, some had their roots in the ACA, and others came from industries as organizational innovations.[32] Following are short descriptions of some of these models.

Patient-Centered Medical Home and Chronic Care Model

A well-known model that preexisted the ACA is the patient-centered medical home (PCMH), which originated in the late 1960s and introduced the concept to create medical homes for pediatric patients with chronic diseases. Since that time, the PCMH has adapted to integrate principles of patient-centeredness by focusing on primary care redesign and a team-based approach to care. The PMCH was historically led by physicians but now NPs are also recognized as PCMH leaders by the National Committee for Quality Assurance, the organization that accredits PCMHs.

The Chronic Care Model (CCM), which is an evidence-based quality improvement approach, includes five elements of the healthcare system that are essential to provide high-quality chronic disease management: community resources, self management support, health system, decision support, and clinical information systems. CCM aims to improve patient outcomes by ensuring the healthcare team is prepared and proactive and then improving the healthcare team's interaction with activated patients.[33]

Nurse-Managed Health Clinics

Nurse-managed health clinics (NMHCs) were authorized and funded through the ACA with the goal to provide comprehensive primary care and wellness services to medically underserved communities. NMHCs must be led by an APRN and be associated with a school, college, university, department of nursing, FQHC, or other not-for-profit healthcare agency.[34] A systematic review of NMHCs found they have had a positive effect on access to care and patient outcomes and are associated with increased patient satisfaction; however, cost-effectiveness has been mixed.[35]

Retail Clinics

Retail clinics are healthcare centers that are designed to manage common acute conditions and are typically located inside retail pharmacies. Examples are the CVS Minute Clinics and the Rite Aid RediClinics; limited healthcare services in these clinics are primarily provided by NPs.[52] An advantage of these clinics is that they provide on-demand care; patients can simply walk in and be seen quickly in most cases, thereby improving access to care. Hoff and Prout[37] conducted a systematic review in 2019 and found that these retail clinics were comparable to other ambulatory settings in terms of lower cost; however, there were few studies that examined quality of care. Retail clinics have also been found to provide more services to underserved patients without primary care providers. They have also been associated with a reduction in ED use for minor acute (5.7%–12%) and preventable conditions (3.3%–13.4%) in a study in the state of New Jersey.[38]

Telehealth/Telemedicine

An estimated 60 million Americans live in rural areas[53] and are more likely to have a greater number of health risk factors and chronic conditions than those living in urban areas.[40] Most rural areas have significant shortages of primary care providers and even fewer specialists, making access to care in rural areas a considerable challenge.[54] Over the past several years, telehealth and telemedicine (referred to as telehealth for this chapter) has been a way to provide care to people without access to care; unfortunately, there were many restrictions to how telehealth could be used, considerable technology challenges, and reimbursement was low compared to office visits.[42] Despite that, telehealth experienced significant growth from the late 1990s through 2019. In 2020, with the COVID-19 pandemic, telehealth growth was exponential; a RAND Corporation study reported a 20-fold increase during the pandemic.[55] Interestingly, much of the growth came not from rural areas, but from wealthier counties and patients in metropolitan areas.

There are three ways in which telehealth can be provided.[56] (a) Synchronously, which is in real time through either telephone or audiovisual communication using a smartphone, tablet, or computer; (b) asynchronously, in which recorded messages can be collected and then reviewed and responded to later; and (c) remote patient monitoring, which allows patient data to be directly transmitted to the healthcare provider.[36] There are several potential benefits from the use of telehealth:

- Access to primary care providers and specialists for chronic health conditions, medication management, and mental and behavioral health
- For coaching patients who need additional support managing chronic health conditions, including weight management and nutrition counseling
- Ability to participate in physical, occupational, or speech therapy as a hybrid approach to in-person care
- Monitoring clinical signs and trends of certain chronic medical conditions (e.g., blood pressure, blood glucose, other remote assessments)
- Performing case management and care coordination for patients who have difficulty accessing care (e.g.,

those who live in very rural settings, older adults, those with limited mobility)
- Regular follow-up with patients after hospitalization
- Delivering advance care planning and counseling to patients and caregivers to document patient preferences if a life-threatening event or medical crisis occurs
- Providing nonemergent care to residents in long-term care facilities (particularly from specialists such as dermatologists and cardiologists)
- Providing education and training for other healthcare providers through peer-to-peer professional medical consultations (inpatient or outpatient) that are not locally available, particularly in rural areas[45]

Obviously, telehealth services were extremely important and useful during the COVID-19 pandemic to prescreen patients who were symptomatic of COVID-19 and to provide low-risk urgent care services for patients without COVID to reduce the risk of exposure.[45]

There are also limitations to telehealth that revolve around interstate licensure issues because clinician licensure is controlled by the state. Although there is some technology that can transmit clinical data and there are some guidelines on physical examination via telehealth, there are limits to the physical examination. Technology challenges include problems with bandwidth, shortfalls in some smartphones or older computers, discomfort with technology for some providers and patients, and cultural expectations of patients who may prefer in-person visits. CMS issued reimbursement waivers during the pandemic, but adequate reimbursement remains a long-term challenge.[45]

NPs are considered appropriate telehealth providers along with a variety of other clinical providers such as physicians, psychologists, and social workers.[56] AGNP students are expected to be prepared to provide telehealth services upon graduation, which would increase access to care, decrease health costs, and improve quality of healthcare in rural settings.[47] However, that requires that NP schools begin to provide the training within the curriculum. The National Organization of Nurse Practitioner Faculties advocated telehealth education for NP programs and provided guidelines for educators in 2018, which is in the early stages of development. The NP Core Competency document includes telehealth and the following competencies, which should be included in NP programs:

- Telehealth etiquette and professionalism while videoconferencing
- Skills in using peripheral equipment, such as otoscope, stethoscope, and ophthalmoscope
- An understanding of when telehealth should and should not be used
- An understanding of privacy/protected health information regulations

- Proficiency in the use of synchronous and asynchronous telehealth technology
- Knowledge of appropriate documentation and billing of telehealth technology
- An ability to collaborate interprofessionally using telehealth technologies
- Proficiency in taking a history, performing an appropriate physical examination, and generating differential diagnoses using telehealth.[48]

Telehealth opportunities for NPs have expanded during the pandemic; however, barriers still exist in the development of standardized telehealth academic preparation, training and education, and standardized competencies across all providers.[49] NP professional and academic organizations will need to continue lobbying efforts to reduce these barriers.

Emergency Department

The ED provides emergent care for older adults who may have cognitive impairment, functional limitations, and frailty. This extremely challenging environment is the perfect setting for an AGNP to collaborate with an interdisciplinary team to identify and intervene on the unique care needs of older adults. Beyond competencies in certification for specialties, emergency NPs need specialized education, task-related practice standards, and additional certifications testing. According to the National Center for Health Workforce Analysis, the non–primary care specialty NP full-time equivalents will grow by 141% over the next 7 years, with the largest anticipated need in areas of physical medicine, rehabilitation, and EDs.[57] EDs that dedicate a team of geriatric specialist NPs, physicians, and pharmacists to evaluate and deliver acute care for older high-risk patients may avoid hospital readmissions and have safer, shorter lengths of hospital inpatient stays.[40]

Innovative emergency care delivery models are being implemented to improve access to care for the uninsured and underinsured in unscheduled convenient walk-in settings.[41] The core mission of ED work is in stabilizing patients with life-threatening illnesses and injuries. Between 28% and 50% of all diagnostic and new-onset illness visits nationwide are evaluated in EDs rather than primary care.[42] According to the National Center for Health Statistics, 7.9% of ED visits nationally ended with admission with less than 20% of patients being outside the AGNP scope of practice (newborns, infants, young children) seen in ED settings. This increase in emergent care supports the need for NPs with AGNP life-span and primary care general knowledge, skills, and competency in this high-volume area.[42]

Older adults who present to an ED and experience a subsequent hospitalization may experience a decline in function and quality of life, along with adverse outcomes, such as iatrogenic infections or medication errors. Having an AGNP who works on an interdisciplinary team allows providers to address potential gaps in care, as well as perform cognitive assessments, medication management, and safe and smooth transitions of care for patients leading to their next level of care.[17, 51]

Post-Acute and Long-Term Care

NPs provide care to residents in skilled nursing facilities (SNFs) in 63% of the nation's nursing homes, despite only 3% of NPs working in institutional long-term care (LTC) settings.[1] In the United States, AGNPs have been working in LTC settings[17] since the mid-1970s. For the AGNP, the primary role on-site in long-term care facilities was to provide early evaluation and treatment to reduce service utilization, thus decreasing unnecessary hospitalizations and unplanned transfers. Care provided by NPs has been found to reduce service utilization by enhancing access to on-site care, maintaining the functional status of patients, and guiding in-home safety through engaging in the patient–caregiver dyad.[21] NPs tend to manage patients with neuropsychiatric conditions such as dementia and acute exacerbation of chronic illnesses in nursing homes when compared with physicians.[58]

Transitions of Care

Older individuals with multiple comorbidities are estimated to use 70% of Medicaid and Medicare funding. One in five Medicare beneficiaries is readmitted to the hospital within 30 days of discharge, which is considered a failed transition of care.[55] More than half of these readmissions occur in patients 65 years of age and older. AGNPs provide safe and smooth transitions of care from one setting to another (i.e., hospital to home or LTC). A systematic review performed by Mora et al. found that transitional care can be enhanced to prevent 30-day readmissions and decrease length of hospital stay by using NP-led protocols that include standardized assessments, home visits as needed, and follow-up phone calls.[56]

The transitional care NP engages the patient and family during an acute illness phase to coordinate care for discharge planning in order to meet the patient's specific needs at the next setting or level of care. When comparing transitional care provided by NPs to usual care, the transitional care provided by an NP was better than usual care provided by physicians alone in 5/6 outcome measures.[21] The NP care was superior for length of stay (4/5, 80%), cost (3/4, 75%), quality of life (3/4, 75%), and satisfaction (3/4, 75%), compared to physician-alone usual care.[21] In addition, the role of the AGNP was shown to provide consistently equivalent or better outcomes compared to physician care alone or usual care in five identified geriatric settings: primary care, home care, LTC, acute care, and transitional care.[21]

In a large national sample of medically complex patients within the Veterans Affairs system, researchers noted greater rates of hospitalizations, ED visits, and higher healthcare spending occurred among patients managed by primary care physicians as compared to those managed by NPs and PAs.[6] These outcomes may be attributed to the emphasis by NPs on coordinated patient-centered care and patient/caregiver engagement in self-management[21] while transitioning between care settings.

Home-Based Primary Care

Homes are another primary care setting that have become more prevalent in recent years. In particular, new models of care have emerged to provide care to homebound older adults. Independence at Home (IAH) has been one of CMS's most successful demonstration projects and was designed to keep frail older adults at home and to prevent them from being admitted to nursing homes. Both physician- and NP-led practices participated in the demonstration project. The project targeted high utilizers of Medicare services, and by the end of the first 5 years of the project, practices were reducing costs by up to 30%, generating more than $100 million in cost savings. Similarly, home-based palliative care provides similar types of services but for shorter periods with a greater focus on goal clarification and care planning.[57]

House call programs are also an emerging practice model that targets patients similar to those in the IAH program. In 2013, about 3,300 NPs provided more than 1.1 million visits to home or domiciliary settings, making NPs the most common health professional providing house call services. Unfortunately, there are several regulatory and reimbursement policy barriers that NPs still face in this setting such as the inability to certify and sign orders for Medicare fee-for-service home health patients or to certify terminal illness for hospice patients.[59]

CONCLUSION

AGPCNPs play an important role in the healthcare team and are uniquely qualified to manage chronic diseases and promote wellness in the aging population. While the ACA expanded the availability of primary care services and innovative models have emerged, primary care provider shortages remain a concern. Additionally, scope of practice along with regulatory and payment policies continue to be barriers for NPs who work in many of these settings, which points to the importance of NP research and policy efforts to change the existing regulations and policies that impact NP care.

REFERENCES

References for this chapter are online and available at https://connect.springerpub.com/content/book/978-0-8261-8414-6/part/part01/toc-part/ch7.

CHAPTER 8

Palliative and End-of-Life Care

Deborah Chapa and Debra Hain

LEARNING OBJECTIVES

At the conclusion of this chapter, the learner will be able to:

➤ Describe epidemiologic information about palliative care (PC) and end-of-life (EOL) care in the United States and globally.

➤ Compare and contrast PC principles to EOL care.

➤ Demonstrate the primary care adult-gerontology nurse practitioner (AGNP) role in providing care for populations with chronic disease and cancer-related diagnosis receiving PC.

➤ Discuss interprofessional partnerships with primary care AGNP and PC team.

INTRODUCTION

This chapter provides an overview of palliative care (PC) and end-of-life (EOL) care for adolescent to older adult populations living with serious chronic illness and individuals with a cancer-related diagnosis who may need PC or EOL care. The information presented will not provide in-depth discussion regarding treatments for specific disease; for that information, please see other chapters in the textbook.

PALLIATIVE CARE

The World Health Organization (WHO) defines "palliative care" (PC) as "a crucial part of integrated, people-centered health services. Relieving serious health-related suffering, be it physical, psychologic, social, or spiritual, is a global ethical responsibility. Thus, whether the cause of suffering is cardiovascular disease, cancer, major organ failure, drug-resistant, tuberculosis, severe burns, end-stage chronic illness, acute trauma, extreme birth prematurity, frailty of old age, palliative care may be needed and must be available at all levels of care.[1] It is estimated that about 14% of people who need PC receive it and that about 78% of adults in need of PC live in low- and middle-income countries.[1]

PC is an essential component of care for noncommunicable disease, yet there remains a substantial gap in government funding allocation for PC. Among many high-income countries, the United States is considered advanced in PC; however, there is still more room for improvement. At this time the U.S. healthcare system does not meet the needs of individuals and families living with a serious illness.[2] The medical community tends to focus on disease-specific treatments instead of taking a person-/family-centered approach to care. About 12 million adults and 400,000 children are living with a serious illness, such as cancer, heart disease, kidney disease, or dementia. Approximately 23% of people with a serious illness reported that hospital staff were not responsive to their needs, and less than 50% stated that they were asked about their personal preferences should a life-threatening situation occur. More than 30% of family caregivers of someone with a serious illness reported increased strain and burden (e.g., emotional and physical stress, financial constraints, and poor health).[2] PC is a specialized team (e.g., physician, nurse practitioner [NP], nurses, social worker, chaplain) approach that can address these issues as well as reduce healthcare costs of unnecessary or undesired care. PC is "appropriate at any age and any stage of illness and can be provided along with curative treatment. Because PC services are based on patient and family need, not prognosis, PC teams respond to the episodic, complex, and long-term nature of a serious illness."[2]

End-of-Life Care

EOL care (comfort care) is an essential aspect of medical/NP care and is part of the continuum of PC. The goals are to prevent or alleviate suffering while improving quality of life and honoring the person's wishes. Hospice care, a model and philosophy of care, focuses on providing PC for an individual with a life-limiting illness. Hospice care provides holistic, person-/family-centered care but is provided when the person has a diagnosis that is considered terminal and meets the criteria for the specific illness prognosis of 6 months or less. Hospice care is provided

Table 8.1: Compare and Contrast Palliative and Hospice Care

Palliative Care	Hospice Care
• Interprofessional team • Symptom management • Promotes effective communication • Provided to individuals of any age or serious illness • Alleviate suffering in all stages of illness (curable, chronic, progressive) • Not limited to EOL • Provided at same time as curative or life-prolonging disease treatments (e.g., dialysis) • Provides family support • Honors person's wishes and preferences for care • Provides physical, psychologic, and spiritual care	• Interprofessional team • Symptom management • Promotes effective communication • Provided to individuals of any age or serious illness • Alleviate suffering • Provides family support, bereavement services for up to 13 months after the death of their loved one • Disease-modifying treatments are no longer beneficial (burden outweighs the benefit) • Prognosis of 6 months or less if the disease follows its usual course through recertification • Honors the person's wishes and preferences for care • Provides physical, psychologic, and spiritual care

by a similar team as PC either directly or by phone 24 hours, 7 days per week in the person's home, nursing home, or residential living facility as well as a dedicated facility such as a hospital inpatient facility (see Table 8.1 for comparisons and contrasts between hospice and PC). Consider hospice care when there is a decrease in physical or cognitive function, psychologic distress, poor quality of life, family or informal caregiver increased stress, increasing frequency of medical and symptom crisis, and/or increasing episodes of hospitalizations or emergency department visits. There are specific criteria that a patient must meet to be eligible for hospice care (see Box 8.1). The main reasons for discharge from hospice include stabilization of the person's index condition, patient or family request, and pursuit of disease-modifying treatments. It is important to note that many patients are not receiving hospice care prior to hospitalization and/ or when death is imminent. Having a hospital-based PC program can help identify patients who may benefit from PC before they have advanced illness with a prognosis of 6 months or less if the disease follows its usual course. The problem is there is a lack of PC programs in many hospitals, particularly rural areas of the country (see Box 8.2). Therefore, it is essential to have conversations about PC and EOL early in the illness trajectory about care options as the disease progresses, especially in those with a serious and life-limiting illness.

🕛 CLINICAL PEARLS

- In the United States, patients are not legally required to have a do not resuscitate (DNR) status to receive hospice care; however, patients and families should understand that enrolling in hospice is a choice to accept that death may occur in the next 6 months and that life-sustaining treatments will not be provided.

- Help patients and families understand that it is a misconception that hospice hastens death.

Box 8.1: Eligibility for Hospice Benefit

Eligibility for Medicare Part A (covers hospice and other care services) requires the following:

- U.S. citizen or legal residents who are eligible for social security or railroad retirement benefits

- Age 65 or younger than age 65 and eligible for Medicare because of a long-term disability for more than 2 years and/or with end-stage kidney disease

- Referral to a hospice that is Medicare-certified

- A statement signed by the patient indicating that they are choosing hospice care instead of regular Medicare for their hospice diagnosis. Medicare allows for reimbursement for incidental medical expenses that are unrelated to the terminal illness. The determination of "relatedness" is complex and is the responsibility of the hospice medical director.

- Certification by both the patient's personal physician and the hospice medical director that the patient has a terminal illness and likely to have less than 6 months to live if the disease follows its usual course

- Treatment priorities are alleviating symptoms of illness and focus on comfort care and quality of life rather than cure or disease-modifying treatments

For more information about Medicare Part A Hospice benefit, see www.medicare.gov/Pubs/pdf/02154 -medicare-hospice-benefits.pdf.

The trajectory of the illness and the need for PC and hospice care is unique to the diagnosis (e.g., terminal cancer, serious life-limiting illness). See Figure 8.1 for the trajectory of someone with PC and Figure 8.2 for comparison of those with cancer, organ failure, frailty, and dementia. See Figure 8.3 for the phases and layers of care; palliative, end-of-life, and terminal.

Box 8.2: Hospitals and Palliative Care Programs

Hospital Palliative Care Grades:

- 2019 Report Card states about three-fourths of states receive an A or B with more than 60% of the hospitals in those states reporting a PC program.

- The states with the highest number of programs are Delaware, New Hampshire, Rhode Island, Vermont, Connecticut, the Dakotas, Utah, and the District of Columbia. The lowest performing states were Mississippi, Alabama, Oklahoma, and Wyoming.

- Only 17% of rural hospitals with 50 or more beds reported PC programs. In contrast, 94% of hospitals with 300 or more beds have PC programs.

Source: Morrison RS, Meier DE. *America's Care of Serious Illness: A State-by-State Report Card on Access to Palliative Care in Our Nation's Hospitals.* Center to Advance Palliative Care and the National Palliative Care Research Center. Published September 2019. Updated May 2020. https://www.capc.org/documents/download/2

PRINCIPLES OF PALLIATIVE CARE

Clinical Practice Guidelines for Quality Palliative Care, Fourth Edition (commonly referred to as NCP Guidelines)[3] provides primary care NPs with a way to establish a comprehensive foundation for providing quality PC for those living with serious illness. The National Consensus Project Guidelines have eight domains of PC (see Table 8.2), including clinical and organizational strategies, screening and assessment elements, practices, examples, tools, and resources (available at www.nationalcoalitionhpc.org/ncp). The domains are interrelated with some being more apparent when caring for patients and their families. These domains are incorporated in the assessment and delivery of care for PC patients.

It is important to note that PC can be an integral part of care delivery in any setting. All clinicians can deliver PC and should have a support team of PC specialists and an interprofessional team (IPT; see Chapter 4 for more information about IPT) with a focus on delivery of patient- and family-centered care. The IPT members

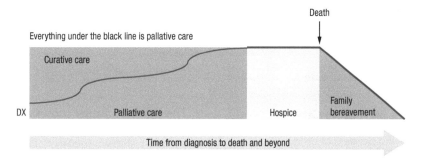

Figure 8.1: Trajectory of palliative care

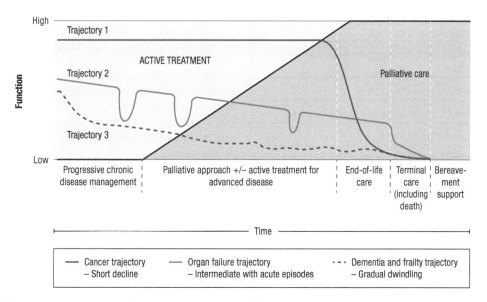

Figure 8.2: Difference in trajectory with cancer, end-organ failure, or serious life-limiting illness

Source: Rawlin M, Jones F, Pond D, et al. *RACGP - Aged Care Clinical Guide (Silver Book): Part A. Palliative and end-of-life care.* Royal Australian College of General Practitioners; 2020: Figure 1. https://www.racgp.org.au/getattachment/55aea74c-fbe9-4d01-8cbc-425948225cb8/Palliative-care.aspx

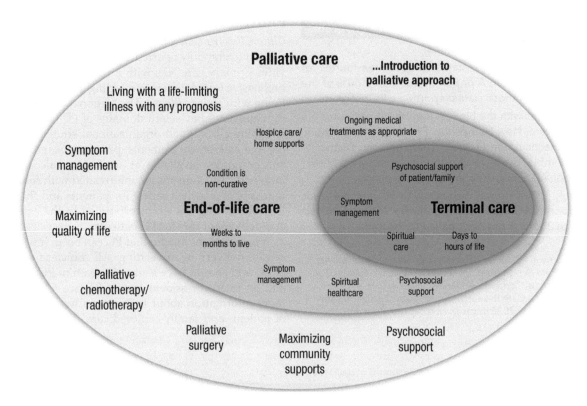

Figure 8.3: The phases and layers of care

Table 8.2: Eight Domains of Palliative Care

Domain 1	Structure and process of care
Domain 2	Physical aspects of care
Domain 3	Psychologic and psychiatric aspects of care
Domain 4	Social aspects of care
Domain 5	Spiritual, religious, and existential aspects of care
Domain 6	Cultural aspects of care
Domain 7	Care of the imminently dying patient
Domain 8	Ethical and legal aspects of care

Source: National Consensus Project for Quality Palliative Care. *Clinical Practice Guidelines for Quality Palliative Care.* 4th ed. National Coalition for Hospice and Palliative Care; 2018. https://www.nationalcoalitionhpc.org/ncp

may be composed of physicians, APRNs, physician assistants, nurses, social workers, and chaplains, as well as other healthcare workers, depending on the needs of the patient and their family. Primary care clinicians may work with interprofessional teams to embed PC in their practice.[4]

The first step in the process of providing PC begins with a comprehensive assessment (see Table 8.3). This assessment should focus on family engagement, communication, care coordination, and continuity of care across healthcare settings. Some key points in this assessment should include, but not be limited to, the patient and family understanding of the illness, goals of care, treatment preferences, and review or completion of advance directives. It is crucial to determine the decision-making capacity of the patient and identification of the person with legal decision-making capacity if the patient cannot make medical decisions. Other key points to the assessment are summarized in Table 8.3. Functional status, advance directives, social determinants of health, and anticipatory grief are vital to the comprehensive assessment.[5]

Functional status is foundational to determining prognosis. Examples of scales to assess functional status are the Karnofsky Performance Scale (KPS),[6] Eastern Cooperative Oncology Group (ECOG) scale,[7] the Palliative Performance Scale (PPS),[8] and the Edmonton Functional Assessment Tool.[9] The KPS is an 11-item scale that ranges from 0% to 100% and is used to assess functional status and prognosis in PC patients. Similar and based on KPS is the PPS, which also is an 11-item scale ranging from 0% to 100%.[6] The parameters evaluated are the patient's

Table 8.3: Assessment Criteria

Patient and family understanding	Illness, goals of care, treatment preferences, advance directives
Decision-making capacity	Patient and/or person with legal decision-making capacity
Physical examination	Symptoms and functional status
Medical records review	Notes, labs, and diagnostic tests
Medical history	Therapies, recommended treatments, and prognosis
Comorbid conditions	Medical, cognitive, and psychiatric disorders
Medication reconciliation	Prescribed medicine, over-the-counter medications, and complementary therapies
Social determinants of health	Financial vulnerability, housing, nutrition, safety, social support
Social and cultural factors	Caregiver support, availability to meet needs of patient
Spiritual and emotional	Patient and family assessment and evaluation of prior trauma
Communication	Health literacy, language, hearing and culture
Grief	Evaluate for anticipatory grief, loss and bereavement
Additional assessment	Eligibility for VA benefits and for pediatric patients' identification of developmental status and understanding of their disease

ambulation from no restrictions to bedridden, activity ranging from normal to inability to perform any activity due to extensive disease, and self-care from fully independent to total care. Oral care ranges from normal to mouth care only, and consciousness from full consciousness to drowsy with or without confusion or comatose. The ECOG is a 5-point general functional assessment tool ranging from ability to walk and care for self as requirements for dependence or hospitalization.[7] More research is needed to determine the appropriate scale for ethnically diverse populations.

Advance directives can be divided into two types and vary from state to state, so it is important to know the laws in the state you practice. Most states combine both types (durable power of attorney and living will) into one document. The durable power of attorney designates who the patient wants to make healthcare decisions for them if they are not able to make those decisions. States also

have laws governing who that would be in the absence of this document. For example, Florida it defaults to the spouse, then the children, followed by the parents and then the siblings. The living will contains wishes about the EOL such as feeding tube, pain medication, and intubation. The DNR wishes may be included in the document. However, separate documents may be required for DNR to be implemented. Some states have different requirements for inpatient and outpatient documentation.[10]

Social determinants of health provide a focus to address the complex relationship between social relationships, economics, health policy, and health (see Chapter 1 for more information about social determinants of health). Since the time of Florence Nightingale, nursing has been aware that the health of the individual is not solely determined by the individual but is influenced by environmental factors, social conditions, and policy that impact health disparities, health equity, and social justice.[11] When completing your health assessment, ask questions about income, occupation, housing, food, transportation, and social support. An assessment of health literacy should be included in this information. This information will be used when discussing goals of care and treatment plans. Knowledge of government, private, and community resources is vital to assist patients when assessing through a lens of social determinants of health.[11]

Advance care planning (ACP) is an important topic and includes more than physical assessment, grief assessment, and advance directives. The primary outcome is to optimize the quality of life for the patients and families as they move through the illness trajectory. It is important to establish a therapeutic relationship with patients and families. Shared decision-making is a key component of ACP. The first step is to meet the families and patients where they are in the process of understanding the illness. From this point, the provider can give health education as needed and support through the grief process that often accompanies chronic illness. Depending on the type of illness—for example, cancer, heart failure, kidney disease, dementia—it may be important for an oncologist or another specialist to present the prognosis to the patient and family. Decisions can be made about the type of treatments by considering and presenting the risk–benefit ratio and the impact on quality of life. There are certain events, such as increased hospitalizations or emergency department (ED) visits or poor quality of life, that the NP should address as the person transitions to a different level of care.[12] The timing of the discussion, providing a comforting environment, and offering compassionate listening will assist the patient and family to make important decisions during their transition process.

Pain and symptom management are key for quality of life in patients. Pain and dyspnea are the most common symptoms people may experience, but others are nausea, vomiting, oral pain, dysphagia, fatigue, constipation, diarrhea, and a decline in physical function. The plan of care should include pharmacologic and nonpharmacologic treatments focusing on achieving established goals, alleviating suffering, and improving quality of life. It is always important to identify the etiology of all symptoms and disease processes in order to develop the best treatment plan. Psychologic factors can trigger and increase physiologic symptoms. PC philosophy supports a holistic approach to a patient's treatment of symptoms. This approach includes an evaluation of spiritual, emotional, cultural, physical, and social determinants of health. Proper management, along the trajectory of PC from one of aggressive treatment to conservative treatment and EOL care, is vital for patients and their families.[4]

There are several issues to consider when evaluating psychiatric and psychologic aspects of care for people receiving PC. Mental health-related issues include (a) anxiety, depression, delirium, and cognitive impairment; (b) family caregiver stress, anticipatory grief, and coping strategies; (c) pharmacologic and nonpharmacologic treatments; and (d) patient/family grief/bereavement (see Chapter 18 for more information about mental health conditions).

Having a serious illness can stimulate a cascade of physiological stress responses. Compounding the physiology changes is the psychologic response to stress.[13] Stress increases the likelihood of anxiety or depression.[21] Some of the treatments for the illness can also cause stress. This, in turn, impacts the body's ability to heal. Early intervention to combat stress is key and should include communication with and education of the patient and the family. Complementary strategies for stress reduction, such as an increase in physical activity, meditation, yoga, and biofeedback, may be helpful. An evaluation of the patient's coping strategies to assist with the stress response is also helpful as is coaching the patient regarding individualized stress reduction strategies.[14,15]

Anticipatory grief is a response a family member or loved one may have when a patient is experiencing an illness that will lead to their passing.[16] The patient experiencing the dying process may also have anticipatory grief over the thought of their death, and what this will mean to family members. This type of grief may appear like depression but is a reaction to the eventual passing of the loved one or patient. The anticipatory grief of the loved one can impact the emotions and decisions of the patient. It is important to assess this in families and provide support as appropriate. Grief before death may increase one's anger and loss of emotional control that can trigger negative interpersonal reactions.[16] Emotional conflict can impair decision-making when the patient is critical, so it is important for the NP to recognize and take the time to be authentically present with the person to support

disclosure of feelings. Anticipatory grief is high in the intensive care unit and, when present, can increase anxiety and depression. Glick and colleagues[17] conducted a cross-sectional study with surrogate decision-makers and identified that when surrogates had anticipatory grief, they experienced more difficulty with problem-solving that could impact their decision-making.[17] Taking a person-/family-centered approach to decision-making while paying attention to anticipatory grief can help surrogates or other decision-makers assure the patient's wishes are honored. The awareness of all the deaths that have occurred during the COVID-19 pandemic has increased the possibilities for anticipatory grief.[18] So paying attention to this can help you be prepared to respond to family members or other decision-makers when a patient is experiencing a decline in health that may result in death. More research is needed to determine the impact of anticipatory grief on the bereavement process during the pandemic.

There are some strategies to assist with anticipatory grief. Communicating with patients and families is vital. It is important to listen to the person's concerns, respond to their concerns, and then utilize validation techniques of their statements and feelings. ACP decisions should occur as early as possible with consideration for anticipatory grief, for this has been shown to help families with bereavement. Connecting patients and families with community resources is an important strategy to assist with anticipatory grief. Many resources now are available online and should be included when educating patients.[19]

The diagnosis of delirium in an inpatient and outpatient setting often is missed and may contribute to cognitive decline that is reversible if addressed early. Signs and symptoms of delirium can be cognitive changes, sleep disturbances, diminished attention span, reduced ability to focus, disorientation, confusion, or hallucinations (see Chapter 18 for more information). The etiology of delirium can be underlying disease processes, infection, uncontrolled pain, constipation, pharmacology-induced, or related to a change in environment. Treatment includes finding the etiology and implementing evidence-based strategies to alleviate the symptoms. Other treatments include time with family, increased daylight, reorientation, and sleep at night and awake during the day.[20]

Advanced directives and designation of a healthcare surrogate are important parts of the social assessment. Functional assessment as discussed earlier also plays a role in the social assessment. The patient may have needs or treatment options that will depend on the functional assessment. An example is in oncology care, where patients must have an adequate performance status to receive many types of chemotherapy. A discussion of intimacy and sexuality should be included in the social assessment as appropriate. Collaborating with a social worker may assist NPs in discovering the best approaches to social issues.

Constructing a family meeting with the patient, healthcare surrogate, and other members of the patient's social network is important. There are tools available to assist with developing goals of care and address shared decision-making (discussed later in the chapter). Setting standards for the meeting ahead of time and goals and questions from patients and families will assist with more productive family meetings.

SPECIAL POPULATIONS

The principles of PC and EOL care are similar across the life span; however, there are some unique issues to address when caring for adolescents/young adults and older adults.

Adolescents/Young Adults

In adolescents and young adults with cancer, there are many things to consider, but one important aspect is their psychologic development. The added stress of having a cancer diagnosis along with normal life transitions can be challenging for adolescents and their families. The desire for independence may be compromised by an increased need for assistance, which promotes more dependence on parents or other family caregivers. As adolescents transition into adulthood, there may be a marked change in personal and spiritual growth.[21] Having a serious illness or terminal diagnosis has a substantial impact on their educational goals, social and familial goals that may result in loss of employment, financial freedom, and the ability to achieve life goals.

It is important to promote autonomy in the decision-making process by involving the adolescent in conversations about goals of care. Sometimes this can be challenging because parents, out of concern for their child, may want to be in control of decision-making. It is important to note that when caring for an adolescent or young adult that you should help parents understand the importance of the adolescent being involved in the decision-making (see Chapter 11 for more information about adolescent care). In addition, NPs should consider issues related to race/ethnicity, gender, religion, immigrant status, education level, socioeconomic status, sexual orientation, and indigenous heritage because these can impact treatment options.[21] Other principles of PC are similar in adolescents and adults; they are to alleviate suffering and improve quality of life. ACP such as alleviating suffering and improving quality of life is essential for those who have cancer and/or other serious life-limiting illnesses. During ACP conversations, it is critical that the adolescent/young adult's wishes and preferences for care be discussed. Voicing My Choices and My Wishes (available at https://fivewishes.org/five-wishes/individuals-families/individuals-and-families/

children-and-adolescents) can help provide direction to parents, caregivers, and healthcare providers in conversations to assure the adolescent's/young adult's voice is heard in the decision-making process.

Older Adults

Geriatric PC integrates the principles of geriatric care and PC to provide comprehensive care for older adults. A major challenge in caring for some older adults in need of PC is their ability to make informed decisions. Communication about PC and EOL care can be complicated by communication barriers, cognitive impairment, tension between a healthcare proxy and the patient, and difficulty interpreting nonverbal behavior of a patient with moderate to advanced dementia. Conflict can occur between family members, which often results in the older adult's wishes and preferences for care not being honored. Some of this can be addressed by using decision aids and ACP. A particular challenge can be caring for those with advanced dementia. Many family members may understand what it means to have a loved one with Alzheimer's disease and related dementias, but there may be a disconnect between the reality that the disease is progressive with physical and cognitive decline until death. When engaged in decision-making regarding life-prolonging treatments, they may not understand the lack of benefit, which sometimes leads to hospitalization. Patients with dementia and their families can benefit from PC when diagnosed and then hospice care when the prognosis is 6 months or less if the illness runs its usual course. Many times, someone with dementia experiences a decline in cognitive and physical function due to an acute illness requiring hospitalization. The decision for hospice care may be made at the time of an acute illness and then, after 6 months or longer, if the person improves and no longer meets the criteria, hospice care is discontinued. This pattern can repeat itself each time the older adult experiences an acute illness until there is a substantial decline with eventual death.

ROLE OF PRIMARY CARE NURSE PRACTITIONER

Individuals receiving PC can be comanaged by PC specialists and primary care NPs. In addition, PC can be provided by clinicians who are not PC specialists, which is called primary or basic PC.[2] This can be beneficial for patients who may not have access to PC specialists. In the United States, most PC specialists are members of hospital-based PC programs and may not have a practice in the community. Patients may not be referred to a PC specialist until late in the illness trajectory, so having a primary care provider who recognizes the need for PC is important. NPs can assess and treat physical symptoms and focus on psychologic, social, cultural, and spiritual aspects of care by evaluating for depression, anxiety, social and financial stressors, and caregiver burden. It is critical that primary care NPs gain knowledge and skills to communicate "bad news" and engage in ACP conversations that elicit the patient's wishes and preferences for care (e.g., aggressive life-sustaining treatment vs. supportive care) as well as identifying a surrogate decision-maker and provide emotional support. There are many tools to use that support having ACP conversations and discussions about PC and hospice care. Singer et al.[22] performed a systematic test of available tools for discussions with the patient and family regarding PC and hospice. The authors identified 23 tools (not all tested in research) for discussions with patients and their families (together or separate), but one that may be useful in primary care is the Conversation Project available at https://theconversationproject.org.

In addition, the Johns Hopkins University Evidence-Based Practice Center under a contract with the Agency for Healthcare Research and Quality conducted a study about assessment tools for PC and the findings can be seen in a report that is available at https://effectivehealthcare.ahrq.gov/sites/default/files/pdf/palliative-care-tools_technical-brief-2017.pdf.

It is also important to know what resources are available in your community.

MODELS OF CARE

As the United States and other countries witness a growing population living with serious illness, the need for PC is substantially increasing. Some newer approaches to PC should include rethinking PC by putting more emphasis on educating healthcare professionals and reimbursement support for community-based PC with subspecialists and non-PC specialists managing patients who can benefit from PC services. The following are some suggestions for new models of care:

- Increasing NP curricula to include PC for non-PC specialists and primary care clinicians
- PC telehealth for consultation in rural areas
- Comanagement of patients by PC specialists, primary care clinicians, and subspecialists (e.g., cardiology, nephrology)

Patient Education

There are many resources for patients and their families (see Box 8.3). It is critical that patients and families have

Box 8.3: Educational Resources for Patients and Families

- National Institute on Aging (NIH) www.nia.nih.org
- Get Palliative Care https://getpalliativecare.org
- Palliative Care-Cancer Net www.cancer.net
- Patient and Family Resources www.capc.org
- Understanding Palliative Care www.caregiver.org

appropriate education to aid in clinical decision-making. Providing decision aids can help, but it is also essential that the AGNP is prepared to have conversations about wishes and preferences for care when a patient is making a decision about PC or EOL care. Taking a person-/family-centered approach can be beneficial (see Chapter 2).[23]

CONCLUSION

PC is a continuum of care that starts when a patient is diagnosed with chronic disease and continues through the end of life. In addition, those with a cancer-related diagnosis at the time of diagnosis who don't meet the criteria for hospice may benefit from PC. A thorough assessment of the patient that includes social determinants of health, psychosocial, physical, spiritual, and other domains of PC along with wishes and preferences of care is essential. ACP should be addressed early in the disease process and reevaluated as needed throughout the disease trajectory. Quality of life is a major focus along the pathway of PC. Receiving appropriate treatment and managing symptoms optimizes the quality of life for many patients. When patients have a life-limiting disease, they no longer want aggressive medical treatment and the focus becomes symptom management and quality of life only, at which point the transition to hospice care may be appropriate. Families have an important role in shared decision-making (if the patient agrees). Effective communication with patients and families is vital to optimize the journey for patients and ensure that patients make informed decisions that reflect their wishes before they may not be able to disclose.

REFERENCES

References for this chapter are online and available at https://connect.springerpub.com/content/book/978-0-8261-8414-6/part/part01/toc-part/ch8.

CHAPTER 9

The Role of AGNPs in Disasters

Gordon H. Worley

LEARNING OBJECTIVES

At the conclusion of this chapter, the learner will be able to:

➤ Understand the epidemiology of disasters and the disaster cycle.

➤ Describe the nature of disaster medicine and how to adapt to providing patient care under austere medical conditions.

➤ Discuss the role of the nurse practitioner (NP) or advanced practice registered nurse (APRN) in disaster planning, preparedness, response, mitigation, and recovery.

➤ Describe how to become involved in disaster preparedness and response and how to prepare for these roles.

INTRODUCTION

Nurses have long played a vital role in the response to disasters, conflicts, and humanitarian catastrophes dating back to Florence Nightingale in the 1850s. Nurse practitioners (NPs) and other advanced practice registered nurses (APRNs) are uniquely prepared to provide care and support in disaster situations and humanitarian responses. This chapter provides an overview of the role of the NP or APRN in disaster planning, preparation, response, mitigation, and recovery. It is based on the core concepts and competencies identified by the National Panel for APRN Emergency Preparedness and All Hazards Response Education,[1] the International Council of Nurses (ICN) Core Competencies in Disaster Nursing (version 2.0),[2] and the *Sphere Handbook: Humanitarian Charter and Minimum Standards in Humanitarian Response,* Fourth Edition.[3]

This chapter discusses the important aspects of disaster preparation and response, but it is not intended to be a substitute for practical, hands-on training. One cannot expect to become proficient in the knowledge and skills needed to be a safe, effective disaster medical responder from a textbook chapter alone. The interested reader is encouraged to seek out additional training and to refer to the listed references.

THE EPIDEMIOLOGY OF DISASTERS

The United Nations defines a "disaster" as "a serious disruption of the functioning of a community or a society causing widespread human, material, economic or environmental losses which exceed the ability of the affected community or society to cope using its own resources."[4] A disaster may be a natural occurrence, such as an environmental event (flood, storm, hurricane, wildfire, drought, famine), a geologic event (earthquake, tsunami, landslide, volcanic eruption), or a biologic event (infectious disease outbreak, epidemic, pandemic). It may also be a human-caused event related to war, conflict, or terrorism; an industrial or transportation accident; a hazardous material (HAZMAT) or chemical, biologic, radiation, nuclear, explosive incident; or the result of political upheaval, infrastructure failure, or economic collapse. The common thread is that the event has a large-scale negative impact on the affected population.

Vulnerable Populations

While disasters are indiscriminate and affect all persons living in the disaster area, certain populations are more vulnerable and often bear the brunt of the adverse effects. These vulnerabilities can be social, economic, health-related, or geographic in nature.

Marginalized groups who face societal discrimination based on ethnicity, religion, gender, income, or other factors are considered socially vulnerable. Economically vulnerable populations include those with limited economic means and those living in economically depressed areas. These populations may not have access to many of the resources available to the more affluent members of society. They often reside in housing that cannot withstand the effects of a hurricane, earthquake, or another catastrophic event. They may have limited or no ability to evacuate from a threatened or damaged area and can lack the resources to shelter in place and be self-sufficient for days or weeks. These populations are also less likely to be able to withstand a loss of wages or employment.

Groups with health-related vulnerabilities include those who cannot care for themselves such as older adults, the very young, residents of long-term care (LTC) facilities, and some individuals with disabilities or chronic conditions. People with comorbidities such as diabetes, respiratory disease, or kidney disease are also considered vulnerable to adverse effects both from the disaster itself and from the resulting lack of access to healthcare or other resources.

Residents of earthquake-prone regions, areas susceptible to hurricanes or floods, and remote or isolated communities can be described as geographically vulnerable. This designation also applies to those living in locales already stressed by drought or environmental degradation and to populations dwelling near industrial sites, dams, or other potential hazards.[3]

A final vulnerable group includes those who have been displaced from their homes by the disaster. This can range from a few families evacuated due to a flood or wildfire to the mass-migrations seen across the world of refugees and others fleeing conflict, famine, and economic collapse.

The Disaster Cycle

Disasters are usually sudden events, but they are not completely unpredictable. The Gulf Coast of the United States will be impacted by hurricanes every year, and the Pacific Rim will continue to have earthquakes and volcanic eruptions. Climate change will result in worsening droughts and floods across the planet, and war and conflict will unfortunately continue to affect many places in the world.

Disasters and disaster management follow a cycle (Figure 9.1). Disaster planning lays the foundation for preparedness for future disasters. Preparedness efforts support the response to disaster events when they occur. The response phase is triggered by the disaster event, with the scope of the response dictated by the nature of the event. Following the initial response phase, the community moves into the recovery phase during which efforts are made to recover from the disaster and mitigate its long-term effects. This, in turn, leads to a review of the disaster response and recovery efforts, and subsequent planning and preparedness for the next disaster based on the lessons learned.[5]

Disaster Preparedness

Disaster planning and preparedness occur at a wide range of levels, including in local communities (counties, cities, towns); regionally (multiple county areas); by state, territorial, or tribal governments; and at the federal level. This preparedness involves developing disaster

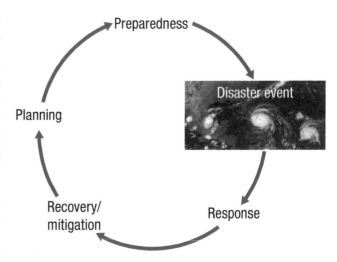

Figure 9.1: The disaster cycle

Inset photo courtesy of National Oceanic and Atmospheric Administration. https://www.jbcharleston.jb.mil/News/Photos/igphoto/2001953480

plans, obtaining and storing supplies and equipment, and constructing or strengthening infrastructure (buildings, levees, dams, bridges, etc.). It also involves training personnel, establishing command structures, designating shelter and casualty collection points, and conducting disaster drills. Another important aspect of preparation is developing mutual aid agreements with other local jurisdictions, which can provide rapid support from adjoining communities when needed.

Hospitals, clinics, LTC facilities, and other health facilities are required to have their own emergency plans. The Centers for Disease Control and Prevention (CDC),[6] the American Academy of Family Practice,[7] and others have developed resources to help individuals, hospitals, clinics, LTC facilities, and communities develop emergency preparedness plans. The U.S. Department of Health and Human Services has a comprehensive online collection of disaster planning resources focused on the needs of LTC facilities.[8]

The Disaster Event

Some disaster events, such as hurricanes or approaching wildfires, may provide the affected community with some warning. This can permit local authorities time to plan, evacuate populations at risk, and stage resources to respond. Other events may occur with no warning (earthquakes, transportation accidents, etc.). The disaster event triggers the activation of the emergency plan and the response phase begins.

Disaster Response

The common wisdom is that all disasters are local. This statement refers to the fact that when a disaster event occurs it is the responsibility of local authorities to evaluate the nature and scope of the incident and manage the initial and ongoing response efforts within their jurisdiction. Once they have evaluated the incident, local authorities can determine if they have sufficient resources to manage the situation or if additional resources are needed.[9]

When it is determined that there is a need for outside assistance, the initial request will be for mutual aid resources from surrounding communities.[10] If these surrounding communities are also affected or if the scope of the incident is beyond what these combined resources can manage, then state, territorial, and other resources may be requested. These resources may include EMS and fire/rescue strike teams, incident management teams, search and rescue (SAR) teams, disaster medical teams, and National Guard assets. Nongovernmental organizations (NGOs) may be requested to augment the medical response, set up shelters, and provide support services for displaced populations. If the incident involves multiple communities or jurisdictions the coordination of the response and requests for outside resources may be transferred to a regional, state, or territorial emergency management agency.

In a large-scale event in which local and regional/state resources have been overwhelmed, the state or territory will call on the federal government for assistance. These requests are often supported by federal disaster declarations, which provide additional sources of funding and access to federal agencies such as the Federal Emergency Management Agency (FEMA), the Department of Defense, and the National Disaster Medical System.

Requests for state and federal assistance take time to communicate and organize, which means local responders and emergency managers may be on their own for up to the first 72 hours. Local disaster plans should take this into account. Plans should also address how outside resources will be integrated into local command and control systems as they arrive. In the case of large-scale incidents, such as hurricanes or other events that can be anticipated, requests for state and federal assistance may be placed prior to the incident. Resources can then be mobilized and prestaged in a safe location to be able to rapidly respond in to the affected communities or regions.

A disaster response is a dynamic and often chaotic environment, and an effective response requires that all local and outside responders operate within a mutually understood structure. The National Incident Management System (NIMS)[11] was developed to provide such a standardized, structured approach for the coordination and management of large-scale incidents. The NIMS identifies key response roles and responsibilities, standardizes terminology and communications systems, and defines consistent operating procedures to permit response agencies from multiple states and jurisdictions to work together efficiently. All disaster responders need to be familiar with the NIMS, and one of its most important tools—the Incident Command System (ICS). NIMS and ICS training courses are offered by FEMA through the Emergency Management Institute.[12]

International disaster response may be provided by governmental agencies and by NGOs. These responses are usually requested by the affected national government and may be general or specific. The *Sphere Handbook* defines the minimum standards for international disaster and humanitarian response.[3]

Disaster Recovery and Mitigation

Once the initial response is concluded, or often while it is still occurring, the recovery and mitigation phase begins. This is a critically important phase but one that often lacks the attention-grabbing headlines of the original event. There is still much to be done, including physical cleanup, restoration of utilities and community services, rebuilding of private homes and public infrastructure, and the reestablishment of the routines of life.

During this period as the community works to return to its predisaster status, the healthcare system plays an important long-term role. There is not only the need to care for those injured or otherwise affected by the disaster event but also the need to continue to manage the physical and mental health of the community and to prepare for the next disaster event.

Disaster Planning

Along with recovery efforts, the disaster response should be reviewed and planning and preparation for the next disaster started using the lessons learned. Tools that can be used to guide future planning include after-action reports and operational debriefings. The goal should be to improve the level of preparedness for future responses and reduce the impact of future events.

DISASTER MEDICINE

The Austere Medical Environment

The medical response to disasters presents many challenges, the most significant of which is the need to provide medical care to large numbers of patients with limited resources. This situation is known as the austere medical environment. Resource limitations may be due to an overwhelming number of injured or ill patients; damage to health facilities or other infrastructure; damage or loss of medical supplies, equipment, and medications; supply chain disruptions; loss of staff availability due to the effects of the disaster; or most often a combination of some or all of these factors.

Operating in the austere medical environment requires a different mindset and a different set of assumptions and goals. Routine healthcare in the developed world is aimed at the prevention and treatment of disease and injury for every individual in the community. During a disaster, this is often not possible. The *Sphere Handbook* states that "the aim of healthcare in a crisis is to reduce excess morbidity and mortality."[3] The focus shifts from providing optimum care for each individual to providing care to meet the needs of the largest number of members of the affected population.

Under austere conditions, it may not be possible to provide comprehensive care for any individual patient. It may be hard to justify devoting scarce resources to care for a single critically ill or injured patient with a low probability of survival at the expense of not treating a larger number of individuals who have a much better chance of recovery if provided with basic care. These situations can create significant professional and ethical dilemmas. A detailed discussion of disaster ethics is beyond the scope of this chapter, but it is important that NPs who may find themselves responding to a disaster event are aware of the possibility of facing this type of issue.

One tool to address these ethical dilemmas is the use of predetermined crisis standards of care (CSC). These CSC provide guidelines for the temporary adjustment of practice standards during disaster situations where it is not possible to provide the usual standard of care, and for the modification of ethical guidelines to emphasize the needs of the community rather than the needs of the individual. One recent example of a CSC during the SARS-CoV-2 (COVID-19) pandemic was the development of protocols for the use of a single ventilator for two patients at the same time to adapt to a critical shortage of ventilators in some locations.[13]

The Institute of Medicine,[14] the American Medical Association,[15] the American College of Emergency Physicians,[16] and other organizations have created guidelines to help providers, health systems, and communities develop CSC policies and protocols as a component of local disaster planning. Another useful resource is the collection of regularly updated clinical practice guidelines published by the Wilderness Medical Society. These guidelines address the management of a wide range of conditions and situations that may be encountered in austere and remote medical settings.[17]

Disaster medical care may be provided in a wide range of locations and environments. If local hospitals and clinics are undamaged, they will be the first choice. If the volume of patients exceeds hospital ED capacity, other areas of the hospital may be repurposed as patient care areas. Most acute care hospitals have surge plans in place to be able to respond to these types of situations that identify what areas will be used for what purpose and how they will be staffed and supplied. If the demand exceeds this capacity, or if the hospital is physically damaged or must be evacuated, field hospitals may be established. These can be set up in locations such as sports arenas, community centers, school gymnasiums, or in tents erected on the hospital grounds or elsewhere. Temporary community clinics may be set up in any available suitable structure. Planning for these eventualities is an important part of hospital and community disaster planning and preparation.

In disaster situations, LTC facilities may be asked to care for more acutely ill patients than they might typically see to reduce the load on acute care facilities. Adult-geriatric nurse practitioners (AGNPs) and other providers may need to manage conditions or situations that are outside their regular practice. Caring for long-term residents may also require a different approach than during day-to-day operations due to loss of utilities, or disrupted access to food, medications, and supplies. Events such as the SARS CoV-2 pandemic may place LTC facility patients and staff at higher risk and require specialized equipment and approaches to care.

Increased mortality and other adverse outcomes among LTC facility patients have been documented following natural disasters.[18] Community disaster plans should include mechanisms to check on LTC facilities and homebound patients following disaster events to ensure their needs are being addressed.

There are other situations that may be described as austere medical environments, particularly for providers who are used to practicing in the setting of plentiful resources. In much of the world, clinicians must make do with chronically limited resources. In otherwise resource-rich nations, resource-limited conditions may exist in remote rural clinics, underserved urban areas, isolated wilderness settings, and other locations. The knowledge, skills, and approaches to problem-solving learned in any of these austere medical situations are applicable to disaster response and to a wide range of other similar situations.

Adapting to the Austere Medical Environment

Providing care under austere medical conditions requires a different approach and thought pattern. It involves doing more with less and refining care down to the absolute necessities. If one is faced with a large group of evacuated patients who all have a need for supplemental oxygen, but the supply is limited, how should they all be managed? There is not one answer, but options could include using the lowest flow possible for each patient, rotating who gets oxygen on a 10-minutes-on, 10-minutes-off cycle (which could double the effective available oxygen supply), and/or monitoring all patients clinically and with a portable oximeter, providing supplemental oxygen only to those who are symptomatic or have worsening hypoxemia.

Two key abilities in adapting to the austere medical environment are creativity and improvisation. What do you need to do and what do you have available to accomplish it? If a specialized piece of equipment is not available, can you improvise an alternative? If not, can you figure out another way to manage the patient that does not require that item? Dr. Kenneth Iserson describes this as the "How can I do this?" mindset in his book *Improvised Medicine*.[19]

A third pillar of adapting to the world of austere medicine is personal predisaster preparation. Learning about disaster medicine and obtaining and studying resources such as Dr. Iserson's book are important aspects of personal preparation. Another aspect of personal preparation is having and carrying one's own basic diagnostic tools (stethoscope, otoscope, pocket pulse oximeter, etc.), other personal equipment (headlamp, trauma shears, etc.), and supplies (personal protective equipment [PPE], etc.).

One should never count on having anything, even basic equipment and supplies, in disaster and other resource-poor settings. This can include one's own clinic or hospital after a major event when you are faced with triaging a large number of patients in the parking lot or lobby or working with no electricity, water, or air conditioning. Additional information on training resources and personal preparation is covered later in the chapter.

Disaster Triage

An important tool in managing large numbers of patients is an effective triage system. Triage systems are used in virtually all EMS systems and emergency departments in North America to establish the severity of illness or injury for individual patients and to prioritize care. In routine operations, those patients who are determined to have the most severe or life-threatening conditions are given top priority, while those with less severe conditions are assigned a lower priority. In a disaster when resources are limited, the prioritization system may need to be different.

As described earlier, the priority becomes population health versus individual patient care, and a patient who has a better chance of survival or recovery may be given a higher priority than a more severely ill or injured patient with a low probability of survival. Situations in which disaster triage may need to be used include initial responder arrival at the scene of the disaster event and at hospitals and other health facilities when large numbers of patients arrive by private transport or by EMS.

There are several multiple casualty incident (MCI) and disaster triage systems. One of the most commonly used systems is the START (**S**imple **T**riage **A**nd **R**apid **T**reatment) system. The START system is based on four basic criteria: the ability to walk, respirations, perfusion, and mental status. Patients are grouped into four categories based on these criteria: minor (the "walking wounded"), delayed, immediate, and deceased/expectant.[20]

When using START with a large number of casualties, all those who are able to get up and walk are separated from the rest and designated as minor. The remaining patients are then evaluated for their ability to maintain their airway and breathing, perfusion by capillary refill or the presence of a radial pulse, and mental status by their ability to follow simple commands. Those who have adequate respirations, adequate perfusion, and are able to follow simple commands are designated as delayed. Patients who have inadequate respirations or perfusion, or who cannot follow simple commands are classified as immediate. Patients who are not breathing or have obviously lethal injuries are classified as deceased or expectant. Depending on the available resources, immediate patients are given top priority.

An important factor in START and other disaster/MCI triage systems is secondary triage. As additional resources become available or after all patients have been assessed and prioritized, nonimmediate patients (delayed, minor, expectant) should be reevaluated for changes in condition and priority. The pediatric version of START is the JumpSTART system.[20]

Triage tags such as the METTAG™ permit easy identification of each patient's category and provide a place to document patient information (Figure 9.2). Those who may need to perform disaster or MCI triage should obtain training in the triage system in use by their agency or jurisdiction.

Resource Assessment and Allocation

Another important aspect of disaster medical response that APRNs may find themselves involved with is the assessment and support of local infrastructure. This usually begins immediately after the disaster event to establish the immediate needs for shelter, water, food, and medical care. As the situation progresses, this assessment will shift to determining what resources are needed and available for the ongoing response and recovery. New needs will often arise, including those created by housing large groups of evacuees in shelters. Specific things that need to be evaluated and addressed include chronic disease management, access to medications and supplies, sanitation, infectious disease management, family reunification, and social services.

Disaster Medical Care

There is not space in this chapter to delve deeply into the tremendous variety of possible medical and trauma conditions one may face during a disaster. We discuss a few important general topics and highlight areas for further study. The interested reader is encouraged to seek out specialized training and to refer to the references. In addition to general disaster response training, it is important to prepare for each individual

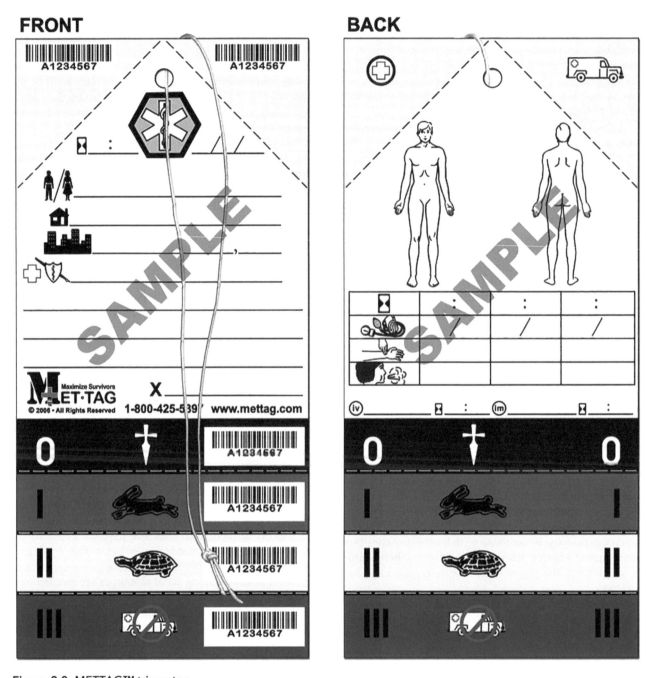

Figure 9.2: METTAG™ triage tag

Source: Image courtesy of the American Civil Defense Association, used with permission

response by educating oneself on the conditions that may be encountered on that deployment, such as crush injuries following an earthquake or waterborne disease after a flood or hurricane.

Trauma and Injury

Trauma and injury management include initial triage, trauma assessment, stabilization to the extent possible, and deciding who needs to be urgently evacuated. Assessment will almost always rely on clinical evaluation and judgment. Compact portable ultrasound devices can be of great value in assessing injured patients in austere settings when they are available, but other advanced tools will often not be accessible. Evacuation priorities should be focused on which individuals would benefit the most from surgical intervention and have the best chance of survival if evacuated. Care of those who cannot be evacuated may involve management of acute wounds and chronic or infected wounds, orthopedic injuries, burns, crush injuries, and blast injuries.

Chronic Illnesses

Patients with chronic illnesses are at high risk for adverse outcomes during disasters, their comorbidities make them more vulnerable to disease, and the disruption in services can exacerbate their underlying conditions. Care should be taken to monitor patients with chronic conditions in shelters or remote settings to be able to detect worsening of their condition and intervene promptly. Many of these patients will initially be stable, but they have a high potential to deteriorate as time goes by. A commonly encountered example is dialysis patients who will be well appearing initially but will become progressively ill as the time since their last dialysis session grows.

Shelter Medicine

While much of the publicity surrounding disaster medical response focuses on the initial response and the care of disaster victims during the immediate phase, the care of affected populations in the days, weeks, and sometimes months or years following the disaster is a major aspect of disaster medicine. Shelter medicine combines managing chronic diseases, caring for acute conditions related to the disaster or from other sources, and preventing disease outbreaks. It also involves doing what is possible to assist the disaster victim in coping with the situation. In situations in which LTC or homebound patients need to be evacuated to shelters, AGNPs would be a valuable addition to the team managing those shelters.

Infectious Disease

The primary infectious disease (ID) concern in disaster settings is communicable disease prevention and control. The nature of the communicable disease prevention requirements will vary according to the characteristics of the incident and can range from treating outbreaks of lice in shelter residents to providing adequate sanitation and the control of waterborne diseases to managing more dangerous outbreaks such as Ebola, SARS-CoV-2, or weaponized infectious agents. The risk of a communicable disease outbreak increases during prolonged disaster responses and with larger displaced populations. Communicable diseases can spread rapidly through populations in shelters and refugee camps, making early identification and control efforts critical. Natural disasters generally do not result in outbreaks of nonendemic diseases, but nonendemic infectious agents may be introduced by disaster responders or others coming in from the outside, such as occurred with the cholera outbreak in Haiti following the 2010 earthquake.[21]

Surveillance and identification of potential or actual outbreaks are necessary in most, if not all, disaster responses. This will typically be coordinated by the local public health agency. If a potential outbreak is identified, then isolation and containment of infected individuals, contact tracing, vector control, and use of proper PPE will need to be put in place quickly. This can be an enormous undertaking and one which can be fraught with unanticipated pitfalls. An understanding of the affected culture and society and how the population views the disease and the need to control it are vital in managing large-scale ID events. Recent experience has brought pandemic disease to the forefront of our awareness and the management of pandemics, isolation/lockdown protocols, and plans for mass vaccination or prophylaxis need to be included in disaster planning, preparation, and training.[22]

Disaster Mental Health

Disaster mental health has been recognized as a vital component of disaster preparedness and response. Victims of disasters face a wide range of stressors that can have significant psychologic effects. They may have witnessed the death of others, been forced to leave their homes, been separated from family or other support systems, lost loved ones, or suffered other traumatic events.

Competency sets have been developed for disaster healthcare, but only a few address disaster mental health. These disaster mental health competencies all focus on the same core elements—a knowledge of the psychologic impact of disasters; the ability to assess and manage mental health issues; an understanding of family-level concerns, such as bereavement, and community-level concerns, such as the promotion of community resilience; and the ability of disaster responders to attend to their own mental health needs.[23] Disaster mental health, including psychologic first aid, should be a component of all disaster medical training.

Psychologic First Aid

The World Health Organization describes psychologic first aid (PFA) as "humane, supportive and practical help to fellow human beings suffering serious crisis events."[24] Psychologic first aid is intended to provide practical care and support for those who are suffering following a disaster or other traumatic event. It involves assessing the individual's needs and concerns by listening and comforting them, helping them address basic needs such as food and water, connecting them to sources of information, and protecting them from further harm. It is not professional counseling or a postevent debrief. The goal is to address the person's immediate needs and to help them to feel safe and able to help themselves.

One does not need to be a mental health professional to provide effective PFA. Most providers of PFA are responders or community members who may encounter people who have been affected by a traumatic event. There are a range of PFA training opportunities available; a link to the American Psychological Association (APA) listing of training programs is contained in Table 9.1.

Culture, Cultural Competency, and Cultural Humility in Disaster Settings

"Culture" may be defined as the system of behaviors, attitudes, and beliefs learned and shared in common by members of a group. This group may be defined by national origin, language, ethnic background, religion, profession, shared identity, or other factors. Cultural competency is an understanding of the differences in language, worldview, attitudes, behaviors, and health beliefs and practices found in different cultural groups.

Cultural humility goes beyond cultural competency by emphasizing a lifelong commitment to self-exploration and a willingness to learn. It seeks to develop a respectful and humble attitude toward people from other cultures. Cultural humility helps each individual to recognize their own individual cultural biases and to realize that they cannot know or understand everything about a culture that is not their own.[25]

It is important to remember that cultural diversity exists everywhere. Each person you encounter in day-to-day life or during a disaster has a mixture of cultural influences that will impact how they will react when faced with a stressful situation. Every culture views health, illness, and the response to calamity in its own way. Depending on the location and culture involved, patients may subscribe to the biomedical model of health and illness or to traditional folk medicine practices, or quite commonly to a hybrid of the two. They may follow an active problem-solving response to misfortune or have a more circumspect "what will be, will be" approach.

The diversity of cultural practices and beliefs is immense but there is one general piece of advice that applies to all cross-cultural interactions, whether in your own facility or on deployment across the globe. Learn about the cultures and cultural practices of the groups you may encounter. This may be accomplished by attending training sponsored by your organization, consulting reference materials, or by meeting with local cultural, religious, or civic leaders who can assist in understanding local health practices and beliefs.

The Dead and Dying

An aspect of disaster medicine that is frequently overlooked is the care of the dead and dying. Palliative care in disaster settings is an important component of disaster medical response and is identified as a priority area in the *Sphere Handbook*.[3] Patients with terminal illnesses will still need to be cared for, and the stress of the situation may cause them to worsen. Resources to provide regular palliative care may be lacking, but every effort should be made to provide comfort to palliative care patients.

Patients who were not considered palliative care patients prior to the disaster may need to be considered for this status due to injuries suffered in the disaster or from worsening of chronic illnesses. This can be another situation where the resources may not be available to aggressively treat patients with a low likelihood of survival when there are many more who could survive if given timely care.

The dead need to be treated with respect and it is important to understand cultural practices and expectations surrounding death and dying. These situations need to be handled with sensitivity, but also in a manner that reduces the risk of disease transmission among the survivors. During the Ebola crisis from 2014 to 2016, one West African funerary ritual involved family members washing the deceased to prepare them for burial, which exposed many more people to the infection.[26] Arrangements need to be made to safely store the deceased to reduce the risk of contagion, even during nonpandemic events. In an ideal situation, refrigerated storage trailers or other methods of safely housing the deceased will be available. This may not be the case in remote locations, early in the course of the response, or if there is an overwhelming number of fatalities.[3]

Other Aspects of Disaster Medical Response

Disaster medical response involves a number of activities outside the direct medical care of disaster victims. Large numbers of evacuated and displaced persons will need to be sheltered, clothed, and fed. Evacuation shelters and the community at large will need to be monitored for infectious disease outbreaks. Secondary health risks to the affected population such as water contamination or carbon monoxide poisoning from generators or charcoal heaters will need to be evaluated and mitigated. Damage to medical and community infrastructure will need to be assessed to determine what will be needed to restore the local healthcare system and when these services can be reestablished.

Patients who have conditions that cannot be managed locally will need to be evacuated to a location with the necessary capabilities. The transportation of these patients will need to be organized, appropriate transport resources secured, and the patients will need to be tracked so that families can be kept up to date on where the evacuated individuals are. Arrangements may need to be made to reunify families who may have been separated by the disaster or in its aftermath.

Communications are often disrupted by the disaster event. Telephone lines may be damaged or destroyed, cellular phone towers may be damaged or without electricity, and internet connections may be disrupted.

Disaster responders need to be familiar with the alternative methods of communication and communications technologies such as radio systems, satellite phones, and satellite messaging devices used by their agency or agencies.

Another aspect of disaster communication that all persons involved in the response must be familiar with is how to respond to questions from the media. In most cases, these questions should be referred to the public information officer or another agency representative who is authorized to talk to the media. Responders must also know what is and is not appropriate to post on social media.

THE NURSE PRACTITIONER IN DISASTER PREPAREDNESS, RESPONSE, AND RECOVERY

Personal Attributes

Disaster response is by its very nature unpredictable and chaotic, and the ability to function effectively in this environment is key. There are many attributes of a successful disaster responder, the most important of which are flexibility, adaptability, and being a team player. Other valuable traits and behaviors are patience, a willingness to learn, creativity, and the ability to gracefully manage stress and change.

The Adult Geriatric Nurse Practitioner in Disaster Planning and Preparedness

Every NP should be involved in disaster planning and preparedness at some level. The most basic level is knowing your own practice site's disaster plan and contributing to the ongoing review and updating of the plan. Other opportunities to contribute include participating in local, regional, or statewide disaster planning, and in disaster drills. The AGNP is well positioned to be an advocate in these settings for residents of LTC facilities and other vulnerable populations to ensure that they are not overlooked in disaster planning.

NPs should also be personally prepared for potential disaster events. A significant factor in many disaster events is the loss of availability of healthcare and other vital personnel due to the impact of the disaster on their personal lives. If the NP can safely take care of their own and their family's needs, they will be better prepared to respond to the needs of their community and workplace.

The Nurse Practitioner in Disaster Response and Recovery

The role of the NP or APRN in disaster response may be broken down into two broad categories. One is when the disaster is in your community, and the other is when the disaster is somewhere else. In the first case, the disaster comes to you and in the second you go to the disaster.

The need to respond either locally or to another community or state can occur during any phase of the disaster. While the initial response often requires the most resources, there will still be ongoing needs that must be met. The initial wave of responders will need to be relieved and damaged local health infrastructure may need external support for an extended period during the recovery phase until it is able to function on its own.

When the Disaster Is in Your Community or at Your Facility

This is the most likely scenario most NPs will encounter. The primary challenges in this situation are managing the chaos of the initial phases of the incident and establishing a structure to respond adequately. Specific issues that may need to be addressed include loss of utilities (power, water, air conditioning/heating, telephone service), disruption of electronic health records and other computer systems, and physical damage to buildings and other infrastructure.

Patient care must still be provided with these limited or damaged resources, potentially for large numbers of patients. There may need to be modifications to the scope of practice of NPs and other healthcare professionals under crisis standards of care or on an ad hoc basis. Normal referral and consultation resources may be disrupted, and alternatives such as telehealth should be considered when developing disaster plans.

In some disaster events, hospitals and LTC facilities may need to be evacuated. The decision whether to evacuate a facility or shelter in place can be a challenging one. It is highly dependent on the nature of the disaster event. If there is significant physical damage to the facility or the threat of imminent danger, such as the flooding following Hurricane Katrina, then evacuation is indicated. If the facility is intact but there is a loss of utilities or disruption of access to food and supplies, it may be appropriate to shelter in place if the duration of the event is expected to be short.

When the Disaster Is Somewhere Else

Many NPs are interested in serving as disaster responders. This section discusses the role of the NP as a disaster responder and how one can become involved in disaster response. There are a couple of important caveats regarding disaster response. The first is that disaster deployments are not vacations, so responders should not expect any free time to see the sights or explore the destination. The second is that disaster response is a team sport. A successful team needs to train and practice together. The time to decide to become a disaster responder is not when one sees a report about a hurricane or earthquake on the news. The time is well before that when one can locate and join an established, reputable response organization and obtain the necessary training to be able to respond safely and effectively.

In every disaster, there are well-meaning individuals who decide they want to help, buy a backpack and a plane ticket, and show up at the scene of the disaster with a stethoscope and good intentions. They often have no arrangements for lodging, transportation, food, security, or a way to find out where to go and what the needs are. These individuals can consume more resources than they contribute. If disaster response interests you, devote the time to finding an agency to work with and learning what you need to know before the disaster occurs.

Response Agencies

Finding a compatible, responsible disaster response agency to join will involve doing some homework. There are many governmental and nongovernmental agencies that are involved in disaster response. One method of finding a response agency is to confer with colleagues who participate in disaster response for ideas or referrals. Another method is to contact established response agencies and find out if they fit your interests and availability. A list of some of the larger response agencies

appears in Table 9.2. There are also many smaller local government, NGO-based, and other teams across North America. Your state, territorial, or municipal emergency management agency can be a good resource in locating these organizations.

Disaster Training and Education

Receiving adequate training is important in all aspects of healthcare and medicine, and disaster medical response is no different. Training may be agency-based or from outside disaster training programs. Training programs can be broken down into a few broad categories. Disaster preparedness and management training are valuable for all who are interested in disaster response. It provides knowledge and tools for both personal and institutional preparedness. Disaster response training can include agency-specific training and nationally recognized courses such as FEMA's ICS classes.

Disaster medical training encompasses a broad range of topic areas. Specialized disaster medicine courses are offered by a number of institutions and professional

Table 9.1: Disaster Training Resources

Disaster Preparedness and Response Training	
Cornell University Emergency Management Program	https://emergency.cornell.edu
FEMA Emergency Management Institute (NIMS and ICS courses)	https://training.fema.gov/emi.aspx
Disaster Medicine Courses	
Stanford Disaster Medicine online training	https://online.stanford.edu/courses/som-y0015-disaster-medicine-training
National Disaster Life Support Foundation	www.ndlsf.org/all-courses
American College of Surgeons–Disaster Management and Emergency Preparedness course	www.facs.org/Quality-Programs/Trauma/education/DMEP
Wilderness Medical Society listing of wilderness medicine conferences and courses	https://wms.org
Hazardous Materials Response Training	
Centers for Disease Control, Agency for Toxic Substances and Disease Registry–HAZMAT Emergency Preparedness Training	www.atsdr.cdc.gov/hazmat-emergency-preparedness.html
National Institute of Environmental Health Sciences–HAZMAT Disaster Preparedness Training Program	www.niehs.nih.gov/careers/hazmat/training_program_areas/hdpt/index.cfm
Psychological First Aid Training	
American Psychological Association list of PFA training resources	www.apa.org/practice/programs/dmhi/psychological-first-aid/training
Academic Electives and Fellowships	
American College of Emergency Physicians -Listing of disaster medicine fellowships and other training programs	www.acep.org/how-we-serve/sections/disaster-medicine/disaster-medicineems-fellowships-and-other-training-programs/

ICS, Incident Command System; NIMS, National Incident Management System; PFA, psychologic first aid.

Table 9.2: Disaster Response Agencies

NGO/Volunteer Disaster Response Organizations	
There are many NGOs and volunteer groups that provide disaster response services. Many of these agencies also participate in other humanitarian medical activities. This is not an exhaustive list and no recommendation is inferred for any agency listed.	
International Medical Corps	https://careers.internationalmedicalcorps.org/volunteer.html
Project Hope	www.projecthope.org/ways-to-help/volunteer
International Volunteer Programs Association (volunteer agency listings)	http://volunteerinternational.org
American Red Cross	www.redcross.org
Canadian Medical Assistance Teams	www.canadianmedicalteams.org
Governmental Disaster Response Agencies	
National Disaster Medical System—DMAT and other teams	www.phe.gov/Preparedness/responders/ndms/ndms-teams/Pages/default.aspx
Medical Reserve Corps	https://aspr.hhs.gov/MRC/Pages/index.aspx
Many states and local municipalities sponsor disaster medical teams or other emergency preparedness programs. Consult your state or territory's emergency management agency.	

NGO, nongovernmental organization.

organizations. The National Disaster Life Support Foundation offers a variety of Basic and Advanced Disaster Life Support courses. Wilderness medicine courses and conferences can be a useful way to become familiar with the austere medical environment and many include disaster medical subject matter. A listing of these and other training resources appears in Table 9.2. Another component of disaster medical training to consider is education on the management of patient populations outside your regular specialty area.

Personal Preparation for Response

There are a number of things that individual responders need to do to be prepared to respond. These include having all of the equipment and supplies necessary to be self-sufficient for 72 hours and to be away from home 2 weeks or longer, having arrangements in place for family and work responsibilities, and making sure that one is mentally and physically prepared for the deployment.

The personal equipment and supplies required will vary depending on the response agency and the nature of the deployment. A basic list of suggested items appears in Table 9.3. The packing system recommended by many disaster response agencies is to divide your gear between a 72-hour bag (also called a "bug-out" bag) and a larger general gear bag. As the name implies, the 72-hour bag contains what you will need to be self-sufficient for the first 72 hours of the deployment. It should be a carry-on-sized backpack that you can keep with you at all times. The rest of your gear will go into the larger bag that can

be checked for air travel. All clothing and other personal property should be labeled with the owner's name and contact information.

A common concern among NPs who are interested in disaster response is how to get support and approval to deploy from their employer and colleagues. It is important to have honest conversations with existing and prospective employers about how this would be handled. Most healthcare employers understand the need for responders to assist when disasters occur. Not everyone is able to serve in this role, but a hospital, practice, or clinic can participate in the response by supporting those providers who are willing and able to respond by covering shifts and other commitments. This allows the responding provider to represent the organization while on deployment.

It is important to keep the leadership of the organization and the other providers informed about on-call schedules and deployment requests. Developing contingency plans to guide how a potential absence would be covered can help ensure that a deployment will cause minimal disruption to regular operations. Family support is also important and how disaster deployments will affect the family needs to be discussed ahead of time and contingency plans developed.

Disaster deployments can be physically demanding, and a reasonable level of physical fitness is important. Each response agency will have policies outlining its requirements. Other health issues that may need to be considered include personal medications, immunizations,

Table 9.3: Suggested Basic Deployment Gear List

72-Hour/Bug-Out Bag (~50 liter backpack, airline carry-on size):	
• Change of clothing, jacket, hat, extra socks, and underwear • Leather work gloves • Raincoat and pants • Basic toiletries kit in TSA compliant pouch • Sunscreen and insect repellent • Hand sanitizer • Personal first aid/emergency survival kit • Personal medications (7-day supply) • Spare glasses and sunglasses • Contact lens supplies • Phone and/or other communications devices • Phone cables, chargers, etc. • Water bottle and/or hydration system • Water purification tablets or filter • Food (24–48 hours)	• Waterproof tarp or poncho • Books, playing cards, recreational items • Earplugs, sleep mask • Headlamp and/or flashlight • Batteries • Map(s) of destination, compass • Reference information about destination • Pens, notepad • Personal medical gear/PPE (stethoscope, pocket mask, isolation masks, goggles or face shield, medical gloves, etc.) • Folding knife or multitool, trauma shears, and other TSA-restricted items in a small pouch that can be easily removed from the carry-on bag and placed into checked luggage
Main Deployment Pack (backpack or duffel bag with pack straps, 80–100 liter):	
• Clothing as dictated by mission • Tent and/or mosquito bed netting (depending on deployment destination) • Sleeping bag, sleeping pad, camp pillow • Personal medications (1-month total, including supply in bug-out bag) • Food (additional 48 hours) • Kitchen pack: plate, cup, bowl, utensils, paper towels, dish detergent • Toiletries bag, camp towels, personal care wipes, shower shoes/sandals	• Spare flashlight & additional batteries • Other medical gear • Pharmacy and medical reference pocket books and/or cards • Laundry pack: collapsible washbasin, detergent, paracord, clothespins • Sanitation pack: small shovel, toilet paper, personal care wipes, zip-lock bags, hand sanitizer • Repair/sewing kit, duct tape, safety pins • Contractor-size garbage bags (2-3, to line packs, emergency shelter, etc.)

TSA, Transportation Security Administration.

travel medical insurance, and personal evacuation insurance. Disasters can also be psychologically and emotionally challenging, and each responder should prepare themselves for this as well, as discussed in the disaster mental health section of this chapter.

Safety and Security

Safe operations need to be the cornerstone of all disaster response missions. This requires the full investment and compliance of all team members. The first priority is the safety of each individual team member and of the entire team. If a team member is injured or incapacitated, the team not only loses that individual's services but also loses one or two others who must care for or evacuate the injured team member.

There are a variety of safety hazards that can be anticipated and planned for. These include weather and other environmental hazards, water and foodborne illnesses, recurrent natural events (earthquake aftershocks, flooding, etc.), transportation accidents, toxic exposure, injuries, endemic/epidemic diseases, wild/feral or displaced domestic animals, and civil or political unrest, criminal activity, and terrorism.

Personal Safety

Each individual is responsible for their own personal safety. This includes learning and following agency safety protocols and maintaining situational awareness of one's surroundings and potential hazards. Recommended personal safety practices include knowing one's personal limitations, following the buddy system (no individual is ever left alone); protecting money, documents, and so on, using money belts, passport wallet/belts, or other methods; and having exit strategies or escape plans in place when in potentially hazardous situations or environments. The ultimate goal of every disaster response mission and every disaster responder is that everyone returns home safely.

CONCLUSION

The NP or advanced practice nurse is uniquely qualified to contribute to disaster planning, preparation, response, and recovery. This may involve helping prepare one's local hospital, LTC facility, clinic, or community for possible disaster events, providing care during a local disaster, or becoming a member of a disaster response organization or team. For those who have an interest in disaster response, it is important to become associated with a reputable, responsible disaster response agency and to obtain the necessary training before deploying as a component of disaster response. Personal preparation for deployment includes obtaining this training, making arrangements with family and employers, and making sure that you are physically and mentally prepared to respond.

REFERENCES

References for this chapter are online and available at https://connect.springerpub.com/content/book/978-0-8261-8414-6/part/part01/toc-part/ch9.

PART III

Population Health

CHAPTER 10

Specific Health Issues for Older Adults

Kathryn Sexson and Hannah Spero

LEARNING OBJECTIVES

At the conclusion of this chapter, the learner will be able to:

➤ Demonstrate an understanding of the common geriatric syndromes presented and the role of adult-gerontology nurse practitioners (AGNPs) in their diagnosis and treatment.

➤ Identify patients at risk for health alterations related to common geriatric syndromes based on their epidemiology.

➤ Construct a plan of care for each of the geriatric syndromes presented including risk assessment, clinical presentation, diagnostic inquiry, and treatment considerations.

➤ Develop treatment considerations, incorporating both pharmacologic and nonpharmacologic interventions, for each of the geriatric syndromes presented.

INTRODUCTION

Older adults are not simply adults who have chronologically aged past 65 but, rather, individuals who undergo physiologic, psychologic, and sociologic changes along a dynamic continuum. As adults age, their organ systems experience a decline in their ability to respond to stressors.[1] This decline is highly individualized based on the person's exposure to multiple risk factors and chronic illnesses).[1,2] In fact, approximately 70% of older adults have either mild or no functional impairments. There are many myths surrounding older adults, and we are learning more and more about the health and resilience of people in this age group as the population increases. Some of the more prominent myths that need to be dispelled by healthcare professionals include depression and loneliness are part of getting older; older people need less sleep; older people are unable to learn new things; if a person lives long enough, they will develop dementia; there is a point where the risks of exercise outweigh the benefits for the older adult; and changing lifestyle is of little value in the older adult.

The 4 Ms of an age-friendly approach guide the approach to practice with older adults. This framework includes the following:

1. **Matters:** What matters to each patient and their family? What are their values and preferences?

2. **Medication:** Is it necessary? If so, is it age-friendly. Does it adversely impact the other 3 Ms?

3. **Mentation:** Does it promote brain health? Does it identify and treat abnormalities (depression, delirium, dementia) effectively?

4. **Mobility:** Does it promote mobility to maintain function so they accomplish what matters?

The "what matters" is arguably the most important piece of quality geriatric care. Understanding what is important to the older adult in their care and what brings them a quality of life should guide all care discussions and decisions. Advanced care planning, including identifying a proxy decision-maker for healthcare and documenting care preferences, is part of this understanding and should be discussed early in geriatric care, but "what matters" goes beyond that. One's preferences during potentially life-threatening situations, as documented through a Physician Orders for Life-Sustaining Treatment (POLST), advance directive, or living will, are still important to complete with older adults, but the provider must explore with the older patient what they want their life to look like outside of those life-threatening circumstances. Do they want to focus on comfort and avoid any painful procedures? Do they want to maintain enough energy to play with their grandchildren? Do they want to take their daily walks around the block? Discussions centered on these priorities in their day-to-day life will direct how you manage any care needs that arise.

In addition to the 4 M approach to care, clinicians need to be aware of the common geriatric syndromes. It is theorized that individuals who develop geriatric syndromes have accumulated impairments in multiple systems associated with significant morbidity and poorer quality-of-life outcomes. These complex syndromes, often seen in frail older adults, present across systems and affect multiple disciplines, creating challenges to the typical approach to care.[3] This chapter focuses on the epidemiology, risk factors, clinical presentations, diagnostic inquiry, and treatment considerations, both pharmacologic and nonpharmacologic, associated with common geriatric syndromes not addressed elsewhere in this edition.

FRAILTY

Frailty is thought of as the geriatric syndrome that underlies all geriatric syndromes. It is characterized by physiologic decline in multiple systems resulting in diminished muscle strength, decreased endurance, and unintended weight loss with emotional, social, and spiritual impacts. It is a dynamic process that occurs along a continuum in which frailty can improve or worsen over time. As decreased resilience to physiologic or psychologic stressors occurs, it may be influenced by multiple modifiable risk factors (e.g., medical diagnoses, home/food/financial insecurity) as well as the presence of more challenging conditions, such as dementia and depression. Frailty increases the risk of hospitalization, and conversely, hospitalization increases the risk of frailty.[4] As this syndrome progresses it often results in increased dependence on both formal and informal caregivers.[5] Because of the increased risk of adverse outcomes for people experiencing frailty, early identification may provide a significant opportunity for modification of risk factors to improve the health of frail older adults.

Epidemiology

Bandeen-Roche and colleagues[6] conducted an analysis of the National Health and Aging Trends Study to calculate weighted estimates of frailty in the United States. They found that in the general population, 15% of individuals 65 and older were frail, and 45% met the criteria for prefrail. Female gender, racial and ethnic minorities, being in a supported residential setting, and lower income were all associated with frailty.

Risk Factors

The presence of chronic disease and environmental factors associated with lower income or underresourced communities place older adults at greatest risk. In addition, those who have undergone hip, back, or heart surgery or experienced a fall within the last year demonstrate greater risk for developing frailty.[6]

Clinical Presentation

Commonly, frail older adults present with at least a 5% unintended weight loss over the past year; express feelings of exhaustion; demonstrate weakness, slowed walking speed, and decreased physical activity; and exhibit less resilience when recovering from medical or surgical interventions.[7]

Diagnostic Inquiry

In busy primary care practices, efficiently establishing the presence of frailty is imperative. The use of either the nine-point Clinical Frailty Scale[8] or the five-item FRAIL scale[9] to identify and quantify frailty is exceedingly helpful. A thorough geriatric assessment should follow to identify modifiable risk factors and assist in comprehensive plan development.

Treatment Considerations

Treatment is primarily nonpharmacologic as pharmacologic interventions typically target underlying conditions rather than frailty itself. The plan of care includes a comprehensive personalized approach involving the patient and family caregiver in the development of patient- and family-centered goals. Interventions require co-creation to be successful and include exercise and nutritional interventions, vitamin D supplementation, reducing polypharmacy, resource activation, and considering palliative care strategies for individuals experiencing advanced stages. Collaboration with the interdisciplinary team, including gerontologic experts, physical therapists, occupational therapists, and a registered dietician nutritionist, can provide important expertise. The provision of caregiver support is also crucial to successfully mitigate the risk of frailty or improve existing frailty.

THE DEMENTIAS

ALZHEIMER'S DISEASE

Alzheimer's disease (AD) is the most common type of dementia, representing 60% to 80% of all dementia diagnoses.[10] There are two types: early onset and late onset. Specific genetic mutations have been linked to each type, including amyloid precursor protein (APP) and Presenilin 1 (PS1) and 2 (PS2) in early onset and apolipoprotein E (APOE4) alleles in late onset. Environmental factors, such as unhealthy diet choices and sedentary lifestyle, also appear to contribute to its development.

Epidemiology

According to the Alzheimer's Association,[10] 13.8 million people older than age 65 are projected to have AD by 2050. It is the fifth-leading cause of death among individuals older than 65 in the United States.[11] Multiple studies have identified racial and ethnic disparities in risk for dementia.[12] Even after adjusting for risk factors, Black persons are two times as likely to be diagnosed with AD or other dementias compared to their White counterparts; Hispanics are 1.5 times as likely compared to their White counterparts.[11]

Pathophysiology

AD pathophysiology involves two major processes. First, beta-amyloid protein plaques accumulate between the nerve cells of the brain. Second, tau proteins develop into tangles within brain cells. The plaques and tangles inhibit neurotransmitter signals in brain neuron synapses affecting nerve transmission within and outside the brain. Typically, these changes start in areas of the brain affecting memory.

Risk Factors

Although there is no cure for AD, researchers have been able to identify multiple risk factors. Increasing age is considered a major risk factor, as well as a family history of AD, particularly in a first-degree relative. Research regarding specific genes related to AD is ongoing, but there are four genes that have been identified as increasing one's risk: *APP*, *PS-1*, *PS-2*, and *APOE4*.[10] The presence of conditions and behaviors damaging to vasculature also increase the risk for AD. These include diabetes, heart disease, atherosclerosis, hypertension, stroke, autoimmune conditions, high cholesterol, high-fat diets, tobacco use, and a sedentary lifestyle. Damage to vessels anywhere in the body is believed to indicate potential damage to vessels in the brain, which can impair the brain's blood flow and contribute to the pathophysiologic changes of AD.

Clinical Presentation

The clinical presentation of AD reflects its pathophysiology. The earliest symptom is often an issue with short-term memory. Patients or their loved ones may report that they remember things that happened years ago but cannot remember what they did yesterday or what is planned for the weekend. They might also report they feel like they are misplacing things more often. It should be noted, however, that a patient may not have insight into the extent of their memory issues, so it is helpful to get collateral information from family members and caregivers. As the disease progresses, more symptoms become apparent as it affects other parts of the brain. The patient may exhibit increased confusion and disorientation, mood changes, and paranoia. As with other dementias, patients exhibiting consistent behaviors that interfere with care may be considered to have "behavior disturbance." In advanced disease, a patient eventually becomes bed-bound and unable to walk, swallow, or speak.

Diagnostic Inquiry

A thorough history including collateral information from those around the patient, in conjunction with a full physical examination, is key to identifying dementia, differentiating the potential dementia type, and identifying reversible conditions mimicking dementia. It is also important to complete a cognitive assessment (Mini Mental Status Exam, the Montreal Cognitive Assessment, or another validated examination). These tests provide insight into the patient's specific types of cognitive deficits, including memory, abstraction, language, new learning, or visuospatial skills. AD is primarily a diagnosis of exclusion; therefore, diagnostic laboratory testing should be completed for HIV, syphilis, vitamin deficiencies (B12), thyroid disorders, electrolyte imbalances, blood glucose abnormalities, hyperlipidemia, hepatic dysfunction (encephalopathy), and infection, among others, to rule out other potential causes of symptoms. When malignancy, costovertebral angle (CVA), trauma, or other structural brain abnormality is suspected, MRI or computed tomography (CT) should be performed. Research evaluating these imaging studies for AD diagnosis is still ongoing. Some specialists may use imaging to see if a patient's beta-amyloid level is elevated, a possible indication of the disease, but this testing is uncommon. The same can be said for a positron-emission tomography (PET) scan. It is far less common in the evaluation for AD, as it typically requires greater patient preparation than MRI or CT scan without providing additional information to that found in an MRI or CT scan. It is also often harder to schedule, as it is more specialized and harder to get approval for as part of a dementia workup. The exception to this would be if a patient is unable to have other imaging or if frontotemporal dementia (FTD) is strongly suspected, in which case a PET scan is more medically necessary. Neuropsychologic testing may also be helpful in identifying specific cognitive deficits that may indicate AD over other dementia types.

Treatment Considerations

Pharmacologic

Unlike other dementias, there are Food and Drug Administration (FDA)-approved drugs available for AD. Cholinesterase inhibitors (CIs) work in the brain to stop the breakdown of acetylcholine, a key neurotransmitter in memory and learning. Increasing the available acetylcholine is thought to slow progression. Donepezil is approved for use in all stages of dementia. Galantamine and rivastigmine are approved for the mild to moderate stages. With all CIs, the most common side effect reported is gastrointestinal upset. In addition to the CIs, patients with moderate to severe AD may be prescribed memantine. This medication regulates glutamate, another neurotransmitter involved in information processing and memory. Memantine is often combined with one of the CIs to improve memory, language, and attention to increase the ability of the person with dementia to complete daily activities. It can also be prescribed as monotherapy. Its common side effects include headache, dizziness, constipation, and confusion. When starting any of these medications for AD, it should be emphasized to the patient and their family unit that these medications will not stop the progression of AD. The intention is to slow its progression; no noticeable decline in mentation would indicate that the medication is working (see Chapter 13 for more information).

Nonpharmacologic

In persons with dementia with behavior disturbance, it is also important to provide the family with support and anticipatory guidance for addressing the behaviors. The Needs-Driven Dementia Compromised Behavioral Theory postulates that nonnormative behaviors occur in response to a specific need the person with dementia is attempting to convey. It encourages caregivers to reframe the way they think about their loved ones to understand distressing behaviors as unmet needs and seek solutions to address the need. In certain situations when behavioral disturbances cannot be managed with environmental changes, low-dose antipsychotics may be considered for management on a temporary basis. When possible, antipsychotics should be avoided in geriatric patients due to their side effects and black-box warning of increased risk of death in persons with dementia (see Chapter 13 for more information). Once a provider has diagnosed a patient with dementia, it is of the utmost importance that the diagnosis be relayed to the patient and their family unit. Although this diagnosis can be devastating, conveying the diagnosis in a direct and timely manner allows the patient and their family to start to cope with the news, learn about the changes to come, and plan for care. Although there are medications that can slow the progression of dementia, there is no cure for the condition. Advance care planning can ensure smoother care as the disease progresses, decreasing caregiving stress.

FRONTOTEMPORAL DEMENTIA

FTD refers to a group of brain disorders impacting the frontal and temporal lobes of the brain. Compared to other types of dementia, its onset is much earlier, with an average age of 50 to 65 years old.[13] Like other dementias, onset can be insidious, with symptoms progressing slowly over multiple years. Although some genetic mutations have been linked to FTD, most patients have no family history of dementia. To further complicate diagnosis, because the condition's primary features are behavioral, patients are often misdiagnosed with psychiatric conditions before the true diagnosis is identified.

Epidemiology

FTD accounts for 20% to 50% of early-onset dementias.[13] The Alzheimer's Association reports that FTD accounts for 5% to 10% of all dementia cases.[10]

Risk Factors

There are no known risk factors for FTD except a family history of FTD or other conditions that cause degeneration in the frontotemporal region of the brain.

Pathophysiology

The pathophysiology of FTD is similar to other dementias, but the affected areas of the brain differ. Abnormal protein clumps fill brain cells in the frontal and temporal lobes, causing the cells to become damaged and unable to communicate well with one another. When the cells become damaged, they shrink or atrophy, which eventually causes the atrophy of the entire lobe. The frontal and temporal lobes are responsible for executive brain functions. This includes decision-making, language, and personality. In rare cases, alterations in movement may also be present. Memory impairment seems to occur in more advanced stages of FTD as the damage extends to other areas of the brain.

Clinical Presentation

When diagnosing FTD, the history often provides the most insight. The signs and symptoms of the condition tend to fall into three different clusters: behavioral changes, speech/language impairment, and movement disorders (Table 10.1). Behavioral changes are the most common cluster. Symptoms in the same clusters tend to present with each other, but some people may exhibit symptoms from more than one cluster. In general, symptoms become progressively worse over a period of years, with average life expectancy ranging from 5 to 13 years from the onset of symptoms.

Diagnostic Inquiry

In addition to a thorough history, several other diagnostic evaluations can crystalize a diagnosis of FTD. Lab tests for liver, kidney, and other conditions should be completed to rule out other causes, similar to the workup in other dementias. A sleep study may be useful as well to rule out obstructive sleep apnea as a cause of the processing or behavioral changes. As with other dementias, neuropsychologic testing is key to identifying specific cognitive deficits to narrow the differential diagnosis. Finally, brain imaging such as an MRI or specific PET scans, like a fluorodeoxyglucose (FDG) PET scan, can also help identify brain abnormalities specific to FTD or other disorders.

Treatment Considerations

Pharmacologic

Antidepressants, such as trazadone or selective serotonin reuptake inhibitors (SSRIs), as well as antipsychotic medications, can help reduce distressing behaviors in FTD.

Table 10.1: Frontotemporal Dementia Symptom Clusters

Symptom Cluster	Examples of Symptom
Behavioral Changes	Lack of judgment
	Inappropriate social behaviors/ lack of inhibition
	Loss of empathy
	Difficulty relating to others
	Decreased personal hygiene
	Compulsions to eat inedible objects or put things in the mouth
	Overeating or new preference for sweet foods or carbohydrates
	Apathy
Speech/Language Impairment	Hesitant speech
	Sentence construction errors
	Difficulty naming things
	Difficult with understanding both written and spoken language
Movement Disorders	Tremor
	Decline in coordination
	Rigidity
	Decrease in strength
	Muscle spasms
	Inappropriate laughing or crying

With antipsychotics, however, it is important to attempt other interventions first to manage behaviors, as this class of medication increases the risk of death in people with dementia.

Nonpharmacologic

Although there is no cure or specific treatment for FTD, there are care interventions to help manage the manifestations of the condition. Multiple interventions can effectively maintain the patient's safety. For example, in patients with FTD with movement disorder symptoms, removing fall hazards or raising toilets may help reduce the chance of injury. Regular exercise may also support the patient's mood and processing, although the disease will continue to progress.

Caregivers may also be able to decrease problematic behaviors by changing the environment to remove triggers for those behaviors, keeping the home environment calm and structured, and identifying effective distraction tactics to redirect the patient away from the behavior. Those with language impairments may benefit from speech therapy, which can help them develop other means of communication.

Given the often-distressing behaviors and early onset of the condition, caregiver support is vital in the care of patients with FTD. The diagnosis and its manifestations can represent an immense emotional and physical burden for caregivers as well as a sense of loss of their loved one. Support groups, such as those through ADRD Caregiver Support and SAVVY Caregiver, should be offered to these caregivers. Identifying respite programs, adult day programs, or home health services will also allow these caregivers a break from what is often 24/7 care. In some circumstances, caregivers may also seek nursing home placement for their loved one when they can no longer manage care in the home. Early in the FTD diagnosis, providers should offer anticipatory guidance to caregivers and families about what to expect and services available so that they can plan for smoother care or transitions of care.

LEWY BODY DEMENTIA

Lewy body dementia (LBD) affects both cognitive and motor function. Studies reveal that the average age of onset is 75 and that it is more common in men than women by a ratio of 4:1.[14] A family history of LBD or Parkinson's disease has also been strongly associated with the development of LBD. An accumulation of misfolded alpha-synuclein proteins, also known as "Lewy bodies," in neurons within the cortex and substantia nigra cause the cognitive and motor decline seen in this condition. Although this is a similar pathologic process to that of Parkinson's disease, the disease that manifests is different. Neurons become less and less functional as Lewy body deposits increase until the person dies; there is no cure for LBD.

Epidemiology

It is estimated that LBD accounts for 5% of all dementia cases in the United States.[15]

Risk Factors

Increasing age, male gender, and a family history of LBD or Parkinson's have all been identified as risk factors for LBD.[14]

Clinical Presentation

The progression of LBD can generally be divided into three stages: early symptoms, middle symptoms, and late symptoms. Early LBD typically presents as fluctuating cognitive impairment. This includes difficulty concentrating, memory issues, changes in wakefulness and sleep patterns, and trouble with problem-solving or simple tasks. Early symptoms may also include autonomic nervous system dysfunction. A person may become dizzy, demonstrate orthostatic hypertension, have increased falls, and develop new bowel or bladder incontinence. In some cases, the early stage may also include psychiatric symptoms, such as depression, anxiety, or hallucinations. Middle symptoms include more motor impairment. In addition to continued cognitive decline, a person may start to have increased falls and great difficulty with speech. As a patient with LBD progresses into late symptoms, motor symptoms manifest even more; it is during this stage that the patient with LBD most resembles patients with Parkinson's disease. A patient with LBD may experience flat affect, resting tremors, muscle rigidity, a loss of coordination and balance, and a shuffling gait. When completing cognitive assessments, particularly the clock-drawing test, a provider may also note that the patient has extremely small handwriting.

Diagnostic Inquiry

The diagnosis of LBD is typically a clinical diagnosis. The patient history, from both the patient and their loved ones, helps establish the pattern of decline seen in this condition, starting with changes in cognition and progressing to include more motor impairment similar to that seen in Parkinson's disease. Certain features, such as the early presence of visual hallucinations and fluctuations in attention/cognition, further help distinguish LBD from Parkinson's disease or other dementias. The workup should include cognitive assessments, such as the Montreal Cognitive Assessment or Mini Mental Status Exam, as well as a full neurologic examination. Some patients may also be referred for neuropsychologic testing to further define their exact cognitive impairments. Although some providers may order brain imaging such as an MRI, CT, or PET scan to support their differential, these studies do not confirm an LBD diagnosis. As with the other types of dementia, diagnosis can typically only be confirmed upon brain autopsy.

Treatment Considerations

Although there is no cure for LBD, there are both pharmacologic and nonpharmacologic interventions that can greatly improve a patient's quality of life.

Pharmacologic

Cognitive impairments in this population may improve with the use of CIs, such as donepezil, memantine, and rivastigmine. These medications may help slow cognitive decline but will not stop it; it is also important with this class of drugs to monitor for weight loss and other side effects. A patient's parkinsonian motor symptoms may also be improved with carbidopa/levodopa combination therapy. If a patient's LBD includes sleep disturbances such as insomnia or excessive daytime sleepiness, melatonin may be an effective intervention in combination with sleep hygiene measures. Although antipsychotic medications may be used to treat visual hallucinations or other behavioral symptoms in LBD, they should be

used with extreme caution in this population given the increased risk of death (see FDA black-box warning). In LBD specifically, antipsychotic medications may worsen parkinsonian motor symptoms or autonomic dysfunction.

Nonpharmacologic

When a diagnosis of LBD is made and throughout the course of the disease, it is vital that providers support the caregiver of the patient. Nonpharmacologic interventions for LBD encompass environmental, physical, and behavioral support for both patients and caregivers. The combination of behavioral changes and functional decline in this disease creates immense emotional and physical strain on caregivers. Providers can support caregivers by connecting them to support groups, providing anticipatory guidance about disease progress, and identifying respite care and other support services for the patient. Triggers for distressing behaviors in the home can be removed to reduce patient anxiety. Complementary therapies, such as aromatherapy, music therapy, pet therapy, and massage, may also reduce anxiety and depression in LBD. This population may also benefit from physical therapy or mobility aids to maintain their function; consistent physical activity may also help reduce depressive symptoms in LBD. Modifications to the home, including ramps, grab bars, shower benches, and elevated toilet seats, may also help prevent falls as motor symptoms progress. For patients with difficulty feeding themselves due to a tremor or poor dexterity, wide-handled utensils, such as those used in Parkinson's, can help a person continue to feed themselves. If a patient develops difficulty swallowing, thickened liquids may be necessary to reduce the risk of aspiration. However, this should be part of a larger goals of care discussion with a patient and their loved ones.

VASCULAR DEMENTIA

Vascular dementia is caused by impaired blood flow to the brain, leading to permanent changes in cognition. As its name implies, the major etiologies of the condition are vascular, be they from an acute event like a cerebrovascular accident (stroke) or over time from a combination of vascular disease risk factors.

Epidemiology

Vascular dementia accounts for roughly 20% of all dementias globally, making it the second-most common type of dementia after AD.[16]

Risk Factors

The same risk factors for heart disease and stroke are also risk factors for vascular dementia. These include a history of stroke or transient ischemic attack, a history of heart attack, diabetes, hyperlipidemia, hypertension, tobacco use, obesity, and atrial fibrillation. Additionally, one's risk for this dementia increases with age, as the effects of vascular disease compound. What this means, however, is that individuals can decrease their risk for vascular dementia through risk factor modification: a low-fat diet, smoking cessation, regular exercise, and treatment of comorbid vascular diseases.

Clinical Presentation

The manifestations of vascular dementia vary depending on areas of the brain with impaired blood flow. It is more common, however, to see impairments in executive function (problem-solving and decision-making) than in memory. This is especially apparent when the dementia is the result of an acute stroke as it often affects cortical function—problem-solving, abstraction, language, and planning, among others. In addition to these cortical functions, a person with vascular dementia may demonstrate other neuropsychiatric impairments, such as depression, uncontrollable laughing or crying, indecision, sensory changes, or depression symptoms. The onset of symptoms can be acute (as with a major stroke) or gradual (as with chronic vascular disease). Symptoms are considered irreversible.

Diagnostic Inquiry

A provider should rule out depression, as this can manifest as mental status changes in older adults specifically. Additional diagnostic testing should aim to rule out other potential causes of the dementia or behavior change, like those discussed in the evaluation of AD. A patient's current blood pressure and blood pressure history can also help identify cardiovascular versus noncardiovascular sources. Brain imaging studies, such as CT and MRI, can also identify cerebrovascular changes that point the provider toward a diagnosis; these studies may show infarcts or white matter lesions. Finally, consider neuropsychologic testing to identify specific cognitive deficits. Individuals with vascular dementia often struggle with problem analysis and planning on these tests, though this can also occur in AD.

Treatment Considerations

Pharmacologic

Currently, there are no FDA-approved drugs for the treatment of vascular dementia. Treatment involves control of cardiovascular risk factors. In addition to lifestyle modifications, it is important to manage vascular disease, including tight glucose, cholesterol, and blood pressure control. Disruptive neuropsychiatric symptoms may be treated symptomatically.

Nonpharmacologic

Nonpharmacologic treatments include regular exercise, social interaction, regular daily routines, familiar spaces, and interventions to maintain safety based on the

patient's specific symptoms. Decisions about treatment should be made through shared decision-making with a patient and their caregivers based on the co-created goals of care.

It is important to educate the patient, family, and caregivers about what to expect. As the disease progresses, the person with vascular dementia may require increasing levels of care. It is unlikely, despite treatment, that a return to previous levels of function will occur. The provider can assist caregivers to connect to resources and to better understand and manage associated behaviors. It is also recommended that the provider discuss advance care planning early in the diagnosis, as life expectancy in vascular dementia is estimated at 3 to 5 years after symptom onset.[11]

DELIRIUM

Delirium indicates acute brain dysfunction and is considered a rapidly progressive neurocognitive disorder. Its pathogenesis is a complex interplay between the neurotransmitter systems and psychoneuroimmunology pathways.[17] It is characterized by altered attention, awareness, and cognition developing over hours to days. Delirium usually falls into one of five types: hyperactive, extreme hyperactive, hypoactive, mixed motoric, or catatonic[18–21,48,49] (Table 10.2). Long-term negative sequelae may result. Early recognition and prevention are key with a rapid implementation of pharmacologic reversal agents and nonpharmacologic interventions. Hyperactive delirium commonly occurs and often manifests with harmful patient behaviors to self and healthcare professionals. The absence of clear psychomotor activity is characteristic of hypoactive and carries a higher risk of mortality and other comorbidities. This is particularly true when it is superimposed on dementia.[22]

Table 10.2: Types of Delirium

Type	Manifestations
Hyperactive	Agitation, rapid cycling mood changes, hallucinations, refusal to cooperate in care, and restlessness
Extreme Hyperactive	Extreme uncontrollable agitation, significant mood changes, anxiety-provoking hallucinations, extreme restlessness
Hypoactive	Inactivity, sluggishness, unusual drowsiness, seemingly in a daze
Mixed Motoric	Cycling between hyperactive and hypoactive, cycles may occur rapidly or slowly
Catatonic	Immobility, stupor, mutism

Epidemiology

Delirium represents the most common psychiatric syndrome experienced by hospitalized patients.[18] Its prevalence ranges from 11% in medical-surgical units to as high as 87% in critical care units.[23] Delirium has been found to be as high as 50% in postoperative patients.[24]

Risk Factors

Risk factors for delirium include sociodemographic factors, comorbidities, high-risk medications, and sensory impairment (Table 10.3). These factors place older adults at significantly greater risk for developing delirium and experiencing subsequent sequelae.

Clinical Presentation

Clinical presentations of delirium vary widely. Disturbances may occur across multiple domains, including memory, language, orientation, perception, and visuospatial ability. Additional features include altered sleep cycle, psychomotor disturbance, and emotional variability.[23]

Diagnostic Inquiry

Rapid identification and treatment are imperative as delirium carries with it an increased rate of mortality for up to 22.7 months post–hospital discharge.[25] A thorough clinical evaluation is considered the gold standard. Confirm the delirium diagnosis with the Confusion

Table 10.3: Risk Factors for Delirium

Sociodemographic	Age >70, male, institutionalization, hospitalization (especially critical care)
Comorbid Conditions	Underlying dementia (5-fold increase in risk), depression, social isolation
	Severe medical illnesses including atypical presentation of urinary tract infection or pneumonia
	Burn patients, ventilated patients, surgical patients, or immunosuppressed patients
	Central pontine myelinolysis
	Electrolyte imbalance, acid-base imbalance, dehydration, hyperammonemia, hypoalbuminemia
	Substance use disorder
High-Risk Medications	Narcotics, hypnotics, anticholinergics, medications that possess serotonergic activity
Sensory Impairment	Highest incidence seen with vision or hearing impairments

Table 10.4: Delirium Assessment Tools

Confusion Assessment Method[26]	4AT[27]
Feature 1: Acute onset or fluctuating course	Feature 1: Alertness
Feature 2: Inattention	Feature 2: Abbreviated mental test
Feature 3: Disorganized thinking	Feature 3: Attention
Feature 4: Altered level of consciousness	Feature 4: Acute change or fluctuating course

Source: Inouye S, van Dyck C, Alessi C, Balkin S, Siegal A, Horwitz R. Clarifying confusion: the confusion assessment method. *Ann Inter Med.* 1990;113(12):941–948. doi:10.7326/0003-4819-113-12-941; MacLullich A. 4AT rapid clinical test for delirium. n.d.. https://www.the4at.com

Assessment Method (CAM) and 4AT rapid clinical tests for delirium (Table 10.4). They are easy to administer and have high sensitivity and specificity.[23] To ascertain severity, the CAM-Severity (CAM-S) is a reliable and valid tool. Collaboration with a psychiatric service to examine neuropsychiatric processes is recommended. Identifying the etiology is extremely important as is assessing for the presence of risk factors. Consider precipitating events such as substance withdrawal, paraneoplastic syndromes, seizure disorders, coagulopathy, stroke, infection, electrolyte imbalances, and myocardial disorders. If focal neurologic symptoms are present, eliciting the expertise of a neurologic consult is recommended.

Treatment Considerations

Once delirium is identified, correcting the underlying cause and managing the symptoms are integral to limiting morbidity and mortality, including sequelae such as cognitive impairment. Educating the family is imperative, including signs and symptoms; their association with an organic cause, usually reversible; and the family's role in management.

Pharmacologic

No conclusive evidence exists to support the consistent use of antipsychotics in delirium. Given their side-effect profile, careful consideration of risks and benefits in collaboration with the patient's decision-makers is necessary. Table 10.5 outlines pharmacologic approaches and considerations.

Nonpharmacologic

Prevention is the best approach. The Yale Delirium Trial demonstrated a reduction from 15% to 9% incidence of delirium in hospitalized patients by implementing a prevention protocol that used risk-based criteria and utilized strategies to target orientation, preserve sleep cycles, mobilize early, evaluate for high-risk medications, address sensory deficits, and hydrate.[28] The protocol has

Table 10.5: Pharmacologic Therapy for Treatment of Delirium

Antipsychotics	Use with extreme caution: Use time-limited trial approach.
	Clinical indications (clearly document in record): Significant anxiety or agitations that meet the following criteria: Causes patient distress AND Patient at risk of harm to self or others AND Unresponsive to nonpharmacologic interventions

	Considerations:
	
	  Choice based on pharmacodynamics and side-effect profile
	
	  Prior to initiation perform ECG to evaluate the QTc.
	
	  Monitor QTc throughout therapy.
	
	  QTc should not exceed 450 msec or 25% of baseline. If this occurs, stop the antipsychotic.
	
	  Use the lowest effective dose when initiating.
	
	  Monitor delirium symptoms.
	
	  If only partial response, titrate up slowly (start low, go slow).
	
	  Reevaluate a minimum of every 4 to 8 hours depending on the level of agitation.
	
	  Evaluate for side effects of the antipsychotic (extrapyramidal symptoms, oversedation).
	
	  Optimize electrolytes to minimize QTc prolongation risks.

	Titration: As the patient improves, titrate slowly back to prn dosing during the day with the bedtime dose being the last to transition from scheduled to prn.
Valproic Acid	Avoid use in significant pancreatic or liver disorders, active bleeding, low platelets, and pregnancy.
	Use with caution: Medications that share the CYP450 2C9, 2A6, and 2B6 pathways—monitor for inhibitory effects as this can elevate valproic acid levels.[41]
	Monitor drug levels, liver functions, and ammonia levels.
Melatonin	Showing promise in small trials for sleep consolidation and maintenance of sleep-wake cycles
	Given the tolerability and side-effect profile, consideration of a 3 mg dose as an empirical trial may be helpful.[23]
Vitamin B1 (thiamine)	Deficiency should be corrected as it is associated with several changes in mental status and should be given in conjunction with magnesium repletion.
	Magnesium is required to convert thiamine to its active form.[23]

now been implemented in multiple settings with good effect. Additionally, as the use of physical restraints increases the risk of persistent delirium by 300%, restraint use mitigation strategies benefit at-risk patients.[3]

Once delirium develops, using nonpharmacologic measures is integral to successful management. Using the ABCDEF bundle[29] has been shown to be effective. These measures include **A**ssessing, preventing, managing pain; **B**oth spontaneous awakening and breathing trials should be completed; **C**hoice of analgesia and sedation (nonbenzodiazepines preferable); **D**elirium assessment (CAM or 4AT), management (identify and correct underlying cause), and prevention; **E**arly mobilization; and **F**amily engagement (inclusion in rounds, decision-making, management).

PAIN

Pain is a common response to injury and disease experienced at all ages, but there are considerations specific to older adults. Understanding pain and pain control in the geriatric population can help this group better fight disease and maintain not only their functional mobility but also their social roles. There are many myths about pain in older adults, including pain as an inevitable part of aging, older adults being less sensitive to pain, or dementia patients not being able to report pain. These ideas are false. Older adults must be assessed for pain and it should be treated as an abnormal finding, independent of their cognitive status.

Clinical Presentation

The first step in understanding the pain of an older adult is identifying the type of pain and its possible sources. Pain is either nociceptive or neuropathic. Nociceptive pain can further be broken down into somatic and visceral pain. Somatic pain comes from the activation of pain receptors in tissue, such as skin, muscles, tendons and ligaments, or bones; it often occurs as a cramping or gnawing sensation. Visceral pain, in contrast, occurs

when the pain receptors in the viscera (or organs) are stimulated. This pain is vague and frequently difficult to localize. Neuropathic pain is the result of damage to neurons, peripheral or central; it might be described as a shooting or burning sensation (Figure 10.1).

Pain can further be classified as acute or chronic. Acute pain is short in duration and can often be related to an identifiable cause; it may be accompanied by tachycardia, elevated blood pressure, or diaphoresis. Pain is considered chronic or persistent when present for more than 3 months. Chronic pain is the result of changes to the nervous system, leading to an increase in pain over time.[30] Pain is commonly associated with depression, fatigue, irritability, issues with sleep, and social isolation. Compared to acute pain, it can be more difficult to identify a cause. When obtaining the pain history, identifying the type and duration of pain are key to treatment. Vital signs usually do not change in chronic pain.

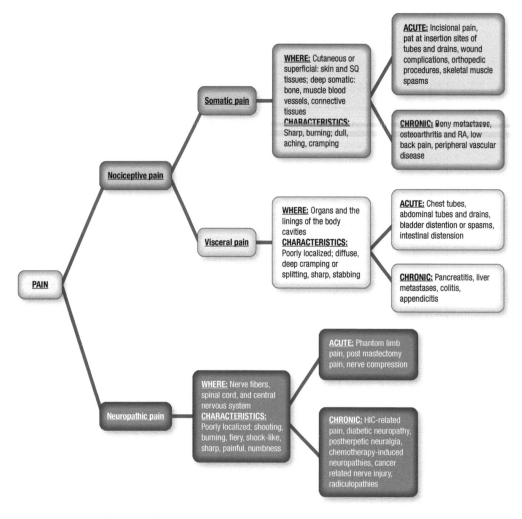

Figure 10.1: Nociceptive and neuropathic pain

Diagnostic Inquiry

The pain history includes similar aspects to other histories of present illness. The provider should assess onset, location, duration, characteristics, aggravating factors, alleviating factors, associated symptoms, treatments attempted and their effectiveness, and severity at its worst, at its best, and currently. Multiple scales are available to have a patient rate their pain severity, such as the Numeric Scale, in which the patient selects a number from 1 to 10, with 10 being the worst pain they have ever experienced. Another commonly used scale in the geriatric population is the FACES-Revised Scale.[31] It consists of six faces depicting pain intensity ranging from no pain to very much pain. When describing it to a patient it is recommended that you point to the first face on the left and state this face shows no pain and then state that each face depicts more and more pain, pointing to each one, up to the last face that depicts very much pain. When scoring the scale, use the numerical indicators below each picture. The physical assessment should further center on identifying any abnormal findings and triggers or relieving factors. For example, the straight leg maneuver can help differentiate neuropathic back pain from musculoskeletal back pain. In patients with dementia who may not be able to express that they are in pain, the provider should look for vocal cues like moaning, facial cues like grimacing, movement changes, or changes in mental status as possible indications the patient is in pain. The provider should also consider if a report of pain in dementia patients could be a way of indicating another need, such as anxiety or fear.

Treatment Considerations

Prior to the initiation of pharmacologic or nonpharmacologic interventions for pain, a nurse practitioner should set goals for pain with the patient. It may be that the pain will never go away completely, so it is important in setting pain goals to discuss an acceptable level of pain for the patient. This might be a numeric rating goal, such a 4 out of 10 or less, or it may be a goal related to function, such as being able to walk around their house each day. Setting a goal for reducing pain with the patient helps evaluate the effectiveness of interventions and provides more realistic expectations for possible pain reduction.

Pharmacologic

Initial pharmacologic intervention should be a nonopioid medication, such as a nonsteroidal anti-inflammatory drug (NSAID), acetaminophen, antidepressant, anticonvulsant, topical therapy, or muscle relaxant. Each of these medications, however, carries its own risks and side effects. When deciding on a pharmacologic therapy, the provider should consider the patient's comorbidities, kidney function, liver function, and risk for falls. Changes in drug absorption and metabolism that come with age may affect drug effectiveness and put the patient at higher risk for drug toxicity. Dosages may be reduced for older adults. In older patients at increased risk for falls, sedating pain medications, such as certain neuroleptics, may put them at even higher risk for falls. Benefits and risks should be weighed with each option. When it comes to opioids, they should not be used as first-line therapy in older adults for several reasons.[32] In addition to their risk of dependence, opioids can cause issues with balance, increase the risk for delirium or mental status changes, and lead to constipation, something older adults are already at a higher risk of experiencing.[32] With all interventions for pain management, a slow, stepped approach, with regular monitoring to determine effectiveness and side effects, is important to effectively treat pain while keeping geriatric patients safe.

Nonpharmacologic

The management of pain, at any age, depends on the type of pain and what is likely causing it, but there are specific considerations to make when managing pain in older adults. In general, nonpharmacologic interventions should be attempted in the geriatric population, with or without pharmacologic interventions. This includes ice or heat, distraction, physical therapy, cognitive behavioral therapy, and meditation, among others. Nonpharmacologic and nonsystemic therapies often present less risk to older patients. Overall, it is important to emphasize, particularly when it comes to chronic pain, that the pain may never go away completely and that the goal of any therapy is to decrease the pain enough to increase quality of life, allowing the older adult to engage in the things they want to do.

CONSTIPATION

Constipation definitions vary, but there are two consistent characteristics. Constipation involves (a) difficulty passing stool and/or (b) infrequent stool passage. Multiple clinical guidelines define "constipation" as having fewer than three bowel movements per week.

Epidemiology

Constipation is one of the most common symptoms in this population. In adults age 65 and older, 26% of women and 16% of men self-report constipation.[33] The prevalence of self-reported constipation is even greater in those age 84 or older, with 34% of men and 36% of women endorsing constipation.[33]

Risk Factors

Constipation should not be considered a normal or expected finding in older adults, but there are several aging-associated physiologic factors that place this group at higher risk. Over one's life span, gut transit time and colonic motility decrease, partially due to gastric wall thickening, a loss of enteric neurons, and changes in the internal anal sphincter and pelvic strength. Older adults are further at risk due to their increased likelihood of chronic disease, immobility, constipating medications, and dehydration. Despite these changes in gastric function with age, constipation in older adults should still be treated as an abnormal finding and worked up by the provider based on the patient's goals of care.

Clinical Presentation

A patient may report multiple days without a bowel movement and/or difficulty with passing hard stools. Constipation may make the older adult feel nauseous and bloated. Depending on the body habitus, a provider may even be able to palpate stool in the colon. In addition to these constipation-specific signs and symptoms, a patient may also demonstrate symptoms specific to whatever is causing the constipation, such as tremors and bradykinesia in the case of Parkinson's disease.

Diagnostic Inquiry

When assessing constipation in older adults, a thorough history can be guided by the symptom's potential etiologies. The interview should start by assessing the constipation itself, including its onset, duration, stool consistency and caliber, defecation patterns, presence of blood or mucus in stool, aggravating and alleviating factors, previous treatments, and associated symptoms. It is also vital to gather additional information about the patient's life and history. The causes of constipation are broad and varied. During the diagnostic process, one can consider the etiologies by category itemized in Table 10.6. It is important to ask about diet, activity, medications, and other disease etiology-related questions.

In addition to assessing the patient's abdomen, the physical examination and diagnostic testing should also aim to rule in or out possible etiologies. For example, does the patient have a normal gait or shuffling gait that could indicate Parkinson's disease? Does the patient report feeling fatigued and have an elevated serum thyroid-stimulating hormone (TSH), raising concerns for hypothyroidism? It is also important that the provider consider the patient's stated goals of care and individual risk level when considering any diagnostic testing. When possible, the nurse practitioner identifies the etiology and creates a plan to address it (e.g., electrolyte replacement in hypokalemia, increased daily activity for a sedentary patient). It is not always feasible to determine the exact cause. In some cases, there may not be a reversible treatment for the cause, or the treatment may be contraindicated or not in line with the patient's goals of care. In either case, there are also symptomatic treatments available.

Table 10.6: Constipation Etiologies by Category

Etiology Group	Examples of Etiology
Daily Living	Low fiber diet
	Dehydration
	Immobility
Medications	Opioids
	Anticholinergic medications
	Laxative abuse
Colorectal Conditions	Tumors
	Irritable bowel syndrome
	Volvulus
	Hemorrhoids
	Anal fissure
Endocrine & Endocrine-Related Conditions	Diabetic autonomic neuropathy (gastroparesis)
	Hypothyroidism
	Hyperparathyroidism
Psychiatric	Depression
Electrolyte Imbalances	Hypercalcemia
	Hypokalemia
Neurologic Conditions	Stroke
	Spinal cord injury
	Multiple sclerosis
	Parkinson's disease

Treatment Considerations

Pharmacologic

Pharmacologic treatments for constipation outlined in Table 10.7 include stool softeners, stimulant laxatives, osmotic laxatives, enemas, and other cause-specific agents. Ideally, when utilizing pharmacologic therapies, interventions can be temporary until the constipation episode resolves. However, in situations of chronic constipation that are difficult to manage in primary care, the provider may consider referral to a gastrointestinal specialist for further treatment as indicated and in line with the patient's goals of care.

Nonpharmacologic

Interventions include increasing dietary fiber, adequate hydration, and regular physical activity, such as walking every day.

Table 10.7: Pharmacologic Treatments for Constipation

Agent Group	Medication Name	Route	Clinical Pearls
Stool Softeners	Docusate sodium	PO	Generally safe for long-term use in older adults Tends to prevent constipation rather than treat it
Stimulant Laxatives	Senna glycoside	PO, PR	First line for opioid-induced constipation Not intended for long-term use Most common side effect: abdominal cramping
	Bisacodyl	PO, PR	Can worsen bowel obstruction Not intended for long-term use Most common side effect: abdominal cramping
Osmotic Laxatives	Lactulose	PO	Created for treatment of hepatic encephalopathy Older adults should stay hydrated while taking Hold for loose stools
	Polyethylene glycol	PO	Well tolerated for daily use in older adults
	Magnesium hydroxide (milk of magnesia)	PO	Caution in renal failure due to high magnesium Most common side effect: abdominal cramping
	Magnesium citrate	PO	Caution in renal failure due to high magnesium Most common side effect: abdominal cramping
Enemas	Warm tap water	PR	Can help soften stool impaction Not first or second line for constipation Considered safer than saline enemas in elders
	Mineral oil	PR	Can help soften stool impaction Not first or second line for constipation Considered safer than saline enemas in elders
	Soap suds	PR	Considered less safe than warm water or mineral oil
	Saline or sodium phosphate	PR	Avoid in elders
Other Agents	Metoclopramide	PO	Promotility Not for long-term use Contraindicated in bowel obstruction Black-box warning: tardive dyskinesia
	Linaclotide	PO	Used in chronic idiopathic constipation or IBS-C Contraindicated in bowel obstruction Most frequent side effect: loose stools Administer on an empty stomach
	Lubiprostone	PO	Works through chloride channel activation Used in chronic idiopathic constipation, IBS-C, or opioid-induced constipation Reduce dose in hepatic impairment Limited studies in elders
	Prune juice	PO	Well tolerated in elders Safe for long-term use Good as adjuvant therapy

PO, by mouth; PR, by rectum.

MALNUTRITION AND WEIGHT LOSS

Malnutrition can be defined as "faulty or inadequate nutritional status; undernourishment characterized by insufficient dietary intake, poor appetite, muscle wasting, or muscle loss."[34] Weight loss is generally considered to be a loss of 10 pounds or more, or 5% of body weight, over a period of 6 months to a year.[35] Often quite insidious, it can signify a variety of pathologies, which can be divided into six groups (see Table 10.8).

Epidemiology

Malnutrition and weight loss in older adults are common phenomena. In Europe and North America, it is estimated that 1% to 15% of older adults in the community and 35% to 65% of older adults in care facilities suffer from malnutrition.[35]

Risk Factors

As people age, there are some physiologic changes that may impact nutritional status and lead to weight changes. Body mass declines, gastrointestinal nutrient absorption changes, energy requirements decrease, and basal metabolic rate decreases. Older adults are further at risk for malnutrition and weight loss because of sensory decline in smell, taste, and vision in addition to environmental, functional, and socioeconomic factors. As one ages, the total number of taste buds decreases, and some taste buds atrophy. Older adults may also produce less saliva. The combination of these factors, in addition to decreases in

Table 10.8: Pathologies Associated With Malnutrition

Chronic Conditions	Examples: liver disease, pulmonary disease, diabetes, cancers, pernicious anemia, AIDS, rheumatoid arthritis, malabsorption syndromes, Parkinson's disease
Psychiatric/ Cognitive Problems	Examples: dementias, depression, anorexia nervosa
Medications	Examples: amphetamines, antibiotics, antacids, analgesics, antidepressants, digoxin, NSAIDs, oral hypoglycemics, steroids
Oral Health	Examples: poor dentition, dry mouth, thrush, oral lesions
Special Dietary Needs	Examples: cardiac diets, renal diets, celiac disease
Functional/Social Issues	Examples: immobility, low income, social isolation, poor dexterity

sense of smell, alters the experience of eating for older adults, making food less pleasurable and often leading to decreased oral intake or a change in foods they want to eat. Studies also correlate social isolation to malnutrition and weight loss.[35] Comorbidities may make preparing or eating a meal physically difficult, leading to a decreased likelihood of adequate intake. It could also be that an older adult does not live near a grocery store with affordable fresh produce. All these factors make older adults at higher risk for insufficient caloric intake, protein malnutrition, nutrient deficiencies, and unintended weight loss.

Clinical Presentation

Older adults with malnutrition and weight loss may have varying presentations with a few hallmarks. Many will demonstrate objective weight loss; they may appear thinner on physical examination. In severe cases, the older adult may also present with a cachectic appearance, with prominent bony features. Temporal wasting is also a good indication of severe malnutrition. In addition to weight-related objective and subjective findings, a patient with malnutrition and weight loss may also exhibit signs specific to their malnutrition, as discussed next in "Diagnostic Inquiry."

Diagnostic Inquiry

Taking a patient history to assess for malnutrition and weight loss should address multiple aspects of nutrition and overall health. It can be helpful to start with a screening assessment. The Mini Nutritional Assessment allows providers to assess nutrition in older adults quickly, asking questions about changes in food intake, weight loss, mobility, acute psychologic or disease-related stress, neuropsychologic problems, and body mass index (BMI).[36] The provider can then pull out more specific information about eating habits to consider potential causes; this might include who they eat with, food preferences, difficulty chewing or handling utensils, and associated symptoms. The physical examination, then, looks for clues pointing to specific types of malnutrition or evidence of weight loss. These findings will vary depending on the type of etiology or deficiency. For example, a vitamin A deficiency might present with ocular symptoms while a vitamin D deficiency might present with multiple fractures after a ground-level fall. Iron-deficiency anemia's only symptom may be a patient report of fatigue. It is also important, with all patients, to examine the patient's mouth, as poor dentition or other oral conditions can impede oral intake.

In addition to a physical examination, weight, and BMI calculations, a provider should consider specific diagnostic testing to identify any nutritional deficiency. Lab tests might include serum levels of vitamins A, B1, B12, D, E, and K in addition to iron or other suspected deficiencies. It can be helpful to also obtain the patient's pre-albumin level, as hypoalbuminemia may indicate protein malnutrition. Other helpful labs include HIV, complete blood count (CBC), complete metabolic panel (CMP), glucose, and thyroid hormone levels. If cancer is a suspected etiology, imaging or cancer marker labs may be indicated. If medications may be contributing to poor nutrient absorption or anorexia, consider obtaining medication levels when appropriate. Tracking changes in diagnostic results will also be important over time.

Treatment Considerations

Pharmacologic

Pharmacologic interventions should focus on treating the underlying cause. Enteral and parenteral nutrition are important adjuncts and may be indicated in certain conditions, although they should be considered in the context of the patient's goals of care given the potential for complications and decreased quality of life. If supplemental nutrition is indicated, consultation with the gastroenterologist, nutrition nurse, dietician, and possibly a psychologist or social worker is recommended.

Nonpharmacologic

Treatment of malnutrition and weight loss in older adults involves multiple approaches and involves an interdisciplinary team. First, if a cause or deficiency is identified, it should be treated. Registered dieticians or nutritionists may be particularly helpful with this in cases resistant to first-line interventions. Second, environmental changes may help slow weight loss and increase intake. This might include eating with others rather than alone or providing adequate light so a person can see their food. Third, a medication reconciliation to consider decreasing or removing medications causing malabsorption or anorexia may be effective. Fourth, special tools or prosthetics, such as wide-handled utensils, may enhance the ability of people with impaired dexterity or tremors to more easily manage eating, or properly fitting dentures in a person with poor dentition may diminish painful mastication; occupational health may also be indicated to assist in the use of some equipment. If mastication or swallowing issues are suspected, the provider may refer to speech therapy. In patients with dementia who forget how to use utensils, frequent snacks or increased "finger food" may encourage increased intake.

Overall, it is a good rule of thumb to encourage adding calories, not volume, to the diet of the older adult. Nutritional supplements may be helpful, but this should be implemented under the supervision of a registered dietician nutritionist. In patients who have been anorexic for longer periods, reintroduction of more food should be gradual to prevent refeeding syndrome. When considering supplemental feeding in older adults via artificial means such as feeding tube or parenteral routes, a discussion should be held with patients and their loved ones to consider the benefits and risks to the patient and consider together what is consistent with the patient's goals of care. In many geriatric patients, tube feeding and parenteral nutrition represent many serious risks with minimal improvement to their quality of life or survival.

URINARY INCONTINENCE

"Urinary incontinence" (UI) is defined as involuntary loss of urine[37] and is not a normal result of aging. Most commonly it is associated with overactive bladder, urinary retention (overflow), stress incontinence, or a mixture of these. It is a complex problem that impacts all aspects of the individual's health. Frequently individuals with UI attempt to manage through self-help strategies rather than enlist the assistance of a healthcare professional. UI is one of the most distressing syndromes for family caregivers and is often a precipitating factor for admission to residential care.

Epidemiology

UI is more common in older adults and represents a significant portion of those experiencing this condition.[37] Stress and overactive bladder UI are the most common. According to the National Association for Continence,[37] rates vary by living quarters with the highest rates occurring among nursing home residents (75.8%) and patients enrolled in hospice (62.1%), followed by community-dwelling older adults (50.9%) and home healthcare patients (45.4%). The lowest rate is reported in residential care facilities (39%). It affects approximately twice as many women as men with men reporting prevalence rates of approximately 15%. The annual financial cost of care is estimated at $20 billion and is a major factor underlying long-term care admissions; quality of life may be diminished, and fall risk is increased.

Risk Factors

The remainder of the discussion in this section focuses on overactive bladder (OAB) and stress UI. OAB, considered a clinical syndrome, encompasses both urge incontinence and symptoms of urgency, frequency, dysuria, and nocturia. Risk factors include problems with the lower urinary tract such as carcinoma, infection, atrophy of the vaginal and/or urethral tissue, and obstruction, as well as central nervous system disorders, such as cerebrovascular accidents, multiple sclerosis, and Parkinson's, in addition to certain classes of medications, including sedative-hypnotics and narcotics. Stress incontinence is precipitated by an increase in intra-abdominal pressure that results in urinary leakage. In women, this may be associated with poor pelvic floor strength or hypermobility of the bladder base most commonly resulting from childbirth or radiation. In men, stress UI is associated with trauma to the prostate or an underactive detrusor. UI is most commonly reported by those who self-identify as White and by those with a BMI of 30 or above.

Clinical Presentation

Older adults, when asked, may describe OAB as a sensation of fullness rapidly followed by urine passage. Stress UI is often related as a loss of urine with coughing, sneezing, laughing, and lifting. Symptoms associated with UI are generally classified as either irritative (frequency, urgency, nocturia) or obstructive (difficulty initiating stream, decreased strength of stream), and complications that raise suspicion of UI include decubitus ulcers, urinary tract infections, sepsis, and renal failure.

Diagnostic Inquiry

A careful history of urine loss or leakage is imperative but may be difficult to obtain due to a variety of factors ranging from cultural considerations to embarrassment, to the belief that "this is just what happens when you get old." Destigmatizing UI is an important first step. You might start with a simple approach, such as "When was the last time you accidentally lost your urine or leaked?" followed by "Does it impact what you do?" The mnemonic TOILETED (Thin, dry vaginal and urethral epithelium, Obstruction, Infection, Limited mobility, Emotional, Therapeutic medication, Endocrine disorders, and Delirium) may be helpful in assisting the nurse practitioner to identify underlying causes of UI.[38] If patients are willing, a bladder diary can be most helpful.

A complete physical examination is imperative and includes assessment of the abdomen; pelvis and genitalia; rectum; neurologic system, including deep tendon reflexes and sharp/dull sensation; mental status; musculoskeletal system; postvoid residual and provocative stress testing; and observation of voiding.

Laboratory testing includes urinalysis with culture, as indicated. If an obstruction is suspected, order blood urea nitrogen and creatinine levels. If polyuria is present, consider either medication or endocrine disorders (fasting serum glucose, serum calcium levels). If hematuria or sudden onset with irritative symptoms, order cytology to rule out malignancy and, in men, consider a prostate-specific antigen (PSA) for men older than age 50 and/or who have increased risk (African American race, family history of prostate cancer, as well as those consuming high-fat diets, low vegetable intake, and cigarette usage).[39,40]

Treatment Considerations

Pharmacologic

Nonpharmacologic approaches are first-line options in the treatment of UI. When medications are needed, the FDA has approved anticholinergics that block the muscarinic receptors and result in detrusor relaxation (e.g., oxybutynin, tolterodine, solifenacin, darifenacin, trospium, fesoterodine). These drugs carry significant side effects for older adults and their benefits should be weighed against the risks including dry mouth (affecting oral health), constipation, mood changes,[41] and cognitive changes. The beta-3 agonist, mirabegron, has similar efficacy with increased tolerability to treat urge symptoms and OAB. As with any medication prescribed to an older adult, start with the lowest effective dose and titrate up slowly to manage symptoms and use in conjunction with nonpharmacologic measures.

Nonpharmacologic

For OAB and stress incontinence, behavior therapies are first-line options. These options include bladder training, habit training (scheduled voiding), prompted voiding, pelvic floor exercises such as Kegel's, vaginal cones, and biofeedback. The physical therapist specializing in pelvic floor strengthening can be an invaluable partner in helping older adults manage UI. Furthermore, consideration of complementary therapies may be advantageous as evidence is emerging for modalities such as acupuncture, guided imagery, yoga, and others. Advanced practice nurses caring for individuals with UI may consider partnering with colleagues in integrative medicine to maximize benefits of alternative therapies.

CHRONIC INSOMNIA DISORDER

This disorder is one of the most common sleep pattern disturbances experienced by older adults. The *International Classification of Sleep Disorders*, Third Edition, diagnostic criteria for chronic insomnia includes (a) difficulty initiating or maintaining sleep, (b) adequate ability and circumstances to sleep exist, (c) experience daytime disruption, (d) occurs for at least 3 months and at least three times in a week.[42]

Epidemiology

An examination of various studies worldwide reveals a prevalence rate between 10% and 30% with some estimates as high as 60%.[43]

Risk Factors

Being female; being alone, especially separated, divorced, or widowed; frequency of alcohol consumption; the use of hypnotics; and concurrent medical or psychiatric disorders increase the risk of developing chronic insomnia. It should be noted that in the past we have often undertreated insomnia working from the premise that if we treated the medical or psychiatric disorder, the insomnia would resolve. We now know there is a bidirectional relationship between insomnia and comorbid conditions such as pain.

Clinical Presentation

Fewer than one-third of people experiencing insomnia seek intervention from a healthcare clinician, choosing instead to self-manage with over-the-counter preparations or other remedies such as the use of alcohol. Older adults are often easily arousable, experience less restorative deep sleep, and encounter less risk evaluation and mitigation strategy (REM) sleep, resulting in a sleep pattern that is often fragmented and variable in duration. Nocturia is often a problem in both males and females older than age 60 resulting in sleep pattern disturbances. Alcohol is frequently used as a hypnotic. Although it may help with sleep onset due to its initial central nervous system (CNS) depression effect (mimicking GABA and inhibiting glutamate), within several hours as GABA is metabolized into glutamate, excitation occurs, leading to frequent periods of awakening.

Diagnostic Inquiry

According to the American College of Physicians, the sleep evaluation should include a detailed sleep history and a detailed medical, psychiatric, and substance use history. An investigation of treatments used (both pharmacologic and nonpharmacologic) and their effectiveness should also be conducted.[44]

Treatment Considerations

The goal of treatment is to improve restorative sleep and improve daytime functioning and associated distress. Nonpharmacologic interventions are considered first line, followed by pharmacologic interventions or a combination thereof.

Pharmacologic

Ramelteon's side-effect profile is minimal, and it is effective for decreasing sleep onset and improving total sleep time; thus, it should be considered first line.[45] Moderate-quality evidence supports the use of suvorexant for improvement of onset latency, total sleep time, and nighttime arousals. There have been some reports of daytime sleepiness so patients should be cautioned. There is low- to moderate-quality evidence to indicate that doxepin helps with sleep onset, total sleep time, and the ability to return to sleep after waking.[44] Considering side-effect profiles in older adults, in the presence of depression, a low-dose sedating antidepressant may be considered. Gabapentin or nortriptyline may be useful in the presence of comorbid neuropathic pain.[45]

There is insufficient evidence to determine the benefits, if any, of benzodiazepines. Considering the risks of benzodiazepines, including interference with attaining REM sleep, increased fall risks, cognitive impairment, and mobility impairment, they should be avoided in older adults.[44,45] Although the nonbenzodiazepine receptor antagonists' side-effect profile is considered better, the adverse effects of dementia, fracture, and serious injury should dictate that they be used with caution.

Diphenhydramine has significant anticholinergic effect and should be avoided in older adults. Patients should be instructed to check all over-the-counter sleep aids for this ingredient. Valerian root and melatonin are also available over the counter. They have been shown to slightly reduce sleep onset and may produce residual sedation. They are not regulated, but if patients choose to take them, they should be encouraged to look for products containing the USP-verified mark to ensure they are receiving the ingredients listed at the quantity and potency indicated; that the product does not contain harmful levels of contaminants such as lead, mercury, microbes, and others; that the product will metabolize as indicated, ensuring its availability to be absorbed; and that it has been created in an environment that is safe and sanitary. This logo can be found on the supplement label.

Nonpharmacologic

Psychologic interventions shown to be effective in older adults (older than 55 years of age) include good sleep hygiene and cognitive behavioral therapy (CBT), brief behavioral therapy, stimulus control, relaxation strategies, and sleep restriction. CBT can be delivered through multiple modalities (individual, group, trained clinicians, web-based applications).[44]

SENSORY LOSS

Declines in sensory function (vision, hearing, taste, smell, peripheral sensation) are associated with aging and affect the way older adults experience and respond to their environment. Significant declines in function have been associated with increased morbidity and mortality.[46] Two of the most common impairments are loss of vision and hearing, which is the focus of this section as they have been correlated with increased mortality.[46]

Epidemiology

Approximately 67% of the older population in the United States is affected by two or more sensory deficits. Approximately 27% report only one deficit. Multisensory deficits are more common among older adults, men, and persons of African American and Hispanic descent.[47]

Risk Factors

Vision

The three most prevalent deficits are cataracts, age-related macular degeneration, and open-angle glaucoma.

Cataract Formation

Cataracts may form due to aging, diabetes, excessive sunlight exposure, tobacco use, obesity, hypertension, prior eye injury or surgical intervention, prolonged use of corticosteroids, and excessive alcohol intake; these conditions place the older adult at risk for cataract formation.

Age-Related Macular Degeneration

Factors associated with increased risk of developing age-related macular degeneration include age over 50, family history, Caucasian descent, smoking, obesity, and cardiovascular disease.

Open-Angle Glaucoma

Because damage may occur prior to the onset of signs or symptoms, it is important to understand and mitigate risk factors. Risks for developing glaucoma are increased when intraocular pressures (IOP) are elevated; age is greater than 60; being of Black, Asian, or Hispanic descent; family history of glaucoma; comorbidities including diabetes, heart disease, hypertension, and sickle cell anemia; history of thinning of the cornea; significant myopia or hyperopia; eye injury; and corticosteroids, especially ophthalmic solutions for an extended period.

Hearing Loss

Hearing deficits commonly occur from damage or loss of the cilia and nerve cells in the inner ear. Aging results in degeneration of these structures over time and represents the culmination of damage from loud noises that has occurred over the years. A history of short bouts of excessive noise (gunfire), genetic factors, occupational exposures to loud noises, recreational exposure (motorcycles, 4-wheelers, snow vehicles), loud music, a history of ototoxic medication use, and a history of high fevers place older adults at risk for increased hearing loss.

Clinical Presentation

Vision

All ocular structures (cornea, pupils, lens, ocular muscles, etc.) undergo changes as we age. Patients will commonly complain of difficulty focusing on items that are closer to the eye, difficulty discriminating fine detail, a loss of peripheral vision and difficulty rapidly adjusting to changes in lighting levels (bright lights/darkness), experiencing dry eyes, seeing "floaters," and having difficulty looking upward.

Hearing

Presbycusis is often reported as difficulty hearing higher pitched sounds (female, child voices), a loss of consonant differentiation, requiring more time to process auditory input, inability to filter background noise (e.g., crowded restaurants), tinnitus, significant cerumen accumulation, and balance impairments. Hearing loss may result in social isolation, significant communication impairment, memory loss, and decreased quality of life.

Diagnostic Inquiry

Vision Loss

More common diagnoses to consider that are not a normal part of aging are age-related macular degeneration, cataracts, and chronic open-angle glaucoma. As with all complaints, a thorough history and examination are warranted. Testing for visual acuity, visual fields, extraocular movements, fundoscopic evaluation, and, when warranted, slit lamp, CT, MRI, and tonometry are all part of the diagnostic evaluation.

Hearing Loss

Screen hearing at the primary care annual wellness visit.[48,50] Abnormal findings should be referred to a hearing specialist. The physical examination should include otoscopy, screening tests (e.g., whisper), and evaluation for sensorineural or conductive hearing loss. If abnormalities are present, additional diagnostic evaluation may include audiogram, CT/MRI, biopsy, and tympanocentesis. Common disorders in older adults include conductive and/or sensorineural hearing loss, central auditory processing disorder, tinnitus, and Meniere's disease.

Treatment Considerations

Collaboration with ophthalmology and encouraging regular eye examinations are important strategies to prevent adverse outcomes from normal aging and to develop appropriate treatment plans for eye disorders. For low-vision disorders, incorporating a low-vision rehabilitation specialist and community resources, such as the Center for the Blind, may be helpful for your patients. The Center for the Blind also helps with low vision and often is able to access grants and resources to help with assistive devices. Collaboration with an audiologist and/or ENT specialist is recommended to address hearing loss. Telephone technology has advanced considerably as the telephone has become the main method of verbal communication among more than 1.7 billion users worldwide. Special telephones are available with closed captioning, volume amplification well beyond that of a standard telephone, voice modifications for high and low voice tones, filters to eliminate background noise, and ringer amplification. Programs exist in almost all states through the Center for the Hearing Impaired to support individuals with hearing loss.

Pharmacologic

Collaborate with ophthalmology for pharmacologic treatment of visual impairment and monitor for side effects. There are no current pharmacologic treatments for hearing loss.

Nonpharmacologic

Risk reduction for cataracts includes healthy weight, healthy diet, sunglass usage to protect from ultraviolet light damage, not smoking, moderation in alcohol intake, ensuring hypertension and diabetes are well controlled, and wearing eye protection to prevent injuries. Risk reduction for age-related macular degeneration includes ensuring cardiovascular conditions are well controlled, abstaining from tobacco usage, maintaining a healthy weight, engaging in regular exercise, and consuming a healthy diet with at least five servings of fruits and vegetables and including omega-3 fatty acids. Risk reduction for glaucoma includes regular eye examinations to help detect glaucoma in its early stages so that vision loss can be minimized. If you are at risk for glaucoma, more frequent screening may be needed. Exercise should be encouraged to promote vascular health and reduce IOP. If patients have increased IOP that does not yet meet the criteria for a diagnosis of glaucoma, encourage them to use the prescribed ophthalmic medication to reduce IOP and mitigate the risk of progression.

Risk reduction for hearing loss including ear protection is recommended to limit deficits and progression.

MOBILITY AND FUNCTIONAL DECLINE

Functional status includes the ability to independently perform either activities of daily living (ADLs) or instrumental activities of daily living (IADLs). It is a sensitive indicator of health in older adults. ADLs include bathing, dressing, grooming, toileting, mobility (transfers), and feeding. IADLs include self-administration of medications, grocery shopping, meal preparation, using the telephone, managing finances, driving, transportation, housekeeping, and laundry. Functional decline is considered when an individual has difficulty performing one or more of these tasks or requires the assistance of one or more individuals to perform one or more of these tasks. The functional assessment has now been incorporated into the annual wellness visit for all Medicare beneficiaries as it is recognized that comparative functional status assessments are needed to accurately identify disability, potential illness, and changes associated with normal aging. Failure to complete this assessment may lead to an increased risk of complications such as hospital admission, nursing home relocation, malnutrition, falls, decreased quality of life, and increased mortality risk.

Epidemiology

Okoro, Hollis, Cyrus, and Griffin-Blake[49] reported approximately one in five older adults are disabled, with an overall prevalence of mobility deficits of 13.7%, vision deficits 6.6%, and self-care deficits 5.5%. Prevalence statistics were higher in women overall except in hearing and self-care. Men reported a prevalence of 19.4% compared to women at 11.3%, with self-care reporting approximately the same. Of older adults reporting by race, 54.9% of American Indians/Alaska Natives, 50.5% of Hispanics, and 49.9% of other race or multiracial identification reported a disability in at least one area. The rate of disability declines as poverty declines. Of those 65 and older, the most common unmet healthcare needs because of cost occurred in hearing (7.3%) and self-care (14%).

Risk Factors

Risk factors for functional decline include existing functional loss prior to a hospitalization, two or more comorbidities, administration of five or more prescription medications, hospitalization or emergency department visit within the last 12 months, depression, delirium, cognitive impairment, pain, malnutrition, self-assessment of independence, and fear of falling.[50]

Clinical Presentation

Clinically, patients present with deficits in gait, hand strength, sensory abilities, cognition, and increased pain levels.

Diagnostic Inquiry

A comprehensive functional assessment is needed to determine the patient's functional status and any potential causes of decline. The comprehensive assessment may include the patient, the family, and any caregivers to ensure accurate assessment data. Evaluation involves ability to perform IADLs (Lawton IADL scale, DAFA [Direct Assessment of Functional Abilities] for persons with dementia), ADLs (Katz ADL Index), and ability to independently engage in social activities as well as sensory abilities, pain level, cognitive status, ambulation abilities (Timed Up and Go Test), degree of frailty (Fried Frailty Scale), cognitive screening (mini-COG, MOCA, clock drawing, three-item recall at 1 minute), depression screening (PHQ-2), and patient perception of health (SF-36 version 2 or SF–6D). Determination of causes or potential risk may be ascertained from the following testing as medically indicated: CBC with differential (anemia, infection), CMP (glucose levels, renal dysfunction, hepatic dysfunction, electrolyte imbalance), urinalysis (infection), B12 levels (anemia), TSH (hypothyroidism), erythrocyte sedimentation rate (ESR)/ C-reactive protein (CRP) (inflammatory process), EKG (arrhythmia), and dual-energy x-ray absorptiometry (DEXA; osteopenia/osteoporosis) and chest x-ray (if suspect pneumonia). Any older adult experiencing sudden loss in abilities should be evaluated for an acute illness.

Treatment Considerations

The key to decreasing functional decline and its complications is prevention, early detection, and early intervention. The goal of any intervention is to preserve or improve mobility and function.

Pharmacologic

Pharmacologic interventions should address any reversible underlying causes that may be contributing to the decline or potential decline. This may include medication for depression (SSRI, serotonin and noradrenaline reuptake inhibitor, tricyclic antidepressant), treatment of hypothyroidism (levothyroxine), anemia (iron, B12, folate), infection (antibiotics), diabetes management, electrolyte replacement, bisphosphonates, calcium, vitamin D, treatment of dementia or Parkinson's, pain management, and others. But the mainstay of treatment for mobility and functional decline is nonpharmacologic.

Nonpharmacologic

Interprofessional approaches to functional decline have been found to be the most effective. Consider referrals to occupational therapy for fine motor strengthening such as improvement of grip strength and assistive device recommendations; physical therapy for muscle strengthening, balance and gait training, and development of a home exercise program; a registered dietician for nutritional evaluation and strategies to address any deficits; social services to mobilize resources and support group referrals; and a mental health provider if counseling is warranted. Weight management is a top priority to reduce the risk of comorbidity and load on weight-bearing joints. Encourage 30 minutes of mild to moderate aerobic activity 5 days a week and strength training 2 days a week as tolerated. The older adult's ability to manage medications should be addressed and consultation with the pharmacist to reduce pill load should be considered. Additionally, if organizational or reminder strategies are needed, consider mediset, medication alarms, or other assistive devices.

PRESSURE INJURIES

Pressure injuries represent the failure of the largest organ system in the body and affect approximately one million people at a cost of $1.6 billion annually.[1] Older adults have multiple risk factors for developing soft tissue injury, including loss of protective layers over boney prominences, alterations in nutrition, perfusion, comorbidities, and medications. The National Pressure Injury Advisory Panel Guidelines[51] describe pressure injuries as localized injury to the skin and/or the underlying tissue, typically over a bony prominence or associated with medical or other devices. The injury may manifest as either intact skin or an open ulcer. It may be painful. The injury results from intense pressure, prolonged pressure, or pressure in combination with shear. The National Pressure Injury Advisory Panel Guidelines[51] offer a clear explanation of staging, prevention, and treatment.

ADVANCING AGE AS A RISK FACTOR

Certain physiologic processes diminish for many individuals as they age (renal blood flow and glomerular filtration rate, glucose tolerance, taste, cellular immunity) while others remain unchanged (e.g., total lung capacity). As discussed throughout this chapter, the way disease manifests (e.g., infection) may be strikingly different, and although chronic disease may occur at any point throughout the life span, there are a number of diseases for which advancing age is a risk factor that are discussed elsewhere in this text. These include arthritis (Chapter 21), hypertension (Chapter 20), asthma (Chapter 19), cancer (Chapter 27), chronic bronchitis (Chapter 19), coronary artery disease (Chapter 20), diabetes (Chapter 26), osteoporosis (Chapter 21), hyperlipidemia (Chapter 20), herpes zoster (Chapter 28), chronic kidney disease (Chapter 23), and cerebrovascular accident (Chapter 17).

According to the National Council on Aging,[52] advancing age, social isolation, disability, and cognitive impairment place older adults at increased risk for abuse and neglect. This includes physical, sexual, and emotional abuse; confinement (isolating); passive neglect; willful deprivation; and financial exploitation. It is estimated that approximately 10% of people older than age 60 have experienced at least one of these forms of mistreatment. The mistreatment is most commonly perpetrated by someone well known to them (spouse, adult child, other family member). As mandatory reporters, clinicians are required to report suspected abuse, but reducing risk should be a priority of care. Interventions that have been shown to be successful are encouraging older adults to seek care for substance use disorders and depression both for themselves and their family members. Providing resources for caregivers and older adults, such as support groups, to learn ways to minimize risks for mistreatment; encouraging older adults to maintain connections to family and friends; advocating older adults have their own means of communication (e.g., phone, computer) rather than relying solely on a family member for connection; supporting the use of direct deposit to avoid potential financial abuse; discouraging the provision of personal information over the phone; and informing them of how to access assistance should they need it are integral to reducing the risk for abuse.

CONCLUSION

Quality of life is the primary goal of care in this population. A patient- or family-centered approach can be invaluable to achieving this goal. If a caregiver is involved, their preparedness should be assessed, and training provided as indicated. Finally, the use of motivational interviewing and shared decision-making approaches are vital to preservation and improvement in quality of life for the elder and those in their social circle.

REFERENCES

References for this chapter are online and available at https://connect.springerpub.com/content/book/978-0 -8261-8414-6/part/part01/toc-part/ch10.

CHAPTER 11

Specific Health Issues for Adolescents

Cathy M. St. Pierre

LEARNING OBJECTIVES

At the conclusion of this chapter, readers should be able to:

➤ Describe the physical and psychologic stages of development for adolescents.
➤ Discuss behaviors and approaches to prevention and early screening of risk-taking behaviors in adolescents.
➤ Conduct appropriate health screenings and assessment of adolescents.
➤ Have knowledge of potential ethical dilemmas when caring for adolescents.
➤ Identify professional resources for health promotion and assessment of adolescents.
➤ Describe the APRN role in the assessment and treatment of adolescents and their parents/caretakers.

INTRODUCTION

Adolescence is a time of complex physical and psychologic development. Adolescents' physical bodies undergo rapid changes as their mind and body mature for functioning as responsible adults. For both parents and teens, it is often an exciting and distressing time. For teens, this is an exciting period of transition toward adulthood and independence. The purpose of this chapter is to discuss multiple aspects of the physical and psychologic development of adolescents as they mature and grow into adulthood. The chapter includes frameworks to utilize in assessing adolescents at wellness visits and provides guidelines for anticipatory guidance. In addition, this chapter focuses on some of the developmental phases that adolescences may experience and a review of at-risk behaviors including experimentation with substances, such as alcohol, cigarettes, and illicit drugs. The chapter also covers potential risks, such as rape trauma, intentional and unintentional pregnancy, and sexual experimentation. Pertinent case studies illustrating some of the complexities that Advanced Practice Registered Nurse (APRN) may encounter as they provide care for

Box 11.1: Top Five Causes of Deaths in Adolescents
1. Unintentional Injuries
2. Homicide
3. Suicide
4. Cancer
5. Heart Disease

Source: Cunningham RM, Walton MA, Carter PM. The major causes of death in children and adolescents in the United States. *N Engl J Med.* 2018;379(25):2468-2475. doi:10.1056/NEJMsr1804754

adolescents will be provided. The top five causes of death in adolescents are presented in Box 11.1.

HEALTHY PEOPLE 2030

Healthy People 2030 is the fifth edition of the Healthy People initiatives and the overarching goals, which are focused on achieving healthy development, eliminating health disparities, and decreasing preventable diseases, disability, and premature death[1,2] (see Chapter 1 for more information about the Healthy People initiative).[3] The current edition, *Healthy People 2030*, includes over 355 objectives, organized by age groups and health conditions. These guidelines can be very useful in working with adolescents and trying to determine what are the most appropriate parameters for each wellness visit.

For example, in the section on adolescents' health goals, the first general goal is to increase the proportion of adolescents who have had a preventative health examination in the past 12 months from 78.7% to 82.6%.[2] This goal is well within the scope and practice of the APRN. It should be the goal of each healthcare provider to offer these annual examinations and to review all findings. This type of annual screening is the perfect time to assess adolescents' progress, assess for risk, and redefine goals/focus for the coming year. This visit provides you with an opportunity to assess how well things are going physically and psychologically for the adolescents

Table 11.1: Top Five General Goals for Adolescents in *Healthy People* 2030

AH-1: Increase the proportion of adolescents who received a preventative healthcare visit in the past year from 78.7% to 82.6%.
AH-2: Increase the proportion of adolescents who speak privately with a physician or other healthcare provider during a preventative medical visit 38.4% to 43.3%.
AH-3: Increase the proportion of children living with at least one parent employed year-round, full time from 77.9% to 85.1%.
AH-4: Increase the proportion of high school completers who were enrolled in college the October immediately after completing high school from 69.1% to 73.7%.
AH-5: Increase the proportion of elementary, middle, and high schools that have official school policies and engage in practices that promote a healthy and safe physical school environment.

Source: Hasbrouck L. Healthy People 2030: an improved framework. *Health Educ Behav*. 2021;48(2):113-114. doi:10.1177/1090198121997812

that you care for. These examinations should be comprehensive and should include an assessment of physical growth and development, vital signs, and height and weight measurements, with documented percentage as well as body mass index (BMI). These objective parameters provide you with clear data and are important indicators of growth when compared to the previous year's assessment. It also provides the opportunity for early intervention, if growth delays, obesity, malnutrition, and at-risk behaviors are detected. In addition, it is important to assess the mental health status of each adolescent who may be at risk for depression, suicidal ideation, or sexual promiscuity. Each visit provides an opportunity for appropriate and timely health education including what to expect in the coming year (anticipatory guidance) for both adolescents and their parents/caretakers. The current 2030 goals/objectives for adolescents are outlined in Table 11.1. More information about *Healthy People 2030* can be found at www.Healthypeople.gov.

ADOLESCENT GROWTH AND DEVELOPMENT

As noted previously, the period of adolescence is a rapid time of growth and development and generally occurs over a 5-year span but can take up to 7 years for complete maturation. During this time, adolescents develop rapidly both physically and psychologically with changes in both the physical body and brain development. The adolescent period is the second-most rapid cycle of growth and development (after infancy) in the human life cycle.

Within these two aspects of development, growth is often divided into stages: preadolescent and adolescents. An APRN needs to be informed regarding both components of growth. It is helpful to utilize a framework as a foundation for understanding psychosocial development. Erik Erikson is a well-known psychologist who developed a framework for understanding psychosocial development. According to theorist Erikson, there are eight stages of psychosocial development which correspond to specific periods of growth and development from infancy through senescence (see Table 11.2).[3] Erikson's[4] theory identifies two stages of psychosocial development during adolescence: Stages 6 and 7. Stage 6 is "Identity vs. Role Confusion," which correlates with puberty and early adolescence, while Stage 7, "Intimacy vs. Isolation," corresponds to late adolescence through young adulthood. In the past, it was believed that developing a sense of identity was a major focus of adolescence, but it is now understood to be an ongoing process well beyond adolescence into adulthood.[5]

During Stage 6, adolescents begin to identify who they are and what their beliefs are. This process involves the development of self-esteem, as well as their beliefs, values, and morals, which may or may not be in congruence with their parents/caretakers' beliefs. These contemplative tasks can often lead to risk-taking behaviors and experimentation. They may want to try out new things and changes such as clothing, mannerisms, physical appearances, and interests or hobbies. Not all experimentation is negative and can be considered a positive step

Table 11.2: Erikson's Stages of Psychosocial Development

Stage	Age	Important Events
1: Trust vs. Mistrust	Infancy (birth–18 months)	Feeding
2: Autonomy vs. Shame & Doubt	Early childhood (2–3 years)	Toilet training
3: Initiative vs. Guilt	Preschool (3–5 years)	Exploration
4: Industry vs. Inferiority	School (6–11 years)	School
5: Identify vs. Confusion	Adolescence (12–18 years)	Social relationships
6: Intimacy vs. Isolation	Young adulthood (19–40 years)	Relationships
7: Generativity vs. Stagnation	Middle adulthood (40–65 years)	Work and parenthood
8. Integrity vs. Despair	Maturity (65–death)	Reflection on life

toward building a sense of self-esteem and comfort in themselves.

During Stage 7, "Intimacy vs. Isolation," adolescents begin to contemplate their own sexual identity and the psychologic capacity for engaging in intimacy with other human beings. This includes sexual experimentation and choices such as developing intimate relationships with members of the opposite sex, the same sex, or both. This period of development can occur during Stage 6 or 7 depending on the adolescent. It is "when experimenting with alternatives" is considered appropriate unless it causes physical or psychologic harm (APA, 2002).[6]

Tanner Stages of Development

Adolescent physical development is often defined as puberty, which generally occurs in females from ages 11 to 14 while their male counterparts mature later, from 14 to 17 years of age. During this period of puberty, males and females begin the development of secondary sexual characteristics, such as the appearance of axilla and pubic hair, breast development, and the onset of menses for females. In males, the development of axilla and pubic hair, penis and testicular growth and changes, voice changes, and increases in height generally occur. On rare occasions, some children begin this development at a much earlier age, between 7 to 9 years, and this is known as precocious puberty. On the other end of the spectrum, some adolescents are delayed in secondary sexual characteristic development, which can be as late as 18 years. Either of these scenarios is a cause for concern and should be further investigated. Family genetics can also play an important part in the onset of puberty for children and a thorough family history assessment should be undertaken in a child who is developing too quickly or too delayed based on age parameters. If family genetics is ruled out as an etiology, a child who begins the development of secondary sexual characteristics earlier or later than the identified norms should be evaluated for possible endocrine dysfunction.

Physical development of secondary sexual characteristics occurs in stages and occurs at different rates for both males and females (Table 11.3). Tanner, a British pediatric endocrinologist, developed a tool known as the Tanner Scale or Tanner Stage of Development Tool that is a very helpful guide for clinicians to be used for assessing the

Table 11.3: Tanner Stages of Development

Female:

Stage	Breast Development	Pubic Development
Stage 1	No change	No change
Stage 2	Breast bud develops under the areola.	Fine downy hair is noted.
Stage 3	No areolar development; palpable tissue is noted around the areola.	Terminal hair begins to develop.
Stage 4	Areola is elevated above the contour of breast, forming a "double scoop" appearance.	Terminal hair fills the entire triangle overlying the pubic region.
Stage 5	Areolar mound recedes into single breast contour with areolar hyperpigmentation, papillae development, and nipple protrusion.	Terminal hair extends beyond the inguinal crease onto the thigh.

Male:

Stage	Genitalia Development (Testicular and Pubic)
Stage 1	No change in testicular size, no hair visible in either pubic or axillae area.
Stage 2	Testicles begin to increase in volume from 4–8 mL, fine downy hair noted in both pubic and axilla region.
Stage 3	Testicles continue to increase in volume to 9–12 mL, terminal hair begins to develop in pubic and axillae area.
Stage 4	Testicles continue to increase up to 15–20 mL, terminal hair fills the entire region. Terminal hair also increases in the axilla area.
Stage 5	Testicles increase to >20 mL, terminal hair extends beyond the inguinal crease into the thigh area.

Source: Emmanuel M, Bokor BR. Tanner Stages. In: StatPearls [Internet]. StatPearls Publishing; 2020.[7] https://www.ncbi.nlm.nih.gov/books/NBK470280.

stages of development in adolescents.[6] This scale has been organized to identify the five stages of development in both males and females (Table 11.3).

Female Development

In Stage 1, the adolescent female begins to develop axilla hair. The hair is still quite fine and sparse. During Stage 2, she will begin to have some changes in nipple architecture as it will begin to be more distinct and erect, and the circumference of the areola begins to become more distinct. In addition, the pubic hair will become more prominent, thick, and coarse. In the third stage, the breasts begin to develop more, and the pubic hair increases. During the fourth stage, the breasts become more prominent, and the pubic hair continues to increase. During Stage 5, the breast development is complete, the nipples are more noticeable, and the pubic hair has fully developed in a triangular shape covering the pubis and extends to the medial aspect of the thighs. Sometime between Stage 3 and Stage 4 development, menarche (age of onset) will usually begin. Menarche signals the onset of a menstrual cycle. By age 15, 98% of all females will have experienced menarche. The average menstrual period lasts from 4 to 7 days and generally occurs every 30 to 45 days. Up to 50% of all female adolescents will have an irregular menstrual cycle for the first 2 to 3 years after menarche.

Male Development

Males during Tanner Stage 1 of development also begin to have some axilla and sparse fair villus hair is noted over the pubis. During Stage 2, the pubic and axilla will continue to develop more hair and the hair in the pubic region is noted to be straight and fine in texture. The testicular sac is noted to be changing to a pink/reddened color and slightly increase in size, and the sac will start to develop folds known as rugae. During Stage 3, the pubic hair will continue to develop and has now become coarser and curlier in its appearance as the penis will begin to elongate. Stage 4 shows hair distribution over the pubis, which will continue to increase, as well as the size of the penis, and the glans of the penis will become distinct. And in the final stage, it will be noted that the pubic hair is denser surrounding the penis and extended onto the medial aspect of the thighs. The penis has reached its full size and width. Testicular growth is complete and the rugae are now evenly distributed over the testicular sack (Marshall & Tanner, 1970).[9]

Discussions About Growth and Development of Adolescents

At each physical assessment visit, you have an opportunity to discuss growth and development and provide appropriate anticipatory guidance. Prepare prior to each assessment visit by familiarizing yourself with the guidelines for the growth and development of adolescents. If

you note on assessment that a female's development is Tanner Stage 2, you should inform the parents/caretakers of their daughter's pubertal progress and suggest that they begin to start the dialogue about menarche and the relationship of secondary sexual development to sexual relationships between the sexes. In males who have reached Tanner Stage 2 or 3, you should also inform parents/caretakers and encourage that they converse about sexual development and the changes that their son may notice. You should also address any concerns that the teenager might have about their own growth and development. Be factual and accurate, but honest. This situation can sometimes escalate to a stressful interaction, especially if parents/caretakers are not comfortable with this type of discussion. It is best to try to initiate this conversation with their parents/caretakers prior to beginning any discussion with the adolescent. You should also ask their permission to discuss growth and development with their teen. It is always important to include parameters for growth and developmental milestones as each child is different and the rate that they achieve development will vary.

The APRN should be astutely aware and in tune to the fact that your adolescent patient may have unspoken concerns about their own development of secondary sexual characteristics. Teens are constantly dealing with a barrage of peer pressures and this pressure can extend to their own rate of pubertal development. Many teens may be teased or bullied based on their too slow or too rapid development. We need to be sensitive to this fact and ask each adolescent about how they feel about their own development and if they have any questions about their bodies or rate of development. Answer their concerns not only with support and empathy but also allow time for them to ask more questions. These unexpressed concerns can be a significant cause for their own low self-esteem and should be addressed. As a healthcare provider, you are an authority figure who has knowledge and expertise to provide factual data that, when shared, may greatly allay their personal anxieties about their bodies. Bear in mind that either precocious or delayed development may also be of great concern to vulnerable teenagers.

Currently, there are many adolescent assessment tools available, in both standard pediatric textbooks and online professional resources, to assist APRNs in providing comprehensive adolescent wellness examinations. Resources such as the American Academy of Pediatrics (AAP)—including one of AAP's products, Brightfutures .Org—and the National Association of Pediatric Nurse Practitioners can provide comprehensive tools to be downloaded and used. It is important to look to professional resources that are evidence-based and current to serve as guidelines for up-to-date health assessments as guidelines can change frequently and often do. As a healthcare provider, you also have an obligation to stay

current by frequently reviewing national resources such as the Centers for Disease Control and Prevention (CDC) for changes in the current guidelines. For example, immunization guidelines change frequently, and what was recommended a year ago may have changed or been eliminated. As evidence continues to emerge, it is important to access professional resources via websites to assist you in determining the best practices for adolescents.

ADOLESCENT RISK-TAKING BEHAVIORS

As noted previously, taking risks can be a normal task of adolescent growth and development. However, when it leads to activities that put their lives at risk, it can become dangerous. Unfortunately, risk-taking is more likely to occur among teens when they are in the presence of their peers.[8] Peer pressure is strong and can lead to adolescents taking chances that they would not have taken if they were alone. With peers, they may also be cajoled into, for example, drinking alcohol in excess, which can lead to dire consequences such as motor vehicle accidents, hospitalization, disability, and even death. Research has indicated that even when the adolescent is aware of the possibility of a negative outcome, they may still take a risk.[8] One of the long-held theories about adolescent risk-taking is that although they may be aware of the negative consequences of a behavior, they feel "it cannot or will not happen to me." In other words, they believe that they are infallible and will be safe from any harm. As healthcare providers utilizing evidence-based principles, we know that this belief is a fallacy and are cognizant of the fact that taking risks can lead to an untimely death and disability for teenagers.

As APRNs, we have an obligation to provide venues for discussions with adolescents regarding risk-taking behaviors and their deleterious effects. We should initiate these conversations often and provide the facts to substantiate potential harm for each type of behavior. Discuss all risk-taking behaviors in a factual manner providing an opportunity for the adolescent to ask questions and verbalize their own feelings or concerns regarding these behaviors. Present information succinctly but do so in an open manner that allows teenagers to feel comfortable talking about these behaviors. We should also encourage adolescents to have this type of open discussion with their parents/caretakers, and they may ask your advice on how to handle these discussions. In addition, their parent/caretakers may also solicit your advice on how to begin this conversation. Having a list of evidence-based resources/guides available for distribution would be helpful.

Risk-taking behaviors include physical and psychologic effects. For example, the ingestion of alcohol/drugs can affect both physical and psychologic changes in the body. Psychologic changes include impaired judgment and can compromise one's ability to act in a safe manner. In addition, physical abilities include poor coordination and an inability to act responsibly. In the case of alcohol ingestion, a teen may try drinking alcohol and do so to "feel a buzz" or lessen their own inhibitions, and this can lead to them experiencing alcohol poisoning, which can lead to permanent disability or death. In illicit drug experimentation, the adolescent may be cajoled into trying an illicit drug substance, by peers, and thus, experience serious side effects, including instant death from this first-time experimentation. Although both scenarios regarding alcohol or drug ingestion are extreme examples, they do occur and can occur the first time that a teen experiments with either of these substances.

According to a research study by Miech, Johnston, O'Malley, et al.,[9] alcohol is the preferred drug of choice as compared to cigarette smoking or marijuana use in teens from ages 12 to 18. In this study, they found that alcohol use among eighth graders was 9.7% as compared to cigarette smoking (3.6%) or marijuana use (6.5%). Alcohol continued to be the drug of choice found in 12th graders with more than a third of them (35.3%) choosing it over cigarettes (11.4%) or marijuana use (21.3%). This study also showed that the use of cigarettes and marijuana had more than doubled in 12th graders as compared to students in eighth grade. Cigarette smoking is a legal habit in this country; currently, marijuana sale and distribution in the United States is legal in 25 states and the District of Columbia (DC). In four of these states and DC, it is legal for use recreationally while 20 of the states allow use for medicinal purposes only.

Cigarette Smoking

It is well documented that long-term cigarette smoking (i.e., nicotine) can cause physical harm to several systems in the body, including the heart, lungs, and vascular system. It is the primary cause of vascular-related problems, such as venous insufficiency and cancer. Scientific evidence regarding the connection between long-term use of cigarettes and disease has identified 14 different types of cancers, including lung, oral, bladder, pancreatic, and cervical, that are connected to smoking.[10] Overall, the rates of smoking in the United States have declined. From 1997 to 2013, the prevalence of smoking declined from 38% to 15% for high school students. But despite this decline in cigarette smoking, we are now seeing more adolescents engaging in alternate forms of nicotine ingestion such as e-cigarettes.[11]

Because it is legal, a plethora of media sources (i.e., movies, social media, YouTube) advertise cigarette smoking as a trendy or glamorous thing to do. This advertisement minimizes the impact or dangers of smoking. Instead, they encourage teens and other adults to purchase and use cigarettes. Although there are laws that ban retailers from selling cigarettes to minors, these restrictions are rarely policed, and the associated fines are also not enforced. Therefore, access to the purchase and sales of cigarettes by minors in the United States is easy.

Nicotine is a drug, and it affects the body in several ways. It acts as both a vasoconstrictor causing an increase in heart rate and blood pressure and it also helps to relax smooth muscle fibers. The effects of nicotine reach the brain within 8 to 10 seconds after smoking inhalation begins. The effect on the brain has similar properties to acetylcholine and causes the smoker to feel a sense of pleasure. Partially this occurs from the direct effect of nicotine on the brain, but it is also believed that one of the other ingredients in cigarettes causes suppression of MAO inhibitors, which allows for an increase in dopamine production.[12] Addiction to nicotine occurs in a short period, from days to weeks. Each cigarette smoked delivers approximately 10 mg of nicotine. Most adults who smoke began experimenting with nicotine during adolescence, before age 18. Over time, as the effect of nicotine takes hold, tolerance is reached and the need to achieve the same effects from nicotine can only be achieved through an increased intake of nicotine (i.e., smoking more cigarettes). Long-term smoking can become a lifelong habit and today is a major cause of death in the United States, as previously discussed. It is also important to be aware that there are many alternative types of smokeless tobacco that teens are utilizing today. These alternatives include chewing tobacco, snuff, bidis, hookahs, and electronic cigarettes.[12] These types of tobacco products are being used by up to 25% of high school students as noted in a study by Singh et al.[13] Although these are alternative types of nicotine, they are not without adverse effects; adolescents need to be counseled regarding these potential carcinogens.

Alcohol Consumption

It is important to recognize that alcohol consumption in the United States, as well as many other countries around the world, is a legal social norm. Much of the U.S. culture is built around the social consumption of alcohol during holidays and other celebrations. Many families may allow their teens and sometimes even young children to "sip or taste" alcohol on special occasions. These events are at the discretion of the parents. In 2019, alcohol sales in the United States totaled $252.2 billion.[14] Currently the rate for an alcohol use disorder (AUD) in this country is over 16 million, and more than 88,00 deaths annually in the United States are attributed to AUD. AUD is the fourth-leading cause of preventable death in the United States.[15] There are several health-related consequences, such as heart disease, hypertension, liver disease, stroke, and cancer,[16] that can occur in anyone who drinks to excess.

Identifying Adolescents With Alcohol Use Disorder

In an effort to decrease illegal consumption of alcohol among teenagers, and its long-term sequelae, the United States has placed restrictions on the consumption of alcohol by designating a legal age for drinking to 18 years and older. It is believed that this is done to protect the health and well-being of these young adults who have not completed their growth and development. As APRNs, our concerns regarding alcohol consumption in adolescents are illegal consumption of alcohol at a critical period in their growth and development. There is also growing evidence that a history of early drinking, as well as a family history of AUD, places them at higher lifelong risk for AUD. In a comprehensive review of scientific research studies on the neurotoxic effects of alcohol on brain development in adolescents, the authors found that there were consistent changes in gray and white matter. These changes resulted in decreases in cognitive abilities for teens with a history of alcohol abuse.[17] These white and gray matter changes in the brain were detectable on functional magnetic resonance imaging (fMRI) and electroencephalogram recordings. Of interest, the review showed that long-term effects due to excessive alcohol intake carried over into adulthood and resulted in increased long-term abuse of alcohol and increased psychopathology. In addition, immaturity due to the incomplete development of the brain is another factor in adolescents that leads to impulsive decision-making in a split second that can forever alter their health and well-being.

The average age of first consumption of alcohol in the United States is 14 years but can occur in children as young as 12.[18] Approximately 11% of all alcohol consumed in America is consumed by 12 to 20 years of age. And in 2015, more than 7 million adolescents between the ages of 12 and 20 admitted to drinking more than "a few sips of alcohol."[19] Another area of concern regarding alcohol consumption in adolescents is binge drinking. Binge drinking, defined as drinking several drinks of alcohol in a short period, is also a significant and growing problem. See Table 11.4 for a summary of the number of drinks by age defined as binge drinking. In 2015, the Center for Behavioral Health Statistics and Quality found that more than 1.3 million teenagers admitted to binge drinking five or more days in the past month.[20] These statistics demonstrate that illicit alcohol intake among adolescents is a serious risk factor that needs to be addressed by teachers, parents/caretakers, and healthcare providers.

Illicit Drug Use

Adolescents have always been at risk for illicit drug use. As discussed previously, their incomplete brain development leads to risky or impulsive behavior choices, and these choices can lead to drug experimentation. More

Table 11.4: Definition of Binge Drinking by Age

Definition: For adults, binge drinking means drinking so much within about 2 hours that blood alcohol concentration (BAC) levels reach 0.08 g/dL, the legal limit of intoxication. For women, this typically takes about four drinks, and for men, about five. But, according to recent research estimates, it takes fewer drinks for children to reach these BAC levels.

For boys:

Age	Number of Drinks Consumed
9–13	About 3 drinks
14–15	About 4 drinks
16–17	About 5 drinks

For girls:

Age	Number of Drinks Consumed
9–17	About 3 drinks

Source: National Institute on Alcohol Abuse and Alcoholism. *Binge drinking.* 2021. https://www.niaaa.nih.gov/publications/brochures-and-fact-sheets/binge-drinkingf

recently, this issue has been propelled to the front page of media sources due to an increase in illicit opioid drug abuse in our country. Drugs such as heroin and cocaine are in increased supply and decreased cost, which has led to more widespread use and, sadly, an increase in untimely deaths due to overdose. According to the Substance Abuse and Mental Health Services Administration, in 2013, 2.4 million Americans had used an illicit drug in the past month.[20] In this survey, over half (54%) were teenagers. It is predicted that between 15% and 40% of teens younger than age 16 have experimented with illicit drugs.[21] These authors conducted a meta-analysis of 22 randomized controlled trials (RCT) looking at parental influences and experimentation with illicit drugs. They found that frequent illicit drug use among teenagers is associated with academic failure and mental health disorders including depression and psychosis. They also found that parental influence may have a potential preventative factor in adolescents' experimentation with illicit drugs. This research highlights the need for parents/caretakers to take several opportunities to discuss illicit drugs with their teenagers and discourage experimentation with them. This type of conversation needs to occur frequently, and parents/caretakers should take the lead by providing an open dialogue with their child, letting them know that it is okay to come and speak with them about drugs or alcohol, whenever needed. This might also be a great time to discuss with their teens an emergency plan if the teen should feel unsafe in any situation. This plan could include giving permission to call a parent day/night for a ride if the child should feel unsafe without any retribution.

As discussed in the introduction, the use of opioids among Americans is increasing. It is approaching epidemic proportions resulting in significant deaths from overdose and escalating addictions. According to the American Society of Addiction Medicine (2016),[24] up to 50% of adolescents between 12 and 17 years old reported using opioids for nonmedical reasons and approximately 460,000 reported an addiction to opioids.[22] From 2005 to 2015, opioid deaths had doubled from 3.4% to 7.1%.[23,24] Most teens revealed that they accessed opioid drugs for free from relatives or friends. However, up to a third have received a prescription for opioids to treat pain. Drugs in the opioid family include oxycodone, morphine, and heroin (see Table 11.5). Heroin, a morphine derivative, is an illicit drug that is sold on the street and has become abundant in supply. The use of heroin causes a euphoric feeling in the body. It acts on endorphin sites and decreases the production of natural endorphins in the body. Because of this decreased natural endorphin production, the body will crave more heroin to continue to experience of euphoria. Pure heroin is not generally for sale but is "cut" with other ingredients before being sold. Up to 200 ingredients have been found in the mix for heroin, and these include caffeine, sugars, and fertilizers containing ammonium chloride. In 2015, the Drug Enforcement Agency (DEA) issued an alert due to a recent surge in overdose deaths related to fentanyl. Fentanyl is a strong synthetic opioid derivative that is believed to be up to 50 to 100 times more potent than heroin. On the street, heroin was being mixed with fentanyl for a stronger effect while decreasing the strength of heroin in the mixture.[25] Users of the drug were not aware that the heroin they were using also contained fentanyl. If they sought help for an overdose, neither the user nor the healthcare provider was aware of the mix of these two lethal drugs. Adolescents also tend to favor inhalant substances such as breathing fumes of household cleaners, lighter fluid, glues, aerosol

Table 11.5: Opioids and Other Commonly Used Illegal Drugs

Prescribed	Illegal
• Fentanyl	• Heroin
• Lorcet (Hydrocodone/ Acetaminophen)	• Cocaine
• Morphine	
• Oxycodone	
• Oxycontin	
• Percocet	
• Vicodin	

Any of the prescribed opioids are illegal when taken by a person who is not prescribed the medication.

sprays, and office supplies (i.e., correction fluid) when they do not have access to other drugs such as alcohol or marijuana.

One drug that is used to reverse drug overdoses is naloxone (Narcan). Naloxone is a safe, non-addicting drug that can reverse an overdose in up to 75% to 100% of the cases, if used quickly (Clark, Wilder, Winstanley, 2014).[26] Currently, three quarters of U.S. states have approved access to naloxone for administration by nonmedical or lay personnel. Efforts have included the distribution of naloxone to users who are at high risk for overdose and/or their family members who may be available to administer this drug. To accommodate this need, intranasal and auto-injection forms of naloxone have been developed and are in stock at most pharmacies. Increasing access and availability of naloxone saves lives. However, this effort has caused a lot of concerns for consumers and healthcare providers.[27] Concerns include that easy access and availability of naloxone will cause an increase in illicit drug use in the community. This concern has not been substantiated and research studies are being conducted to support or refute this belief. Another option in treating opioid use disorder (OUD) is the use of a medication, buprenorphine (Suboxone). Buprenorphine is an opioid agonist that was approved for treating opioid disorders in 2002.[28] This medication has been used successfully to help decrease the desire for opioids in people addicted to the illicit drug. This drug has been found to be effective in treating adolescents.[29] The prescribing of Suboxone requires that the provider (MD or APRN) complete 8 hours of educational training and apply for a waiver to prescribe. Recent legislation, in 2021, proposes that physicians will be able to prescribe without a waiver. However, this has not been enacted yet.[30] However, at this time, nurse practitioners (NPs) are still required to complete the education and apply for the waiver. Drug addiction is a major concern for all Americans and multiple efforts are being undertaken to decrease the sale and distribution of illicit drugs, as well as legislation enacted to provide oversight and close monitoring of prescribers who write for narcotic pain prescriptions.

Discussions Regarding Risk-Taking Behaviors

It is important for APRNs, parents/caretakers, and teachers to stay informed and be aware of trends in risk-taking behaviors so they can proactively address them with all teenagers. As healthcare providers, we have an obligation to discuss the pros and cons of these behaviors, as well as the dire consequences that can happen because of experimentation with illicit drugs and legalized drugs such as alcohol, nicotine, and marijuana, or other medications that are prescribed but not for the adolescent. Early intervention and primary prevention should be the shared goal of all adults who can influence teens.

SEXUALITY AND SEXUAL HEALTH

As previously discussed, the normal growth and development of adolescents include the development of secondary sexual characteristics. These changes are due to hormonal influences such as estrogen, progestin, and testosterone in the body. With the development of secondary sexual characteristics comes the desire for sexual contact. It is a normal desire to want to be sexually active with another human being. However, physical development and psychologic development do not always occur simultaneously. So, although an adolescent has reached physical sexual maturation, they may not have reached psychologic sexual maturation and may not be ready to have sex. This dichotomy between the physical and psychologic maturation for adolescents is not uncommon and can lead to risky behaviors when some adolescents are ready for sexual contact with another person and others are not. Therefore it is important to have a conversation about sex (see Box 11.2 for possible questions to ask). Development and sexual maturation occur at different rates between males and females. In general, males desire for sexual contact occurs much earlier than females. This fact can lead males to aggressively approach females for sex. It can also lead to peer pressure by males to coerce females to engage in sexual activity before they are ready. This can lead to the trauma of rape either from a stranger or within the

---

Box 11.2: Conversation About Sexual Activity

During physical examination, review physical changes that have occurred:

- ▪ Use open-ended questions.
- ▪ Provide a safe place to make them feel comfortable when asking sensitive questions.
- ▪ Start with the statement, "Our discussion during this time is considered confidential unless you reveal any information that places you at risk for harm. Although I would encourage these conversations with your parents/caretakers, I know this is not always possible."
- ▪ Then, begin with general questions regarding physical body changes that occurred in the past year and move forward with more specific questions:
  - "Some teenagers your age are having sex. Have you heard about this or do you know anyone like this? What are your feelings/thoughts about this? Have you had any thoughts or feelings about becoming sexually active yourself?"
- ▪ If necessary, you may need to explicitly define what is meant by *sex* as there has been an increase in oral sexual activities among younger adolescents.

context of what is known as "date rape." Rape trauma and the types of rape are discussed later in the chapter.

Sexually Transmitted Infections

In 2017, the Youth Behavioral Risk Survey found that of the high school teens who were surveyed, 40% had experienced intercourse and 56% had not used any birth control method while engaging in sexual activity. And of those who engaged in sex, approximately 10% had sex with four or more partners. Approximately 34% of these high schoolers admitted to using drugs or alcohol prior to sexual intercourse.[28] All these risk factors put adolescents at greater risk for developing a sexually transmitted infection (STI). The spectrum of sexual health encompasses many things, including sexual development and maturation, psychologic maturation that accompanies this phase of life, and preventing STIs and unintended pregnancy, which are discussed over the next few paragraphs.

Half of the 20 million cases of new STIs reported each year occur in adolescents between the ages of 15 and 24.[31] If left undiagnosed and untreated, lifelong infections can occur leading to infertility and cancer of the sexual organs such as the cervix, vagina, or penis. In addition to unintended pregnancy, not utilizing any self-protecting methods such as condoms or barrier contraceptive methods can also lead to contracting human papillomavirus (HPV), hepatitis B, and/or human immunodeficiency virus (HIV). If not detected or treated, these three viruses can cause serious health problems, including liver disease, cancer, and immunodeficiency infections.

The APRN taking care of adolescents should take an active lead on the discussion of STIs focusing first and foremost on prevention and then early screening and detection of any STI. It is important to be cognizant of the fact that sex and sexually transmitted infections are often considered taboo subjects for general discussion between parents/caretaker and their teenage son/daughter. Discussing STIs needs to become an integral part of an annual health visit for adolescents or during any visit where you suspect that the adolescent may be sexually active. The APRN can take the lead by discussing current trends in the incidence and prevalence of STIs in the adolescent population. Presentation of this type of information may lead a teen to ask questions about how these infections are transmitted and what is the best prevention against them. You might also probe them with more general questions such as if they are aware of anyone who has been diagnosed with an STI. These types of questions provide a platform for you to discuss STIs and the consequences of untreated infections. In addition, discussion of STIs needs to include the fact that some of these infections may not produce any symptoms, and therefore, a potential sexual partner may not even know that they have an infection until it is discovered years

later during a gynecologic visit or, even more frightening, on an initial infertility evaluation in both males and females. This fact helps highlight the importance of taking precautions such as wearing condoms or delaying sexual activity until both partners have been tested for STIs and negative results are found. Another important factor to be discussed is that most STIs are treatable; however, there are some evolving bacteria that are resistant to the current recommended treatment, and this can further complicate eradicating an STI.[32]

If this adolescent is sexually active, the healthcare provider will also need to determine whether they are in a monogamous relationship or having sex with multiple sexual partners. Even if the teen states that they are in a monogamous relationship, the APRN should probe whether they know if their sexual partner is also only having sex with them. It is important to elicit a thorough sexual history particularly if the adolescent reports being sexually active. The information in Box 11.3 can guide education about "safe sex" and the use of some type of consistent barrier contraception. It is important to discuss the type of contraception being used and whether it is used to only prevent conception or whether it is also protective against transmission of an STI. Often, females believe that if they are using oral contraceptives such as "the Pill," an intrauterine device (IUD), or a 3- to 5-year implantable contraceptive device, such as Norplanon, they are not at risk of STIs. However, these methods do not protect against STIs. A more comprehensive discussion regarding contraceptive methods is discussed in a later section.

Contraception

First and foremost, in their roles as healthcare providers working with adolescents, APRNs must encourage health promotion and wellness, which includes sexual health. Contraception is an important topic to include in the discussion of sexual health. The artificial method of contraception prevents implantation of an ovum by interfering with either ovulation, fertilization, or implantation. There are currently 23 different contraceptive methods, and their effectiveness varies from 80% to 99.7% effective[33] (see Table 11.6). As more evidence becomes available, these methods of contraceptives continue to evolve, and more options are becoming available frequently. For example, in the past, the most preferred method of contraception was combined oral contraceptives (COCs) because of the effectiveness and ease of administration. However, with the addition of implantable devices such as Nexplanon or Implanon and the evolution of IUDs, such as Copper T or Mirena type, COCs are not considered as one of the most effective methods of contraception anymore. It is now considered easier to have an implantable device versus the daily ingestion of

Box 11.3: Questions to Consider When Interviewing About Sexual Health

■ Reassure about privacy and confidentiality

■ Consider interviewing separate from the physical exam

■ Always face the adolescent and pay attention to what is being said and what is not being said

■ Ask developmentally appropriate questions

■ Establish a rapport and trusting relationship

■ Ask permission before giving advice and providing information

■ Use reflective listening

■ Avoid

- "Why" questions
- Assumptions about gender identity, sexual orientation, sexual identiy and sexual behaviors
- Judgmental comments
- Medical jargon or technical terms the adolescent may not understand

■ Having the conversation

- "I am going to ask some personal questions that will help me provide the best care possible and give you specific information and/or advice as needed."
- "When it comes to discussion related to sex everyone is different, so I would like to find out a little more about you, is it ok with you for us to discuss sexual matters?"
- "My goal is to make you feel comfortable and I will not be judgmental. I will respect your thoughts, feelings, and experiences you choose to share with me."

■ Questions to ask

- "What gender pronouns do you prefer I use when I talk with you? He or she? His or her? Or some people want 'them'?"
- "When people are born, they are assigned a gender, but the person may feel different inside, what gender do you identify with? How comfortable are you with your gender? Do you ever feel confused about your gender? If yes, is there someone you can talk to about these feelings?" And ask if their parents are aware of the feelings.
- "Some young people your age find themselves attracted to boys, girls, or both, and some are not sure. This is normal and can change as you get older. Who do you find yourself sexually attracted to?"
- "What is your understanding of sexual identity (sexual orientation) What do you consider your

sexual identity to be? (gay, straight, bisexual, asexual, queer, or another)?"

- "Have you had a sexual partner or partners? If yes, tell me about your past and current sexual partners?" Ask the patient to tell you at what age they became sexually active.
- If the patient has been sexually active, ask about oral sex and do they use protection against STI or pregnancy? Are their parent(s) aware that they are sexually active?
- You can ask them if they ever felt pressured to have sex and if someone has ever touched them inappropriately.

It is best to ask open-ended questions and truly be present by maintaining eye contact and not taking a lot of notes or paying too much attention to the computer if you are using electronic medical records.

Source: Pfeffer B, Ellsworth TR, Gold MA. Interviewing adolescents about sexual matters. *Pediatric Clinics of North America.* 2017;64:291-304.

a "pill," because once they are implanted by a medical professional the patient does not have to worry about remembering to take a pill every day or returning every 3 months for a repeat injection. The effectiveness rates for these two methods are as high as fewer than 1 woman out of 100 will get pregnant as compared to 6 to 12 out of 100 with the COCs.

Special Considerations in Contraception for Adolescents

There are many factors to consider in recommending a type of contraception for adolescents (see Box 11.4). These factors include the adolescent's accurate knowledge about pregnancy prevention and use of contraception, concerns about confidentiality and parental notification, age and maturity of the adolescent, ease of use/application of contraceptive methods, and costs.[34] There is an abundance of choices in contraceptive methods, but all these factors need to be discussed, analyzed, and considered before recommending the best contraceptive choice for each adolescent. For example, if you have a 14-year-old female who is being seen for contraceptive counseling and she is known to be unreliable and forgetful in her daily routines, making a recommendation of a COC may not be the best choice for her. An implantable device such as Norplant rods or a Mirena IUD may be a better and more reliable choice for her. Once either implantable device, is inserted by a healthcare provider, this method remains effective for several years (5 years) and requires minimal monitoring by the adolescent herself. However, a female who uses either one of these devices needs to be educated that the use of a condom may still be necessary to prevent transmission of STI or HIV infections.

Table 11.6: Types of Contraception and Efficacy

Contraceptive Classification	Type	Perfect Use Efficacy	Typical Use Efficacy
Short-Acting Reversible	1. Combined oral contraceptives (COCs)	99.7%	93%
	2. Progestin-only pill	99.7%	93%
	3. Combined vaginal ring	99.7%	93%
	4. Combined contraceptive patch	99.7%	93%
	5. Monthly injectable	99.8%	96%
Long-Acting Reversible (LARC)	1. Implant	99.9%	99.8%
	2. IUD–Copper	99.4%	99.2%
	3. IUD–Levonorgestrel	99.5%	99.3%
Barrier Methods	1. Male condoms	98%	87%
	2. Female condoms	95%	79%
	3. Spermicide only	84%	79%
	4. Condoms & spermicide	99%	
	5. Diaphragm with spermicide	84%	83%
	6. Cervical cap	73.1%	67.5%
Ovulation Methods		97%	87%
Withdrawal Method		96%	80%
No Method		15%	15%

Source: Festin MPR. Overview of modern contraception. Best Pract Res Clin Obstet Gynaecol. 2020;66:4–14. doi:10.1016/j.bpobgyn .2020.03.004

When evaluating the various types of contraceptives, two values are usually associated with each type of birth control method in the literature: perfect use versus typical use. These two values are generally represented as a percentile; perfect use is the percentage effective if used exactly as directed and consistently, whereas typical use percentage indicates the success rate in prevention of pregnancy in the average person utilizing this method. Perfect use is a higher percentage of success versus typical use. For example, withdrawal is a popular contraceptive method in up to 57% of adolescents.[35] Perfect use of withdrawal results in two pregnancies out of 100 women versus typical use, which is 18 out of 100 women during the first year of use. There are several factors that negatively impact this method of contraception. Scientific evidence demonstrates that the withdrawal method of contraception can be a less reliable method of contraception for two reasons: (a) Sperm can still be released into the reproductive canal prior to a male ejaculation, and (b) this method provides no protection against STIs or HIV infections. However, the popularity of this method may be related to a lack of forethought and has no cost associated with it.

Barrier methods of contraception are popular among adolescents and include male and female condoms, contraceptive sponge, and the use of spermicide alone.[36] The most popular method identified was male condom use (see Box 11.5). Approximately 53% of those surveyed admitted to using a condom during their last act of sexual intercourse. The ease of convenience in purchasing condoms and the ability to obtain them without a prescription are factors that favor this method.

Certain types of contraceptive methods may be more appropriate and effective for use in the adolescent population. Contraceptive methods that are less dependent

Box 11.4: Discuss the Pros and Cons of Contraceptives for Each Individual

- Efficacy and ease of use
- Prevention of STIs
- Benefits and risks
- Contraindications and adverse events
- Any special considerations of adolescent females

Include the parent/caretaker when possible and according to the state laws where you practice (particularly in those who are younger than 18 years).

Box 11.5: Safety Issues

- Make sure the male adolescent knows how to properly use a condom.
- Use of a spermicide along with the condom is best.
- Use a new condom with each episode of sexual encounter.

Source: Festin MPR. Overview of modern contraception. *Best Pract Res Clin Obstet Gynaecol.* 2020;66:4-14. doi:10.1016/j .bpobgyn.2020.03.004

on user compliance are recommended for adolescents. The contraceptive rates of failure are much higher in adolescents using birth control pills, ring, or the patch as compared to the longer acting reversible contraception (LARC).[37] Hormonal contraceptives are a popular choice for adolescents and include combined oral contraceptives (COCs), injectable such as Depo-Provera, hormonal patches such as Ortho-Evra, and chemically treated vaginal rings. The effectiveness rates of these types of contraception result in a failure rate of seven pregnancies per 100 women in 1 year.[33] More than 50% of sexually active female teenagers are using a COC for contraception.[35] All hormonal contraceptive methods require a baseline physical examination and screening and can be prescribed by a healthcare provider such as an APRN. The hormonal contraceptive choices are divided into two categories: short-acting and LARC (see Table 11.6). COCs also provide some noncontraceptive benefits such as regulation of menstrual cycle, decreased blood loss and cramping with menses, and an improvement in acne.[35]

The final category of reversible contraception is the use of an implantable device such as an IUD. There are two types of devices currently available: a copper T-shaped IUD or a 52-mg levonorgesterol IUD. An IUD works by causing thickening of the cervical mucus, creating an environment within the uterus to inhibit implantation. In the past, IUDs were not recommended for nulliparous females. It was believed that this method could lead to infertility and would not be a choice for any female who was planning on becoming pregnant later in life. However, research has demonstrated that this method of birth control can be reversed with removal and that there is a quick return of fertility after its removal.[35] There is also a concern that the presence of an IUD in the uterus can place a female at increased risk for pelvic inflammatory disease (PID) due to an STI. Research has demonstrated that although a small risk is in effect for up to the first 20 days after insertion, an IUD does not increase the risk for PID. Depending on the type of IUD inserted, it remains effective for 3 to 10 years. This method has become a more popular type of birth control in the past few years and up to 5.8% of sexually active females from 14 to 19 years of age currently use an IUD for contraception as compared to only 2.2% in 2009.[38] Box 11.6 provides some resources to consider for STI prevention.

Discussion Regarding Contraceptive Use and Recommendations for Adolescents

Contraceptive conversations with adolescents are important. The APRN may be the only knowledgeable adult that the adolescent is conversing with regarding their sexuality. It is important to elicit screening questions that may reveal their knowledge or lack thereof regarding the risks of unprotected intercourse. As noted previously in this section, general questions regarding their current sexual behaviors are nonthreatening and can create a platform for launching a conversation regarding sex and the inherent risks associated with it. Having initial conversations with the adolescent, even if they elect not to reveal any pertinent history with the APRN, is a good way to "open the door to this topic," and they will know that the APRN is open to discussing sex with them and will also maintain confidentiality in doing so.

Intended/Unintended Pregnancy

Teenage pregnancy has far-reaching negative effects on the teenage mother, her child, and society at large.

Box 11.6: Resources

APRNS must remain up to date regarding knowledge and management of STI contraceptives. The following resources can help you:

- CDC annual updates in *Morbidity and Mortality Weekly Reports*
- American College of Obstetrics and Gynecology
- American Academy of Pediatrics

Other helpful resources for screening:

- www.BrightFutures.org
  - All **Bright Future** questionnaires can be downloaded and used for screening specific age groups. The questionnaires provide a choice of three answers for each question—Yes, No, or Unsure—and the best answer is selected and circled.
  - An adolescent could complete this questionnaire prior to seeing the healthcare provider and bring it into the examination room with them for review. This type of screening tool can be valuable in helping to introduce topics to teenagers who are uncomfortable asking about sexual activity topics and guide your intervention.

- www.uptodate.com
  - A large evidence-based medical information site
  - Requires an annual subscription but many hospitals, academic centers, and large healthcare organizations have access

Teenage mothers are more likely to not finish high school and have high-risk pregnancies.[39,40] In 2010, the United States spent more than $9 billion in costs associated with teenage pregnancy. In recent years, a number of national initiatives have been implemented to try to decrease the rates of teenage pregnancy. As a result, there was a reduction of 428,000 fewer births to teenage mothers, resulting in a savings of over $4.4 billion.[41] Although this is good news, there are still far too many teenagers giving birth before they turn 18 years old, and in 2015, more than 220,000 babies were born to teenage mothers.[38] From 1999 to 2013, there was a 57% decrease in teenage pregnancy in the United States. However, the rate of U.S. teenage pregnancy is still one of the highest in the developed world at 57/1,000 as compared to the lowest rates of teenage pregnancy in Switzerland at 8/1,000.[39,42] It is well documented that unintended pregnancy rates are high and correlate with higher infant morbidity and mortality rates.[42] In some cases adolescents may consider emergency contraceptives. This is not the recommended method of prevention, but it is important to understand the safety issues (see Box 11.7). It is hopeful to note that the rates of teenage pregnancy decline with age and inversely correlate with the rates of contraceptive use. In other words, older adolescents are more likely to use some form of contraception as compared to their younger cohorts. From 17 to 19 years of age, in those who use some form of contraception versus those who do not use contraception, there was a 2% versus 11% rate of pregnancy at age 17.[43] In fact, by age 19, at least 93% of all sexually active females and 99% of sexually active males reported using some type of contraception at least once while having sex. Of all types of contraception available,

Box 11.7: Safety Issues

- **Emergency Contraception:** Hormonal contraception used up to 120 hours/5 days post-coital to prevent pregnancy
  - Progestin-only (Plan B) or insertion of a copper IUD or high-dose combination of estrogen-progestin oral contraception
  - Female weight is considered in prescribing; if the female is more than 165 lb, then the EC-levongesterol method is not recommended.
  - Some versions of emergency contraception such as Plan B are available over the counter for women over 17 years of age (proof of age is not required).
- **Permanent Sterilization** (not recommended for adolescents)
  - Vasectomy for males
  - Tubal ligation or use of Essure for females

condoms are the most preferred method. Condoms are convenient, can be purchased without a prescription, are portable, and can be disposed of after use. They require no preparation to be used and are expandable to accommodate a variety of penis sizes.

Some have speculated that the decrease in teenage pregnancy from 2013 to 2015 is due to the efforts of the Office of Adolescent Health (OAH), a department under the umbrella of the Health and Human Services (HHS) agency. This office opened in 2010 with the mission to lead our nation in ensuring that American adolescents thrive and become healthy, productive adults. The OAH was mandated by HHS to designate $10 million of its budget to support efforts to develop an evidence-based teen pregnancy prevention program.[44] These efforts were aimed, in part, at delaying the onset of sexual activity in teenagers and encouraging the use of contraception.[45] Forty-four programs were selected for funding and were required to collect performance measures and report them annually. An important outcome of the program was 94% of high school seniors participating in the program graduated in their senior year as compared to 51% of young females who have a baby and did not earn a high school diploma until the age of 22.

Rape Trauma

Rape is a serious crime that creates significant physical, emotional, and psychologic harm to anyone who experiences this violent act. Adolescent females appear to be most at risk for rape. According to the CDC, out of 7 million young women, 6% will experience rape and 2% will experience attempted rape. It is important to assess for possible rape or inappropriate touching (see Box 11.8). In comparison, 6% of males will experience rape.[42] "Rape" is defined by the CDC under the term "sexual violence" and is defined as "a sexual act committed against someone without that person's freely given consent.[46] "Rape," in general, is defined as nonconsensual vaginal, anal, or oral penetration that involves threat or force.[47] The nation's largest antisexual violence prevention network, The Rape, Assault & Incest National Network, states that a rape occurs every 108 seconds, and it occurs every 8 minutes in children.[48] In the adolescent population, defined as ages 14 to 17, up to 28% of adolescents report being victims of sexual abuse.[49] From 1993 to 2014, there was a decrease overall in the number of rapes in this country. The rates declined from 4.3/1,000 in 1993 to 1.1/1,000 in 2014.[48] However, the fact that rapes occur at all is unacceptable, especially considering the fact that only 16% of all rapes are ever reported.

Questions directed toward identifying possible rapes, sexual assaults, or incest should be posed at each wellness visit for all children including adolescents. Three types of sexual assault or rape have been defined: stranger, acquaintance, and date rape. Stranger rape occurs

---

Box 11.8: Safety Issues

- Ask specific questions about personal risk for forced sex or threats:
  - "Has anyone tried to force you to have sex with them?" If they answer yes, you need to ask them to explain in more detail.

- Ascertain the need for more specific gynecologic questions and testing for sexually transmitted infections.

- If it appears that a rape or sexual assault has occurred, APRNs must contact local authorities for guidance. The local police department and/or the Department of Social Services (depending on the age of the patient and the details of the potential crime) are good resources.

- It is important to first elicit a detailed history from each patient before deciding how quickly to proceed. If this potential crime has occurred recently, the local authorities need to be contacted right away. However, if the incident occurred months ago, it still needs to be reported, but the window of time to report this potential crime is extended.

It is always best to stay informed regarding the current rules and regulations in your community pertaining to sexual assault and rape.

---

between two people who do not know each other, whereas acquaintance rape occurs between two people who know each other but may not be dating. "Date rape" is defined as nonconsensual sexual penetration that occurs between two people who are in a romantic or causal relationship.[47]

Date rape is a serious problem in our culture as up to 80% of these rapes go unreported.[50] Date rape can occur while the victim is alert, sleeping, or drugged with alcohol or drugs. Among adolescents, up to 50% of all sexual assaults involve alcohol consumption. A small group of drugs have become known as the "date rape" drugs and include rohypnol, ketamine, and GHB. These drugs are often slipped into an alcoholic drink and may be odorless and tasteless. This type of drug-laced alcohol is another reason to discourage teens from drinking alcohol and especially from accepting a drink from someone at a party. The effects of these drugs are serious and are considered a central nervous system depressant that can lead to visual disturbances, depression, and delirium.[47] In 2017, a survey done on youth risk behaviors found that approximately 7% of high schoolers admitted that they had been physically forced to have intercourse against their will at some time during their lifetime.[36] Date rape can take place in several places including cars, apartments, fraternity houses, dormitory residences, or in private homes. Other factors implicated in date rape are related to the location, such as being alone with a date in their place; or having an expensive meal that they paid for as an underlying context of what the intent of the date is for. Nonetheless, date rape can occur in many places while dating someone who is known to the victim and with whom they may have had previous consensual sex. Suggestions for prevention of date rape can be found in Box 11.9.

Rape Crisis Management

Rape is a serious event/trauma, and a comprehensive assessment needs to be done by a certified health professional such as a sexual assault nurse examiner (SANE). These nurses have specialized training and are certified in the medical forensic care of sexual assault victims. If a rape has occurred involving a minor, it becomes a legal matter, and the police will need to be contacted. If an adolescent admits to you that they have been raped or experienced attempted rape, your discussion has now become information that may be used in legal proceedings. More detailed information for this type of questioning is beyond the scope of a general physical examination, and you will need to refer them to the nearest SANE who may be located at the local emergency department (ED). If the rape has recently occurred, it may become necessary to enlist the help of a rape crisis team and a trained rape advocate for the adolescent. Also, if the rape occurred recently, this patient should be transferred by ambulance to the nearest ED for further assessment. This action may be necessary for preserving evidence and providing immediate care for the adolescent.

In addition, the legal guardian will need to become involved. You can help the teenager by being supportive and offering guidance while conforming to your legal duties that are defined by the state that you are practicing in. In some acute situations, such as the fact that this assault has taken place in the past few days, you may need to stop what you are doing, provide for the patient's immediate needs, stabilize them, wrap them up in blankets and package up any potential evidence items, such as underwear, clothing, and so on, using gloves in an effort not to contaminate the evidence and send it with the patient. Bear in mind that it is not unusual for a young female to have been raped by someone they know such

---

Box 11.9: Date Rape Prevention

- Encourage adolescents to trust their gut and get out of any uncomfortable situation.
- Have a safety plan with friends when going out. Develop a code word to use if they feel unsafe and want to leave.
- Discuss what to do in these situations.
- Being proactive and making a pact to watch out for each other can be the best safeguard against rape or sexual trauma.

as a casual friend, boyfriend, parent, stepparent, uncle, or even a male sibling. It is currently estimated that up to 66% of all rapes occur with someone already known to the victim. It is also possible that this was not the first occurrence of rape for this adolescent.

Primary prevention is the optimal approach to preventing these crimes. Healthcare providers can support efforts in sexual violence prevention by actively educating all adolescents about sexual violence and providing support to empower adolescents to engage in assertiveness training and self-esteem building efforts. One such effective program is known as Striving to Reduce Youth Violence Everywhere.[51]

MENTAL HEALTH SCREENING IN ADOLESCENTS

It is important to screen for mental health disorders in adolescents. This section will provide an overview of mental health disorders in adolescents; please see Chapter 18 for more detailed information. Screening for mental health disorders in adolescents is paramount as up to almost 47% of adolescents will experience a mental health disorder during their lifetime.[52] Fifty percent of all mental health disorders begin by age 14 and increase up to 75% by age 24 in adolescents. In addition, 50% of all adolescents with mental health disorders will drop out of school and up to 70% of youths in the juvenile justice system today have a mental health disorder.[57] Awareness of the rapid physical, emotional, and psychologic changes that occur for adolescents places them at an increased risk for mental health disorders. However, the average time from the presence of a mental health disorder to treatment is a lag time of 8 to 10 years. These statistics highlight the need for early mental health screening and intervention.

The four most common mental health diagnoses affecting adolescence are depressive disorders, anxiety disorders, substance abuse/dependence, and attention-deficit hyperactivity disorder (ADHD).[53] An occasional occurrence of anxiety is considered a normal experience in short-term situations such as taking a test, awaiting a medical test result, or, in the case of an 18-year-old teenager, waiting to find out what college you have been accepted into. These are common examples of an occasional anxiety situation that are generally short term and resolve when the test results are known. However, anxiety disorders under the realm of mental health disorders are a more significant problem related to excessive worry and/or concern about real or imagined problems/situations for the person involved. Anxiety disorders are increasing in the adolescent population and it is believed that the increased focus in our society on materialism may be a contributing factor.[54]Approximately 20% of the adolescent population will suffer from anxiety disorders. Adolescent females are at higher risk for anxiety disorders at a rate as high as 30%.[55]

Suicide is a devastating event that can occur because of depression and anxiety. Suicide among adolescents currently rates as the second-leading cause of death in this age group.[56] In 2019, the CDC conducted a survey on adolescents and found that 8.9% of at-risk teens had contemplated suicide in the past year, and 18.8% of ninth through 12th graders surveyed during that year had thoughts of attempting suicide. This survey revealed that 15.7% of the teenagers who contemplated suicide had a plan and 8.9% of them had attempted suicide. Of those who had made a serious attempt at suicide, 2.7% had self-inflicted injuries requiring medical attention.[53] In the analysis of the CDC's survey data, some gender differences emerged. Although females were almost twice as likely to think about committing suicide as their male cohorts (24.1% vs. 13.3%), males were five times more likely to commit suicide as compared to females. Over 50% of males who commit suicide will use a weapon whereas females are more likely to poison themselves. It has also been determined that 90% of all teens who committed suicide had an underlying mental health illness.

Recommendations for Discussion and Screening for Mental Health Disorders

The importance of mental health assessments has been substantiated in the previous paragraphs. Mental health screenings as part of the health and wellness visits are essential for early case findings. Screening for these serious disorders should be an ongoing discussion at every annual visit and any episodic visit of an adolescent whose physical presentation or complaints may indicate mental health symptoms. General approaches to mental health screening can include general questions such as: "How have you been feeling in the past 2 to 4 weeks?" Another question asked may be, "Has anything happened to you recently that was upsetting and caused you to lose sleep or feel angry or depressed?" There are also several validated depression and anxiety screening tools that are available for use in general practice. Screening tools such as the Beck Depression Inventory (BDI) or the State Trait Anxiety scale (STAI) can be used to quickly assess a client's risk for depression or anxiety (see Chapter 18). These screening tools can be given to the adolescent when they check in, requesting that they complete this questionnaire prior to being seen for their visit. These types of tools have been utilized for several years and have been validated as reliable tools to be used in a clinical setting. They are easy to complete and can be quickly evaluated to ascertain a client's risk.

If an adolescent score is above the normal range for these tests, further questions will need to be asked, such as, "Have you thought about harming yourself? If so, have you thought about how you would do this, and do you have a plan to carry this out?" These types of questions are helpful in making a judgment on how quickly the APRN must act in seeking mental health expertise for the adolescent. Symptoms such as a flat or depressed affect, avoidance of eye contact, disheveled or unkempt appearance, tearful behavior or direct verbal comments regarding depression or anxiety, a loss of appetite, poor school performance, or a loss of interest in daily activities may be signs/symptoms of a significant mental health disorder. In situations in which the adolescent presents with any of the previously mentioned symptoms, the APRN should focus on performing a quick depression/anxiety screening to take rapid action. If this client is found to exhibit serious signs of depression, anxiety, or suicidal ideation, they should be immediately referred to a mental health provider for further evaluation. If the APRN is practicing in a setting that has mental health services available within the same setting, a "warm handoff" may be necessary. A warm handoff is done when an APRN assesses the adolescent for risk and, if found to be high risk, escorts the person to the mental health clinic/provider for immediate care. This is important in an acute situation in which the adolescent may be at risk for self-harm or trauma. If a mental health provider is not available in the setting that you work in, you will need to coordinate the patient being transferred to a tertiary facility such as a hospital or ED setting where they can be cared for and monitored. The transfer of this person may include engaging an ambulance service if no other option is available or appropriate.

In less acute situations, an adolescent can be referred for mental health services to another agency. Coordinating this referral is important and should be done to ensure that the person has an established appointment and contact information of the mental health provider/service that they are being referred to. In addition, the APRN should review with each person at risk of suicide an action plan for them to evaluate if the symptoms are improving or worsening.

There are also several other health assessment questionnaires/resources that are available and comprehensive and include mental health questions for a comprehensive adolescent health assessment. For example, the Bright Futures.org screening tool for adolescents from 15 to 17 includes a series of quick questions to be checked off by the teen. Bulleted questions such as

- Depression: Yes or No, and if yes, when _____?
- Anxiety: Yes or No and if yes, when _____?

And the format continues to include suicidal ideation. These types of questionnaires are comprehensive and well organized to assist the APRN in completing a comprehensive review of each adolescent in a reasonable period of time.

ETHICAL DILEMMAS IN CARE OF THE ADOLESCENT

APRNs providing care to adolescents may encounter ethical dilemmas. Ethical dilemmas are situations that require review and a decision about the most effective way to deal with a situation. Although most healthcare settings have policies in place that outline the steps to be taken when dealing with an ethical dilemma, these policies are often more focused on specific aspects of care such as end-of-life care. However, it is common for a healthcare provider to encounter a myriad of ethical dilemmas that are not as clearly defined. It is important to consider these situations individually, gather all the facts of the case, and then seek input from other designated professionals within your organization. These individuals may include your immediate supervisor(s), collaborating healthcare providers, members of your healthcare team with expertise in the area of concern, or a specially appointed ethics committee to determine an appropriate course of action. The most effective way to assess each situation is to first determine if this is a minor or major ethical dilemma. For example, a minor ethical dilemma may be your decision to not provide direct care for an adolescent you know personally outside of your APRN role. If a situation makes you feel potentially uncomfortable, you need to first acknowledge this feeling and then seek assistance in making your decision. Part of your action needs to include finding another provider willing to see the adolescent who does not have a conflict of interest.

A more difficult dilemma may be when you are caring for an adolescent who is underage (age 16 or younger) and is seeking contraception when their parent/caretaker has informed you that the adolescent is not sexually active. This situation can create many stressors for you, and you will need to seek professional guidance on how best to approach this situation. A major ethical dilemma can occur when an adolescent is refusing medication or a treatment that may help them to eradicate or reduce the outcome of a serious illness or disease. This is a very difficult situation and needs to be comprehensively reviewed by a designated ethics committee or designated ethics consultant for support and guidance on what to do.

In caring for the adolescent population, there is great potential for APRNs to encounter ethical dilemmas. The following case studies, which are based on real cases, can provide you with an opportunity to explore some of these potential situations and what your action plan will include.

CONCLUSION

Adolescence can be a challenging time because of the rapid physical and psychologic changes adolescents experience. Often they have to make choices that will impact their adulthood, but because of peer pressure and other factors, they may not make the best decision. So having a caring and competent NP who has the knowledge and capability to engage in conversation regarding the pros and cons of the many life choices is essential. This chapter provided an overview of many of the challenges this population faces along with evidence-based recommendations for APRN practice.

CASE STUDY
UNDERAGE PATIENT REQUESTS COMBINED ORAL CONTRACEPTIVE WITHOUT LEGAL GUARDIAN

Kelly, a 17-year-old female, and her family are well known to your practice. Many of the family members, including Kelly's mom, have seen you for healthcare. Kelly makes an appointment to see you and requests that you prescribe an oral contraceptive for her. Your discussion includes an assessment of her sexual activity, her knowledge about the various methods of contraception, and her parents' knowledge (or lack thereof) regarding the fact that Kelly is sexually active. Kelly reveals to you that her parents have no knowledge of her sexual activity and that she has no intention of informing them about this. You complete your history and physical examination of this client and prescribe a COC for this client. You also provide her with information regarding how to take this medication and what she is to expect with it. Twenty minutes later, the in-house pharmacist contacts you and informs you that she has just presented Kelly with her COC prescription when Kelly's mom arrives and demands that the pharmacist tell her what has just been prescribed for her daughter. This mom then proceeds to grab the bag and rip it open, noting the prescription for COCs and who wrote it.

The pharmacist informs you that this mom "is very angry and upset and is coming to your department to demand to see you!"

Case Study Questions
- How would you handle this situation?
- What are your legal responsibilities in this situation as Kelly is underage and her mother is her legal guardian?

CASE STUDY
PATIENT EXPERIENCING BULLYING

Randy, a 16-year-old male, comes in to be seen for an episodic visit. During the visit, he reveals to you that he has been bullied at school for months. You further assess this situation while noting that Randy has not reached full sexual maturation. Your discussion with him includes suggesting that you would like to notify his parents about this situation. Because his father is in the waiting room, you suggest that you invite him into the visit and that both you and Randy inform him of what is going on at school. Randy adamantly refuses to let you tell his father or mother about what is going on and says that he has been "handling it himself."

Case Study Questions
- How would you handle this situation?
- What is your responsibility in this situation?
- Would you seek any other professional consultation regarding this, and who would you consult with?

CASE STUDY
PATIENT WITH URINARY BURNING AND DYSURIA

Taylor, a 15-year-old female, accompanied by her mom comes in for an acute visit. Taylor is complaining of urinary burning and dysuria. You complete a history assessment and have been told by both Taylor and her mother that she has not ever been sexually active. You request a urine specimen for lab testing. This specimen is sent off to the laboratory for a stat urinalysis examination. You inform Taylor that you would now like to have her get undressed to perform an examination of her. You ask her if she would like her mom present or to step out of the room. Her mother quickly responds that she will step out of the room. You complete an examination on Taylor focusing on the abdomen and external genitourinary inspection. Now, the laboratory technician calls to inform you that she has examined Taylor's urine under the microscope and has found "active sperm swimming in her urine."

Case Study Questions
- How will you proceed in this situation with Taylor?
- Do you have a responsibility to inform Taylor's mom that her daughter is having sex?
- Do you need to perform another physical examination? What will you do?

REFERENCES
References for this chapter are online and available at https://connect.springerpub.com/content/book/978-0-8261-8414-6/part/part01/toc-part/ch11.

PART IV

Preparation for Practice

CHAPTER 12

Physical Examination

Gerald Kayingo, Vasco Deon Kidd, and Joshua Anderson

LEARNING OBJECTIVES

At the conclusion of this chapter, the learner will be able to:

➤ Summarize the fundamental physical assessment skills and concepts necessary to care for older adults.

➤ Describe correct techniques in performing focused and comprehensive physical examinations with attention to the geriatric patient's comfort, modesty, and cultural values.

➤ Present a systematic approach to examining the geriatric patient from head to toe.

➤ Discuss common physical examination abnormalities or features frequently associated with the aging patient.

➤ Integrate surface anatomy landmarks, physiologic principles, and the aging process when approaching a physical examination in older adults.

➤ Discuss how appropriate physical assessment skills, knowledge, and attitudes play a critical role in the improving health of older adults.

INTRODUCTION

Older adults display heterogeneous changes in anatomy and physiology. These changes often lead to atypical presentation of diseases, a loss of function, and an increased risk of disability. Older adults are also most likely to have multiple comorbidities;[1] they often overestimate healthiness and underestimate the severity of disease. It is important that healthcare professionals develop competencies and skills necessary for a comprehensive assessment to prevent or reduce disability while maximizing function in older adults. Health professionals should be able to perform geriatric-tailored physical examinations and measure physical, cognitive, psychologic, social, and environmental domains of health. This chapter presents an overview of a systematic and sequential physical examination of older adults and describes various techniques commonly performed in primary care settings. Both comprehensive and focused examinations are covered using the four cardinal techniques of examination: inspection, palpation, percussion, and auscultation. Unlike a traditional physical examination in other populations, assessment of older adults calls for enhanced focus on functional assessment during the physical examination.

GENERAL SURVEY, VITAL SIGNS, AND ASSESSING FUNCTIONAL STATUS

A systematic approach to examining older adults should start with evaluating the general appearance and assessing functional status. Examiners should note the apparent state of health, level of consciousness, signs of distress, skin color changes, or any obvious lesions. It is also important to note how the older adult is dressed, along with their grooming and hygiene. During this general survey, also note facial expression, any odors of body or mouth, posture, gait, and motor activity, as well as height, weight, and body mass index (BMI). General appearance can signal an underlying medical condition. For example, flat or impoverished affect may signal depression, Parkinson's disease, or Alzheimer's disease.

Assessment of functional status in older adults addresses the individual's ability to perform tasks and fulfill social roles associated with daily living. It provides a baseline around various aspects of health such as cognitive abilities, mobility, bowel and bladder function, nutritional status, and vision and hearing. Several validated tools are available to assess functional status; a commonly used performance-based assessment tool is the 10-Minute Geriatric Screener.[2] This tool covers three important areas of geriatric assessment: cognitive, psychosocial, and physical function. The tool asks about vision, hearing, leg mobility, urinary incontinence, nutrition/weight loss, memory, depression, and physical disability. Additionally, examiners should screen for fall risk among older adults through a detailed history, medical review, and assessment of gait and balance.

Vital Signs

Similar to a traditional physical examination, assessing vital signs in older adults includes measuring temperature, heart rate (HR), respiratory rate (RR), and blood pressure (BP). In addition to determining the HR, the examiner should also assess the rhythm for irregularities. A regularly irregular heart rhythm may suggest premature ventricular contractions (PVCs) or premature atrial contractions (PACs), while an irregularly irregular heart rhythm is classically associated with atrial fibrillation. Evaluate pulses for their intensity or amplitude, as well as their contour. The amplitude is generally rated on the following scale:

0 = absent
1 = faint or weak
2 = normal
3 = strong
4 = bounding

When assessing the BP, ensure that the BP cuff is the proper size and that the patient is appropriately positioned sitting in a chair with feet flat on the ground and relaxed. When assessing vital signs in the ambulatory office, have the patient sit for 5 minutes prior to measuring the BP and pulse to avoid getting a false high reading. It is very important for older adults to determine orthostatic vital signs, commonly referred to as "orthostatics." With the patient in the supine position for 5 to 10 minutes, measure HR and BP, and then have the patient stand up for 3 minutes and measure HR and BP again. Orthostatic hypotension is a drop in systolic BP of 20 mmHg or more or diastolic BP drop of 10 mmHg or more from supine to standing position. Orthostatic hypotension may signal dehydration, medication side effects, or other systemic causes.

SKIN EXAMINATION

Skin examinations in older adults are particularly important to screen for skin cancer. The examiner should inspect and palpate the skin, noting color, moisture, texture, and turgor. Assess for any lesions: anatomic location/distribution, patterns/shapes—linear, clustered, annular (ring-shaped), aciform (in an arc), geographic, serpiginous, or dermatomal. Pay attention to the ABCDs of melanoma (**A**symmetry, Irregular **B**order, Variation in **C**olor (mixtures of black/blue/red), **D**iameter >6 mm). During the skin examination, inspect and palpate the hair, noting for quantity, distribution, and texture. Hair loss may signal endocrine abnormalities or alopecia. In addition to skin and hair, inspect and palpate the fingernails and toenails, noting for lesions, and any changes in color or texture.

HEAD, EARS, NOSE, SINUSES, MOUTH, THROAT, NECK, AND THYROID EXAMINATIONS

Examination of the Head

Among older adults, serious pathologies such as basal and squamous cell skin cancers manifest on the head. Endocrine disorders such as hyperthyroidism, as well as head trauma, should always be assessed in this population.

Inspection

Clinicians should examine the hair quantity, distribution, texture, and pattern of loss (if any). The presence of coarse or fine hair may signal hypothyroidism and hyperthyroidism, respectively. Hair loss/patches may indicate lupus or alopecia areata. The clinician should examine the scalp for lesions or scaliness as seen in older adults with seborrheic dermatitis, psoriasis, or fungal infections. Inspection should also note the skull size, contour, and if there are any lumps or deformities. Inspect the face for any asymmetry, twitches, swelling, or lesions. Note the patient's facial expression (a depressed stare may signal Parkinson's disease or other neurologic disorders).

Palpation

Palpate the head for any tenderness, lumps, depressions, or any skull irregularities.

Examination of the Ears

Hearing in older adults can be impacted by a variety of disorders such as cerumen impaction, ear infections, ruptured tympanic membranes, cholesteatoma of the middle ear, as well as sensorineural and conductive hearing loss.

Inspection

Clinicians should start by examining the external ear for any erythema, scaliness, swelling, deformities, skin lesions, or lumps. The inspection should note if there is any discharge or bleeding.

Palpation

Assess for any tenderness with movement or palpation of tragus, auricle, or mastoid process. Tenderness may indicate otitis externa, otitis media, or mastoiditis.

Otoscopic Evaluation

Using an otoscope, the clinician should inspect the inside ear for erythema, discharge, edema, cerumen, or foreign bodies. Inspect the tympanic membrane for color, contour, scarring, the presence of tympanostomy tubes, or perforations. The otoscopic inspection also helps in identifying any fluid or pus in the middle ear as well as assessing membrane mobility.

Evaluation of Hearing

Start with a gross evaluation by assessing the individual's ability to hear a whispered phrase such as "99" or "baseball." If deficits are noted, it is a good idea to assess whether the individual has conductive or sensorineural hearing loss. Two special tests are commonly performed to help differentiate the form of hearing loss.

1. **Weber Test for Lateralization:** Administered by holding a vibrating tuning fork (128 Hz) on the vertex of the patient's head. The patient is asked to report in which ear the sound is heard louder. In normal hearing, the patient will hear the sound equally in

both ears. In a conductive hearing loss, the sound is lateralized to the impaired ear. With a sensorineural hearing loss, the sound is heard better in the nonimpaired ear.

2. **Rinne Test:** Test for comparison of air conduction versus bone conduction hearing loss. Place the stem of the vibrating tuning fork (typically 512 Hz) initially on the mastoid process behind the ear until the sound is no longer heard. Then, without restriking the fork, place the prong end of the fork quickly just outside the ear and ask the patient to report when the sound is no longer heard. In normal hearing, the sound should still be heard when the tuning fork is moved to air near the ear, indicating that air conduction (AC) is equal or greater than bone conduction (BC). Normally, AC is greater than BC; in conductive hearing loss, BC equals AC or BC is greater than AC; and in sensorineural loss, AC is greater than BC (Rinne is not ideal in distinguishing sensorineural hearing loss from normal hearing).

Examination of the Nose and Sinuses

Inspection

Gross inspection of the nose and sinuses will identify any swelling, obvious deformities, bruising, lesions, and skin color. In older adults, skin cancers are commonly on the nose. Rhinophyma (a large, red, bumpy nose) may be seen in older adults with rosacea or alcohol abuse.

Palpation

Assess for patency of the nares. Palpation of the frontal and maxillary sinuses may reveal tenderness.

Visual Examination With Otoscope

Inspect the nasal mucosa, color, and inflammation and compare bilaterally. Inspect for discharge and note amount, color, consistency, or blood. A clinician should evaluate for structural abnormalities, such as a deviated nasal septum or nasal polyps. Older adults who have a history of intranasal drug use may have a perforated nasal septum. Transillumination of the sinuses can be helpful to elucidate fluid-filled sinuses that may occur with sinus infection or trauma.

Examination of the Mouth and Throat

Even though many disorders of the throat and mouth are common in older adults, this area is frequently less emphasized in primary care offices. Healthcare professionals should pay more attention to mouth examinations to screen for disorders related to dentition, gum disease, xerostomia (dry mouth), and oropharyngeal cancers.

Inspection

Inspect the lips for color, moisture, and ulcers. Oral mucosa should be moist and without lesions. Identify Stensen's and Wharton's ducts and the location of submandibular and parotid glands. Inspect the condition of the teeth and gums (you may need to remove dentures). Inspect the tongue for lesions, contour, color, texture, and papillae. Inspect hard and soft palate for color and lesions. Inspect the throat, including the uvula, for erythema, swelling, or deviation. Inspect the tonsils, which may be surgically absent. If present, note any swelling, erythema, or exudates. Clinicians should also inspect the pharynx for color, drainage, and swelling. Common disorders of the mouth and throat include pharyngitis, tonsillitis, thrush, oropharyngeal cancers, aphthous ulcers, herpes simplex virus, leukoplakia, Kaposi's sarcoma (immunocompromised individuals), and hairy tongue.

Examination of the Neck and Thyroid Gland

Inspection

Inspect the neck for symmetry, masses, or scars. Look for enlargement of the parotid glands or any visible lymph nodes. Look at the trachea and inspect for any obvious deviation from the midline. Inspect the thyroid for any obvious enlargement. If an enlargement is noted, be sure to measure and further investigate any other related abnormalities. One quick trick to estimate the size of the thyroid is to apply a wide paper tape over the thyroid and outline the thyroid on the tape, making it easier to measure. Write the measurement on the tape. Take pictures and upload into the chat or, if still using a paper chart, print the picture and adhere it to the paper chart.

Palpation

Palpation of the neck should focus on lymph nodes, noting their size, shape, mobility, consistency, and any tenderness. Palpate the trachea, noting any deviation, tenderness, or masses. Palpate the thyroid gland, feeling enlargement, nodularity, or tenderness.

Auscultate the Thyroid Gland

Listen for any bruits. Common disorders of the neck and thyroid gland include goiter, hyperthyroidism/Graves' disease, hypothyroidism, thyroid cancer, thyroiditis, cystic hygroma, lymphadenopathy, and lymphadenitis.

Examination of the Eyes

Eye disorders are among the most prevalent disorders in older adults, with approximately one person in three having some form of vision-reducing eye disease by the age of 65.[3] Common age-related eye problems include cataracts, glaucoma, presbyopia, dry eyes, macular degeneration, and retinopathy. These vision changes can dramatically affect the quality of life of older adults, leading to an increased risk for falls and an increased risk for mortality. It is important that the healthcare professional develop competencies in screening for these eye-related problems. The three vital signs of ophthalmology are visual acuity, pupils, and intraocular pressure.

Inspection

Inspect the external eye, noting the position and alignment of the eyes. Examine the eyebrows looking for hair distribution and scaliness. Next, inspect the eyelids, looking for edema, discoloration, lesions, eyelashes, and the adequacy with which eyelids close (lid lag, ptosis). Inspect the conjunctiva and sclera for color, vascular pattern, nodules, or swelling. Note the lacrimal ducts and if there is excessive tearing, dryness, or swelling. Next, inspect the pupils for size, shape, symmetry, and reaction to light (direct and consensual). Note the color of the iris and inspect the limbus surrounding the iris. For the cornea and lens, look for opacities, lesions, and corneal reflection. Next, assess extraocular muscles, looking for deviations, nystagmus, lid lag, or paralysis. There is a special test for convergence of the eyes. You may perform the cover test to assess for weak eye muscles and ocular deviations. In the cover and uncover test, one eye is covered with the occluder for approximately 1 to 2 seconds. During this time, the uncovered (unoccluded) eye is observed for any shift in fixation.

Visual Acuity

Assess visual acuity by using the Snellen or Rosenbaum eye chart.

Visual Fields

Assess visual fields through the technique of confrontation. In this technique, ask the patient to look directly at your (examiner) nose, and then test each quadrant in the patient's visual field by having them count the number of fingers or say yes when they first see a wiggling finger (or a moving target).

Ophthalmoscopic Examination of the Eye (Fundoscopic Examination)

To conduct a successful examination of the fundus, the examining room should be semi-darkened or completely darkened so that the pupil can become as dilated as possible. For examination of the patient's right eye, sit or stand at the patient's right side and vice versa. Clinicians should pay attention to the correct positioning of the patient as well as the correct technique when using the ophthalmoscope.

Note the optic cup and disc. The outline of the optic disc should be clear. It should be light yellow with a reddish-pink background. The optic disc represents the optic nerve head. The optic cup is the central portion of the disc. Normally, it should be less than half the diameter of the disc and be flat. Pallor of the optic disc may indicate optic nerve disease. Blurred disc margins or an elevated/edematous disc may indicate hypertensive retinopathy or papilledema. An enlarged or elevated cup may indicate hypertensive retinopathy, glaucoma, or papilledema. The presence of new blood vessels growing on the disc surface may indicate diabetic retinopathy.

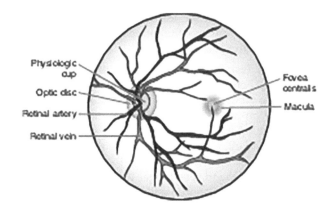

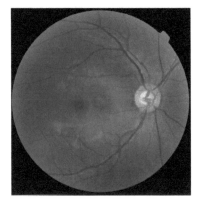

Figure 12.1: A normal ocular fundus

Source: **Chiocca EM.** *Advanced Pediatric Assessment.* Springer Publishing Company; 2020.

Examine the retina, which typically is red/orange in color with the macula being dark and avascular temporally (toward the ear). Prominent flame hemorrhages of the retina may indicate hypertensive or diabetic retinopathy, papilledema, neoplasm, increased intracranial pressure (ICP), or trauma. The presence of cotton wool spots (fluffy white patches of the retina) can signify hypertension, diabetes, AIDS, or blood dyscrasias.

Examine the blood vessels of the retina, where the arterial–venous ratio is typically 2:3 (i.e., the veins are larger). The arteries appear bright red, the veins a slight purplish color. Dilated vessels, engorged veins, tortuosity, A-V nicking, and copper and silver wiring are all associated with long-standing hypertension and diabetic retinopathy. A normal eye fundus is shown in Figure 12.1.

CARDIOVASCULAR EXAMINATION

Cardiovascular disease continues to be a leading cause of mortality and morbidity among older adults.[1,2] Both the anatomy and body physiology change with aging. For example, the stiffness of large arteries increases, and age-related changes in the contraction of myocardial tissue and the electrical system may lead to arrhythmias.[3] Given

Table 12.1: Basic Elements of the Cardiovascular Examination

Examining the Heart: Patient Laying at 30° to 45° and Then Flat
Measure height of JVP.
Palpate carotid arteries bilaterally.
Auscultate carotids bilaterally.
Palpate precordium/PMI (when patient is sitting & lying).
Auscultate heart using diaphragm (when patient is sitting & lying).
Auscultate heart using bell (sitting & lying).
Auscultate for S3, S4, & mitral murmurs–supine & left lateral decubitus position.
Auscultate for aortic regurgitation murmur–with patient leaning forward.
Examining Lungs and Thorax: Patient Sitting
Inspect anterior–posterior diameter of thorax.
Inspect and palpate posterior chest.
Perform tactile fremitus posteriorly.
Test posterior chest expansion.
Percuss costovertebral angle tenderness bilaterally.
Percuss posterior chest.
Percuss diaphragmatic excursion bilaterally.
Auscultate lungs posteriorly at least 3 areas bilaterally.
Inspect/palpate anterior chest.
Perform tactile fremitus anteriorly.
Percuss anterior chest at least 3 areas bilaterally.
Auscultate lungs anteriorly at least 3 areas bilaterally.

JVP, jugular venous pressure; PMI, point of maximum impulse.

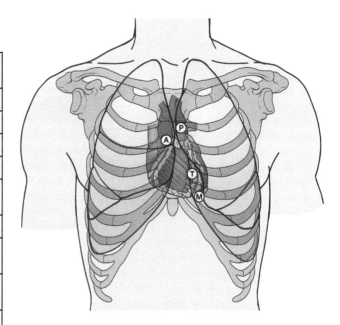

Figure 12.2: Anatomic locations for auscultating heart sounds associated with specific valves. A, aortic; M, mitral; P, pulmonary; T, tricuspid

Source: Tkacs N, Herrmann L, Johnson R, eds. *Advanced Physiology and Pathophysiology: Essentials for Clinical Practice.* Springer Publishing Company; 2020.

these epidemiologic and pathophysiologic factors, it is important that health professionals improve their competency in cardiovascular assessment, diagnosis, treatment, and appropriate referrals. Typically, the cardiovascular examination should include neck vessels, the heart, peripheral, vascular, and lymphatics systems (Table 12.1). The anatomic positioning of the heart is shown in Figure 12.2.

Examination of the Neck Vessels

Examining the Carotid Arteries

The clinician should start with inspecting the neck for pulsations. This is followed by palpating each carotid artery separately. During palpation, assess the amplitude of the pulse in the carotid arteries and compare both sides. A decreased pulsation may be reflective of decreased stroke volume or atherosclerotic narrowing of the carotid arteries. After palpation, auscultate for bruits using the bell of the stethoscope. In addition to atherosclerotic narrowing, carotid artery bruits may signal external carotid disease, aortic stenosis, hypervascularity of hyperthyroidism, or external compression from thoracic outlet syndrome.

Estimating the Jugular Venous Pressure

Estimating the jugular venous pressure (JVP) provides an estimate of the pressure in the right atrium. A JVP greater than 6 cm at 30° or greater than 4 to 5 cm at 45° above the sternal angle is abnormal and suggests right-sided heart failure (most common). Other causes of increased JVP may include pulmonary hypertension, pericardial tamponade, and pericarditis. The patient should be positioned with their head elevated 30° or 45° and turned slightly away from the side of the examiner (Figure 12.3). The examiner should use tangential (oblique) lighting to maximize visualization of the venous pulsations. With the patient properly positioned, identify the highest point of pulsation in the internal jugular vein. With a centimeter ruler, measure the vertical distance between this point and the sternal angle.

Examination of the Heart

Inspection

Assess for skin color changes that may indicate abnormal blood supply. With the patient in a supine position or

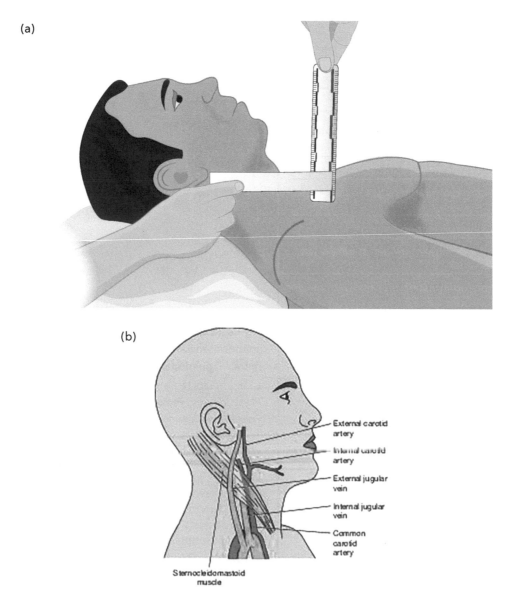

Figure 12.3: Estimating the jugular venous pressure (JVP): Patient should be positioned with head elevated 30° or 45° and head turned slightly away from the side of the examiner

Sources: (a) Gawlik KS, Melnyk Mazurek B, Teal AM, eds. *Evidence-Based Physical Examination: Best Practices for Health and Well-Being Assessment.* Springer Publishing Company; 2021; (b) Myrick K, Karosas L, Smeltzer S, eds. *Advanced Health Assessment and Differential Diagnosis: Essentials for Clinical Practice.* Springer Publishing Company; 2021.

at a 30° or 45° angle, inspect the precordium and chest for any deformities and for the point of maximum impulse (PMI), which is usually in the fourth or fifth intercostal space at the midclavicular line (see Figure 12.2).

Palpation

Palpation of the heart should focus mainly on three things:

1. **Palpate for the PMI:** This provides an estimate of the heart size and it is best assessed in the left lateral decubitus position. Examiners should assess the location, diameter, amplitude, and duration of the impulse. Palpation for the apical impulse can provide clues on strength of LV contraction and stroke volume. Patients with chronic obstructive pulmonary disease (COPD) may have a displaced PMI due to right ventricular hypertrophy. Lateral displacement from cardiac enlargement is seen in heart failure, cardiomyopathy, and ischemic heart disease.

2. **Palpate for Heaves/Lifts:** These are palpable movements of localized areas of the precordium due to increased intensity of the sustained systolic contraction.

3. **Palpate for Thrills:** Assess for any palpable murmur. A thrill is best felt through bone, so examiners should use the ulnar surface of their hands to increase the sensitivity of the examination. A palpable thrill is more likely to be present if a murmur is grade IV or above.

Percussion

Not routinely performed but may be done to estimate heart size.

Auscultation

Cardiac auscultation determines the HR, rhythm regularity, murmurs, rubs, gallops, and clicks. It is important for the examiner to identify the normal heart sounds, S1 and S2, which represent ventricular systole and ventricular diastole, respectively. The examiner should auscultate at the following locations:

a. Right second interspace close to the sternum (aortic)

b. Left second interspace close to the sternum (pulmonic)

c. Along the left sternal border at each interspace from the third to the fifth (tricuspid)

d. At the apex (mitral)

The examiner should also listen at each site with the diaphragm of the stethoscope, then with the bell.

a. **Diaphragm:** Able to hear S1 and S2 better, which are relatively high-pitched sounds. Also, murmurs due to mitral and aortic regurgitation and pericardial friction rubs are heard best with the diaphragm.

b. **Bell:** Able to better hear S3 and S4, if present, with the bell. Also, the murmur of mitral stenosis is a lower-pitched sound heard better with the bell. The examiner should use light pressure when using the bell because it allows better appreciation of S3 and S4. It is important to note that certain patient positions may help to bring out abnormal heart sounds, which may not otherwise be heard. For example, leaning forward can be helpful in accentuating the murmur of aortic insufficiency.

Auscultatory Sounds
Normal Heart Sounds

1. S1 heart sound indicating closure of the mitral (and tricuspid) valves

2. S2 heart sound indicating closure of the aortic (and pulmonic) valves

3. Physiologic split S2 can be heard during inspiration only.

Abnormal Heart Sounds

Split S1 may be physiologic or could indicate a right bundle branch block. Increased intensity of S1 could indicate hypertension, hyperthyroidism, and mitral stenosis. Diminished S1 may occur with weak ventricular contraction, first-degree heart block, aortic insufficiency, and/or calcified mitral valve leaflets. "Splitting of S2 may be harder to hear in older people as its pulmonic component becomes less audible."[4] Increased intensity of S2 may occur with ascending aortic aneurysm or pulmonary hypertension. Diminished S2 can indicate arterial hypotension, aortic stenosis, or pulmonic stenosis.

Gallops

1. S3 gallop commonly associated with mitral regurgitation

2. S4 gallop commonly associated with left ventricular hypertrophy

Other Sounds

1. **Friction Rub:** Caused by inflammation of the pericardial sac (pericarditis, cardiac tamponade)

2. **Opening Snap:** Can be heard in mitral stenosis

3. **Mid-systolic Click:** Significant for mitral valve prolapse

Murmurs

Murmurs are categorized by timing (early, mid, or late systolic vs. diastolic), location on precordium, intensity (Grade II–-XI), pattern (crescendo–decrescendo, holosystolic, etc.), pitch (high, low), and posture (supine, erect, left lateral decubitus). The common murmurs follow:

1. Mid-systolic murmur of aortic stenosis

2. Early diastolic murmur of aortic regurgitation

3. Mid-diastolic murmur of mitral stenosis

4. Holosystolic murmur of mitral regurgitation

5. Late systolic murmur of mitral valve prolapse

6. Continuous murmur of patent ductus arteriosus

Systolic Murmurs

■ **Systolic Ejection Murmurs:** May indicate vascular atherosclerosis

■ **Aortic Valve Sclerosis:** Common in the older adult and not hemodynamically significant. Peaks during early systole and does not radiate to the carotids. May develop into aortic stenosis causing outflow obstruction of the left ventricle.

■ **Aortic Stenosis:** Peaks in late systole, pulse pressure narrowed. May see slowed carotid upstroke, but this is not always the case, especially in the older adult, due to diminished vascular compliance.

- **Mitral Regurgitation:** Holosystolic, loudest at apex, radiates to axilla
- **Hypertrophic Obstructive Cardiomyopathy (HOCM):** Intensifies with valsalva
- **Diastolic Murmurs:** Pathologic and indicate some alteration of normal structure or function of the cardiovascular system.
- **Aortic Regurgitation:** Aortic valve leaflets fail to close completely during diastole. A blowing decrescendo murmur is best heard with the patient sitting and holding breath after exhalation.
- **Pulmonary Regurgitation:** Pulmonic valve fails to completely close during diastole. Commonly associated with hypertension and can be asymptomatic.
- **Mitral Stenosis:** Mitral valve fails to open completely in diastole. Can hear decrescendo murmur, opening snap.
- **Tricuspid Stenosis:** Narrowing of the tricuspid valve which may limit blood flow from the right atrium to the right ventricle. Commonly caused by rheumatic fever.

THE PERIPHERAL VASCULAR AND LYMPHATIC SYSTEMS

Examining the Peripheral Vascular System in the Upper Extremities

The clinician should start with inspecting both arms from the fingertips to the shoulders for size, symmetry, swelling, venous patterns, color, and other skin, nail, and hair changes. Assess capillary refill (should be less than 2 seconds) to evaluate perfusion. This is followed by palpating the brachial, radial, and ulnar pulses. The ulnar pulses are not always palpable. Pulses should be assessed for amplitude, contour, and intensity. Remember, pulses are graded on a scale of 0 to 4:

0 = absent
1 = diminished
2 = normal
3 = increased
4 = bounding

Perform the Allen Test if you suspect arterial insufficiency in the radial or ulnar arteries.[4]

For the lymphatic system, palpate the epitrochlear lymph nodes, which are located distal to the medial epicondyle. If a node is present, note its size, consistency, and tenderness.

Examining the Peripheral Vascular System in the Lower Extremities

The clinician should start with inspecting both legs from toenails to the hip for size, symmetry, swelling, venous patterns, color, and other skin, nail, and hair changes, as well as assessing capillary refill.

This is followed by palpating femoral pulse in each leg. The examiner should then palpate the popliteal pulse behind the knee (in the popliteal fossa), then palpate the dorsalis pedis (sometimes congenitally absent) and the posterior tibial pulses in each foot. Palpate the legs for tenderness and palpable cords that might signify a thrombosis.

Lymphatic System

Palpate the superficial inguinal nodes for size, consistency, and tenderness. The clinician should assess for edema in the extremities, which could be localized (e.g., trauma, tumor, local lymphatic, or venous obstruction) or systemic (heart failure, renal disease). Sometimes the degree of edema can lead to pitting of the skin (pitting edema). As shown in Figure 12.4; the degree of pitting edema is based on a 4-point scale:

1+ = trace pitting (2-mm depression)
2+ = mild-moderate (4-mm, depression)
3+ = significant (moderate-severe, 6-mm depression)
4+ = marked (severe, 8-mm depression)

The presence of edema may signal peripheral vascular system abnormalities such as a recent or ongoing deep venous thrombosis, chronic venous insufficiency due to incompetent valves or history of DVTs, or lymphedema.

Examining the Peripheral Vascular System in the Abdomen

The clinician should start with inspecting the abdomen for abnormal or hyperdynamic pulsations. This should be followed by palpating the aortic and femoral pulses. Try to approximate the size of the aortic pulsation. For auscultation, the examiner should listen for bruits over the abdominal aorta, renal, iliac, and femoral arteries.

THORAX AND PULMONARY EXAMINATION

Anatomic and physiologic changes related to the respiratory system commonly occur with aging; therefore, your physical examination should be tailored toward these changes. For example, exercise capacity typically decreases with age. The chest wall can become more rigid, respiratory muscles may weaken, and the lungs may lose some elasticity. Lung mass reduces while residual volume increases. Older adults are at increased risk for atelectasis, respiratory infections (such as pneumonia), COPD, lung cancer, interstitial lung disease, and pulmonary embolism.[5] Coughing becomes less effective at removing toxins and irritants from our airways and the speed of breathing out with maximal effort

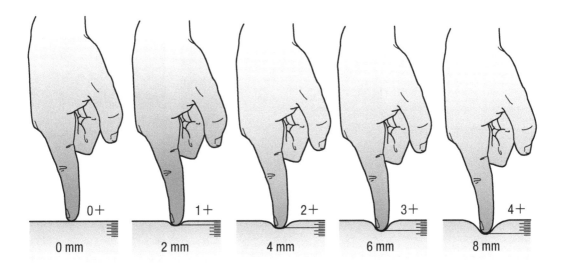

Figure 12.4: Assessing edema

gradually diminishes with age. A thorough lung examination should include anterior, posterior, and lateral fields (Table 12.1). It is helpful to examine the posterior field with the patient seated and with their arms crossed in the front.

Inspection

Examination of the thorax should start with an assessment of breathing effort, noting if the patient is in respiratory distress. Accessory muscle use typically indicates difficulty breathing and may be present in the patient with respiratory distress. Patients with COPD may also be found in a tripod position with lips pursed during exhalation to relieve dyspnea. Inspection should also include assessment for asymmetry or deformities, as well as noting AP diameter. Barrel chest (enlarged AP diameter of the chest) may indicate COPD. Inspect both anterior and posterior aspects of the chest wall. Spinal deformities such as kyphosis should clue you in to the potential for osteoporosis and vertebral fractures. Both kyphosis and scoliosis may diminish lung volumes and lead to breathing difficulties. The clinician should inspect for blue/gray discoloration of the skin, nails, and lips, as cyanosis can indicate hypoxia. Nail clubbing (loss of the normal angle between the fingernail and nail bed) may be noted in older adults with bronchiectasis, congenital heart disease, pulmonary fibrosis, cystic fibrosis, lung abscess, and malignancy.

Palpation

Palpate for any tenderness or masses of the chest. Tenderness at the costosternal joints may aid in the diagnosis of costochondritis. The clinician should evaluate for tactile fremitus (Figure 12.5), which are palpable vibrations transmitted to the chest wall during speech. The examiner places the ulnar edge of their hands on the patient's anterior and posterior thorax and asks the patient

to say, "Ninety-nine," in various lung fields, noting any dissimilarities in the vibrations. Decreased tactile fremitus may be found with COPD, pleural effusion, fibrosis, or tumors. During palpation, the clinician evaluates the ability of the chest to expand and contract (Figure 12.6), which may be diminished in aging individuals or if pathology is present. Unilateral decrease of chest expansion could hint toward lobar pneumonia, pleural effusion, and/or chronic fibrosis.

Percussion

Percussion is useful to determine whether underlying structures are air-filled, fluid-filled, or solid (Table 12.2). Examiners should percuss both the anterior and posterior lung fields in at least three areas bilaterally. The examiner places the left hand firmly on the chest wall and hits the distal interphalangeal joint of the left middle finger with the tip of your right middle finger with a striking wrist motion to elicit a percussive sound. Healthy lungs will produce a resonant sound with percussion. Dullness to percussion could indicate lobar pneumonia, pleural effusion, hemothorax, or empyema. Hyperresonance with percussion is typically found in hyper-inflated lungs and can be indicative of COPD or asthma.

Auscultation

Auscultation of the lungs is a key part of the respiratory physical examination. We typically use the diaphragm of the stethoscope. Patients should preferably be in the seated position with their arms crossed. Auscultation should be done directly to the skin rather than through clothes or a gown. A systematic approach should include auscultation of all lung fields bilaterally in at least three areas, comparing left and right as well as upper and lower lung fields in the anterior, lateral, and posterior aspects.

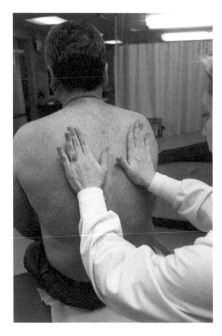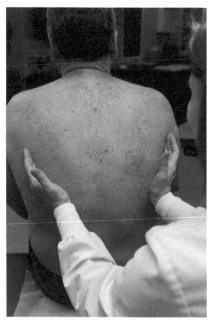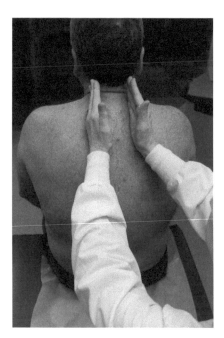

Figure 12.5: Tactile fremitus technique

Source: Gawlik KS, Melnyk Mazurek B, Teal AM. *Evidence-based Physical Examination: Best Practices for Health and Well-Being Assessment.* Springer; 2020.

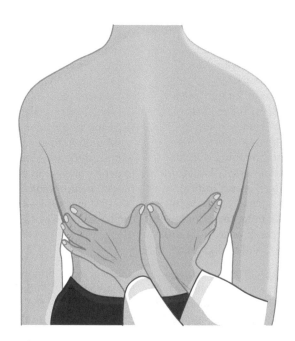

Figure 12.6: Assessing chest expansion

Source: Gawlik KS, Melnyk Mazurek B, Teal AM. *Evidence-based Physical Examination: Best Practices for Health and Well-Being Assessment.* Springer; 2020.

Table 12.2: Percussion Notes and Characteristics

	Relative Intensity	Relative Pitch	Relative Duration	Location	Potential Pathology
Flat	Soft	High	Short	Thigh	Pleural effusion
Dull	Medium	Medium	Medium	Liver	Lobar pneumonia
Resonant	Loud	Low	Long	Healthy lung	Chronic bronchitis
Hyper-resonant	Very Loud	Lower	Longer	Usually none	COPD, pneumothorax
Tympanic	Loud	High	Longer	Gastric air bubble	Large pneumothorax

Abnormal (adventitious) lung sounds may include the following:

- **Rales (Crackles):** Basilar rales may be auscultated in a healthy individual but typically resolve after a few deep breaths. Rales could also point toward atelectasis, lung pathology (pneumonia, fibrosis, early heart failure), or airway disease (bronchitis, bronchiectasis).
- **Rhonchi:** These coarse and low-pitched breath sounds are found when there are secretions in the larger airways.
- **Wheezing:** This can be expiratory or inspiratory and typically found in asthma, COPD, and bronchitis.

ABDOMINAL EXAMINATION

Abdominal complaints are very common in older adults and may include acute or chronic conditions such as constipation, organomegaly, small/large bowel obstruction, inflammatory bowel diseases, diverticulitis, cancers, and abdominal aortic aneurysm (AAA), among others.[6] Unlike other organ systems, the sequence of the abdominal physical examination is as follows: inspection, auscultation, percussion, palpation. Auscultation is now performed before palpation because palpation may alter what was auscultated. It is preferred that the abdominal examination is performed with the individual in a supine position with the knees flexed as this relaxes the abdominal muscles and allows for a more accurate examination (Table 12.3).

Inspection

The clinician should inspect the abdomen for hernias, deformities, scars, skin color changes, and masses. Common abdominal hernias include epigastric, incisional, and umbilical.

Auscultation

First, the clinician will auscultate for bowel sounds in all four quadrants. The absence of bowel sounds may indicate small bowel obstruction or ileus. Next, the clinician will auscultate the abdominal aortic, renal, iliac, and femoral arteries for bruits. Older adults with atherosclerotic arterial disease may present with abdominal bruits. A

Table 12.3: Examining the Abdomen: Patient Lying Flat With Knees Flexed

Inspect abdomen (comment on three things).
Auscultate for bowel sounds in all four quadrants.
Auscultate aortic, iliac, renal, and femoral bruits.
Percuss over abdomen in all four quadrants.
Percuss liver span in midclavicular line (MCL) and note liver size.
Percuss spleen for dullness.
Palpate abdomen superficial in all four quadrants & epigastrium.
Palpate abdomen deep in all four quadrants & epigastrium.
Palpate kidneys bilaterally.
Palpate liver edge.
Palpate spleen tip.
Palpate aortic width.
Palpate inguinal lymph nodes bilaterally.
Palpate femoral arteries bilaterally.
Elicit abdominal reflex.
Perform rectal/pelvic examination as needed.

renal artery bruit may suggest renal artery stenosis while a bruit over the liver suggests hepatic carcinoma or alcoholic hepatitis.

Percussion

With the individual in a supine position and the knees flexed, the examiner percusses the abdomen in all four quadrants. A diffuse tympanic sound can indicate intestinal obstruction while dull areas can indicate things like ovarian tumors, hepatomegaly, or distended bladder. Next, percuss the liver span at the midclavicular line (normally 6–12 cm) and the midsternal line (normally 4–8 cm). Percussion can be particularly useful for evaluating liver masses and ascites (accumulation of fluid in the peritoneal cavity). Ascites can be seen with cirrhosis, heart failure, constrictive pericarditis, or inferior vena cava or hepatic vein obstruction, nephrotic syndrome, ovarian cancer, and malnutrition. In addition to percussing the liver, the examiner should percuss the spleen to estimate the size.

Palpation

There are some important points to remember when palpating the abdomen. We first start with light (superficial) palpation then progress to deeper palpation in all four quadrants, leaving tender areas for last. Next, palpate the kidneys, bilaterally. Following this, palpate the liver edge and the spleen tip for tenderness, masses, and estimation of size. If organomegaly is noted, it could suggest infection, tumor, metabolic disorders, and/or alcohol abuse. Palpation of the abdomen can reveal weak abdominal musculature, which is a risk factor for hernia development. Involuntary guarding (rigidity) is typical with peritoneal inflammation. Palpate the abdominal aorta for aortic width. A widened diameter (≥3 cm) and/or pulsatile mass may indicate aneurysm, of which age older than 65 is a risk factor. Other risk factors for AAA include a history of smoking, male gender, and a first-degree relative with a history of AAA repair.

If a clinician suspects AAA, patients should be recommended for imaging and/or referred to a specialist for further evaluation.[7]

EXAMINING THE MUSCULOSKELETAL AND NERVOUS SYSTEM

Aging is associated with significant changes in the structure and function of the musculoskeletal and nervous systems. Muscle weakness, reduced motor performance, poor coordination, and gait abnormalities are all very common in older adults.[8–10] A common approach to the musculoskeletal examination includes the following: (a) inspecting surrounding skin, color, swelling, deformity, muscle atrophy, alignment, symmetry, size, spasms, limb length, and circumference; (b) palpating muscle tone, heat, tenderness, swelling, crepitus, underlying structures, and ligament laxity; (c) assessing the active and passive range of motion (ROM) of joints bilaterally; (d) testing for muscle strength bilaterally (0–5 scale); (e) performing special tests as indicated for a given patient encounter. It is advisable to always examine the joint above and below the affected area. A systematic and sequential approach to the physical examination of the musculoskeletal and nervous systems of older adults is summarized in Tables 12.4 to 12.7 and Box 12.1.

Table 12.4: Examining the Musculoskeletal System: Patient Sitting/Standing

Assess active range of motion in the neck (in four positions).
Inspect and palpate upper extremity joints.
Assess shoulder flexion/extension.
Assess internal/external rotation shoulder.
Assess abduction/adduction shoulder.
Perform shoulder strength testing (in four positions).
Assess flexion/extension elbow strength.
Flexion/extension, ulnar, radial deviation wrist (+ wrist extension strength).
Assess supination and pronation of wrist.
Evaluate for grip strength.
Evaluate abduction of finger strength.
Elicit biceps reflex bilaterally.
Elicit triceps reflex bilaterally.
Elicit brachioradialis reflex bilaterally.
Inspect and palpate lower extremity joints.
Assess active range of motion in the hip (in six positions).
Perform strength testing of the hip (four positions).
Assess flexion/extension/internal rotation of the knee.
Perform strength testing of the knee (quadriceps and hamstrings).
Assess active range of motion ankle (dorsi/plantar/inversion/eversion).
Perform strength testing of ankle (dorsi/plantar).
Assess flexion/extension first toe.
Elicit patella reflex bilaterally.
Elicit Achilles reflex bilaterally.
Elicit plantar reflex bilaterally.

The Shoulder Examination

The shoulder bony anatomy consists of the humerus, scapula, and clavicle. Rotational strength and range of motion of the shoulder are supported by the rotator cuff muscles (supraspinatus, infraspinatus, teres minor, and subscapularis). Shoulder pathologies are very common in the older adult and include, but are not limited to, rotator cuff arthropathy, adhesive capsulitis, impingement syndrome, and bicipital and calcific tendonitis.

Table 12.5: Examining Cranial Nerves

Test sense of smell bilaterally (CN I)
Assess visual acuity bilaterally (CN II)
Extra-ocular movements (verbalize CN III, IV, VI)
CN V (sensory on face)
CN V (motor—TMJ, masseter muscles)
CN VII (comment: taste of ant 2/3 tongue)
CN VII (motor: facial expressions: raise eye blows, flown)
CN VII (resist opening eyes, show teeth, smile, puff cheeks)
Test auditory acuity bilaterally (CN VIII)
CN IX and X (gag and/or swallow)
CN XI (shoulder shrug + head turning against resistance)
CN XII (tongue movements)

CN, cranial nerve; TMJ, temporomandibular joint.

Table 12.6: Examining Mental Status

Registration short-term recall (three words)
Attention and calculation (WORLD backward)
Language naming (name three words)
Language three-step command
Language repetition (no ifs, ands, or buts)
Language construction (what does that mean?)
Written command (perform a written task)
Language writing (write sentence)

Table 12.7: Sensory and Cerebellar Testing

Rapid alternating movements in upper extremity bilaterally
Rapid alternating movements in lower extremity bilaterally
Finger to nose bilaterally
Heel to shin bilaterally
Proprioception upper/lower bilaterally hands and feet
Vibration sense upper/lower bilaterally hands and feet
Sensory: light touch C5-T1, L3-S1
Sensory: sharp/dull C5-T1, L3-S1—alternating different spots

Box 12.1: Gait Examination

- Gait assessment
- Heel-to-toe walking
- Walk on heels and then on toes
- Shallow knee bend/hop on one foot
- Romberg (articulate 30 seconds)
- Pronator drift (articulate 20-30 seconds)
- Inspect curvatures of the spine
- Range of motion in the spine (six positions)

Figure 12.7 shows the three key joints in the shoulder:
- The glenohumeral (GH) joint, often referred to as a ball-and-socket joint
- The acromioclavicular (AC) joint
- The sternoclavicular (SC) joint

Inspection

Examine the shoulder for swelling, deformity, asymmetry, or muscle atrophy.

Palpation

Beginning medially at the SC joint, the clinician should trace the clavicle laterally with fingers. Palpate the scapula, acromion, the acromioclavicular joint, and the coracoid process. The clinician should also palpate the greater tuberosity, biceps tendon in the bicipital groove, the deltoid and four rotator cuff muscles, and bursae. During palpation, the clinician should note any tenderness, muscular weakness, warmth, effusion, crepitus, deformities, and shoulder instability.

Range of Motion

The ROM of the shoulder is assessed as shown in Figure 12.8. When performing passive or active ROM, it is

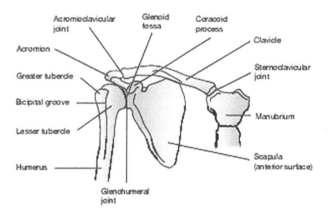

Figure 12.7: Shoulder joints

Source: Myrick K, Karosas L, Smeltzer S. *Advanced Health Assessment and Differential Diagnosis: Essentials for Clinical Practice.* Springer; 2020.

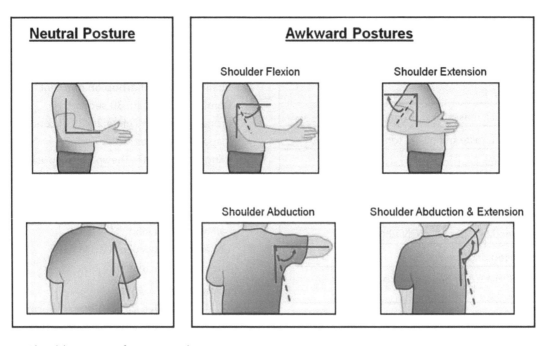

Figure 12.8: Shoulder range of motion technique

Source: Moore SM, Torma-Krajewski J, Steiner LJ. *Practical Demonstrations of Ergonomic Principles.* U.S. Department of Health and Human Services; 2011. https://www.cdc.gov/niosh/mining/userfiles/works/pdfs/2011-191.pdf

recommended to assess shoulder forward flexion, extension, internal rotation (determined by the highest spinal level reached by the thumb), external rotation, abduction, and cross-body adduction. Perform shoulder strength testing in at least four positions.

The Hand and Wrist Examination

The wrist and hands are a complex network of bones, muscles, nerves, tendons, and joints. The bony anatomy of small, ring, long, and index fingers are comprised of distal phalanx, middle phalanx, and metacarpals. However, the thumb is comprised of a distal phalanx and metacarpal. The joints of the fingers include the distal interphalangeal joint (DIPJ), proximal interphalangeal joint (PIPJ), and the metacarpal phalangeal joint (MCPJ). The thumb is composed of the interphalangeal joint (IP), metacarpophalangeal joint (MP), and the carpometacarpal (CMC) joint.

The hand is innervated by the median, ulnar, and radial nerves. The radial nerve supplies the first dorsal web space of the thumb and radial aspect of the dorsum of the hand. The small finger and ulnar half of the ring finger are supplied by the ulnar nerve. The median nerve supplies the index long fingers, the radial side of the ring finger, and the skin on the palmar side of the thumb.

The wrist has eight carpal bones: the scaphoid, pisiform, trapezoid, trapezium, hamate, triquetrum, lunate, and capitate. Proximal to the carpal bones are the radiocarpal joint and distal radial ulnar joint, and these are synovial joints that connect to the radius and ulna bones.

Inspection

Observe for any lesions, excoriations, bony asymmetry, scars, malrotation, and scissoring of the digits. Assess the nail plates for any pitting, spooning, clubbing, or discoloration. Assess intrinsic, thenar, or hypothenar atrophy.

Palpation

When palpating, start distally and move proximally assessing the bony anatomy with corresponding joints. Note any bony or soft tissue irregularities. Assess grip strength.

Range of Motion of Digits

Recommend goniometer when assessing the ROM of digits (Table 12.8). As shown in Figure 12.9, instruct the patient to form a full composite fist. Assess for popping, triggering, or tenderness of the digits.

Provocative Testing

Phalen's test is performed by applying compression over the median nerve or instructing the patient to perform volar flexion of the wrist for 30 to 45 seconds. Tinel's test over carpal tunnel is performed by applying percussion over the median nerve; a negative test does not exclude

Table 12.8: Range of Motion

Range of Motion of the Wrist Is Expressed in Degrees, Right/Left/Normal
Flexion: 60/60
Extension: 60/60
Ulnar deviation: 35/35
Radial deviation: 20/20

carpal tunnel syndrome. Tinel's over cubital tunnel is performed by applying percussion over the ulnar nerve just proximal to the cubital tunnel. Assess sensation in the median nerve distribution using a 2-point discrimination wheel or paperclip. Finkelstein's test is performed by having the patient tuck in the thumb (with clenched fist) coupled with ulnar deviation of the wrist. A positive test will solicit irritation of the abductor pollicis longus (APL) and extensor pollicis brevis (EPB) tendons, indicating de Quervain's tenosynovitis.[11]

Knee Examination

The bony anatomy of the knee is composed of the patella, distal femur, and proximal tibia. Additionally, the knee includes the medial, lateral, and patellofemoral compartments. The four collateral ligament structures supporting the knee are the anterior cruciate ligament (ACL), posterior cruciate ligament (PCL), medial collateral ligament (MCL), and lateral collateral ligament (LCL). The nerve innervation to the knee joint is complex and branches from the femoral, tibial, common peroneal, and obturator nerves; it is responsible for sensory/motor function of the extremity.[12]

Inspection

Observe for effusion, skin lesions, or abrasions. While in the standing position, assess the patient for excessive varus or valgus alignment. Assess gait pattern.

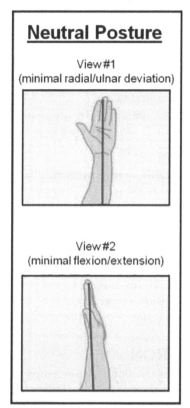
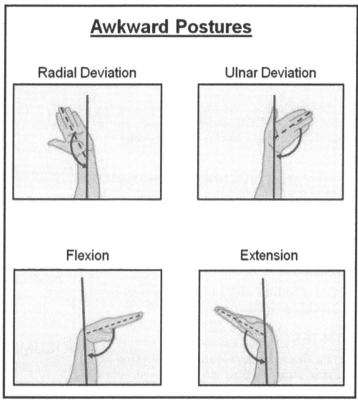

Figure 12.9: Wrist range of motion technique

Source: Practical Demonstrations of Ergonomic Principles. U.S. Department of Health and Human Services; 2011. https://www.cdc.gov/niosh/mining/userfiles/works/pdfs/2011-191.pdf

Palpation

Palpate the anterior lateral and anterior medial joint lines (front of the knee), which may indicate meniscal pathology. Palpate the patella, tibial tubercle, and patellar tendon. Palpate the distal quadriceps muscle, which attaches to the patella. Palpate the posterior knee, the MCL, and the LCL for tenderness and soft tissue swelling.

Range of Motion

Assess knee (ROM), which is from 0 degrees of knee extension to 140 degrees of knee flexion. If available, use a goniometer when assessing ROM. Assess for patellofemoral crepitus.

Provocative Testing

The Lachman's test is used for assessing ACL insufficiency; a positive test is when the tibia moves anteriorly without an abrupt endpoint. The Apley compression test is used to assess meniscal pathology. The patient is placed in a prone position, with the knee flexed at 90 degrees coupled with axial loading and rotation of the knee. A positive test is pain with this maneuver.

Spine Examination

The adult spinal column is composed of 24 vertebrae, 7 cervical vertebrae, 12 thoracic vertebrae, and 5 lumbar vertebrae. Spinal nerves control motor and sensory function of the extremities, including the bowel and bladder. Compression or irritated nerve roots can lead to radicular symptoms affecting the extremities.

Inspection

Assess for cutaneous lesions, bruising, swelling, atrophy, and costovertebral angle (CVA) tenderness. Assess spinal alignment (excessive lordosis, kyphosis, or scoliosis).

Palpation

Assess for midline spinal tenderness, paraspinal tenderness, and sacroiliac joint tenderness, and spasm. Assess sensation to light touch and 2-point discrimination in L3–S1 dermatomes. Assess reflexes in the patellar and the Achilles. Assess the bulbocavernosus reflex (BCR) if spinal injury or spinal shock is suspected.

Range of Motion

Assess the ROM of both the neck and the spine according to Boxes 12.2 and 12.3.

STRENGTH TESTING

Strength testing should be done during the physical examination of any extremity. Strength testing is stratified based on the following criterion (Box 12.4).[13]

Grade 0: No movement is observed.
Grade 1: Only a trace or flicker of movement.
Grade 2: Muscle can move only if the resistance of gravity is removed.

Box 12.2: Cervical Range of Motion Is Expressed in Degrees, Actual/Normal

Flexion: 50/50 Bend neck forward to touch sternum with chin.
Extension: 60/60 Bend neck backward so chin points upward.
Rotation (R/L): 80/80 Turn head with chin pointing right and left.
Lateral Tilt (R/L): 40/40 Tilt the head so the ear bends toward shoulder.

Box 12.3: Lumbosacral Spine Range of Motion Is Expressed in Degrees, Actual/Normal

Flexion: 90/90 Bend the body forward, bending at the waist.
Extension: 30/30 Bend the body back without bending the knees.
Lateral Bend Right: 40/40 Bend the body to the right side, bending at the waist.
Lateral Bend Left: 40/40 Bend the body to the left side, bending at the waist.

Grade 3: Movement against gravity but not resistance.
Grade 4: Movement against at least some resistance supplied by the examiner.
Grade 5: The muscle contracts normally against full resistance.

Provocative Testing

Spurling's Test (Highly specific with only mild to moderate overall sensitivity):[14] The examiner has the patient extend the neck and laterally bends to the affected side as axial compression is applied. A positive test is suggestive of cervical radiculopathy.
Straight Leg Test (High sensitivity but low specificity):[15] The patient is supine while the examiner stands on the affected side. The examiner lifts the patient's leg in full knee extension, causing flexion of the hip. A positive test is suggestive of lumbar radiculopathy.

DOCUMENTATION

Once the physical examination has been completed, it is critical to document it as soon as possible. Delays in documentation may lead to errors in the documentation. Documentation serves as a permanent record of your examination, which can be used by subsequent providers to understand the patient's physical status at that point in time. It also records that you performed the comprehensive examination.

Box 12.4: Motor Examination/Lower Extremities, Actual (Right/Left)/Normal

Hip Flexion: 110–130/110–130 Flex knee to bring the thigh closer to the abdomen.

Hip Extension: 30/30 Move thigh backward without leaning trunk forward.

Abduction: 45–50/45–50 Move thigh away from the midline.

Adduction: 20–30/20–30 Move the thigh inward and across the midline.

Internal Rotation: 40/40 With flexed knee, swing lower leg away from midline.

External Rotation: 45/45 With flexed knee, swing lower leg toward midline.

Knee Flexion: 130/130 Bend knee with calf toward hamstring.

Knee Extension: 15/15 Straighten knee to the maximum possible.

Internal Rotation: 10/10 Twist the lower leg toward the midline.

Ankle Flexion: 45/45 Bend the ankle so toes point up as far as possible.

Ankle Extension: 20/20 Bend ankle so toes point down as far as possible.

Ankle Eversion: 20/20 Bend ankle so bottom of foot faces out away from midline.

Ankle Inversion: 30/30 Bend ankle so bottom of foot faces toward the midline (see Figure 12.10).

Documentation can be through a written document or, more likely now, as part of an electronic health record. In most office practices, whether paper or electronic, there is a template for the physical that helps the provider to document appropriately. There are times that you cannot complete all elements of the examination due to extenuating circumstances. In those cases, you should document "not examined" for the elements that were not examined.

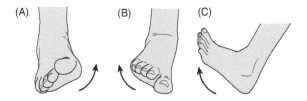

Figure 12.10: Ankle and foot range of motion technique (A) Inversion: Movement of the sole of the foot medially at the intertarsal joints; (B) Eversion: Movement of the sole of the foot away from the midline at the intertarsal joints; (C) Dorsiflexion: Flexion of the ankle, which brings dorsum of foot closer to leg, as when walking on the heel.

Source: Tkacs N, Herrmann L, Johnson R, eds. *Advanced Physiology and Pathophysiology: Essentials for Clinical Practice.* Springer Publishing Company; 2020.

CONCLUSION

The physical examination is a key component in the clinician's toolbox for assessing a patient's health, in offering preventative advice, making a diagnosis, and formulating management plans. Adult-gerontology nurse practitioners (AGNPs) need to master this skill and be able to correlate physical examination findings with the patient history and laboratory tests. Older adults display heterogeneous changes in anatomy and physiology, which affect the sensitivity and specificity of various physical examination techniques. AGNPs should develop a systematic approach to examining older adults starting with evaluating the general appearance and assessing functional status while maximizing function in older adults. Geriatric-tailored physical examinations should assess physical, cognitive, psychologic, social, and environmental domains of health. Irrespective of a patient's complaints, assessment of the older adult calls for enhanced focus on functional assessment during the physical examination.

REFERENCES

References for this chapter are online and available at https://connect.springerpub.com/content/book/978-0-8261-8414-6/part/part01/toc-part/ch12.

CHAPTER 13

Medication Use in the Older Adult

Shannan Takhar, Noelle Nelson, Demetra E. Antimisiaris, Ashley Trask, Paul MacDowell, and Timothy W. Cutler

LEARNING OBJECTIVES

At the conclusion of this chapter, the learner will be able to:

➤ Identify pharmacokinetic and pharmacodynamic changes in the older adult that increase their risk for medication-related issues and adverse drug events (ADEs).

➤ Define medication reconciliation and describe the steps used to perform an accurate medication reconciliation.

➤ Use medication reconciliation as a means to identify and address medication discrepancies and concerns.

➤ Recognize the impact of polypharmacy and identify strategies to reduce polypharmacy in older adults.

➤ Recognize the difference between an ADE and an adverse drug reaction (ADR).

➤ Provide examples of strategies that reduce the occurrence of medication errors.

INTRODUCTION

Ensuring safe and effective medication management in older adults is critical to provide optimal care for this growing population. Older adults are more likely to have multiple chronic illnesses (multimorbidity) and, as a result, experience polypharmacy (taking five or more medications). Additionally, with increased age comes changes in medication pharmacokinetic and pharmacodynamic properties that affect how this population responds to medications. These factors combined put this group at very high risk for adverse drug events (ADEs) and adverse drug reactions (ADRs). Employing strategies such as performing a thorough medication review and reconciliation, avoiding potentially inappropriate medications (PIMs), and deprescribing whenever possible can help to improve the medication use practices for these patients. This chapter describes risks associated with medication use in the older adult population, and strategies that can be used to combat these risks, in greater detail.

POLYPHARMACY, MULTIMORBIDITY, AND MEDICATION RECONCILIATION

Older adults are one of the most unique and diverse of all age cohorts. The diversity of this population is increasing with projections that the share of older adults that are non-Hispanic White will drop from 77% to 55% between 2018 and 2060.[1] While not making up a large part of the population, this demographic is growing at an exponential rate.[2] As a result, older adults need care delivered in a patient-centered manner, taking into account their unique characteristics.

One of the most important considerations for this age cohort is their use of prescription drugs and multimorbidity. Older adults are the age cohort most likely to have taken a prescription drug in the past 30 days and take significantly more prescriptions than younger individuals.[3,4] Older adults purchase 33% of all prescription drugs, a number that is expected to increase to 50% by 2040, despite this group making up only approximately 14.5% of the U.S. population.[5]

The increased use of medications in this age group puts them at risk for polypharmacy. Polypharmacy is defined as taking five or more medications, and it has been estimated to affect about one-third of patients older than age 65.[5] Many older adult patients are at risk for drug–drug interactions as a result of polypharmacy secondary to the treatment of multiple comorbidities and/or poorly coordinated care.[5,6] Polypharmacy increases the risk of ADEs and preventable hospital admissions and is associated with the development and worsening of cognitive impairment, weight loss, falls, frailty, delirium, and urinary incontinence.[5] In addition to using a greater number of prescription drugs, older adults are more likely to have multiple chronic illnesses, a situation commonly referred to as multimorbidity. Specifically, multimorbidity describes the coexistence of two or more chronic conditions. While the prevalence is highest among adults older than 85 (81.5%), most older adults have multimorbidity (67%). The presence of multimorbidity is also associated with increased risk of ADEs.[7]

Another factor that can lead to ADEs is the lack of communication between sites of care and the poor reconciliation of the patient's medications. Deficiencies in reconciling a patient's medications contribute to medication-discrepancy-related adverse events.[8] The risk of medication-related adverse events is increased by the prevalence of low health literacy, which affects more than one-third of American adults, and is highly associated with poor health outcomes.[9] Medication reconciliation is a patient-centered process used to reduce medication errors and ADEs in all populations but is especially important when caring for older adults.

Per The Joint Commission (TJC), medication reconciliation is the process of comparing a patient's medication orders to all the medications that the patient has been taking and resolving any discrepancies. A critical step in this process is to assess the way the patient takes medications compared to what is documented in the electronic health record or presumed by the prescriber. This process is completed to avoid medication errors and should be done at every transition of care.[10] Examples of transitions of care include hospital admission, transfer within the organization, discharge, and follow-up in the outpatient setting, regardless of whether these transitions occur within the same health system.[11] As patients transition between sites of care, the risk for improper medication use and medication errors increases. It has been estimated that 60% of all medication errors occur during transitions of care, and thus focused efforts must be made to ensure proper medication use to reduce adverse outcomes.[12] Table 13.1 shows the steps included in the medication reconciliation process.

When approaching the medication history portion of medication reconciliation, one interactive technique to consider using is the three prime questions model, which was developed by the Indian Health Services.[14] The three prime question model, like other counseling techniques, emphasizes open-ended questioning and active listening. The aim of the three prime questions is to assess the patient's understanding of the purpose, directions, and side effects/monitoring for each of their medications. An example of each prime question follows:

Question 1: What are you using this medication for?

Question 2: How do you take this medication?

Question 3: What have you noticed since starting this medication?

Using this questioning technique has led patients to be more positive, engaged, and receptive, and can work as a "door opener" to help patients share more information. However, on occasion, a lack of engagement could impede the success of this method.[13]

Table 13.1: Steps to Medication Reconciliation

1. Collect a medication history: An accurate list of the medications the patient reports taking
   - Be sure to include the name of the medication, the dose, and how frequently the patient reports taking it
   - Include prescription medications, over-the-counter medications, vitamins, herbal supplements, ear drops, eye drops, injectables, infusions, topical products, etc.
   - Use at least two sources to confirm (ex. patient, refill history from pharmacy, medical record, pill bottles)

2. Compare medication history to prescribed medications and/or medications that are planned to be prescribed during the encounter

3. Clinical decisions regarding the appropriateness of each medication should be made prior to finalizing the list.
   - Ask yourself:
     - Is there an indication for this medication?
     - Is the medication dosed appropriately?
     - Is the patient using the medication correctly?
     - Do I have an opportunity to deprescribe? (see subsequent section)
     - Are the patient's disease states adequately controlled on their current medications?
     - Is the patient reporting any side effects that could be correlated with one of their medications?
     - Do any of these medications have drug-drug interactions?

4. Updated reconciled list should be shared with the patient and/or caregiver

Source: The Joint Commission. Sentinel Event Alert 35: using medication reconciliation to prevent errors. https://www.jointcommission.org/resources/patient-safety-topics/sentinel-event/sentinel-event-alert-newsletters/sentinel-event-alert-issue-35-using-medication-reconciliation-to-prevent-errors

Additional Considerations With Medication Reconciliation

Keeping an up-to-date list of prescription and over-the-counter medications a patient takes will help providers identify potential drug interactions and improve the medication reconciliation process. Prescribers should make an effort to run all medications through a drug interaction database (e.g., Lexicomp, Micromedex, Liverpool, etc.) at regular intervals or request assistance with this process through pharmacist review.[6] Results of this interaction report should be discussed with patients and they should be included in the clinical decision-making process to keep them engaged in care and help them to understand the rationale behind medication changes.

The medication reconciliation process also presents a good opportunity to ask the patient about other important issues such as allergies to medications, adherence rates, and if they experience any medication cost or access barriers. Adherence rates to medications in regular

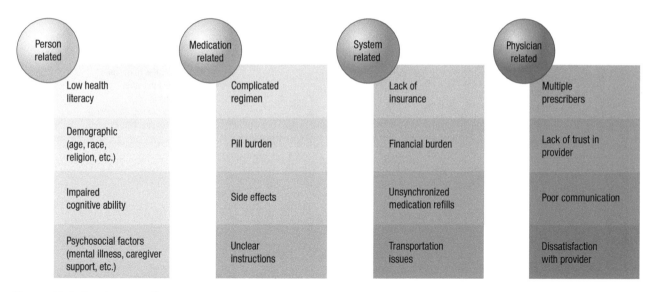

Figure 13.1: Barriers to adherence

Source: Data from Gellad WF, Grenard JL, Marcum ZA. A systematic review of barriers to medication adherence in the elderly: looking beyond cost and regimen complexity. *Am J Geriatr Pharmacother.* 2011;9(1):11-23. doi:10.1016/j .amjopharm.2011.02.004; Yap AF, Thirumoorthy T, Kwan YH. Systematic review of the barriers affecting medication adherence in older adults. *Geriatr Gerontol Int.* 2016;16(10):1093-1101. doi:10.1111/ggi.12616

use can be as low as 50%.[14] The simplest way to assess adherence is to ask a patient how often they miss doses of their medications.[15] Once adherence issues are identified, further investigation can be carried out, and potential solutions can be developed.

Systematic reviews of barriers to medication adherence in the older adult and solutions to address these barriers are listed in Figures 13.1 and 13.2.[16,17] There has been inconsistent data to support the use of one adherence improvement strategy over another, but in general, a human-based, multidisciplinary approach should be employed to increase medication adherence in the older adult.[18,19] Motivational interviewing (see Chapter 2) is an important technique that can increase medication adherence rates and should be incorporated into patient care interactions to improve adherence.[18]

Adverse Drug Events/Adverse Drug Reactions, Prescribing Cascade, and Deprescribing

Medication reconciliation also allows the care team to identify side effects, duplication in medications, and other PIM use. Older adults are more likely to suffer from ADEs. In fact, older adults are almost seven times as likely to have an ADE that requires hospitalization when compared to younger people.[20] One study found that more than 50% of ADE-related hospital admissions were considered preventable.[21] Another study found that almost two-thirds of ADE-related hospitalizations were

due to unintentional overdoses with the most implicated medications being warfarin, insulins, oral antiplatelet agents, and oral hypoglycemic agents.[20] Promoting the safe use and management of antithrombotic and hypoglycemic agents can lead to a significant reduction in risk and medication-related harm in this older adult population.[20]

National quality measures designate certain medications as high-risk or potentially inappropriate in older adults. The most common criteria used are the Beers Criteria for PIM Use in Older Adults (Table 13.2) and STOPP/START criteria (Screening Tool of Older Persons Prescriptions/Screening Tool to Alert doctors to the Right Treatment).[22] The Beers Criteria are used by the American Geriatrics Society (AGS) to improve medication selection, provide education to patients and clinicians, and reduce ADEs. The Beers Criteria are also used as a tool for assessing quality of care, cost, and patterns of drug use among older adults. The 2019 update to the Beers Criteria sorts medication recommendations based on five categories: PIMs in older adults, medications that may exacerbate a specific disease, medications to use with caution in older adults, medications that should be avoided or doses reduced based on renal function, and medications with strong anticholinergic properties (an addition to the 2019 AGS Beers Criteria).[23] A common category of inappropriate medications to avoid in the older adult are anticholinergics. While the Beers list is a very useful tool for the clinician, it is not a prescriptive tool,

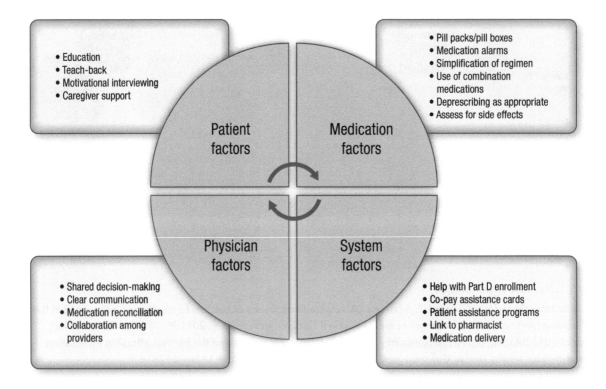

Figure 13.2: Mitigating adherence issues

Source: Data from Gellad WF, Grenard JL, Marcum ZA. A systematic review of barriers to medication adherence in the elderly: looking beyond cost and regimen complexity. *Am J Geriatr Pharmacother*. 2011;9(1):11-23. doi:10.1016/j .amjopharm.2011.02.004; Yap AF, Thirumoorthy T, Kwan YH. Systematic review of the barriers affecting medication adherence in older adults. *Geriatr Gerontol Int*. 2016;16(10):1093-1101. doi:10.1111/ggi.12616

meaning that there may be times where the use of a PIM in an older adult is medically justified. In this circumstance, it is important to document the reason for the use of the medication and have a discussion of the risks and benefits with the patient. An individualized, patient-centered, and measured approach should be taken when evaluating the medications on the Beers list. Pocket guides for the 2019 update of the Beers Criteria are available for a nominal fee at the AGS website: https://geriatricscareonline.org/ProductAbstract/ 2019-ags-beers-criteria-pocketcard/PC007.

The STOPP/START criteria approach inappropriate prescribing (IP) differently than the Beers Criteria. The STOPP/START criteria recognize that IP can consist of both prescribing PIMs as well as potential prescribing omissions (PPOs). The list of PIMs is the STOPP criteria while the list of PPOs is the START criteria. Research has shown that medications included in the STOPP criteria are significantly associated with more ADEs medications than are not.[24] Also, utilizing STOPP/START criteria for medication intervention during hospitalizations for acute illnesses has been shown to significantly

improve medication appropriateness for six months postintervention.[24]

ADRs in older individuals can be difficult to identify. Older adults may present with nonspecific symptoms such as falls, fatigue, cognitive decline, or constipation, all of which can be caused by medications or multimorbidity. As a result, it can be difficult to determine if the symptom is due to one of their chronic conditions or one of their many medications. As a result, the possibility of the symptom being medication-related should be considered in every differential diagnosis for older patients.[22] If an ADR is misclassified as a new medical condition, an additional drug may be prescribed to treat the original drug-induced event. This phenomenon is defined as a prescribing cascade.[25] An example of a potential prescribing cascade is when amlodipine is prescribed for hypertension, and the patient subsequently develops lower extremity edema. Then, instead of recognizing that the edema may be a side effect from amlodipine, a diuretic such as furosemide is prescribed to manage the edema leading to increased polypharmacy and a higher risk of ADRs. Identifying the prescribing cascade and actively

Table 13.2: Example of PIMs from the 2019 Beers Criteria

Therapeutic Category	Example of Medications in Category	Rationale
Anticholinergics	• Diphenhydramine • Doxylamine • Hydroxyzine • Meclizine • Promethazine • Prochlorperazine • Chlorpheniramine • Brompheniramine	• Risk of confusion, dry mouth, constipation, and other anticholinergic effects or toxicity
Antiparkinsonian agents	• Benztropine • Trihexyphenidyl	• Not recommended for prevention or treatment of extrapyramidal symptoms with antipsychotics • More effective agents available for treatment of Parkinson disease
Peripheral alpha-1 blockers for treatment of hypertension	• Doxazosin • Prazosin • Terazosin	• High risk of orthostatic hypotension • Alternative agents have superior risk/benefit profile
Antidepressants	• Amitriptyline • Clomipramine • Desipramine • Doxepin >6 mg/day • Imipramine • Nortriptyline • Paroxetine	• High anticholinergic properties • Sedating • Risk of orthostatic hypotension

Source: Fick DM, Semla TP, Steinman M, et al. American Geriatrics Society 2019 Updated AGS Beers Criteria for potentially inappropriate medication use in older adults. J Am Geriatr Soc. 2019;67(4):674-694. doi:10.1111/jgs.15767

working to deprescribe is an important opportunity to improve the safe use of medications in older adults.[25]

Deprescribing is the process of supervised medication discontinuation or dose reduction to reduce potentially harmful or unnecessary medication use. The key feature of deprescribing is the focus on relative benefit and harm. This requires a holistic review of a patient's medication list, medical conditions, clinical situation, and life circumstances. Figure 13.3 outlines some scenarios that provide opportunities for deprescribing.

The process of deprescribing should be patient-centered involving shared decision-making, informed patient consent, and close monitoring of effects.[26] Figure 13.3 outlines steps to approach deprescribing. Some potential barriers to deprescribing for both the patient and the provider include limited consultation time, fragmented care among multiple prescribers, incomplete information, unclear care goals, and fear of adverse drug withdrawal effects. Some strategies to assist providers with deprescribing include asking patients whether they are experiencing any side effects from their medications or having any problems taking their medications. Also, utilizing a pharmacist to conduct a comprehensive review of a patient's medication list to identify medications

more likely to be unnecessary or harmful can guide deprescribing decisions.[26]

Medication Cost and Access Issues

Prior to the implementation of Medicare Part D supplemental insurance for prescription drug coverage, cost-related medication nonadherence (CRN) was shown to affect 13% to 29% of Medicare patients annually.[27] Although the implementation of Medicare Part D in 2006 reduced the prevalence of CRN, this form of nonadherence is estimated to affect between 6% to 12.6% of patients annually, causing 2.2 to 2.7 million Americans to be non-adherent to their medications secondary to cost concerns every year.[28–31] These CRN concerns lead patients to take lower doses of medication than prescribed, take fewer doses than prescribed, or delay medication refills.[29]

Prescribers can play an important role in ensuring their patients are able to afford their medications to reduce the incidence of CRN. Some strategies prescribers can employ to mitigate drug costs and improve CRN include prescribing generic medication, deprescribing unnecessary medications, engaging patients in clinical decision-making, assessing cost and access barriers at every

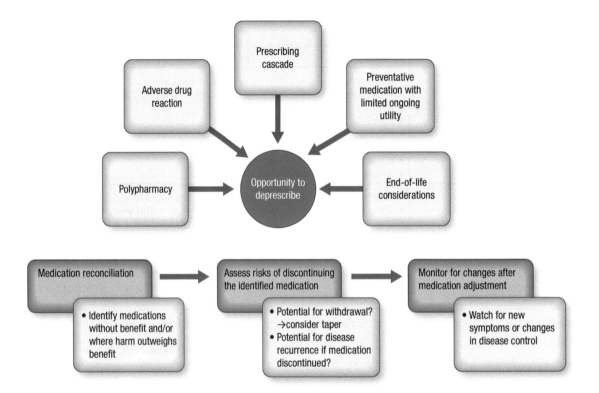

Figure 13.3: Approach to deprescribing

Source: Data from Scott IA, Hilmer SN, Reeve E, et al. Reducing inappropriate polypharmacy: the process of deprescribing. *JAMA Intern Med.* 2015;175(5):827–834. doi:10.1001/jamainternmed.2015.0324; Krishnaswami A, Steinman MA, Goyal P, et al. Deprescribing in older adults with cardiovascular disease. *J Am Coll Cardiol.* 2019;73(20):2584–2595. doi:10.1016/j.jacc.2019.03.467

visit, linking patients to pharmacists for insurance-based access issues (e.g., prior authorizations, patient assistance programs, Medicare Part D enrollment), and using combination products when possible.[30,32]

Multidisciplinary Approach to Medication Management

Although system-based approaches are available to assist in reducing mistakes at each step of the medication use cycle, unforeseen issues can arise during these processes, leading to medication errors. Therefore, multidisciplinary team-based approaches to identifying and mitigating medication errors have been implemented in many healthcare settings.

It has been well documented that a multidisciplinary team approach to medication management can help to reduce medication errors and ensure at minimum the "five rights" of medication administration are followed.[33,34] The "five rights" has been expanded to "nine rights" and may change again in the future; practitioners should stay current with these changes.[35] As part of the

multidisciplinary team, pharmacists' interventions have been shown to improve proper medication use and adherence.[19] In 48 states and the District of Columbia, pharmacists have the ability to work through collaborative practice agreements (CPAs) with prescribers to provide a variety of clinical and medication-management services.[36] However, even without the extended scope of practice a CPA can provide, pharmacists play a pivotal role in an interdisciplinary team to ensure safe and effective medication use.

Similar to the role of physicians and advanced practice providers, including nurse practitioners and physician assistants, pharmacists collect and assess clinical information to develop and implement a plan while subsequently evaluating the outcomes of that plan. However, unlike other providers, pharmacists receive two to three years of didactic education specifically focused on medication efficacy and safety. As such, their approach to this patient care process focuses primarily on optimizing medication therapies.

With increasing emphasis placed on the appropriate use of medications, many organizations have released recommendations about the importance of medication reconciliation.[37] As a result, pharmacists often see patients more often than their primary care physicians to follow-up on the impact of medication use. Based on their systematic review, Tsuyuki et al. found that primary care pharmacists see patients between 1.5 to 10 times more frequently than their primary care physicians.[38] Additionally, this increased interaction between a pharmacist and their patient seems to be more pronounced in older adults over 65 than younger patients, suggesting the high level of complexity of medicine management required for the chronic conditions experienced by older adults.[38,39] When addressing the needs of a geriatric patient population, it is therefore crucial to leverage the higher number of patient touches and expertise of a pharmacist to improve medication appropriateness, adherence, and outcomes.

A team approach is required to improve the care of older adults given that this population is diverse, complex, and unique from all other age cohorts. The unique qualities of this population including polypharmacy, multimorbidity, and pharmacokinetics (PK) and pharmacodynamics (PD) characteristics make medication use a complex issue. Medication reconciliation and deprescribing are some opportunities to reduce ADEs and ADRs in this population. When armed with the appropriate background for the issues that affect older adults, prescribers and other health professionals are in a unique position to care for this vulnerable population.

Pharmacokinetics and Pharmacodynamics in Older Adults

The National Center for Health Statistics reported in 2016 that persons 65 years of age and older represented 35.1% of all hospitalizations, despite representing only 15% of the U.S. population. The National Center for Health Statistics reported in 2018 that persons 65 years of age and older represented 33% of all hospitalizations, despite representing only 15.6% of the United States population.[40,41] Older adults are seven times as likely as younger people to have ADEs leading to hospitalization.[42] Hospitalizations due to ADEs are highly preventable with improved prescribing and monitoring.[43] A major challenge in managing medications in older adults is meaningful interpretation of literature and guidelines which are based primarily on studies of younger patients.[44] Applying medication use skills to older adults is complicated by an increased incidence of polypharmacy, comorbidities, altered PK, and altered PD.

Despite the limitations with the existing literature, the United States-based Beers Criteria and the European Union-based START-STOPP Criteria, take into consideration altered PK and PD in older adults.[23,24,45] As previously mentioned, these criteria help guide the clinician to make informed decisions based on characteristics and principles unique to the older adult. In addition, clinicians can further improve prescribing, monitoring, and medication management by applying basic principles of geriatric PK and PD.

Aging is accompanied by the disruption in homeostatic mechanisms and diminished capacity to maintain homeostatic balance. Therefore, older adults are at elevated risk of impaired capacity for activities of daily living and adverse events due to altered PK and PD. The burden of multimorbidity, as well as polypharmacy, contributes to altered PK and PD in older adults. Disease states, such as cirrhosis of the liver, malabsorption syndromes, and heart failure, are examples of comorbidities that may alter medication outcomes in addition to that anticipated with normal aging. Unintentional weight loss and cachexia may result from underlying chronic diseases common to aging such as cancer, chronic heart failure, chronic obstructive pulmonary disease, and rheumatoid arthritis.[46] It is thought that chronic inflammation linked to chronic disease plays a part in altered metabolism, muscle loss, and cachexia.[47] Cachexia can lead to altered body structure and altered protein function, altered metabolic enzymes, and reduced renal function. Examples of altered body structures include altered gut function and decreased subcutaneous tissue, which may alter absorption of oral and subcutaneously administered medications.[47]

The effects of age on various medication outcomes are highly individualized and not well studied due to study exclusion criteria limiting participation of older adults.[48] Clinicians therefore need to apply principles of the physiology of aging, combined with altered PK and PD implications for each clinical medication management situation. With the goal of helping clinicians strengthen skills in medication management in older adults, some age-related physiologic changes will be discussed along with common age-related alterations in PK (absorption, distribution, metabolism, and excretion or ADME) and PD (effect of the drug on target site).

Age-Related Physiologic Changes Potentially Impacting Pharmacokinetics and Pharmacodynamics

Body composition and biomarkers change with advanced age and disease burden. These changes are significant, resulting in a progressive loss of muscle mass with a relative increase in body fat (35%), a decrease in total body water (17%), a decrease in plasma volume (8%), and a decrease in extracellular body fluid (40%).[49] Alterations in body composition in older adults result in PK that differs from the PK data reported in drug monographs (prescribing information). Drug monograph data is predominantly based on the drug application process that uses Phase 1 to 3 studies in younger adults. Therefore, most drug monograph data do not reflect the altered PK and PD of older adults. Post–marketing experience is generally when we learn about PK and PD challenges in older adults.

Common PK changes due to body composition include altered protein binding of medications (decreased serum albumin due to frailty, increased 1-glycoprotein due to increased inflammatory status and conditions such as cancer), as well as shifts in lipid-soluble medication volumes of distribution (increased) and water-soluble volumes of distribution (decreased).[50] Changes in body composition are more relevant based on frailty rather than an age cutoff. In this case, even middle-aged adults (on an individual basis) who are frail may have significant body composition changes.[49] Changes in body composition may lead to the accumulation of lipophilic drugs (such as haloperidol and diazepam) and increased side effects. In addition, hydrophilic drugs have a smaller volume of distribution (Vd) which can lead to higher-than-expected concentrations of drug in the body (e.g., digoxin).

Cardiovascular changes that result in less cardiovascular compliance and reduced cardiovascular elasticity are common in aging. Often older adults experience reductions in intrinsic heart rate and increased sinoatrial node conduction time. For older adults, tachycardic response during exercise is reduced compared to younger people. The tachycardic response to postural changes is diminished and reliance on stroke volume occurs.[51] In younger people, homeostasis of cardiac output is maintained by increasing heart rate, while older adults must rely on increased stroke volume. When cardiovascular compensation is less robust (as with increased frailty) cardiovascular oxygenation capacity is reduced.[52,53]

Changes at the level of cell signaling also contribute to altered cardiovascular responses in older adults. Diminished beta-adrenoreceptor sensitivity, baroreceptor sensitivity, reduced cardiac muscarinic receptor activity, less beta-1-receptor density, and an affinity for beta agonists are observed with advanced age. With altered postural compensatory response and altered receptor activities, the use of beta-blockers, calcium channel blockers, renin-angiotensin drugs, diuretics, and other cardiovascular medications may lead to unexpected outcomes. This may include a higher risk of orthostatic hypotension and sensitivity to certain antihypertensives (especially direct vasodilators like hydralazine and alpha blockers).[54]

Age-related alterations in cardiovascular physiology make older adults more vulnerable to the side effects of cardiovascular medications, as well as any medications that may affect the cardiovascular system, such as antidepressants that may prolong the QT interval.[55] Common medications that can impact cardiovascular compensation (heart rate, heart rhythm, blood volume, heart contraction, heart conduction, alter blood pressure) may have unpredictable pharmacodynamic effects.

Medications with strong anticholinergic effects pose a particular cardiovascular risk in the older adult population. A recent observational study of 21,636 older adults using anticholinergic medications found an increased risk of mortality and cardiovascular events, with higher anticholinergic exposure relative to linear dose and additive effects.[56] We often think of anticholinergic drugs as being risky for cognition, for persons with dementia or at an increased risk of falls, but do not consider their impact on cardiovascular function. When you consider that anticholinergic medications can be pro-arrhythmic and disrupt normal parasympathetic control of the cardiovascular system, it is reasonable to expect adverse cardiac effects in vulnerable older adults.[57] In addition, diminished cardiovascular reserve makes older adults vulnerable to outcomes not typically seen in younger people.

Renal function and renal mass can decrease with age due to a reduction in the number of nephrons and comorbid conditions. The blood flow to the kidneys can decrease with age and comorbidities, which slows glomerular filtration rates (GFRs). Aging itself has a minor effect on kidney function, and in the absence of disease, kidney function is not decreased as much as was previously thought.[58] From the age of 30 to 70, normal kidney function decreases approximately 35% (without kidney disease). Additional kidney functional loss occurs because of the impact of multimorbidity, including high blood pressure, diabetes, glomerulonephritis, polycystic kidney disease, lupus and autoimmune conditions, and obstructions, such as kidney stones and enlarged prostate, repeated urinary infections, and other conditions.[59] Despite the decline in kidney filtration rate, there may not be a coinciding increase in plasma creatinine. Because serum creatinine is a measure of the kidneys' ability to clear muscle by-products, age-related loss of muscle mass may impact the lab measurement of blood levels of serum creatinine.[60] Therefore, clinicians should be cautious regarding renal dosing in older patients despite "normal" serum creatinine levels. Calculation of GFR using the Cockcroft & Gault (C&G) creatinine clearance equation and a serum creatinine value of not less than 1 mg/dL may be recommended for older adults if the patient is very frail. The biomedical literature is polarized on the topic; the INCHIANTI study on biomarkers of aging found that normal serum creatinine levels underascertain impaired kidney function when measured against the gold standard of 24-hour urine collection, and a literature review of retrospective studies on rounding serum creatinine concluded that rounding leads to inaccurate kidney function estimates and dosing errors.[61,62] C&G is a conservative GFR estimation but used for older patients because it considers age and body mass and is the standard to date (2020) for Food and Drug Administration (FDA) drug monograph renal adjustment unless otherwise specified (e.g., eGFR, Modification of Diet in Renal Disease). See Exhibit 13.1, which contains the C&G equation.[63]

Exhibit 13.1: Cockroft & Gault Equation

CrCl (male) = ([140 − age] × weight in kg)/(serum creatinine × 72)

CrCl (female) = CrCl (male) × 0.85

CrCl = Creatinine Clearance, kg = Kilograms

Source: National Coordinating Council for Medication Error Reporting and Prevention. *Contemporary View of Medication-Related Harm. A New Paradigm.* Published April 15, 2015. https://www.nccmerp .org/sites/default/files/nccmerp_fact_sheet_2015-02-v91.pdf

All calculations err at the extremes and therefore should be balanced with the patient's comorbid conditions as well as their level of frailty. If renal function is critical to drug excretion, it is important to reduce the dose or interval of the medication in older adults. When possible, measuring the drug level is the best option to determine the patient's ability to adequately clear the medication.

Alterations in renal function also include altered ability to regulate acid–base balance, concentrate urine, and respond to water loading. Reduced thirst with water deprivation is possibly due to reduced sensatory response as well as increased renin–angiotensin–aldosterone system activation with age.[64] As a result, older adults may be more susceptible to dehydration and the impact of diuretic use.

Gastrointestinal system changes in aging include diminished gastrointestinal blood flow, delayed gastric emptying, and diminished gut motility.[65] Gastric acid production may diminish with aging, as well as alterations in active absorption of some nutrients such as vitamin B12, calcium, and iron.[66] Phase I metabolism (also known as the first-pass effect or oxidation) occurs when an enzymatic system (cytochrome p450, known as CYP P450) oxidizes medications in the gut and liver. This phase of metabolism is intended to make medications more hydrophilic in the blood by preparing it for excretion. As for liver function, diminished liver mass and blood flow are a part of aging that may affect some phase I metabolism. Some drugs that require first pass (Phase I) activation to activate metabolites (pro-drugs) such as tramadol or enalapril may have a lower active drug serum level when the first-pass effect is diminished in the older adult. Likewise, drugs inactivated (metabolized) by Phase I (CYP P450) to inactive drugs may be cleared slower in older persons, potentially leading to toxicity.[67] The section on drug–drug interactions will provide further discussion of the impact of altered Phase I metabolism. Phase II metabolism leads to additional hydrophilicity (glucuronidation, acetylation, sulfation) and is not changed with aging to any significant extent.[51]

There is increasing awareness that the composition of a person's microbiota influences medication efficacy and toxicity. At least 30 medications are known substrates for gut bacterial enzymes, with alterations in gut microbiota linked to toxicity.[68] Older adults, especially frail persons, have been found to have significantly altered intestinal microbiota compared to younger persons, such as reduced lactobacilli with increased *Enterobacteriaceae.*[69] The use of medications, like antibiotics, can alter a person's microbiota.[70] A person's diet can alter intestinal flora as well. A diet high in animal protein and low in plant protein can favor microbiota species, such as bacteriodes, alistipes, and bilophila, which are noted for intestinal drug deconjugation, thiazole-ring opening, phosphorylase, and azo-reductase activity on substrate medications, which may alter therapeutic drug levels by impairing active drug absorption.[71] Also, altered microbiota can promote the conversion of a chemotherapeutic prodrug to a toxic metabolite potentially harming the host.[72]

The central nervous system (CNS) changes with advanced age may lead to increased sensitivity and unpredictability when using CNS medications. Alterations in neurotransmitters and their receptors in the CNS, such as dopamine, ϒ-aminobutyric acid (GABA), and N-methyl-D-aspartate (NMDA), have been identified as well as changes in noradrenergic, serotonergic, and muscarinic systems. These changes are caused by numerous pathologic influences including infection, blood flow, metabolic health, chronic inflammation, hypometabolic states (decreased glucose uptake), and more.[73] Alterations in CNS function and health can place older adults at increased risk of exaggerated pharmacodynamic response to CNS medications, such as benzodiazepines, antipsychotic agents, sedative hypnotics, antidepressants, antiepileptic drugs, pain medications, and medications with anticholinergic properties. Medications not designed to cross into the CNS via the blood-brain barrier (BBB) may indeed cross the BBB due to weakened P-glycoprotein activity in older adults. P-glycoprotein is a protein located in various tissues, including the intestines, the kidneys, and the BBB, and P-glycoprotein's function is to pump out xenobiotics (foreign substances).[74] The result of this would be an unintentional increase in medications crossing the BBB which would increase their effects, including unwanted side effects. The BBB, when intact, keeps polar (water-soluble) substances out of the brain, which is why, for example, antibiotics are difficult to get into the CNS. The BBB allows lipid-soluble substances into the brain and CNS; thus, psychoactive and pain medications are lipid-soluble.[75] Generally, you can identify lipophilic medications by reading prescribing information and drug databases, which often state lipophilic or hydrophilic status. If not listed specifically as lipophilic or hydrophilic, in general, medications with a large Vd are lipid-soluble (fat-soluble) and medications with a small Vd are hydrophilic (water-soluble).

Diminished or altered CNS function may also impact physiologic functions thought of as non-CNS physiologic functions, adding additional risks of adverse medication effects. Examples include constipation, xerostomia, tremor, arrhythmias, and extrapyramidal symptoms, which can all be impacted by altered CNS function.

PHARMACOKINETICS IN OLDER ADULTS

Drug absorption, distribution, metabolization, and elimination (traditional "ADME" or PK parameters) can be impacted by the physiology of aging, comorbid conditions, and polypharmacy, making medication management in older adults a challenge and highly individualized. Common PK parameters are altered in older adults and are summarized in Table 13.3.[66,70,76-78]

Adding polypharmacy to the PK and PD equation requires clinicians to be aware of drug–drug interactions. Drug–drug interactions that inadvertently move

Table 13.3: Common Pharmacokinetic Parameter Alterations in Older Adults

PK Parameter	Effect on Drug Disposition	Considerations
Absorption	• Normal absorption of passive transport medications • Potential reduced absorption of medications requiring active transport • Reduced Phase I metabolism	• Medications that slow the GI tract are a larger influence on absorption than normal aging. • The use of proton pump inhibitors may alter gastric pH from 1.4 (normal) up to 6-7, impacting absorption of some nutrients and possibly medications.[77] Also, people with past gastric reduction surgery may experience therapeutic failures with oral dosage forms due to altered gastric pH and surface area.[78] • Reduced Phase I: higher plasma levels of high clearance drugs; lower plasma levels of drugs converted from prodrugs
Distribution	Altered volumes of distribution (Vd) • Larger Vd for lipophilic drugs • Smaller Vd for hydrophilic drugs (such as antibiotics) Altered blood-brain barrier permeability Altered plasma protein binding • Higher α-1-glycoprotein-drug binding • Lower albumin-drug binding	• Larger Vd means longer half-life for lipophilic drugs. • Medications not designed to enter the central nervous system may cause altered mental and neurologic status. • Higher free fraction of albumin-bound drugs (thus larger Vd) • Lower free fraction of α-1-glycoprotein bound drugs (thus lower Vd)
Metabolism	• Slow clearance of some Phase I (cyp) drugs • Delayed prodrug activation to active drug entity	• If no drug response, or status change (potential toxicity), be attentive to CYP P450 pathway, interactions, and prodrug status. • Use of a point of care database to perform a drug interaction checker analysis may help identify potential CYP interaction risks (e.g., Epocrates, Lexicomp, Micromedex, Drugs.com).
Excretion	• Prolonged half-life of elimination for renally cleared (water-soluble) drugs.	• *Always* consider renal dose adjustments in older adults. • Use Cockroft & Gault (C&G) creatinine clearance estimation (point of care apps) for dose adjustment (FDA drug monograph standard as of the year 2020, some discussion of change to eGFR)[79] • Recommend rounding serum creatinine levels lower than 1 mg/dL up to 1 mg/dL and use ideal body weight or actual body weight, whichever is less, in C&G creatinine clearance calculations. • Use a stable serum creatinine level.

Source: Adapted from ElDesoky ES. Pharmacokinetic-pharmacodynamic crisis in the elderly. *Am J Ther.* 2007;14(5):488-498. doi:10.1097/01.mjt.0000183719.84390.4d; Merchant HA, Liu F, Orlu Gul M, Basit AW. Age-mediated changes in the gastrointestinal tract. *Int J Pharm.* 2016;512(2):382-395. doi:10.1016/j.ijpharm.2016.04.024

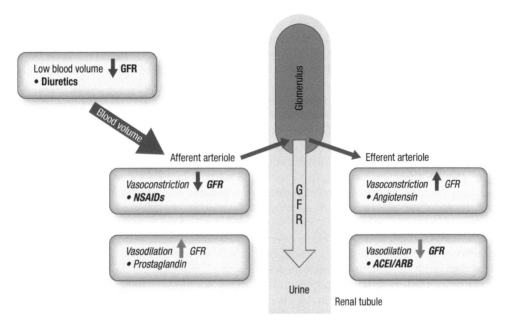

Figure 13.4: Combined use of diuretics, nonsteroidal anti-inflammatory drugs (NSAIDs), angiotensin-converting-enzyme inhibitors (ACEIs), and angiotensin-receptor blockers (ARBs) may precipitate acute kidney failure and additively these drug classes increase serum creatinine and decrease glomerular filtration rate (GFR). Prostaglandins mediate vasodilation of afferent renal arterioles, whereas angiotensin mediates afferent renal arterioles. When prostaglandins are inhibited by NSAIDs and angiotensin is inhibited by ACEIs or ARBs, combined with low blood flow conditions (such as diuretic use or congestive heart failure), the risk of acute renal impairment is elevated.

patients toward toxic PK and PD pathways or exacerbate their remaining physiologic reserve are of great concern in older adults. One example called the "triple whammy" is illustrated in Figure 13.4. The combined use of (a) diuretics (diminished blood volume to kidneys), (b) ACEI or ARB agents (diminished angiotensin support for low volume kidney blood flow), plus (c) nonsteroidal anti-inflammatory agents, or NSAIDs, including aspirin (diminished prostaglandin support for low volume kidney blood flow) additively impairs GFR and increases serum creatinine levels. The result is avoidable chronic kidney impairment and elevated risk of acute kidney failure.[79]

Serotonin syndrome is another example of a PK and PD polypharmacy syndrome, due to combinations of serotonergic medications that result in a heavy serotonin load. Combining medications such as fluvoxamine, fentanyl, olanzapine, and tramadol can result in tremor, balance instability, parkinsonian presentation, autonomic instability, confusion, and significant morbidity and mortality.[80,81] Fluvoxamine can inhibit the metabolism of fentanyl via inhibition of the CYP3A4 metabolic pathway, leading to high fentanyl levels. Fentanyl has serotonergic activity, as does fluvoxamine, olanzapine, and tramadol.[80] Serotonergic and dopaminergic systems have

a reciprocal relationship. Serotonin excess may inhibit dopamine secretion that may exacerbate motor dysfunction and rigidity which may be early signs of serotonin toxicity.[81]

Hyponatremia is a risk often linked to the use of antidepressant agents in older adults. But hyponatremia typically does not develop with antidepressant use alone and is an example of complex PD dynamics in older adults. Older adults have multiple risk factors for hyponatremia, including the use of diuretics, NSAIDs, heart failure, impaired kidney function, endocrinopathies, and even proton pump inhibitor use.[82,83] The reason antidepressants are associated with hyponatremia is that in addition to increasing serotonin levels, some, such as selective serotonin reuptake inhibitors and serotonin-norepinephrine reuptake inhibitors, increased norepinephrine levels, which stimulate alpha-1 receptors, in turn stimulating antidiuretic hormone release. NSAIDs cause the kidney's response to antidiuretic hormone to be enhanced.[84]

Phase I CYP P450 metabolic activity in the gut and liver may be diminished with age. When patients receive polypharmacy, they may experience drug-induced inhibition of CYP P450 enzymes, leading to impaired metabolism and toxic medication blood levels, or the opposite, CYP

P450 enzyme induction (increased metabolic activity and insufficient medication blood levels). CYP P450 inhibitors and inducers can significantly interfere with the normal metabolization of substrates and alter clinical outcomes.

An example is the combination of fluoxetine and tramadol. People with this combination may not experience any pain relief with tramadol, because tramadol is a prodrug that must be converted through the CYP 2D6 pathway to active O-desmethyltramadol, which is 200 times more potent than tramadol. Fluoxetine dramatically inhibits the 2D6 metabolic pathway. PK alteration resulting from polypharmacy has endless potential outcomes, and it is difficult to memorize the inducing or inhibitory character of various medications.

As discussed, the use of drug interaction tools is essential in clinical practice, and these are featured in common point-of-care databases, such as Lexicomp, Micromedex, and Liverpool Lexicomp. These databases can give you a lead regarding CYP P450 drug interactions, although they typically do not explicitly focus on CYP P450 interactions or always explain specific interactions.

To find specific CYP P450 activity, you must reference the FDA drug monograph, drug database monographs under the PK section, or other online resources such as the "Flockhart Table."[85] The Flockhart Table is a comprehensive open-source list of drug interactions from Indiana University's School of Medicine and includes CYP P450 substrates (drugs metabolized by CYP P450 pathways including 1A2, 2B5, 2C8, 2C9, 2C19, 2D6, 2E1, 3A457), CYP P450 inhibitors (including 1A2, 2B6, 2C8, 2C9, 2C19, 2D6, 2E1, 3A457), and CYP P450 inducers (including 1A2, 2B6, 2C8, 2C9, 2C19, 2D6, 2E1, 3A457). Table 13.4 provides a sample list of medications that need to be used with caution to limit CYP P450 interactions.

Variable additional factors can influence PK and PD in older adults besides the basic principles of geriatric PK and PD. For example, specific disease states may disproportionately influence PK and PD, such as heart failure. Medication Vd is reduced in heart failure due to compensatory peripheral vasoconstriction.[86] As a result, loading doses should be smaller for drugs with low therapeutic indexes to prevent unintentional high concentrations of medications. In heart failure, renal excretion and hepatic clearance may be impaired due to hypoperfusion of the liver and kidneys. Most heart failure patients are older adults, making this complex disease state more difficult to

Table 13.4: Select Phase I CYP P450 Substrates, Inhibitors, and Inducers

	Inhibitors	Inducers	Substrates
CYP 2D6	Fluoxetine Sertraline Paroxetine Amiodarone Haloperidol Bupropion	None	Donepezil Metoprolol Oxycodone Carvedilol Citalopram/Escitalopram Metoprolol
CYP 3A4	Fluconazole Grapefruit juice Amiodarone Cimetidine Esomeprazole Norfluoxetine	St. John's wort Carbamazepine Glucocorticoids Pioglitazone Rifampin Modafinil	A majority of medications are metabolized through CYP 3A4 pathway Dextromethorphan Diazepam Codeine (morphine prodrug) Citalopram/Escitalopram
CYP 2C19	Ketoconazole Lansoprazole Omeprazole Pantoprazole Topiramate Voriconazole Fluoxetine	Carbamazepine Prednisone Rifampicin St. John's wort Ritonavir Letermovir Efavirenz	Citalopram/Escitalopram Indomethacin Omeprazole Carisoprodol

Source: Shammas FV, Dickstein K. Clinical pharmacokinetics in heart failure. *Clin Pharmacokinet.* 1988;15:94–113. doi:10.2165/00003088-198815020-00002

predict and manage when added to the basic considerations of altered PK and PD in aging.

Another disease state, dementia, is associated with diminished BBB and p-glycoprotein function. Many medications may enter the brain–CNS and alter the mental status of persons with dementia, even those not typically able to cross the BBB.[76,87] Thus, medications such as trospium (for urinary incontinence), which is highly anticholinergic and used to target bladder relaxation, are designed to be polar (water-soluble) so as not to cross into the brain and cause cognitive impairment. Nonetheless, it can cross into the brain in people with a weakened BBB and cause marked confusion.[88] Additional age-related changes that may impact PK and PD include reduced rate of absorption of subcutaneous or intramuscular administered drugs, which may occur due to reduced blood perfusion or decreased absorption of inhaled drugs because of reduction in chest well compliance and alveolar surface area.[50,89] Transdermal absorption is not significantly different between young and older adults despite altered skin hydration and lipophilic content of an older person's skin.[90]

Prolonged elimination half-lives are the major concern of PK for older adults, potentially leading to undesirably high plasma concentrations when doses are not adjusted. The elimination half-life depends on whether the patient's clearance and Vd are altered. The prolonged half-life of elimination also means a prolonged time to steady state when starting a new medication. Although caution in the older adult is important when dosing medications, it is also important to individualize dosing and recognize that medications have a therapeutic window. If the concentration is too low, the intended effect level will not be reached. However, if the unintended effect window is reached, undesirable side effects are observed. Drugs with a small difference between their therapeutic effect and toxic effect are known as having a "narrow therapeutic index." Examples of narrow therapeutic medications include warfarin, chemotherapy medications, opioids, and so on. Because of the PK and PD changes seen in the older adults, drugs with a narrow therapeutic index should be used in caution in older adults. Thus, conventional wisdom when prescribing for older adults regarding starting dose and titration of dose is to "start low and go slow." However, because medications need to reach their therapeutic targets, the addition to that adage is to "start low, go slow, but go somewhere."

MEDICATION SAFETY

As one can see, there is immense complexity involved in prescribing medications for older adults. Along with this complexity comes the risk of ADEs and medication errors. In this section, we briefly review some strategies for recognizing and mitigating these risks, as well as provide key medication safety terminology and historical context related to the incidence of medical errors.

Scope and Background

It can be challenging to understand the difference among the terms "ADE," "medication error," and "ADR." The National Coordinating Council on Medication Error Reporting and Prevention has created the following graphic (Figure 13.5) to explain the relationship between medication errors and ADEs.

A "preventable ADE" is harm caused by the use of a drug as a result of an error (e.g., patient given a normal dose of drug, but the drug was contraindicated in this patient). A "nonpreventable ADE" is drug-induced harm occurring with appropriate use of medication (e.g., anaphylaxis from penicillin in a patient and the patient had no previous history of an allergic reaction).[91]

Medication errors have long been an unfortunate presence in the health system. However, it wasn't until the Institute of Medicine (IOM) published a groundbreaking report in 1999, *To Err Is Human: Building a Safer Health System*, in which the incidence of medical errors was described in the literature—causing as many as 98,000 deaths annually.[92] Subsequent analyses show error rates up to 2.5 times higher than that reported by the IOM, with medical errors listed as the third-leading cause of death in the United States.[93] Although the IOM report may have underestimated the number of preventable deaths attributed to medical errors, it amplified the scope of the problem and caught the attention

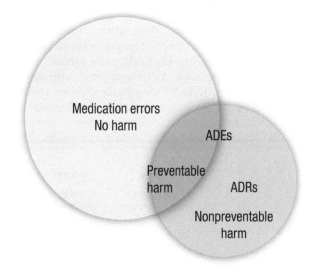

Figure 13.5: Relationship between medication errors and ADEs

ADE, adverse drug events; ADR, adverse drug reactions

Source: Adapted from National Coordinating Council for Medication Error Reporting and Prevention. *Contemporary View of Medication-Related Harm. A New Paradigm.* Published April 15, 2015. https://www.nccmerp.org/sites/default/files/nccmerp_fact_sheet_2015-02-v91.pdf

of those within and outside the medical profession, inciting a call to action. *To Err Is Human* resulted in healthcare reform that built infrastructure around patient safety.

Creating a Culture of Safety

Improving patient safety requires organizations to adopt a "just culture." A just culture is a learning culture that is constantly improving with shared accountability between the user and the system.[94] Goals of a just culture are to evaluate why errors occurred through root-cause analysis and to understand an individual's motivations and if a "workaround" safety system was pursued. Actions focus on consoling, learning, coaching, and designing safe systems which minimize human error. Chapter 3 provides an overview of patient safety and quality improvement.

Error Prevention Strategies

Leveraging Technology

Two technologic advances in error prevention are computerized physician order entry (CPOE) and clinical decision support systems (CDSS). "CPOE" refers to a medication order entered into a patient's record electronically, as opposed to handwritten on paper. "CDSS" are systems that access current and past electronic health record data, such as patient allergies or medications recently prescribed in order to guide decision-making at the point of care. These systems are typically embedded within a single electronic health record platform. These electronic tools are particularly important given their influence on the ordering phase of the medication use process, where a majority of preventable ADEs associated with serious medication errors occur.[95,96] One study showed that the use of CPOE, which includes standardized order sets with typical doses, routes, and frequencies in combination with clinical decision support such as dose-checking,

allergy screening, and drug–drug interaction evaluations, resulted in a 55% reduction in serious medication errors.[97] An additional technology to leverage is context-based ordering, which limits order selections based on predetermined rules using electronic health record data. For example, context-based ordering would prohibit the ordering of morphine for a patient with poor renal function. This is an example of a more sophisticated clinical-decision support tool that can be leveraged to further prevent ordering errors.

Other technologies proven to be useful tools in reducing errors in different phases of the medication use process are depicted in Figure 13.6. These technologies include pharmacy barcode scanning, barcode scanning during medication administration, and an electronic medication administration record.[98]

Low Tech

There are other simple error-prevention strategies that do not rely on technology but are still crucial in preventing harmful errors. The use of enhanced communication, including the use of structured "Situation–Background–Assessment–Recommendation" (SBAR) and closed-loop communication, can be effective strategies to improve the safe use of medications. In fact, the Risk Management Foundation of the Harvard Medical Institutions Incorporated (RMF) found that a lack of or poor communication was a factor in 30% of malpractice claims over a 4-year period.[99] These techniques may be found in a variety of environments and industries (other than healthcare) to control hazards in the workplace.

SBAR is a tool developed by the military to provide concise, relevant information using four key elements: situation, background, assessment, and recommendations. The first letter of each of the sections spells the acronym "SBAR." A recent review of available literature examined the use of SBAR communication tools and

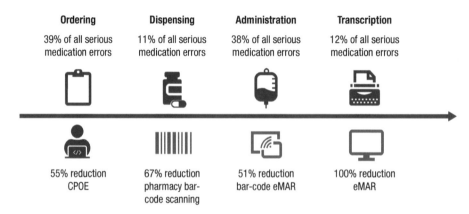

Figure 13.6: Effect of health information technology at key stages in the medication use process.
Source: Adapted from Poon EG, Keohane CA, Yoon CS, et al. Effect of bar-code technology on the safety of medication administration. *N Engl J Med.* 2010;362(18):1698-1707. doi:10.1056/NEJMsa0907115

found a positive impact on patient safety.[100] Closed-loop communication, whereby the recipient of the information repeats what was communicated, is another technique used to validate information provided. This technique is used throughout trauma and emergency medicine and is an effective strategy to enhance information handoff and reduce errors.

Clear communication is also important when writing medication orders and may help avoid an unintended outcome. For example, when ordering a medication that may be confused with a similarly named drug, providing an indication may be warranted. For example, an intended order for "hydrALAzine 20 mg IV x1" might be confused with "hydrOXYzine 20mg IV x1." By adding an indication to the order, "hydrALAzine 20mg IV x1 for hypertension," confusion is reduced. Indications also have value when included in outpatient prescriptions. One study examining more than 4 million prescriptions found that an appropriately entered indication was missing 92% of the time.[101] Including indications for use as part of outpatient prescription labeling may be particularly valuable for older adults taking multiple medications or for caregivers trying to assist with medication administration.

A final strategy to improve clear communication is avoidance of nonstandard or error-prone medical abbreviations. A list of terms to be avoided is published by TJC, a hospital accreditation group.[102] The "Do Not Use" list includes several error-prone abbreviations, such as use of "U" meaning "units," and use of symbols indicating greater or less than, such as "<, >."

Early in this chapter, the importance of medication reconciliation as a strategy for improved patient care was discussed. Incorporating this fundamental practice, along with adopting risk mitigation strategies highlighted in this section such as clear communication, avoiding "Do Not Use" abbreviations, and adding indication to a prescription, are encouraged to promote safe and high-quality patient care.

As highlighted throughout this chapter, older adults are a unique and extremely diverse population. To properly care for older adults, it is critical to use a patient-centered approach that takes into account their unique characteristics, gather relevant medication information using medication reconciliation, evaluate the PK and PD principles specific to this population, reduce polypharmacy and the use of unnecessary medications, and use technology and communication to reduce medication errors. These strategies may not eliminate unintentional harm to this vulnerable population, but it will mitigate and reduce ADEs and improve the safe use of medications in older adults.

CONCLUSION

Caring for the aging patient is complex and requires an individualized approach. This population is particularly sensitive to ADEs and ADRs. To minimize these events, it is critical for the clinician to understand the importance of a good medication review and medication reconciliation, the physiologic changes that happen with aging, the importance of deprescribing, and the need to minimize polypharmacy. Each medication used to treat a condition should be scrutinized to ensure it has the intended effect and does not have risks greater than the benefits. Even with this knowledge, the clinician should review the therapeutic plan regularly to ensure the medications are still relevant and not causing harm. Some medications (known as PIMs) should be avoided in older adults if possible. Incorporating this knowledge and using an individualized approach will help reduce ADEs and ADRs in this population.

REFERENCES

References for this chapter are online and available at https://connect.springerpub.com/content/book/978-0-8261-8414-6/part/part01/toc-part/ch13.

CHAPTER 14

Approach to Billing, Coding, and Documentation for AGNPs

Laura L. Van Auker and Deb Bakerjian

LEARNING OBJECTIVES

At the conclusion of this chapter, the learner will be able to:

➤ Understand the principles behind coding and appropriate documentation for evaluation and management (E&M) services in primary care.

➤ Differentiate among levels of E&M codes for various healthcare settings relevant to primary care.

➤ Locate up-to-date resources to ensure appropriate billing for E&M services.

INTRODUCTION

Adult-gerontology nurse practitioners (AGNPs) are reimbursed for the care of insured patients by submitting a bill for their services to insurance companies. The bill contains a series of codes that represent the setting and level of care provided along with another set of codes that indicate the diagnosis and procedure if one was done. AGNPs are responsible for ensuring that the correct information is submitted and, therefore, must be familiar with both the Current Procedural Terminology (CPT) and the International Classification of Diseases (ICD) 10th Revision manuals that provide guidelines for how to select the correct codes that align with the care provided to the patients. AGNPs must also document their care in the medical record that substantiates the care provided and aligns with the CPT and ICD-10 code submitted for billing.

The American Medical Association (AMA) is the owner of the CPT manual and updates the contents annually. The AMA released significant changes in the CPT coding scheme in 2021 that improved upon and clarified the previous CPT manual guidance. These changes allow providers to code based on time or medical decision-making (MDM) and eliminated the history and physical elements as a basis for code selection. This chapter provides AGNPs fundamental information about insurance billing, with specific emphasis on Medicare billing in the ambulatory care setting.

HOW HEALTHCARE PROVIDERS ARE PAID IN THE UNITED STATES

Primary care providers (nurse practitioners [NPs], physicians, physician assistants [PA], and clinical nurse specialists [CNS]) are paid for their professional services through a system of reimbursement for services, which entails that the provider deliver the services up front and then get reimbursed after the fact. For decades, providers have been paid on a fee-for-service (FFS) basis; in other words, they were paid for any and all services provided without restriction. Under an FFS, providers make more money by seeing more patients, whether the patient needs the care or does not need the care. Providers then are incentivized to see the patients more frequently and for more types of services.

In the early 1970s, in response to significant rising costs of healthcare, the federal government backed the development of health maintenance organizations (HMOs) that have a business model designed to limit costs by limiting where patients could obtain care, emphasizing preventive care, and requiring preapproval for certain types of procedures. The HMOs contract with providers at a reduced cost in exchange for a guaranteed minimum number of patients and assurance of regular monthly income under a system called capitation, which pays the provider a fixed amount each month for each patient *whether or not* the patient was seen in that month.[1] In exchange for this regular payment, the providers agree to deliver care to the patients whenever it is needed for that group of patients. Capitated payments are given to the providers in advance of the care and typically are based on the age of the group of patients. For example, infants often take more time so the provider will receive a higher capitation rate for them than a school-age child. Under a capitation system, the provider is incentivized to reduce or minimize the number of patient visits because they will be paid even if they do not provide care to patients in any given month. Preventive care is strongly emphasized in a capitation system, with the goal of keeping patients healthy so that they do not need to be seen as frequently.

In the late 1980s, further efforts were initiated to reduce costs by developing a resource-based relative-value fee schedule (RBRVS), which is still the current standard used by the Centers for Medicare and Medicaid Services (CMS) and most private insurers and by which most providers are reimbursed.[2] The RBRVS system is centered on the notion that payments for services should be based on the resource costs (provider time, office costs, equipment leases, etc.) of providing that specific service. The goal is to stabilize and standardize the payment system throughout the United States. The AMA brings together the RVS Update Committee, or RUC, to work with physician professional societies to make recommendations to the CMS on what the relative values are for the various services. The payment system assigns a resource cost in three areas, including physician work, practice expense, and professional liability insurance; there is also a geographic cost variance integrated into the system. Medicare, as a large purchaser of medical services, sets a standardized payment schedule based on the RBRVS system in 1992.[1] These values are updated annually.

Sources of Provider Income and Insurance Types

AGNPs can receive income from a variety of sources when providing patient care. The majority of income will come from either federal, state, or private sources. In each of those categories, there are several different types of payers.

Governmental Sources of Revenue

Federal sources include Medicare; Medicaid; Children's Health Insurance Plan (CHIP); the military programs, which are TRICARE and the Veteran's Health Administration; and the Indian Health Services.

Medicare

Medicare covers individuals 65 years of age and older and patients who have end-stage renal disease or younger individuals with certain disabilities. To qualify for Medicare, patients must either be a U.S. citizen or a permanent legal resident who has resided in the United States for at least 5 years. In addition, they must be receiving or eligible to receive Social Security benefits or railroad retirement benefits. Patients, or their spouses, who are current government employees or retirees who have had Medicare payroll taxes deducted are eligible, even though they have not paid into Social Security. Medicare has four distinct parts:

- **Medicare Part A**, which covers inpatient hospital care and limited skilled nursing care, hospice care, and limited home healthcare.
- **Medicare Part B**, which covers medical services by physicians, NPs, PAs, and other providers. It also covers outpatient care, diagnostics, medical supplies, and some preventive services.

- **Medicare Part C or Medicare Advantage** is an integrated plan that covers Medicare Part A, B, and C. This typically requires the patient to use a provider and hospital within the network of the insurance plan.
- Medicare Part D is the prescription drug coverage plan.

Medicaid

Medicaid is a federal–state government partnership to provide health insurance to people with a lower income; the household income cannot exceed a certain percentage of the federal poverty level based on the size of the family. Beneficiaries must meet eligibility standards, which include being a resident of the state in which the patient applies for Medicaid.

Children's Health Insurance Program

The CHIP program provides healthcare coverage to children. This program is also jointly funded between the federal and state governments and covers almost 10 million children who would not otherwise be able to receive routine and preventive healthcare.[3]

Military

The military provides comprehensive healthcare services to active-duty military personnel and their families through TRICARE. There are a variety of different plans available that cover healthcare provided outside of active military healthcare organizations.

Indian Health Services

For individuals of qualified American Indian and Native Alaskan heritage, the Indian Health Services Agency, a division of the federal Health and Human Services Department, partners with state Indian health services to fund health, dental, and social services through a system of local clinics. These clinics may also provide low-income services for non–American Indian members of the community.

Private Insurance

There were a little more than 900 private health insurance companies in the United States in 2021.[4] Most individuals get private insurance through an employer or by paying out of pocket for monthly premiums. Some of the largest insurers include Anthem, Centene, UnitedHealth, and Humana, and most offer similar types of insurance coverage. Some insurers also provide Medicare Advantage plans, like Humana, or HMO plans, such as Kaiser Permanente. Almost all private insurance companies align closely with the federal programs in general service definitions.

The Affordable Care Act

The Affordable Care Act (ACA), also known as "Obamacare," was signed into legislation in 2010 and has been the most significant overhaul of the federal healthcare insurance coverage system since 1965 when

Medicare and Medicaid were enacted. Most of the major provisions of the ACA became effective in 2014 and, over the next few years, made a major impact on the uninsured population, reducing it from about 50 million people (16.3% of the population) to about 24 million in 2016. The ACA has been a hotly debated, controversial piece of legislation politically, but most Americans have appreciated some of the key features that expanded coverage for families, removed the preexisting conditions clause that allowed insurance companies to refuse coverage, and made health insurance affordable by expanding eligibility for Medicaid and creating healthcare exchanges in the states that wanted to participate. The ACA also had provisions to improve healthcare quality, convert FFS payments to bundled payments, and create accountable care organizations or ACOs. More specific information can be found on the U.S. Health and Human Services website (www.hhs.gov/healthcare/about-the-aca/index.html).

Value-Based Billing

One of the goals of the ACA was to align the quality of care, healthcare costs, and value of care while improving population health, which all aligns with the "Triple Aim."[5] These goals resulted in requirements of the federal government to focus on improving the value of care while minimizing costs of care. There are three value-based purchasing strategies: (a) pay-for-performance (P4P), (b) ACOs, and (c) bundled payments, which are each designed to achieve value by reducing costs while improving quality of care based on performance standards that have been predetermined and agreed on.[6] Several initiatives and innovative processes were developed through a variety of demonstration projects and public–private partnerships. The concept of applying quality performance standards to reimbursement and financial incentives is now firmly implanted in hospital systems and is gaining ground in ambulatory care, which will impact how AGNPs practice in those environments.

OVERVIEW OF BILLING, CODING, AND DOCUMENTATION

CPT codes are a uniform system of numbers assigned to all services and tasks performed by medical providers as medical, surgical, and diagnostic procedures.[7,8] These codes provide for uniformity of billing and universal definitions of care for the purpose of reimbursement. CPT codes are used as a standardized shorthand to describe the type of E&M patient visit or a specific procedure and were first published in 1966 by the AMA soon after the Medicare and Medicaid programs were authorized by the federal government. CPT codes are reviewed and updated annually by the AMA, a 17-member advisory panel composed of physicians,

hospitals, insurance representatives, and two non-physician medical representatives.[9]

There is another coding scheme, called the ICD, that AGNPs must learn to use. The ICD codes are used to describe the purpose for the patient's visit.[10] Typically, the ICD codes are associated with a specific type of disease, but there are also codes for conditions like poisoning and nonintended injuries or injuries that are not inflicted purposefully, such as falls or motor vehicle accidents. The combination of CPT (procedure codes) and ICD (diagnostic codes) is used to transmit the type of clinical visit and the reason for the visit in a standardized way to payers. The following section describes these two coding systems in more detail. AGNPs must understand the fundamentals of billing, coding, and documentation to ensure that the practice is reimbursed for the services provided to patients. All insurance companies and the federal and state governments use these two coding schemes for this purpose. A complete description of the CPT and ICD codes is beyond the scope of this chapter; however, some key factors follow.

Current Procedural Terminology Coding

As mentioned, CPT codes are used to describe the services provided to patients to the payer of those services, typically the insurance company. The CPT codes have three main categories of coding:

1. **Category I:** procedures, services, devices, drugs, and vaccines
2. **Category II:** performance measures aligning with the quality of care
3. **Category III:** procedures and services that use emerging technologies

As mentioned, CPT codes are developed, maintained, and copyrighted by the AMA and have been adopted universally by private insurance exchanges and governmental payers such as the CMS, the Veteran's Health Administration, and TRICARE for military personnel and their families.

CPT procedure or patient visit codes are numbered in a way that indicate not only the level and complexity of care but also the setting of care. The codes are organized in a similar pattern with lower numbers (e.g., 99202) within a set representing less complexity or time spent with the patient and higher numbers (e.g., 99204) representing greater complexity. CPT codes are always five-character codes, either five numerical or one alphabetical with four numbers. The codes most commonly used by AGNPs are the E&M codes, which all start with the number "99," range from 99202 to 99499, are clustered together in one chapter of the CPT manual, and are listed by setting type in Table 14.1.

Table 14.1: Frequently Used Categories of Evaluation and Management CPT Codes by Setting

99202-99215	Office or Outpatient Visits
99221-99226	Hospital Inpatient Services
99241-99255	Consultation Services
99304-99318	Nursing Facility Services
99324-99337	Domiciliary, Boarding Home, or Custodial Care Services
99339-99340	Domiciliary, Assisted Living, or Home Care Plan Oversight Services
99341-99350	Home Services
99354-99417	Prolonged Services
99366-99368	Case Management Services
99381-99429	Preventive Medicine Services
99439-99491	Care Management Evaluation and Management Services

These codes are used to delineate the time and complexity of clinical visits. For example, a recheck of a toddler after otitis media has been treated is not the same level of complexity as an older adult with heart failure. A brief follow-up visit may each be approximately the same time (15 minutes), but managing a patient with heart failure is much more complex and requires more thoughtful decision-making. Greater detail is provided later in the chapter about specific levels of codes.

General Principles for Evaluation and Management Coding

For CPT services, E&M codes have been described as the bread-and-butter generators of revenue in the outpatient healthcare setting. These codes provide a uniform translation of time and patient complexity to a standardized reimbursement based upon documentation by the clinician. Successful clinical practice requires not only a knowledgeable medical clinician, but also a skillful coder to capture appropriate codes for billing and payment purposes while avoiding risk to postbilling audits and penalties. The 2021 E&M coding guidelines altered the previous approach to billing that was based on the completion of a proscribed number of examination and history-taking tasks, simplifying the billing for providers.

2021 Changes to Current Procedural Terminology Guidelines

Beginning in 2021, the AMA CPT guidelines provided significant changes targeted at lowering the clinician time required for documentation and simplifying coding for services provided in the ambulatory environment. Emphasis was placed on primary care services to promote

high-quality, complex patient care and management; promote preventive services, and coordinate and manage care transition to optimize patient care outcomes. Many of the 2021 changes were influenced by emergency guidelines implemented in response to the COVID-19 pandemic of 2020–2021 and the public health emergency (PHE) status allowing for licensure flexibility and reimbursement for services provided remotely.[11] During the PHE, a certain scope of practice and place of service definitions were relaxed as well as reimbursement for services through telehealth, allowing for virtual face-to-face remote services. These changes proved highly successful in efficiency, quality, patient satisfaction, and cost-effectiveness.[11,12]

The new AMA 2021 CPT guidelines seek to integrate some of the PHE policies (particularly around the use of telehealth) into permanent status.[13] If PHE-implemented relaxation of scope and place of practice policies become permanent policy following the pandemic, this will broaden reimbursement for qualified healthcare professionals (QHPs). The term "QHP" refers exclusively to NPs, CNSs, certified nurse-midwives (CNMs), and PAs in the outpatient care setting. QHP clinicians are recognized as providing primary care services billable under the same CPT coding mechanisms as physicians.

During the COVID-19 crisis, CMS 1135 (Coronavirus) waivers were implemented within states for expanded services by NPs, permitting full practice authority within their scope of practice. For example, within skilled nursing facilities (SNFs), most previously mandated in-person physician services could be provided by a QHP without restriction in timing and sequence to related physician visits but while remaining under physician supervision. The waivers allowed NPs to perform patient care and seek CMS reimbursement as primary providers of care without proscribed intervals of physician face-to-face visits.[14] In addition, the CMS waived the requirement that all mandated physician visits to SNFs be made by the physician personally with some exceptions. Now any required physician visit can be delegated to a QHP who is not employed by the facility, is working in collaboration with a physician, and is appropriately licensed in the state and working in the state's scope of practice laws. This waiver additionally provides CMS reimbursement services to home-based care by physicians, with allowable delegation of services to the same nonphysician providers as SNF facilities.[15] These 1,135 waivers will extend until the withdrawal of the declared PHE for the COVID-19 pandemic, with current discussions taking place to consider making the waivered changes permanent.

Modifiers

There are several 2-digit modifier codes available that designate various modifications for a related CPT code. For example, modifier 26 indicates the charge is for the professional component of a particular procedure, such as an electrocardiogram, in which a clinician is charging for interpreting the test, not conducting the test. Modifier 25 is a commonly used code that describes a significant, separately identifiable E&M service by the same physician (or QHP) on the same day of the procedure or another service. CPT modifier 25 should also be used when the E&M service is above and beyond the usual pre- and postoperative work of a procedure tied to a global fee period. For example, when the Medicare Annual Wellness Visit (AWV) is provided, conditions might be identified that require a separate E&M service. If a painful ingrown toenail is identified during this visit, the clinician may provide treatment and procedural care for removal of the toenail, adding a separate E&M visit with the modifier 25 attached. If a woman is seen for her postpartum visit provided under a global fee schedule and receives a separate service of an implantable contraceptive device during the same visit, this may be submitted for reimbursement as a separate nonglobal E&M service with modifier 25. While additional documentation is not required to be submitted with a modifier-25 code, in all instances, separate and sufficient documentation within the patient chart must be provided to justify the E&M-visit level selected. There are many other modifiers available; current policy and practice guidelines for use of modifiers can be found in the CPT and the Healthcare Common Procedure Coding System (HCPCS) codebooks.[16] Modifiers are inserted in the appropriate place on the standardized billing form; this is mostly done electronically now.

Current Procedural Terminology G-Codes

CPT G-Codes are used for procedures for which no CPT code has been identified. Many of the G-codes cover a variety of different issues—cancer screening, immunizations, diagnostic testing, oversight of home healthcare, therapy services, specified home healthcare services, or transitional care, among many other processes. These codes were initially used as temporary procedures or professional services, but many of them have been used for several years.

International Classification of Diseases

In addition to the CPT coding system developed for visit reimbursement, a system of coding is also used by clinicians to classify and code all diagnoses, symptoms, and procedures associated with inpatient and outpatient healthcare in the United States. Developed as the ICD, the disease coding system was first adopted in the United States as ICD-9, or the ninth edition of the ICD.[15] ICD codes had been used internationally prior to that time.

Medical diagnostic coding dates to the 17th century in English medicine, but the system was first used in the United States solely on death certificates to classify mortality statistics until adopting ICD-9. Physicians were not required to code diagnoses associated with hospital utilization until 1994 when the CMS published ICD-9 coding and reporting requirements to ensure correct coding. During the United States healthcare reforms in 2009, the Department of Health and Human Services replaced ICD-9 with ICD-10-CM/PCS within the Health Insurance Portability and Accountability Act (HIPAA) transactions. The CMS fully implemented ICD-10 coding requirements on October 1, 2015, which greatly expanded ICD-9 codes by adding greater clinical detail, specificity, and terminology to avoid narrative addendums, as well as to provide the potential for ICD-10-CM coding to track quality of care. By the 2021 edition of the ICD-10-CM Official Guidelines for Coding and Reporting, 72,606 codes were available for diagnoses. This represents the biggest change in billing codes in 20 years.[16]

While correct coding is important for providing valid claims, the ICD-10 diagnosis codes themselves do not generate billing; instead, when used with CPT E&M coding, they provide an alphanumeric (letters and numbers) association with medical terminology describing the patient experience of disease, disorders, and other medical conditions identified by the medical clinician. The ICD-10 classification system consists of two parts:

- ICD, 10th Revision, Clinical Modification (ICD-10-CM).
- ICD, 10th Revision, Procedure Coding System (ICD-10-PCS)- Hospital-based procedures.

The ICD-10-CM coding classification system provides current and potential access to enhanced data for clear diagnostic communication but additionally allows for broader individual and population health surveillance and evaluation (Table 14.2).

ICD-10-CM diagnosis codes follow a specific structure using three to seven alpha and numeric characters which classify the diagnosis to the highest possible descriptive specificity. The first character is always alphabetic, the second is always numeric, and a decimal is always placed after the third character. The first three characters represent the category code with additional characters adding specificity such as laterality, anatomic location, and, in some cases, timing. Code extensions to the seventh character are used primarily in obstetrics and the injuries and poisoning chapters of the ICD-10-CM coding guidelines to provide additional specificity. A dummy placeholder (X) is used to fill empty characters to complete a 7-character code, which allows for future code expansion or further description when the current diagnosis is incomplete or unclear. The elements of ICD-10-CM structure are further divided into:

- Conventions and Guidelines
- Alphabetical Index to Diseases and Injuries (Alphabetic Index)
- Table of Neoplasms

Table 14.2: ICD-10-CM Classification System Enhancements to ICD-9

ICD-10-CM Classification System Provisions
• Measuring the quality, safety, and efficacy of care
• Reducing the need for attachments when processing claims to explain patient's condition
• Designing payment systems and processing claims for reimbursement
• Conducting research, epidemiologic studies, and clinical trials to track outcomes of care
• Setting health policy
• Operational and strategic planning
• Designing healthcare delivery systems
• Monitoring resource use
• Improving clinical, financial, and administrative performance
• Preventing and detecting healthcare fraud and abuse
• Tracking public health and risks
• Codes for unspecified conditions are available when specific codes are insufficient for documentation in the medical record

- Table of Drugs and Chemicals
- External Cause of Injuries Index
- Tabular List of Diseases and Injuries (Tabular List)

Within the ICD-10-CM structure are coding conventions, which provide the general rules for the classification system. These provide details within the Alphabetic Index and Tabular List as instructional guidelines. These conventions include guidelines on acceptable abbreviations such as NEC (Not Elsewhere Classifiable) and NOS (Not Otherwise Specified). NEC provides for "other specified" diagnosis from the Alphabetic Index, which directs to coding in the Tabular List. NOS represents an "unspecified" condition. In the case where a condition has both an underlying etiology and multiple body system manifestations, the ICD-10-CM etiology/manifestation convention dictates that the underlying condition be sequenced first, followed by the manifestations.

For the new clinician, ICD-10 diagnostic coding may seem daunting; however, many electronic health record (EHR) programs provide coding cues and prompts to successfully reach a billable level of coding. There are also several "cheat sheets" available that provide the most common categories of ICD-10 codes used in a particular type of practice and setting. Appropriate diagnostic

coding must begin with the clinician in the clinical visit, but in many organizations, the billing is the responsibility of trained billing and coding specialists who determine compliance with all required conventions and guidelines prior to submission of the service for reimbursement. This requires a cooperative relationship between the clinician and the in-office or contracting coding professionals who review documentation to align with the clinician-selected diagnostic codes for adequacy. Upon initial hire, it is common for healthcare organizations to provide clinicians with the relevant coding training using current CMS guidelines. Resources for clinician training and support are available both electronically and in hard copy versions of ICD-10-CM/PCS and CPT codes. Resources are available as noted in Table 14.3.

The CMS developed and annually updates the National Correct Coding Initiative (NCCI), which promotes correct coding methodologies to reduce improper coding

Table 14.3: Resources for ICD-10-CM Codes and Guidelines

Resources for ICD-10-CM Codes and Guidelines	
National Center for Health Statistics (NCHS)	ICD-10-CM Browser Tool https://icd10cmtool.cdc.gov
Centers for Disease Control & Prevention	www.cdc.gov/nchs/icd/icd10cm.htm
Centers for Medicare & Medicaid Services (CMS) 2021 ICD-10-CM	www.cms.gov/medicare/icd-10/2021-icd-10-cm
The American Medical Association (AMA) Member Bookstore (also sold on Amazon)	www.ama-assn.org/practice-management/cpt/need-coding-resources
ICD-10 Code Lookup-Free website	https://icdcodelookup.com/icd-10/codes
Medicare Learning Network-Publications & Multimedia (Excellent web-based training)	www.cms.gov/Medicare/Coding/ICD10/Medicare-Fee-For-Service-Provider-Resources
Hospice and Palliative Care Toolkit	www.cms.gov/Medicare-Medicaid-Coordination/Fraud-Prevention/Medicaid-Integrity-Program/Education/Hospice
Medicare Learning Network: Medicare wellness visits, components of examinations, billing and coding, resources to optimize benefits	www.cms.gov/Outreach-and-Education/Medicare-Learning-Network-MLN/MLNProducts/preventive-services/medicare-wellness-visits.html

and to minimize payment for incorrectly coded services. One focus of this initiative is to provide clinician training to promote correct coding using the Clinical Concept Series (www.cms.gov/Medicare/Coding/ICD10/ICD-10Resources). The guides include common ICD-10 codes, clinical documentation tips, clinical scenarios, and links to a variety of educational multimedia resources for primary care and specialty practices. The Clinical Concept Guides are provided for the following:

- Family Practice
- Internal Medicine
- Cardiology
- OB/GYN
- Orthopedics
- Pediatrics

The Clinical Concept Series lists the most common conditions found in Family Practice with their ICD-10-CM codes. All ICD-10-CM codes may be found in the annually updated ICD-10 codebook, and CPT codes are fully explained in the CPT book, which is frequently provided as a clinician resource in hardcopy in the clinic setting. Coding cheat sheets may be downloaded from the CMS at www.cms.gov/Outreach-and-Education/Medicare-Learning-Network-MLN/MLNProducts/MLN-Publications-Items/ICN900943.

SPECIFICS ON TYPES AND SETTINGS OF VISITS

As mentioned earlier in the chapter, CPT codes are specifically set to align with the type of service provided as well as with a specific setting of care, such as an ambulatory care office or skilled nursing home or in the patient's home.

Common Codes for Primary Care in Ambulatory Care Offices

Beginning January 1, 2021, the CMS released its CPT E&M billing and coding policies derived from the AMA guidelines, with the adoption of two approaches using either time-based codes or codes based on the level of MDM required for the patient visit. Coding includes identifying a patient as new to the practice or as an established patient, which is defined as having been seen in a face-to-face visit within the prior 36 months and billed by the same medical group number. Prior to the 2021 CPT revisions, billing by time was only allowable when physician or QHP face-to-face time provided the patient with counseling and/or coordination of care comprising more than 50% of the encounter time. For 2021, the visit may be coded by the typical time range and allows for non-face-to-face time occurring on the day of the encounter and not provided by staff as noted in Table 14.4.

Table 14.4: Mandatory New E&M Time-Based Billing Rule: Time-Based Billing: 2021 vs. 2020 Rules

Changes Apply to Office Visit Codes Only		
CPT	Code visit based on time when:	Time is defined as:
2020	Counseling and/or coordination of care comprises more than 50% of encounter time	Face-to-face time between patient and physician and/or non-physician provider (QHP)
2021	Visit meets code's typical time range—or you can use medical decision making—it's your choice (not limited to 2020 counseling/coordination criteria)	Not just face-to-face- include items listed below
2021 Time-Based Billing: Document minutes and performance of the following activities.		
Prep-Work		
• preparing to see the patient (e.g., review of tests)		
• obtaining and/or reviewing separately obtained history		
Examination		
• performing a medically appropriate examination and/or evaluation		
• counseling and educating the patient/ family/caregiver		
• ordering medications, tests, or procedures		
Follow-Up		
• documenting clinical information in the electronic health record (EHR)		
• referring and communicating with other healthcare professionals (when not separately reported)		
• independently interpreting results (not separately reported) and communicating results to the patient/ family/caregiver		
• care coordination (not separately reported)		

Table 14.5: Office Visit Minutes Comparison 2020 to 2021

New Patient	2020 Minutes	2021 Minutes	Established Patient	2020 Minutes	2021 Minutes
99201	10	Deleted	99211	5	Not Specified
99202	20	15–29	99212	10	10–19
99203	30	30–44	99213	15	20–29
99204	45	45–59	99214	25	30–39
99205	60	60–74	99215	40	40–54

Table 14.6: Patient Visit Levels and Prolonged Visit Time

Visit Level	Established Patient Visit	New Patient Visit
LEVEL 2	99212 10–19 minutes	99202 15–29 minutes
LEVEL 3	99213 20–29 minutes	99203 30–44 minutes
LEVEL 4	99214 30–39 minutes	99204 45–59 minutes
LEVEL 5	99215 40–54 minutes	99205 60–74 minutes
99417 x 1	+ 99215 55–69 minutes	+ 99205 75–89 minutes
99417 x 2	+ 99215 70–84 minutes	+ 99205 90–104 minutes
99417 x 3 (or more for each additional 15 minutes)	+ 99215 >84 minutes	+ 99205 >104 minutes

Time-Based Billing

Time-based E&M visits must document the encounter in minutes and align with typical visit times. Normal time code descriptors are based upon an average amount of time to complete all components of a visit at the chosen level (Table 14.5). Billing by time may be beneficial when the MDM may be low complexity, but the time required for counseling and/or care coordination is more complex, and time is the major contributing factor to justify the E&M level when typical time is exceeded. Examples of this might include an "at-risk" adolescent requiring initial family planning and sexually transmitted infection (STI) prevention counseling, a developmentally delayed adult requiring nutritional counseling for obesity, or a patient and family requiring education and care coordination for a new diagnosis of Alzheimer's.

While office staff often may support this type of visit, staff time may not be included as an element in the time-based billing documentation. Prior to 2021, billing by time could document only clinician face-to-face counseling and/or care coordination. Documentation of the performance of designated activities occurring on the same day as the encounter now may include prep work, including reviewing tests and obtaining or reviewing a separate history. Elements of the visit examination must include appropriate examination and/or evaluation, as well as counseling and educating the patient/family/caregiver and ordering medications, tests, or procedures. Follow-up may be included in the encounter time to include proper documentation in the EHR, referrals, and communication with other health professionals, independently interpreting results, communicating results to the patient/family/caregiver, and further coordination of care. The activities on follow-up must not have been reported and billed separately as independent services through medical decision-making E&M codes.

Prolonged Services

Prolonged time services are provided for in the 2021 E&M coding template. When service time exceeds the basic level of service time provided, additional coding indicated as prolonged time can be added to Level 2 through

5 visits to reflect the appropriate time and reimbursement levels. The CPT code 99207 or 99217 should be billed in increments of 15 minutes beyond the time provided in 99215. The CMS has adopted prolonged time in the 2021 Medicare Physician Fee Schedule as HCPCS code G2212 for prolonged services for Medicare patients when the total time on the date of service exceeds the maximum time for a Level 5 visit by 15 minutes or more. A guideline for CPT for prolonged services is listed in Table 14.6.

Coding by Medical Decision-Making

Rather than billing by time, the AGNP may choose to code using MDM E&M codes, which utilize three factors of complexity. Two of the three factors are required to determine coding level using:

1. Problem: the complexity of problems addressed

2. Data: amount and/or complexity of data to be reviewed and analyzed

3. Risk: risk of complications and/or morbidity or mortality of patient management

The highest level reached by at least two out of three elements is used to determine the overall level of the office visit.[17] Table 14.7 provides a summary of the new guidelines for outpatient services, which no longer require specific elements of a history and physical examination to determine E&M level.

Medically appropriate history and examination are expected, but their documentation is not used in code

Table 14.7: Major E&M Revisions for 2021. Revisions for 2021: Comparison of Outpatient/Office E&M Services and Other E&M Code Settings

Component(s) for E&M Visit Level Code Selection	History and Examination Requirement	Code by Time	Code by Medical Decision-Making (MDM)	Documented MDM Elements
In office or outpatient services E&M level selection 1. New patient: No services by same provider/ or associate in same group & specialty within 3 years 2. Established: Seen within 3 years by provider/ associate same group & specialty	No longer used in code selection. Elements required only as medically indicated	Option: Total time on date of encounter **OR** use MDM	Option: MDM **OR** Total time on date of encounter	• Number and complexity of problems addressed at encounter • Amount and/or complexity of data to be reviewed and analyzed • Risk of complications and/or morbidity or mortality of patient care
E&M level selection In other settings: • Hospital • Observation • Hospital Inpatient • Consultations • Emergency Department • Nursing Facility • Domiciliary • Rest Home • Custodial Care Home	*** Requirements remain: Document Key Components: • History • Examination • MDM	*Time not descriptive component for emergency department.* May use face-to-face time at bedside and on patient's floor or unit when counseling and/or coordination of care dominates time	*** Requirements remain: Document Key Components: • History • Examination • MDM	• Number of diagnoses or management options • Amount and/or complexity of data to be reviewed • Risk of complications and/or morbidity or mortality

*** CMS Evaluation and Management Services Guide MLN006764 February 2021. https://www.cms.gov/Outreach-and-Education/Medicare-Learning-Network-MLN/MLNProducts/MLN-Publications-Items/CMS1243514

selection. These changes apply *only* to office visit and outpatient E&M services (CPT codes 99202–99205 and 99211–99215). In other clinical sites such as in emergency departments (EDs), hospital inpatient, and skilled nursing homes, services remain under the 2020 E&M guidelines that do require documentation of the appropriate history and physical examination.

The CMS has provided a summary table, "CPT E&M Office Revisions, Level of MDM," which has been adopted for coding (Table 14.8). A full list of definitions can be found in the "CPT® E&M Office or Other Outpatient (99202–99215) and Prolonged Services (99417) Code and Guideline Changes."

As in billing by time, patients are determined to be new or established. Coding for MDM is determined to be straightforward, low, moderate, or high based on two of the three elements of MDM. CPT provides specific definitions for the level of risk of complications for MDM, which are defined and summarized in Table 14.9.

Skilled Nursing Homes

Nursing home E&M codes are primarily divided into three types of visits: new admissions, discharges, and established patients. Brief descriptions of the most typical reasons for these codes follow; however, to fully understand these codes, NPs are encouraged to read the E&M guidelines in detail. The E&M standards take into consideration the complexity of the problems, the extent of the examination required, the risk to the patient, and the level of MDM by the clinician. Table 14.10 summarizes the routine E&M codes in SNFs.

Table 14.8: 2021 Revisions to Office E&M CPT Codes

CPT E&M Office Revisions Level of Medical Decision-Making (MDM) ***				
Code	Level of Mdm (Based on Two out of Three Elements of Mdm)	Elements for Mdm by Number & Complexity of Diagnoses or Management Options	Amount and/or Complexity of Data to be Reviewed (*Category 1, Each Unique Test, Order, or Document Contributes to Combinations of Two or Three Elements)	Risk of Significant Complications, Morbidity, and/or Mortality From Patient Management
99211	N/A	N/A	N/A	N/A
99202 99212	Straight-forward	**Minimal:** • One self-limited or minor problem (e.g., cold, insect bite, tinea corporis)	**Minimal or none**	**Minimal risk of morbidity from diagnostic testing or treatment** • Laboratory tests requiring venipuncture • Chest x-rays • EKG/EEG • Urinalysis • Ultrasound (for example, echocardiography) • KOH prep ***Treatments such as:*** • Rest • Gargles • Elastic bandages • Superficial dressings
99203 99213	Low	**Low:** • Two or more self-limited or minor problems • One stable chronic illness (e.g., well-controlled hypertension, non-insulin-dependent diabetes, cataract, BPH) • Acute uncomplicated illness or injury (e.g., cystitis, allergic rhinitis, simple sprain)	**Limited:** (Must meet the requirements of at least one of the two categories) **Category 1: Tests and documents** **Any combination of two from the following:** • Review of prior external note(s) from each unique source* • Review of the result(s) of each unique test* • Ordering of each unique test* ***OR*** **Category 2: Assessment requiring an independent historian(s)** (*For the categories of independent interpretation of tests and discussion of management or test interpretation, see moderate or high*)	**Low risk of morbidity from diagnostic testing or treatment** • Physiologic tests not under stress (for example, pulmonary function tests) • Noncardiovascular imaging studies with contrast (for example, barium enema) • Superficial needle biopsies • Clinical laboratory tests requiring arterial puncture • Skin biopsies ***Treatments such as:*** • Over-the-counter drugs • Minor surgery with no identified risk factors • Physical therapy • Occupational therapy • IV fluids without additives

(continued)

Table 14.8: 2021 Revisions to Office E&M CPT Codes (*continued*)

CPT E&M Office Revisions Level of Medical Decision-Making (MDM) ***				
99204 99214	Moderate	**Moderate:** • One or more chronic illnesses with mild exacerbation, progression, or side effects of treatment • Two or more stable chronic illnesses • Undiagnosed new problem with uncertain prognosis (e.g., lump in breast) • Acute illness with systemic symptoms (e.g., pyelonephritis, pneumonitis, colitis) • Acute complicated injury (for example, head injury with brief loss of consciousness)	**Moderate:** (Must meet the requirements of at least one out of three categories) **Category 1: Tests, documents, or independent historian(s)** **Any combination of three from the following:** • Review of prior external note(s) from each unique source* • Review of the result(s) of each unique test* • Ordering of each unique test* • Assessment requiring an independent historian(s) *OR* **Category 2: Independent interpretation of tests** • Independent interpretation of a test performed by another physician/other qualified healthcare professional (*not separately reported*); *OR* **Category 3: Discussion of management or test interpretation** • Discussion of management or test interpretation with external physician/other qualified healthcare professional/ appropriate source (not separately reported)	**Moderate risk of morbidity from additional testing or treatment such as:** • Physiologic tests under stress (for example, cardiac stress test, fetal contraction stress test) • Diagnostic endoscopies with no identified risk factors • Deep needle or incisional biopsy • Cardiovascular imaging studies with contrast and no identified risk factors (e.g., arteriogram, cardiac catheterization) • Obtain fluid from body cavity (e.g., lumbar puncture, thoracentesis, culdocentesis) ***Treatment such as:*** • Minor surgery with identified risk factors • Elective major surgery (open, percutaneous, or endoscopic) with no identified risk factors • Prescription drug management • Therapeutic nuclear medicine • IV fluids with additives • Closed treatment of fracture or dislocation without manipulation • Diagnosis or treatment significantly limited by social determinants of health (SDOH)
99205 99215	High	**High** • One or more chronic illnesses with severe exacerbation, progression, or side effects of treatment	**Extensive:** (Must meet the requirements of at least two out of three categories) **Category 1: Tests, documents, or independent historian(s)Any combination of three from the following:** • Review of prior external note(s) from each unique source* • Review of the result(s) of each unique test*	**High risk of morbidity from additional diagnostic testing or treatment:** • Cardiovascular imaging studies with contrast with identified risk factors • Cardiac electrophysiologic tests • Diagnostic endoscopies with identified risk factors • Discography

(continued)

Table 14.8: 2021 Revisions to Office E&M CPT Codes (*continued*)

CPT E&M Office Revisions Level of Medical Decision-Making (MDM) ***		
• Acute or chronic illnesses or injuries that pose a threat to life or bodily function (for example, multiple trauma, acute MI, pulmonary embolus, severe respiratory distress, progressive severe rheumatoid arthritis, psychiatric illness with potential threat to self or others, peritonitis, acute renal failure) • An abrupt change in neurologic status (for example, seizure, TIA, weakness, sensory loss)	• Ordering of each unique test* • Assessment requiring an independent historian(s) **OR** **Category 2: Independent interpretation of tests** • Independent interpretation of a test performed by another physician/other qualified healthcare professional (*not separately reported*) **OR** **Category 3: Discussion of management or test interpretation** • Discussion of management or test interpretation with external physician/other qualified healthcare professional/ appropriate source (*not separately reported*)	***Treatment such as:*** • Elective major surgery (open, percutaneous, or endoscopic) with identified risk factors • Emergency major surgery (open, percutaneous, or endoscopic) • Parenteral controlled substances • Drug therapy requiring intensive monitoring for toxicity • Decision not to resuscitate or to de-escalate care because of poor prognosis

*** CMS Evaluation and Management Services Guide MLN006764 February 2021. https://www.cms.gov/Outreach-and-Education/Medicare-Learning-Network-MLN/MLNProducts/MLN-Publications-Items/CMS1243514

Table 14.9: Definitions for Levels of Risk for CPT Medical Decision-Making

Self-limited or minor problem	A problem that runs a definite and prescribed course, is transient in nature, and is not likely to permanently alter health status.
Acute, uncomplicated illness or injury	A recent or new short-term problem with low risk of morbidity with little to no risk of mortality with treatment, and full recovery without functional impairment is expected. A problem that is normally self-limited or minor but is not resolving consistent with a definite and prescribed course is an acute uncomplicated illness. Examples may include cystitis, allergic rhinitis, or a simple sprain.
Stable, chronic illness	A problem with an expected duration of at least a year or until the death of the patient. • Conditions are chronic whether or not stage or severity changes (e.g., controlled and uncontrolled diabetes are a single chronic condition). • "Stable" in categorizing medical decision-making is defined by the specific treatment goals for an individual patient. A patient not at their treatment goal is not stable, even if the condition has not changed and there is no short-term threat to life or function. For example, a patient with persistently poorly controlled blood pressure for whom better control is a goal is not stable, even if the pressures are not changing and the patient is asymptomatic. The risk of morbidity without treatment is significant. Examples may include well-controlled hypertension, non-insulin-dependent diabetes, cataract, or benign prostatic hyperplasia.
Chronic illness with exacerbation, progression, or side effects of treatment	A chronic illness that is acutely worsening, poorly controlled, or progressing with intent to control progression, and requiring additional supportive care or requiring attention to treatment for side-effects but does not require consideration of hospital level of care.
Undiagnosed new problem with uncertain prognosis	A problem in the differential diagnosis that represents a condition likely to result in a high risk of morbidity without treatment. An example may be a lump in the breast.

(continued)

Table 14.9: Definitions for Levels of Risk for CPT Medical Decision-Making (*continued*)

Acute illness with systemic symptoms	An illness-causing systemic symptom with a high risk of morbidity without treatment. Has systemic general symptoms such as fever, body aches, or fatigue in a minor illness that may be treated to alleviate symptoms, shorten the course of illness, or prevent complications (see definitions for "self-limited or minor" or "acute, uncomplicated"). Has systemic symptoms in a single system. Examples may include pyelonephritis, pneumonitis, or colitis.
Acute, complicated injury	An injury requiring treatment that includes evaluation of body systems not directly part of the injured organ, the injury is extensive, or the treatment options are multiple and/or associated with risk of morbidity such as a head injury with brief loss of consciousness.
Chronic illness with severe exacerbation, progression, or side effects of treatment	The severe exacerbation or progression of a chronic illness or severe side effects of treatment that have significant risk of morbidity and may require hospital level of care. Examples include heart failure exacerbation or worsening diabetes requiring close monitoring and acute treatment.
Acute or chronic illness or injury that poses a threat to life or bodily function	An acute illness with systemic symptoms, or an acute complicated injury, or a chronic illness or injury with exacerbation and/or progression or side effects of treatment, that poses a threat to life or bodily function in the near term without treatment. Examples may include acute myocardial infarction, pulmonary embolus, severe respiratory distress, progressive severe rheumatoid arthritis, psychiatric illness with potential threat to self or others, peritonitis, acute renal failure, or an abrupt change in neurologic status.

Table 14.10: Routine E&M Codes in Skilled Nursing Facilities

	CPT E&M Code	History and Examination	Medical Decision-Making	Problem Severity	Time in Minutes
Initial Assessment	99304	Detailed/Comprehensive	Straight forward/Low	Low	20
	99305	Detailed/Comprehensive	Moderate	Moderate	45
	99306	Comprehensive	High	High	75
Subsequent Visits	99307	Prob focused	Straight forward	Minor	10
	99308	Expanded Prob focused	Low	Low/Mod	15
	99309	Detailed	Mod	Mod	25
	99310	Comprehensive	High	High unstable	35
Discharge Visits	99315				30 min or less
	99316				>30 min
Annual H&P	99318	Detailed	Low/Mod	Low/Mod	30

CPT, Current Procedural Terminology; E&M, evaluation and management.

There are additional codes that can be used as well, such as AWV, chronic care management, advanced care planning, and transitional care, that are discussed in later sections.

Other Settings of Care

There are several other settings that AGNPs may also provide patient visits such as home care, assisted living, and residential care. It is important that the appropriate codes be used for each of these sites, which are available in the CPT manual. There are two areas of care particularly relevant to many AGNPs: hospice and transitions of care.

Hospice

Hospice programs are elective services that focus upon comfort care (palliative care) providing end-of-life care for terminally ill patients. The goals for hospice care are holistic services to provide pain relief and symptom management as well as support for families through a team-based approach. Interprofessional teams are typically composed of a hospice physician, hospice nurses, social workers, chaplains, home health aides, and, increasingly, hospice NPs. Services are typically covered for patients with Medicare when patients are certified by their primary care doctor or hospice physician as having a medical diagnosis of a 6 months or less life span based on the normal course of illness. Documentation by a physician of this prognosis and supporting evidence are required to initiate CMS reimbursement for hospice. Documentation must also include an individualized written plan of care (POC) developed by the hospice physician or NP, the patient and/or a representative, and appropriate members of the interdisciplinary patient care team. Subsequent certification for a second 90-day plan may be done by an NP or physician but requires a face-to-face visit. AGNPs that choose to work in the hospice environment can expect support from the hospice agency for documentation and reimbursement requirements based upon daily Medicare rates for the hospice level of care.

The hospice level of care is divided into four care levels, ranging from maintenance, during which care may not be needed or provided on some days, to general inpatient care, during which the patient requires hospitalization for pain management or chronic disease management. More in-depth criteria for clinician coding and documentation are best accessed through the hospice agency billing and coding department and the CMS.gov website: www.cms.gov/Medicare/Medicare-Fee-for-Service-Payment/Hospice. Available provider resources may be found for the following: "Hospice Booklet for Providers," "Hospice Checklist for Providers," and other "Palliative Care vs. Hospice" at the Hospice Benefit Toolkit: www.cms.gov/Medicare-Medicaid-Coordination/Fraud-Prevention/Medicaid-Integrity-Program/Education/Hospice.

Transitions of Care

Transitions of care has become an important area for managing patients as they transition from one setting to another.[18] The CMS has stated in the past that a more expected ratio for transitional care management services is three moderate-complexity visits for every one high-complexity visit.

The requirements for code 99495 are as follows:

- Communication (direct contact, telephone, or electronic) with the patient or caregiver within 2 business days of discharge
- MDM of *at least moderate complexity* during the service period
- A face-to-face visit within *14 days* of discharge

The requirements for code 99496 are as follows:

- Communication (direct contact, telephone, or electronic) with the patient or caregiver within 2 business days of discharge
- MDM of *high complexity* during the service period
- A face-to-face visit within *7 days* of discharge

Much of the work of transitional care management is done by clinical staff supervised by a physician or advanced practice provider. Transitional care management has grown over the past decade with greater attention on the care of patients as they are discharged from the hospital to home or skilled nursing homes as this is a time associated with significant adverse events. NP-led transitional care management has been shown to improve communication, decrease readmissions,[18,19] improve some health outcomes,[16,22] and improve patient satisfaction.[21]

To use the transitional care codes, a staff member must call the patient within 2 business days of discharge, open the template on the day of the face-to-face visit, and provide coordination or educational services as directed by the physician or advanced practice provider. By capturing these codes, the physician or advanced practice provider is awarded additional work RVUs for the direction and oversight, and the practice is paid for work it previously did for free or for a lesser rate. Note that the CMS now allows the physician or advanced practice provider to bill the transitional care management code on the day of the face-to-face visit rather than waiting until 30 days after the discharge. This change should make billing for this service easier.

Chronic Care Management

Chronic care management applies to patients who have multiple (two or more) chronic conditions expected to last at least 12 months, or until the patient's death, that place the patient at significant risk of death, acute exacerbation/decompensation, or functional decline. There is a single code: 99490. The three key requirements for billing chronic care management are

1. having a scanned, signed patient agreement;
2. having a patient-centered care plan; and
3. having a monthly log showing at least 20 minutes of staff contact time.

Staff are key to managing these tasks. (For downloadable tools to help you meet these requirements, see "Chronic Care Management and Other New CPT Codes."[20]

Annual Medicare Wellness Visits

The work of the Medicare AWV is twofold:

1. Screening for depression, ability to perform activities of daily living, health risk assessment, and safety at home and giving personalized advice based on the responses. All screening and data collection are staff work. Giving personalized advice is physician or advanced practice provider work.

The Medicare AWV is a more recent procedure code that has been approved for payment by the CMS for the wellness visit for beneficiaries who have been on Medicare at least 12 months.[23] The clinician education tool, provided on the Medicare Learning Network

(MLN), provides clear definitions of components of each type of examination covered and examination elements that may be denied reimbursement (www.cms .gov/Outreach-and-Education/Medicare-Learning -Network-MLN/MLNProducts/preventive-services/ medicare-wellness-visits.html).

Within the first 12 months of Medicare enrollment, the enrollee is eligible for a single free "Welcome to Medicare" visit, which provides a baseline review of current health and addresses the screening questions with a preventive health focus. Unlike the AWVs that occur after the first 12 months of enrollment, there are allowable physical examination screening components provided free once in a lifetime during this Initial Preventive Physical Examination (IPPE). It is valuable for the AGNP to be familiar with the allowable elements and limitations of this IPPE to both enhance the value of the visit for the patient and to avoid misunderstandings in future AWVs when physical examination components are not covered by Medicare. Table 14.11 provides an example of the "Welcome to Medicare" IPPE components, such as allowing a baseline electrocardiogram (ECG), and has the list of G-codes to be used for these services.

Unlike most other types of visits and procedures, the AWP has no deductible if the provider only focuses on those activities covered by the wellness visit. The purpose of the wellness visit is to address health risks and develop a prevention plan. Patients must fill out a "health risk assessment" and participate in developing a prevention care plan. Providers can do cognitive screening, review the history, perform vital signs, and discuss advance care planning (ACP). Activities related to diagnosing or managing diseases or injuries are not covered in this visit. Providers may combine this visit with a regular E&M visit, but then the deductible and coinsurance may apply to the portion of the visit beyond the preventive services and must be separately documented or clearly designated and described as a separate procedure within the visit note. Routine annual physical examinations are specifically prohibited for reimbursement by Medicare, but positive examination findings tied to a condition identified during the AWV may be billed under Medicare Part B and coded as an E&M visit. Additionally, any medically indicated laboratory screening or diagnostics would fall under the patient's deductible, coinsurance, and copayment requirements and must be a medically necessary and reasonable service. More detailed information is available on the CMS website.[27]

Well Woman Screening Breast and Pelvic Examination

The screening pelvic examination benefit covered by Medicare is a stand-alone billable service. Specific elements are required with seven of 11 elements performed and documented for the Breast and Pelvic Exam (Code G0101) as noted in Table 14.12. It is separate from the IPPE or the AWV. Medicare beneficiaries may obtain a screening pelvic examination at any time following Medicare Part B enrollment, including during their IPPE or AWV encounter or once every 24 months, for all asymptomatic females. Individuals with high-risk factors for cervical or vaginal cancer are allowed a covered women's health examination once every 12 months with a documented history of

- early onset of sexual activity (under 16 years of age),
- multiple sexual partners (five or more in a lifetime),
- history of an STI (including human immunodeficiency virus [HIV] infection),
- fewer than three negative or any pap smears within the previous 7 years, or
- DES (diethylstilbestrol)-exposed daughters of women who took DES during pregnancy.

Cervical screening for cancer such as the Pap test may be performed and billed during the same encounter with procedure codes for the examination and the Pap test listed separately. Federally qualified health centers (FQHCs), rural health clinics (RHCs), and non–primary care sites such as SNFs and inpatient care may have different billing guidelines. Additional information for POS codes is available on the CMS website at www.cms.gov/ Medicare/Coding/place-of-service-codes.

Advance Care Planning

ACP is a voluntary face-to-face service provided by a Medicare physician or other QHP including AGNPs. These services are reimbursed by the CMS either when provided during the Medicare AWV or as a separate Medicare Part B medically necessary service. The focus is to determine the patient's healthcare wishes if they become unable to make decisions about their care. A common document to discuss is the advance directive (AD) form, which is provided by each state's attorney general's office website as well as the Physicians Orders for Life-Sustaining Treatment (POLST) form.

Examples of ADs include

- living wills,
- instruction directives,
- healthcare proxy, and
- healthcare power of attorney.

The discussion during the ACP does not require completion of any legal forms to obtain reimbursement but completed forms should be added to the patient medical record if appropriate and the visit content must be clearly documented. This visit can be billed more than once, without limit, if the change in the patient's health status and/or wishes about end-of-life care are noted. The ACP services may be provided in facility and nonfacility

Table 14.11: Medicare Annual Wellness (AWV) Health Risk Assessment (HRA)

Initial Preventive Physical Examination (IPPE) Components	
1. Review the patient's medical and social history	At a minimum, collect information about: • past medical and surgical history (experiences with illnesses, hospital stays, operations, allergies, injuries, and treatments) • current medications and supplements (including calcium and vitamins) • family history (review of medical events in the patient's family, including hereditary conditions that place them at increased risk) • diet • physical activities • history of alcohol, tobacco, and illegal drug use Get more information about Medicare substance use disorder (SUD) services coverage in the Screening, Brief Intervention, & Referral to Treatment (SBIRT) Services booklet.
2. Review patient's potential depression risk factors, including current or past experiences with depression or other mood disorders	Select from various standardized screening tools designed for this purpose and recognized by national professional medical organizations. Find more information on depression screening on the Depression Assessment Instruments website.
3. Review patient's functional ability and safety level	Use direct patient observation, or appropriate screening questions or standardized questionnaires recognized by national professional medical organizations, to review, at a minimum, these areas: • ability to perform activities of daily living (ADLs) • fall risk • hearing impairment • home safety
4. Examination	Measure: • height, weight, body mass index (BMI; or waist circumference, if appropriate), and blood pressure • visual acuity screen • other factors deemed appropriate based on medical and social history and current clinical standards
5. End-of-life planning, on patient agreement	End-of-life planning is verbal or written information offered to the patient about: • their ability to prepare an advance directive in case an injury or illness prevents them from making healthcare decisions • if you agree to follow their wishes expressed in an advance directive This may be provided in a subsequent CMS visit billed under Advanced Care Planning
6. Review current opioid prescriptions	For a patient with a current opioid prescription: • Review their potential opioid use disorder (OUD) risk factors. • Evaluate their pain severity and current treatment plan. • Provide information on non-opioid treatment options. • Refer to a specialist, as appropriate.
7. Screen for potential substance use disorders (SUDs)	Review the patient's potential risk factors for SUDs and, as appropriate, refer them for treatment. A screening tool isn't required but you may use one. Find more information on the National Institute on Drug Abuse Screening and Assessment Tools Chart.

(continued)

Table 14.11: Medicare Annual Wellness (AWV) Health Risk Assessment (HRA) *(continued)*

Initial Preventive Physical Examination (IPPE) Components	
8. Educate, counsel, and refer based on previous components	Based on the results of the review and evaluation services in the previous components, give appropriate education, counseling, and referral.
9. Educate, counsel, and refer for other preventive services	Includes a brief written plan, such as a checklist, for the patient to get: • a once-in-a-lifetime screening electrocardiogram, as appropriate • appropriate screenings and other preventive services Medicare covered in the AWV
IPPE and AWV HCPCS Codes and Descriptors:	
G0402	Initial preventive physical examination: face-to-face visit, services limited to new beneficiary during the first 12 months of Medicare enrollment
G0403	Electrocardiogram, routine electrocardiogram with 12 leads; performed as a screening for the initial preventive physical examination with interpretation and report
G0404	Electrocardiogram, routine electrocardiogram with 12 leads; tracing only, without interpretation and report, performed as a screening for the initial preventive physical examination
G0405	Electrocardiogram, routine electrocardiogram with 12 leads; interpretation and report only, performed as a screening for the initial preventive physical examination
G0468*	Federally qualified health center (FQHC) visit, IPPE or AWV; an FQHC visit that includes an initial preventive physical examination (IPPE) or annual wellness visit (AWV) and includes a typical bundle of Medicare-covered services that would be furnished per diem to a patient receiving an IPPE or AWV
G0438	Annual Wellness Visit, Initial (AWV)—Annual wellness visit, including a personalized prevention plan of service (PPPS), first visit.
G0439	Annual Wellness Visit, Subsequent (AWV)—Annual wellness visit, including a personalized prevention plan of service (PPPS), subsequent visit. Annual wellness visits can be for either new or established patients as the code does not differentiate.

Source: Centers for Medicare and Medicaid Services. Medicare wellness visits. n.d. https://www.cms.gov/Outreach-and-Education/Medicare-Learning-Network-MLN/MLNProducts/preventive-services/medicare-wellness-visits.html

Table 14.12: Well Woman Breast and Pelvic Guidelines: Code G0101

Documentation Guidelines: At least seven of 11 elements must be included and documented and may be provided in Internal Medicine, Family Practice, or OB/GYN office settings.
1. Inspection and palpation of breasts for masses or lumps, tenderness, symmetry, or nipple discharge
2. Digital rectal examination including sphincter tone, presence of hemorrhoids, and rectal masses
3. External genitalia (e.g., general appearance, hair distribution, or lesions)
4. Urethral meatus (e.g., size, location, lesions, or prolapse)
5. Urethra (e.g., masses, tenderness, or scarring)
6. Bladder (e.g., fullness, masses, or tenderness)
7. Vagina (e.g., general appearance, estrogen effect, discharge, lesions, pelvic support, cystocele, or rectocele)
8. Cervix (e.g., general appearance, lesions, or discharge)
9. Uterus (e.g., size, contour, position, mobility, tenderness, consistency, descent, or support)
10. Adnexa/parametria (e.g., masses, tenderness, organomegaly, or nodularity)
11. Anus and perineum

Table 14.13: Advanced Care Planning CPT Codes and Descriptors

99497	Advance care planning including the explanation and discussion of advance directives such as standard forms (with completion of such forms, when performed), by the physician or other qualified healthcare professional; first 30 minutes, face-to-face with the patient, family member(s), and/or surrogate
00498	Advance care planning including the explanation and discussion of advance directives such as standard forms (with completion of such forms, when performed), by the physician or other qualified healthcare professional; each additional 30 minutes (List separately in addition to code for primary procedure)

Medicare waives the ACP coinsurance and the Part B deductible when the ACP is

- delivered on the same day as a covered MWV (HCPCS codes G0438 or G0439),
- offered by the same provider as a covered MWV, and
- billed with modifier 33 (Preventive Services).

ACP, advance care planning; CPT, Current Procedural Terminology

Table 14.14: Requirements for Cognitive Impairment Assessment Visit and Plans

Cognitive Impairment Assessment Visit and Plans Using CPT Code 99483
• Perform a detailed history and physical examination with focus on cognition.
• Record and review the patient's history, reports, and records.
• Conduct a functional assessment of basic and instrumental activities of daily living, including decision-making capacity.
• Use standardized instruments for staging of dementia, such as the Functional Assessment Staging Test (FAST) and Clinical Dementia Rating (CDR).
• Reconcile and review for high-risk medications, if applicable.
• Use standardized screening instruments to evaluate for neuropsychiatric and behavioral symptoms, including depression and anxiety.
• Conduct a safety evaluation for home and motor vehicle operation.
• Identify social supports including how much caregivers know and are willing to provide care.
• Address advance care planning and any palliative care needs.
Written Initial Care Plan to Address Positive Findings
• neuropsychiatric symptoms
• neurocognitive symptoms
• functional limitations
• referral to community resources as needed (for example, rehabilitation services, adult day programs, support groups) shared with the patient or caregiver with initial education and support
Resources: Testing Tools–NIH National Institute on Aging Alzheimer's and Dementia Resources for Professionals https://www.nia.nih.gov/health/alzheimers-dementia-resources-for-professionals

Source: https://www.cms.gov/cognitive

CPT, Current Procedural Terminology

settings. If it is provided outside of the MWV, inform the patient that Part B cost sharing applies as it does for other AGNP services. For these visits use CPT codes 99497 and 99498 as noted in Table 14.13.

Cognitive Impairment Assessment

Cognitive impairment should be assessed during the AWV. When a patient shows signs of cognitive impairment during the AWV or other examination, Medicare provides for a separate visit to evaluate cognitive status using standardized tools and the development of a care plan under CPT code 99483. The goal of the separate cognitive impairment assessment (CIA) visit is to detect dementia, Alzheimer's disease, or other cognitive disorders, and to identify other conditions such as depression or anxiety that may respond to early intervention and treatment. The CMS provides resources for the CIA at www.cms.gov/cognitive. Effective January 1, 2021,

Medicare increased reimbursement for these services and has been included in the definition of primary care services. Telehealth was permanently added to in-person services, which may be provided in office or outpatient settings, private residences, care facilities (SNFs), or rest homes such as assisted living. Telehealth became a much more common patient visit process during the COVID-19 pandemic when many of the initial restrictions were lifted to reduce the risk of COVID-19 transmission.

The CIA may be provided by the physician or AGNP and should include direct observation as well as information offered by the patient, family, friends, and caregivers as independent historians. A typical provider visit for CIA using code 99483 would spend about 50 minutes in face-to-face time with the patient and independent historian with suggested visit components and appropriate plans for follow-up found in Table 14.14. A Medicare resource for the CIA visit can be found at www.cms.gov/cognitive.

DOCUMENTATION REQUIREMENTS

AGNPs and other QHPs are held to the same standards and the same consequences as physicians when it comes to billing, coding, and documentation of their E&M and procedural visits. AGNPs should not be lulled into a false sense of security because they are employed by a physician group or hospital that may be doing the medical billing. Medicare holds each practitioner responsible for their own billing, coding, and documentation. Familiarity with using the CPT *Manual of Medical Procedures* and the ICD manual that provides diagnostic and procedure codes is valuable for AGNPs to avoid visit reimbursement denials. Both the CPT and ICD (current version 10) manuals are updated annually, often with significant changes, so AGNPs must stay current with the changes. It is the responsibility of the AGNP to review the new codes each year, which are generally available in October. NP must document accurately and appropriately to substantiate the billing code for each E&M visit.

Many healthcare organizations have developed EHRs that facilitate meeting the billing and coding standards by allowing providers to create predefined templates for their charting. In these cases, it is important that the AGNP ensures that the resultant chart note accurately reflects the care that was provided. In the EHR, it might be easy to overstate the level of review of systems or physical examination that was completed because the electronic tools available are designed to improve the quality of clinical documentation but also increase the efficiency. It is incumbent on the AGNP to ensure the accuracy and integrity of the medical record and to include only those elements that were completed and not all the possible elements that are available in the EHR template.[21]

Failure to understand and comply with current billing, coding, and documentation standards may result in charges of insurance fraud that carry a fine and, in the case of federal reimbursement, a loss of Medicare and Medicaid privileges. Accurate documentation does the following:

- Provides evidence of the medical necessity of each visit, which is a CMS requirement.
- Demonstrates the appropriateness of patient care.
- Substantiates the quality of care provided.
- Enhances communication between providers and the facility staff.
- Offers verification of Medicare compliance with codes used for billing.
- Facilitates utilization review.
- Aids in data collection for research and education.

AGNP ETHICAL AND LEGAL RESPONSIBILITIES

AGNPs are responsible for ensuring that the correct billing code is applied to each E&M visit they make and that the appropriate ICD-10 diagnostic code is applied. AGNPs should bill for all services provided and bill at the appropriate level. It is not uncommon for AGNPs to undervalue their services, particularly those that are not provided routinely, such as the higher level office codes, transitional care, and the AWV.[22] AGNPs should work with the billing manager in the practice to evaluate their productivity compared with others and then compare the billing to the medical record to make sure that they are optimally billing for their services. Using EHR templates can be helpful and improve efficiency and save time; however, they have been known to lead to ethical dilemmas and legal challenges due to the tendency to code the visit at a higher level than is allowed. Having someone in the office who reviews the codes for accuracy can be helpful to avoid over- and underbilling.

Billing Audits

All billing is subject to audit, which can be initiated at any time. Audits are random, but there are several actions that can trigger an audit. For example, if the AGNP consistently submits higher level codes for all visits, an audit will likely get triggered. Another audit trigger is when the AGNP submits a consistently higher than average number of visit claims in a single day. If the average number of daily visits of all AGNPs in a region is 18 per day and an AGNP consistently submits 24 or 25 claims per day, that will likely trigger an audit. Medicare claim audits are time-consuming, and if the provider is found guilty of overbilling the federal government, it is charged as Medicare fraud, and the penalties are substantial.

Additional information is available at https://www.cms.gov/Outreach-and-Education/Medicare-Learning-Network-MLN/MLNProducts/Downloads/Fraud-Abuse-MLN4649244.pdf.

AGNPs can avoid problems with Medicare by following the Medicare guidelines for billing, coding, and documentation. If the AGNP practice is audited, be sure to take the letter seriously, read the audit letter, and respond appropriately and in a timely manner. Provide all the information requested—typically this is medical records and related diagnostics, medications, consult letters, or any other related forms for a given set of visits that will substantiate your billing claims. If it is a large amount of money or there are records missing, it might be appropriate to obtain legal services.

IMPROVING HEALTH EQUITY AND PATIENT ACCESS

In addition to the COVID-19 pandemic, 2020–2021 highlighted several other long-standing issues in primary care. The pandemic revealed serious issues with inequities in healthcare and the problems related to access to care for underserved communities, including communities of color, rural communities, and the urban underserved. In the upcoming years, the CMS will be focused on improving data collection on health equity, which will require providers to report on race, ethnicity, LGBTQ+, disabled, and rural populations. Efforts may include significant expansion of telehealth to these communities, particularly in the areas of behavioral health and mental health services. Proposals include CMS reimbursement for mental health visits for RHC and FQHCs, expanding the Medicare Diabetes Prevention Program, and additional incentives for providing high-quality care that has value to beneficiaries. AGNPs must participate in this work to advocate for their patients who need these services.

CONCLUSION

AGNPs are eligible to submit insurance claims so they can be reimbursed for care provided to insured patients. The federal government is one of the largest payers of claims and a common insurer for AGNP patients. Because they are such a large payer, many other insurance companies follow their billing standards and fee schedules identified as the Medicare Reimbursement Level. It is critical for AGNPs to submit the correct billing code and diagnostic code for each patient visit and to document the visit appropriately in the medical record.

CASE STUDY
PRACTICE IN CODING

Clinical Scenario: Follow up in internal medicine clinic following ED visit for respiratory distress

Chief Complaint: "Seen in the ER last week."

History: Mr. Haddad is a 57-year-old male, with a history of morbid obesity, type 2 diabetes, peripheral nephropathy, and asthma. He was seen in ER 7 days ago for shortness of breath and is here for follow-up for his diagnosis of bronchitis and asthma flare. He was given albuterol MDI and beclomethasone 80 mcg inhaler prescriptions, along with a 5-day course of azithromycin (Z-Pak). and a 6-day taper prednisone dose pack. He is no longer wheezing, and cough now produces minimal white sputum improved from the frequent yellow-green sputum from the prior week. His current concern is his morning blood sugars which are over 200 each morning. The ED warned him the prednisone might raise his blood sugars, but he has not been this poorly controlled in years.

- Patient has long-standing asthma with two to three exacerbations per week and daily need for rescue inhalers. Patient is still smoking half a pack a day. He is compliant with his inhalers when he is not feeling well.
- Patient has had asthma for 8 years and requires use of his rescue inhaler two to three times per week and whenever he has exertion with physical activities.
- Patient has diabetes with proteinuria, last creatinine 1.9 mg/dL about 9 months ago.
- Hypertension (he does not home monitor)
- Morbid obesity
- Tobacco use disorder: 1ppd x 35 years

REVIEW OF SYSTEMS, PHYSICAL EXAMINATION, AND LABORATORY TESTS

- BMI 43; notable central adiposity; able to speak in full sentences without respiratory distress, occasional non-paroxysmal cough
- BP 144/74, HR 92 RR, 14 Sats: 98% on RA
- HEENT: TMs clear; conjunctiva no injection, redness, or discharge; nose with boggy turbinates, scant clear nasal discharge, sinus nontender; throat—uvula midline, tonsils non-enlarged, mild erythema, no discharge
- Neck: no notable nodes, trachea midline, thyroid non-tender, normal size and consistency, carotids without bruit
- Heart: RRR, without murmur, clicks, gallops, lifts, or bruits
- Lungs: scattered wheezing, no rales or rhonchi; no consolidation with percussion, noted prolonged expiratory phase
- Ext: no edema, normal cap refill, pedal pulses normal

ASSESSMENT AND PLAN

- Tobacco use disorder
- Asthma: moderate persistent, with acute exacerbation
- Bronchitis
- Diabetes type 2 poorly controlled hyperglycemia secondary to prescribed use of steroid medication and diabetic peripheral neuropathy

Summary of ICD-10-CM Impacts

Clinical Documentation Recommendations (Clinical Concept Series [www.cms.gov/Medicare/Coding/ICD10/ICD-10Resources])

- Choosing the first-listed diagnosis in this scenario is determined by the Section IV Guidelines of ICD-10-CM found in Volume 2 of ICD-10-CM
- Section IV. Diagnostic Coding and Reporting Guidelines for Outpatient Services
- Selection of first-listed condition
- In the outpatient setting, the term-first-listed diagnosis is used in lieu of principal diagnosis.
- ICD-10-CM code for the diagnosis, condition, problem, or other reason for encounter/visit
- List first the ICD-10-CM code for the diagnosis, condition, problem, or other reason for the encounter/visit shown in the medical record to be chiefly responsible for the services provided. List additional codes that describe any coexisting conditions. In some cases, the first-listed diagnosis may be a symptom when a diagnosis has not been established (confirmed) by the physician.
- Asthma was chosen as first listed in this scenario.
- Asthma is classified as mild, moderate, and severe with additional detail as intermittent, persistent, and severe; include if there is acute exacerbation or status asthmaticus. Bronchitis was not specified as "acute" so the assignment is made to not specify as acute or chronic. In ICD-10-CM both bronchitis and asthma are reported separately.
- Bronchitis is reported separately from asthma per ICD-10-CM guidelines. Bronchitis was not specified as acute or chronic and the default code would be J40. Conditions involving infectious processes will have "acute" versus "chronic" choice. Providers should document whenever possible "acute" or "chronic."

(cont.)

- Guidelines require reporting of tobacco use or exposure for respiratory, vascular, and some other chronic illnesses such as oral and esophageal cancer codes. The guideline message for using these codes is found at the beginning of Chapter 10 in this scenario.

- Diabetic manifestations are incorporated into the primary code for diabetes mellitus (combination codes). In this case diabetes with nephropathy is a combination code.

- "Uncontrolled" diabetes is no longer a concept in ICD-10. Diabetes that is poorly controlled should include whether hyperglycemia or hypoglycemia is present; whenever either is present it should be coded accordingly. This patient would also have hyperglycemia reported as the recorded blood sugars show hyperglycemia.

- Adverse effects of prescribed medications are reported from the Table of Drugs and Chemicals and then a final code assignment is made from the Tabular List for the seventh character. Identify which medications are causing adverse reactions and go to the Table of Drugs and Chemicals found in Volume 3 of ICD-10-CM. Along the left side of that table, find the drug (or drug class if the individual drug is not found). Then the seventh characters are found at the beginning of the T38 category in Volume 1 (Tabular List) of the ICD-10-CM.

- The choices for seventh character for this table are: A = initial encounter; D = subsequent encounter; S = Sequela.

- In this scenario, it would be an initial encounter as this is the first time this provider is evaluating the patient for this adverse effect.

- Hypertension and obesity are documented as comorbid conditions and reported when treatment is given for those affected by these conditions. Instructions found at the obesity code instruct clinicians to also report the BMI if documented.

- Note: In ICD-10-CM "Nephritis" is not referenced in the diabetes complication codes with nephropathy.

ICD-10-CM DIAGNOSIS CODES

J45.41   Moderate persistent asthma with (acute) exacerbation

J40   Bronchitis, not specified as acute or chronic

F17.210   Nicotine dependence, cigarettes, uncomplicated

E11.21   Type 2 diabetes mellitus with diabetic nephropathy

E11.65   Type 2 diabetes mellitus with hyperglycemia

T38.0x5A   Adverse effect of glucocorticoids and synthetic analogues, initial encounter

I10   Essential (primary) hypertension.

E66.01   Morbid (severe) obesity due to excess calories

Z68.41   Body mass index (BMI) 40.0-44.9, adult

SUGGESTED CURRENT PROCEDURAL TERMINOLOGY EVALUATION AND MANAGEMENT CODING LEVEL BY MEDICAL DECISION-MAKING VERSUS TIME

Mr. Haddad is new to you as a client for initial visit of follow-up for an ED visit. He presents with multiple chronic uncontrolled (unstable) health conditions requiring extensive diagnoses or management options. His multiple conditions, recent exacerbations, and negative effects of his treatment, including hyperglycemia with use of prednisone, increase his risk. Additional risk factors include his use of tobacco and the presence of diabetic nephropathy as sequelae from his chronic unstable diabetes. An E&M code of 99205 is appropriate if properly documented either by time (high complexity 60 to 74 minutes) or by MDM based on problem complexity, number of problems addressed, and risk of complications and/or morbidity of patient management.

Two of the three factors are required to determine coding level using:

- **1-Problem:** The complexity of problems addressed
- **2-Data.** Amount and/or complexity of data to be reviewed and analyzed, and
- **3-Risk:** Risk of complications and/or morbidity or mortality of patient management

High Complexity: 60 to 74 minutes: 50 minutes direct patient care and management, 15 minutes EHR documentation, 10 minutes accessing patient education resources and referrals

Risk: Chronic illness unstable, effects sequelae from treatment; chronic illness with exacerbation, progression, or side effects of treatment: a chronic illness that is acutely worsening, poorly controlled, or progressing with an intent to control progression and requiring additional supportive care or requiring attention to treatment for side effects, but that does not require consideration of a hospital level of care.

Source: CMS Clinical Concept Series for Diagnosis and CPT E&M Level.

REFERENCES

References for this chapter are online and available at https://connect.springerpub.com/content/book/978-0-8261-8414-6/part/part01/toc-part/ch14.

PART V

Common Health Conditions

CHAPTER 15

Common Skin Disorders Encountered in the Primary Care Setting

Rhonda Goodman

LEARNING OBJECTIVES

At the completion of this chapter, the learner will be able to:

➤ Conduct a thorough medical history of the integumentary system.

➤ Perform a thorough physical examination and assessment of the skin, hair, and nails.

➤ Correctly describe and document the morphology of skin lesions.

➤ Develop differential and working diagnoses.

➤ Choose the appropriate pharmacologic and nonpharmacologic care and treatment for skin conditions; choose care that is culturally sensitive and age-appropriate.

➤ Provide culturally sensitive and age-appropriate health promotion and counseling.

INTRODUCTION

This chapter introduces the basics of the physical dermatology assessment for the APRN, with the focus on the late adolescent through the continuum to the older adult patient. Basic anatomy of the skin is reviewed, along with an introduction of examination techniques, primary and secondary lesions, and common skin disorders seen in this population.

OVERVIEW OF THE DERMATOLOGIC SYSTEM

The skin is composed of three layers: the epidermal layer, the dermal layer, and the subcutaneous, or adipose, tissue (Figure 15.1). The superficial epidermis is composed of two layers. The outermost layer is the stratum corneum, made up of dead keratinocytes, while the innermost layer is the stratum basale and stratum spinosum. The stratum spinosum provides the location for the production of melanin and keratin. These substances migrate to the stratum corneum in a month's time.

The epidermal layer is devoid of an adequate blood supply, which is provided by the dermal layer. This layer is composed of connective tissue, such as collagen, elastic tissue, and the reticular fibers, as well as hair follicles, sweat glands, and sebaceous glands. This dense layer provides the nutrition for the epidermis.

Finally, the subcutaneous, or fatty adipose, layer is responsible for homeostasis for body temperature, skin mobility, protection of underlying bodily structures, and the storage of energy created by metabolism.

Four pigments account for the color of skin. The melanin is a brown substance dependent on genetics and by the amount of exposure of the skin to sunlight. Carotene is the yellow pigment found in the subcutaneous layer. Carotene is concentrated in the palms of the hands and in the soles of the feet where the epidermal layer is thickest at approximately 1.5 mm. At the thinnest areas, such as the eyelids, the epidermis is a mere 0.5 mm. Another pigment found in the subcutaneous layer is hemoglobin, which carries oxygen while attached to the red blood cells. Oxyhemoglobin is found in oxygenated blood in the arterial circulatory system, and its red-pigmented color gives the skin a reddish hue. Deoxyhemoglobin circulates in unoxygenated blood in the venous circulatory system and gives the skin a bluer color known as cyanosis.

Also included in the examination of the integumentary system are the hair and scalp, nails, and glands, also known as the adnexa or appendages of the skin. Adolescents and adults have two types of hair. The vellus hair is short, fine, and unpigmented and found on most of a person's body. The terminal hair is thicker, longer, and pigmented and is found on the scalp and eyebrows. After puberty, terminal hair is also found in the genital area.

The nails provide protection for the distal portions of the fingers and toes (Figure 15.2). The nail bed is vascular, providing a pinkish color to the nail plate. A compromise in the circulatory system can result in a bluish, or cyanotic, hue to the nail beds. Chronic circulatory disease may result in nail clubbing, which is visible if the angle of attachment of the nail is greater than 180° (Figure 15.3).

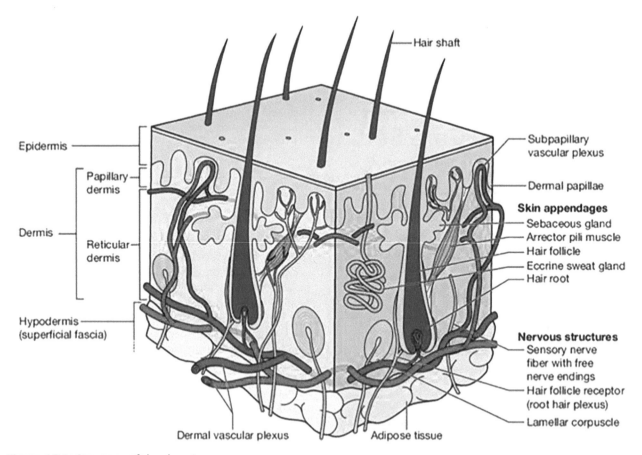

Figure 15.1: Structure of the dermis

The dermis is largely composed of collagen fibers. The cellular components of the dermis consist of mast cells, histiocytes, vascular channels, and nerves. The appendages of the skin are also found well into the dermal matrix.

Source: Myrick KM, Karosas LM, eds. *Advanced Health Assessment and Differential Diagnosis.* Springer Publishing Company; 2021:Figure 5.7.

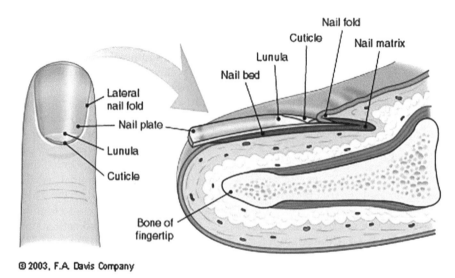

© 2003, F.A. Davis Company

Figure 15.2: Anatomy of the nail

Source: Campo T, Lafferty K. *Essential Procedures for the Emergency, Urgent, and Primary Care Settings: A Clinical Companion.* Springer Publishing Company; 2020.

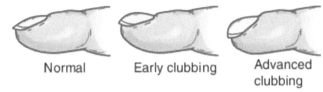

Figure 15.3: Finger clubbing

Source: Chiocca EM. *Advanced Pediatric Assessment.* Springer Publishing Company; 2020.

FUNCTIONS OF THE INTEGUMENTARY SYSTEM

The skin is the largest and heaviest organ, and it carries out multiple bodily functions. The skin provides protection against microorganisms and radiation, tactile sensations, temperature regulation, boundaries for bodily fluids, homeostasis, and vitamin D synthesis. The hair and nails also provide protection and tactile sensations; in addition, they are important guides to the diagnosis of many systemic disorders. Sebaceous glands are found on all skin surfaces with the exception of the palms of the hands and the soles of the feet and produce sebum, a fatty substance composed of wax esters, triglycerides, squalene, and cellular metabolites. Sebum is secreted through hair follicles and helps keep the skin waterproof and lubricates the skin and hair. If the opening is blocked, a pimple may result from the obstruction of sebum secretion. Sweat glands are either eccrine or apocrine and serve the major function of controlling body temperature through the secretion of sweat, which is mostly water and salts. The eccrine glands, in addition to thermoregulation, also allow the excretion of electrolytes and are distributed over the body. The apocrine glands are located in the axillary and genital areas and secrete through hair follicles. Body odor may be the result of bacterial decomposition of the sweat excreted by apocrine glands.[3]

OBTAINING A DERMATOLOGIC HISTORY

A thorough medical history is of utmost importance in establishing a diagnosis for a dermatologic complaint. Many lesions have a similar morphology and distribution, and often, it is the information elicited from the history that guides the development of the differential diagnoses. As in any medical history interview, begin with open-ended questions to gather the data. Move to closed-ended questions in order to clarify or expand the patient's answers. The examiner should begin with questions about the general health of the patient and then move into a more focused interview to address the skin complaint (Boxes 15.1 and 15.2).

Box 15.1: Questions to Ask to Elicit a Skin Health History

- Have you experienced any hair loss?
- Have you noticed changes in your hair, nails, or skin?
- Have you noticed new moles, bumps, rashes, or lesions?
- Have you noticed any changes in your moles (changes in size, shape, color, or borders)?
- Is there a family history of any disease involving the skin, hair, or nails?
- What medications are you taking, both prescriptive and over the counter?
- Are you taking vitamins, supplements, herbals, or "borrowed" medications?
- Are you taking oral contraceptives?
- Are you taking nonsteroidal anti-inflammatory medications (NSAIDs)?
- Do you have any allergies to drugs, foods, or environment?
- If you have allergies, what type of reaction do you have, and what medication or treatment is used for it?
- Do you use sunscreen? Do you use tanning booths?
- What is your occupation? Are you exposed to any chemicals?
- Do you work with young children?
- Describe your living conditions.
- Do you travel? If so, where and how frequently?

Box 15.2: Questions to Ask if Patient Complains of a Lesion or a Rash[3]

- When did you first notice the lesion/rash?
- Where did you first notice the lesion/rash? (It is helpful to ask the patient to point to the area of the body.)
- How many lesions/bumps have you seen?
- Did the lesion/rash spread from the primary site?
- Is the lesion/rash always there, or does it come and go?
- What are the characteristics of the lesion/rash (itching, burning, stabbing pain, aching)?
- If the lesion/rash is painful, what is the pain level on a scale of 1 to 10?
- Are there other symptoms, such as swelling, drainage, odor, blisters, cold, flu, fever, headache, chills, fatigue, weakness, or loss of appetite?
- Have you used any medication or treatment on the lesion/rash? If so, was relief obtained?

- Is there anything that makes the lesion/rash better? Worse?
- Have you ever had a rash like this before? If so, what medication or treatment was used, and was relief obtained?
- Have you been exposed to any illness?
- Does this happen in cold weather? Hot weather?
- Have you been exposed to any chemicals?
- Have you been exposed to any plants?
- What do you do for a living?
- Have you used any new soaps, lotions, perfumes, bath wash, or laundry detergent?
- Are your immunizations up to date?
- Has this lesion/rash had an impact on your sleep, appetite, work, school, or social activities?

SOCIAL DETERMINANTS OF HEALTH FOR THE OLDER ADULT

There will be a myriad of reasons why the adolescent, adult, and/or older adult may not have access to appropriate care. They might live in an underserved area with few primary care clinics or healthcare providers. Low-income neighborhoods might be missing grocery markets, retail venues, or restaurants offering healthy-eating options. A lack of accessible transportation would be an obstacle to accessing care, as would work hours, home responsibilities, and comorbidities. Then there are the obvious barriers to adequate healthcare: age, gender, ethnicity, socioeconomic status, disability, immigration status, and inadequate or no insurance coverage. Availability of community-based resources, such as social workers and/or case managers, would be extremely helpful if utilized to assist the patient to access necessary care, food, and transportation.

The cost of medications for certain skin conditions can be limiting, and if it is not covered by insurance and the patient cannot afford to pay out of pocket, the prescription is likely not to be filled. The provider can access many coupon and discount programs on the patient's behalf in order to make some medications more affordable. In addition, many pharmacies have a published list of low-cost medications, if a substitute medication is available. The older adult will especially need assistance in navigating the many options of Medicare Part D prescription plans. Providers need to stay informed of the annual changes in coding, especially for Medicare visits and examinations.

MORPHOLOGY OF LESIONS

"Morphology" is the description of the presentation of a skin lesion. The characteristics of the lesion are detailed, including the size, shape, color, arrangement, location, distribution, and type of lesion.[15]

Primary Lesions

A primary lesion is the initial eruption of a basic lesion from previously unaffected skin.

Macule: A macule is a flat, circumscribed lesion less than 1 cm in diameter. It may be hypopigmented, or brown, blue, or red, usually involving only the epidermis. Examples of macules are freckles, café-au-lait spots, tinea versicolor, vitiligo, and lentigo (Figure 15.4).

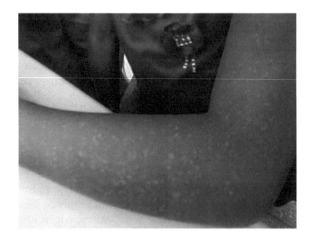

Figure 15.4: Macules
Source: Rhonda Goodman

Patch: A patch is a flat, circumscribed lesion greater than or equal to 1 cm in diameter. Examples of a patch are a birthmark, Mongolian spot, vitiligo, and tinea versicolor (Figure 15.5).

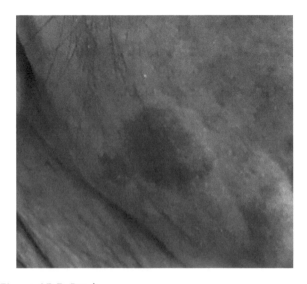

Figure 15.5: Patch
Source: Rhonda Goodman

Papule: A papule is a palpable, elevated lesion less than 1 cm in diameter with variant colors. Raised lesions usually involve not only the epidermis but also the dermis and subcutis. Examples are elevated nevi, basal cell carcinomas, seborrheic keratosis, and molluscum contagiosum (Figure 15.6).

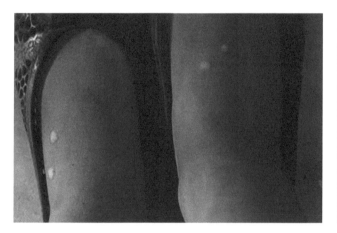

Figure 15.6: Papules
Source: Rhonda Goodman

Plaque: A plaque is an elevated, superficial lesion that is 1 cm or larger and most often is the result of the confluence of multiple papules. Examples are eczema, psoriasis, seborrheic dermatitis, pityriasis rosea, and tinea corporis (Figure 15.7).

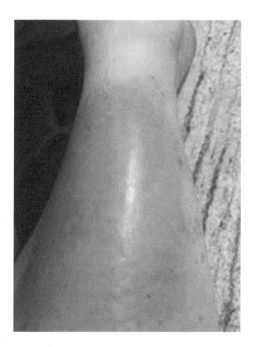

Figure 15.7: Plaque
Source: Rhonda Goodman

Vesicle: A vesicle is an elevated lesion, less than 1 cm, which is filled with serous fluid. Examples are blisters and the lesions of herpes simplex, varicella, and herpes zoster (Figure 15.8).

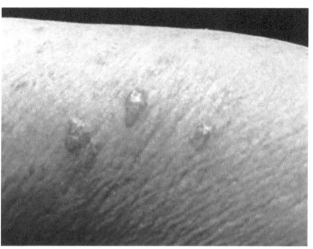

Figure 15.8: Vesicles
Source: Rhonda Goodman

Bulla: A bulla is a large vesicle, greater than 1 cm, and filled with serous fluid. Examples are blisters, impetigo, and herpes zoster (Figure 15.9).

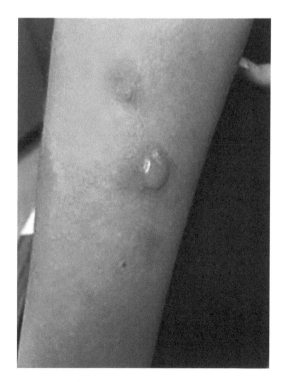

Figure 15.9: Bulla
Source: Erin Bishop

Pustule: A pustule is a vesicle that has become infected. It is filled with free fluid and leukocytes. Examples are acne, impetigo, varicella, and folliculitis (Figure 15.10).

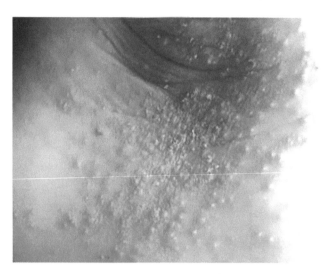

Figure 15.10: Pustules
Source: Rhonda Goodman

Nodule: A nodule is an elevated, solid, and circumscribed lesion, usually larger than 0.5 cm, and firmer than a papule. Examples are lipoma, cyst, melanoma, basal cell carcinoma, and squamous cell carcinoma (Figure 15.11).

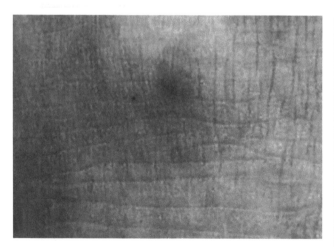

Figure 15.11: Nodule
Source: Rhonda Goodman

Wheals: Wheals, also called hives, are firm edematous plaques that are the result of the dermis being infiltrated with fluid. These lesions may be exposure-related and transient, lasting minutes to hours, and may come and go. Examples are angioedema, allergic and nonallergic contact dermatitis, and urticaria (Figure 15.12). [3,9,10]

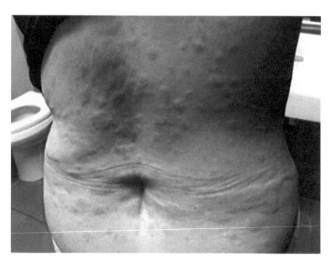

Figure 15.12: Wheals
Source: Rhonda Goodman

Secondary Lesions

Secondary lesions develop from primary lesions as a result of overtreatment, inappropriate treatment, excessive scratching and excoriation, and infection/inflammation.

Scale: Scale is caused by an accumulation of excess dead epidermal cells caused by abnormal keratinization and shedding. Examples of scale are psoriasis, ichthyosis, and eczema (Figure 15.13).

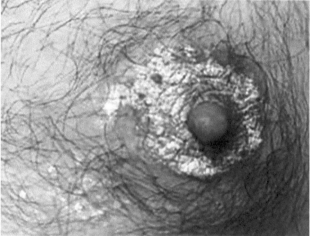

Figure 15.13: Scale
Source: Rhonda Goodman

Crust: Crust is the collection of cellular debris and dried serum, such as a scab. Examples are impetigo, tinea capitis, and atopic dermatitis (Figure 15.14).

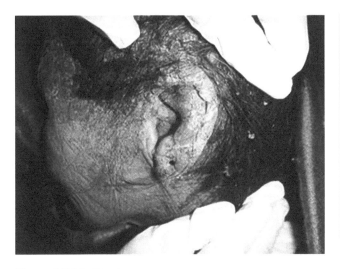

Figure 15.14: Crust
Source: Rhonda Goodman

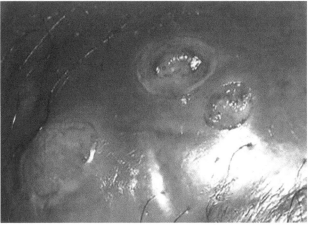

Figure 15.16: Ulcer

Erosion: Erosion involves the loss of epidermis and usually does not penetrate below the dermoepidermal junction. This lesion will usually heal without scarring. Examples are tinea pedis, candidiasis, eczema, and herpes simplex (Figure 15.15).

Fissure: A fissure is a lesion with a linear loss of both epidermis and dermis. Examples are tinea pedis, chapping of hands and feet, and intertrigo (Figure 15.17).

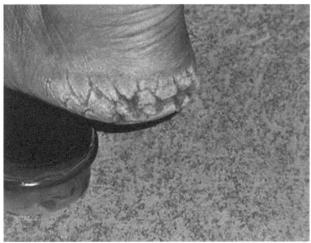

Figure 15.17: Fissure

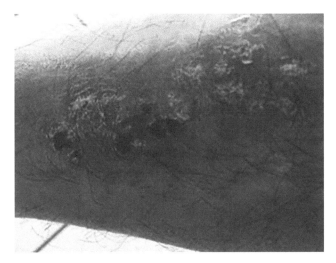

Figure 15.15: Erosion

Atrophy: Atrophy is the thinning of the epidermal or dermal layers and results in a depression in the skin. This may be caused by topical and intralesional steroids. Examples are discoid lupus erythematosus and age-related skin changes.

Scar/Keloid: After surgery or injury to the dermis, scars form from connective tissue; they are initially thick and red or pink, and gradually they atrophy and become pale. Examples are burns, varicella, and herpes zoster. Keloids result from hypertrophic scarring (overgrowth of granulation tissue) with borders extending beyond the initial injury (Figures 15.18 and 15.19).

Ulcer: An ulcerated lesion will have a loss of both epidermis and dermis, and will usually scar with healing. Examples are decubitus, stasis ulcers, and neoplasms (Figure 15.16).

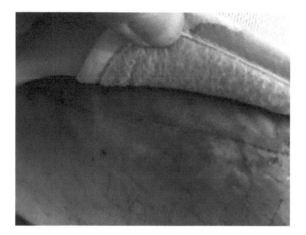

Figure 15.18: Scar

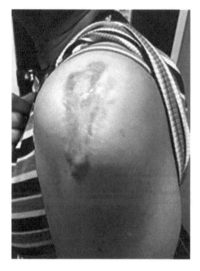

Figure 15.19: Keloid
Source: Erin Bishop

Excoriation: Excoriation is caused by excessive scratching and produces linear or punctuate erosions (Figure 15.20).

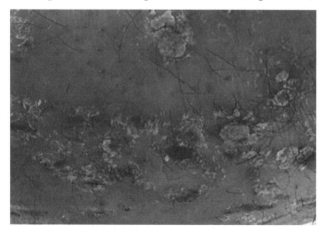

Figure 15.20: Excoriation

Lichenification: Lichenification is caused by chronic and excessive scratching and results in the thickening and roughing of the skin (Figure 15.21).

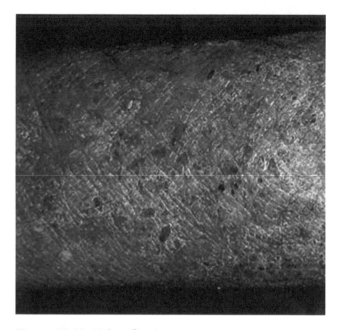

Figure 15.21: Lichenification

Shapes

Annular: round or oval, with raised border and central clearing, as in tineas and impetigo

Reticular: a lacy rash as in the lesions of erythema infections, or fifths disease

Targetoid: a bull's-eye center surrounded by concentric rings, as in Lyme disease

Guttate: teardrop-shaped, separated

Linear: lesions are in a straight line, as in Rhus dermatitis, or excoriation

Serpiginous: snake-line or wavy patterns, as in helminthic diseases

Umbilicated: has a "belly button" depression in the middle, as in molluscum

Discrete: lesions are well circumscribed, not confluent, and separated

Grouped or Clustered: lesions are arranged in groups, as in herpes zoster

Confluent: initial lesions have coalesced into a larger lesion, as in plaque psoriasis

Location

Extensor Areas: surface of an extensor muscle; arm and shoulder, forearm and elbow, hand and wrist, fingers, thigh and hip, leg and knee, toes

Flexor Areas: inside of the elbow, back of the knee

Anterior or Ventral: the front of the body, including chest, abdomen, and pelvis

Posterior or Dorsal: the back of the body, including the cranium and spine

Superior or Cranial: the upper body; toward the head

Inferior or Caudal: the lower body; away from the head

Medial: toward the middle of the body

Lateral: away from the middle of the body

Proximal: the part of the body nearest the trunk or the point of origin of a part

Distal: the part of the body farthest from the trunk

Unilateral or Bilateral: on one side or both sides

Dermatomal: following along a dermatomal pattern

Intertriginous: between the folds of the skin, such as axilla or groin

Symmetrical or Asymmetrical: each side is the same or they are different

Distribution

Diffuse: dispersed or spread out over a large area

Scattered: covering all or most of the body; not concentrated in one place

Localized: contained within a part of the body

Generalized: spread over the entire body

CASE STUDY
CUTANEOUS LARVA MIGRANS

HISTORY

A 16-year-old male presented with complaints of a rash on his right foot. He reported a burning pain, rated 10/10, accompanied by intense itching. He could walk only with help. He first noticed the rash 5 days prior, beginning as one bump which then developed into blisters and spread on the top of his foot. He remembered that, several days prior to the onset, he had played an outdoor game with bare feet in wet dirt in his neighbor's backyard. His neighbor had several pets, including dogs and cats. He had no other symptoms, and he had not used any medication for relief.

PHYSICAL EXAMINATION

Assessment of the foot revealed serpiginous, vesicular tunnels on the dorsal surface of the right foot. The lesions had an erythematous base and had evolved and spread from the top of the foot to the base of the toes (Figure 15.22).

DIAGNOSIS

Due to the history, the presentation of lesions, and the presence of animals, a diagnosis was made without biopsy: cutaneous larva migrans (hookworm or creeping eruption).

TREATMENT

An antihelminthic medication, thiabendazole, was prescribed orally. In addition, an oral antihistamine and topical corticosteroid were used to relieve the intense itching. The patient was instructed to avoid being barefoot, especially on wet soil where animals defecate. Good handwashing was stressed as was the application of cool, moist compresses for comfort and itch relief. It was also advised that the neighbor have the animals checked for hookworm ova in the feces. The lesions were cleared within a month.[8]

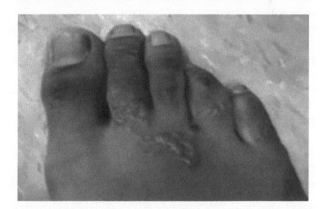

Figure 15.22: Cutaneous larva migrans

PERFORMING A SKIN EXAMINATION: INSPECTION AND PALPATION

The hair, nails, and glands (both eccrine and apocrine) form the adnexa of the skin and are included in the history and examination. If the physical examination is to be focused solely on the integumentary system, a head-to-toe sequence would be the most seamless for the examiner and more comfortable for the patient. For the older adult, most of the examination could be conducted with the patient sitting in a comfortable and safe chair with arms to prevent falls. For the adolescent, the examination could be conducted with the patient sitting on an examination table or even standing. If the assessment of the skin is only a part of a complete physical examination, then it would be more convenient to conduct the skin assessment by system. For example, the examiner would first examine the exposed skin of the head, neck, arms, hands, and lower extremities. Then, as the examination progresses to include the anterior thorax, posterior thorax, and abdomen, the skin would be assessed during the examination of those systems. This would avoid exposing the patient's entire body all at the same time.

Prior to beginning the examination, the examiner should provide a comfortable setting for the patient. Provide privacy by exposing only small areas of the body at a time. Check the temperature of the room, especially for the older adult, whose temperature regulation may have been affected by the aging process. The older adult may have a lower body temperature and a lower tolerance for extreme temperatures, since thermoregulation is affected not only by the skin but also by the declination of the cardiovascular and respiratory systems. Adequate lighting is absolutely necessary, and natural lighting is best. A good lighted magnifying lens is helpful, as well as a clear ruler.

The physical examination of the skin requires two techniques: inspection and palpation. First, the examiner will inspect the skin and identify characteristics of any lesions and differentiate between what is normally expected and what is not. The examiner should feel comfortable touching the patient's skin as touching is not only a caring and assuring approach to the patient; it is also an efficient technique for eliciting data about the skin.[12]

Hair and Scalp

Color: Note the color, dullness or shininess, cleanliness, and quantity of the hair. Examine both the vellus and the terminal hair.

Texture: Note if the hair is fine or coarse, straight, brittle, wavy, or curly.

Distribution: Note the hairline's symmetry or asymmetry. Examine for areas of hair loss, as in alopecia or trichotillomania. Note the presence of dandruff. Is the hair thick or thinning?

Scalp mobility: Assess the mobility of the scalp by moving the scalp horizontally and vertically against the occipital bone. Scalp mobility affects the movement of the facial nerve. Assess for deformities, depressions, lumps, nevi, scale, and areas of tenderness.

Presence of infestation, inflammation, lesions, excoriations, or tinea capitis: Part the hair into small segments and examine closely for the presence of pediculosis (head lice), in the form of eggs (nits) or adult lice. Assess behind the ears and the nape of the neck for signs of scratching from infestation by lice (Figure 15.23).

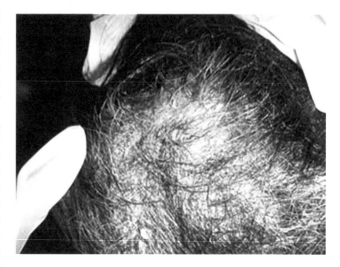

Figure 15.23: Tinea capitis

Nails

Color: Note the color of the nail and whether the nail bed is cyanotic.

Shape: Note the shape of the nail—rounded or squared.

Attachment: Assess for onycholysis (separation of the nail from the nail bed). Assess for onychomycosis (a fungal infection of the nail bed that causes the nail to thicken and yellow; Figure 15.24). Note the angle of

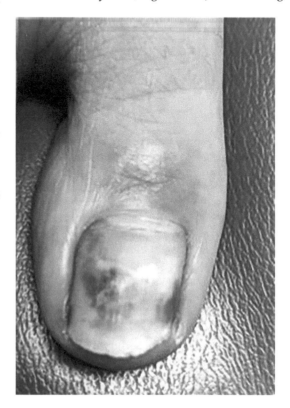

Figure 15.24: Onychomycosis

attachment; it should be less than 180°. Otherwise, if clubbing is present, there may be an underlying circulatory compromise.

Capillary Refill: Place pressure on a fingernail and note blanching. When the pressure is removed, the nail should have a capillary return in 2 to 3 seconds.

Presence of Lesions/Abnormalities: Note any lesions, pitting, and ridging of nails. Also, inspect for any edema, erythema, warmth, and/or tenderness along the proximal and lateral nail folds as this could indicate a paronychial infection. Check for fungal onychomycosis. Palpate the distal interphalangeal (DIP) joints for Heberden's nodes and the proximal interphalangeal (PIP) joints for Bouchard's nodes.[16]

Skin

Color: Note the color of the skin: pink, olive, tan, mahogany, and so on, noting hypopigmentation or hyperpigmentation. Look for redness, pallor, cyanosis, or yellowing. Oxyhemoglobin provides a reddish color best seen at the fingertips, lips, and mucous membranes. In persons with darker skin, look at the palms and soles. Erythema, or a reddish color, would be caused by increased blood flow. Central cyanosis would affect the lips, oral mucosa, and tongue as a result of a low oxygen level in the blood. Peripheral cyanosis would be the result of a decrease in cutaneous blood flow from anxiety or cold temperatures. Look for jaundice in the sclera and assess for carotenemia (yellow hue) on the palms, soles, and face (the sclera will be white, as carotenemia is caused by a diet high in carrots and yellow vegetables). Note the presence of bruising and question the patient about the cause, as this could indicate an underlying medical condition or potential abuse. Also, note the presence of scars and/or keloids and cherry angiomas.

🛈 CLINICAL PEARLS

▧ Many systemic conditions present with dermatologic manifestations. For example, central cyanosis might be present in congenital heart disease, advanced pulmonary disease, and hemoglobinopathies. Peripheral cyanosis might be present in congestive heart failure, pulmonary embolism, and venous obstruction. Jaundice might be present in liver disease and in excessive hemolysis of red blood cells. Pallor is caused by anemia and reduced blood flow, arterial insufficiency, and fainting. Bruising could be not only the result of abuse but also the sign of a clotting disorder or high levels of anticoagulants.

- **Moisture:** Palpate the skin, noting whether the skin is dry, moist, or oily.
- **Texture:** Palpate the skin and note roughness or smoothness.

🛈 CLINICAL PEARLS

▧ The texture and temperature of the skin may be indicative of an underlying disease process.

Localized warm skin may be the result of inflammation or cellulitis. Hyperthyroidism may produce a warm skin temperature with a velvety texture, while hypothyroidism may cause the skin to be cold and rough (a decrease in the speed of natural exfoliation of dead cells).[4]

- **Temperature:** Using the backs of the fingers, palpate the skin, noting whether the skin is cool, cold, warm, or hot.
- **Turgor and Mobility:** In the older patient, lift a fold of the skin at the sternal area, a place less affected by the effects of aging. While examining the adolescent patient, use the dorsal surface of the hand. Note the mobility or the ease with which the skin lifts up, and the turgor, the speed with which the skin returns to its place. Check the back of the hand for "tenting." Mobility would be deceased in edema and scleroderma, and turgor would be decreased if the patient is dehydrated.

▧ **Presence of Lesions:** Thoroughly inspect the skin, noting any lesions.

- Measure the lesions and document the morphology, size, location, arrangement, distribution, color, associated symptoms, and shape.
- Assess the face and the lower extremities for signs of edema, which could indicate an underlying medical condition.

ABUSE

The incidence of elder abuse has increased, and with the heightened awareness and screening by providers, the reporting of elder abuse has also become more common. It is important that the provider elicit information about the patient's living situation and conditions. With whom does the patient live? Does the patient feel safe at home? Is the patient forthcoming with answers when a caregiver is in the examination room? Examine and inquire about all unexplained injuries (Figure 15.25). If there is a possibility of abuse, report this to the authorities. If the injuries are serious, have the patient transported to the nearest emergency department for further evaluation and diagnostics. A nurse navigator or case manager, a psychologist, and a social worker can contribute to the interdisciplinary team to help a patient in this situation.

Quality and Safety Alerts

▧ While the nurse and nurse practitioner are federally mandated to report allegations of abuse, it is not within their practice scope to determine the veracity of the

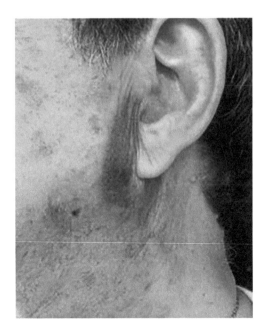

Figure 15.25: Elder abuse

allegations. They are to report what the patient reveals during a history interview and what they observe during a physical examination. The local authorities will determine the truth of the allegations.

ACNE

While patients of all ages may experience acne, it is more common among the adolescent population. If the acne is severe and/or persistent, this can be detrimental in an age group where peer approval and self-esteem are very important, thus producing a serious psychosocial impact. Therefore, counseling for the affected adolescent would be added to the plan of care.

Acne vulgaris is one of the most common reasons for a visit to a healthcare provider, affecting almost 50 million people annually in the United States. Puberty is usually the precursor of the appearance of acne; therefore, girls usually experience it earlier than boys, around the ages of 10 to 12 years. Boys usually have more severe acne but girls experience acne more chronically. The age of onset is higher in persons of color.

In the older patient, adult-onset acne (aged mid-20s–40s) may accompany other medical conditions, such as polycystic ovarian syndrome, Cushing syndrome, hyperandrogenism, hormonal changes, stress, and endocrine disorders. Medications may also be a catalyst for the onset of acne in older adults.

Acne is the result of the combination of many factors beginning with the subclinical inflammation of the skin and an increase in the production of sebum and aggravated by an increased presence of androgens. Pores are enlarged and ultimately plugged with shed epithelial cells

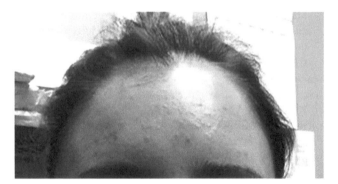

Figure 15.26: Acne
Source: Erin Bishop

Box 15.3: Levels of Severity in Acne Vulgaris

Mild: Mostly involves only the face. Presence of noninflammatory open and closed comedones.

Moderate: May involve the face, chest, and back. Presence of comedones, inflammation, papules, and pustules. May have presence of scarring.

Severe: Usually involves the face, chest, and back. Presence of inflammation, comedones, papules, pustules, cysts, and nodules. Usually involves scarring.

---

which block the opening of the follicles (Figure 15.26). The colonization of *Propionibacterium* acnes then leads to microcomedone development, further blocking the pore. The follicle wall ruptures, and thus begins the development of papules, pustules, and cysts. The resulting lesions are called comedones and may be open or closed. A closed comedone, or whitehead, is not open to air whereas an open comedone, or blackhead, has darkened due to the oxidation of the amino acid, tyrosine, to melanin.

For the adolescent to the older adult, there are three levels of severity for acne vulgaris (Box 15.3).

Approach to Diagnosis

Because diagnosis is usually based on symptoms and appearance, lab testing is not often conducted. However, to discover any endocrine system involvement, it may be necessary to test for free testosterone and dehydroepiandrosterone sulfate (DHEAS), the index of adrenal androgen levels. This may necessitate an endocrinology referral, especially in the presence of associated symptoms, such as hirsuitism and obesity in the female patient with irregular menstrual cycles.

Management

Treatment for acne can be complex, but the objective is to prevent potential scarring, changes in pigmentation, and disfigurement and minimize inflammation. The most common treatments for mild acne are topical retinoids (Retin-A), adapalene gel (Differin), azelaic acid, antimicrobial, and salicylic acid. The patient should be informed of potential adverse effects, such as dryness, photosensitivity, erythema, burning, scaling, and possibly skin atrophy.

If the initial therapy is not successful, or if the level of severity is moderate, use topical and/or oral antibiotics (erythromycin, clindamycin, doxycycline, minocycline), oral contraceptives for females, spironolactone (especially for older females with hirsuitism), benzoyl peroxide, and topical combinations of benzoyl peroxide and antibiotics. Potential side effects of these combination topicals are burning and erythema. The tetracyclines are contraindicated in pregnant women.

Finally, for severe acne, the provider should begin therapy, including topical retinoids, benzoyl peroxide, oral antibiotics, and possibly oral contraceptives in females. However, at this point, a referral to a dermatologist is necessary, as the patient may need oral isotretinoin, which is teratogenic.

🏠 Quality and Safety Alert

▓ If monitoring a patient who is taking oral isotretinoin it is imperative to conduct a monthly pregnancy test. Also, the patient will need education concerning birth control and the potential consequences if a pregnancy should occur.

Patient Education

Patient education is of great importance. The patients should be educated on skin hygiene, using nonabrasive cleansers. The provider should feel confident that the patient understands the appropriate dosage, applications, and side effects of medications. Finally, but very important, the patient should have access to counseling and encouragement, and referral to a psychologist, if needed.

ALOPECIA

While normally associated with the scalp, hair loss may occur wherever there is hair on the body. The most common type of hair loss is male-pattern baldness, or androgenetic alopecia, which occurs over the generalized area of the scalp. Alopecia areata, however, presents with patches of baldness, which may be temporary or permanent, and may be associated with immune system compromise. Causes of hair loss include genetics, emotional stress, levels of hormones (estrogen, testosterone, growth hormone, thyroid hormone, androgens), glucocorticoids, prolactin, and medications.

Approach to Diagnosis

Diagnostic testing, such as antinuclear antibodies (ANA), erythrocyte sedimentation rate (ESR), and rheumatic factor,

may be needed to rule out autoimmune disorders. These disorders may include systemic lupus erythematosus, Hashimoto's thyroiditis, pernicious anemia, Addison's disease, and scleroderma. Other testing may include iron, total iron-binding capacity, complete blood count (CBC), serum testosterone, dehydroepiandrosterone, and thyroid function tests. In some cases, a scalp biopsy might be obtained.

Management

The plan of care is not an easy one with guaranteed results, especially since hair loss might cause a loss of self-esteem and confidence and an increasing feeling of stigmatization. There are medical treatments for the maintenance of regrown hair, but the patient needs to use the medication or treatments daily. Commonly used oral medications are minoxidil (Rogaine) and finasteride (Propecia), while topical minoxidil is also used. As with most medications, these also come with adverse effects and should be monitored cautiously. Finasteride is contraindicated for use by women of reproductive age. Some patients may be candidates for surgical hair transplantation, while others may choose other options, such as wigs, weaves, and toupees.

ANGIOEDEMA

Etiology

Angioedema is a swelling of the dermis and subcutaneous layer of the skin and may also involve the mucosa of the respiratory and gastrointestinal systems (Figure 15.27). The cause is an increase in the vascular permeability of the subcutaneous layer of the skin and respiratory

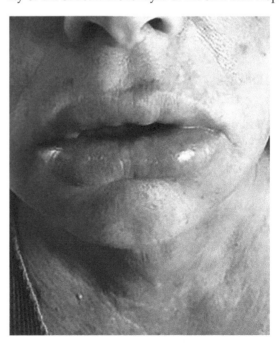

Figure 15.27: Angioedema

and gastrointestinal (GI) mucosa and submucosa. Interstitial fluid collects in these areas producing diffuse swelling. It may or may not occur with urticaria or hives and is usually an allergic reaction. The most commonly affected areas are the lips, face, throat, GI mucosa, palms, soles, extremities, and genitals. The patient will complain of burning pain, swelling, and, sometimes, itching.

Causes of angioedema may be idiopathic or immunoglobulin E (IgE)–mediated. The idiopathic type of angioedema is the most common, occurs at any age, and has an unpredictable pattern of recurrence. Antihistamines and glucocorticoids are used as prophylactic therapy. The severe allergic type I of the IgE-mediated allergic reactions is another cause of angioedema, as well as urticaria. Due to the histamine release, this type of angioedema is often accompanied by hives, or wheals, as well as other allergic symptoms and anaphylaxis.

Approach to Diagnosis

The patient will present with diffuse swelling of the skin and mucosa. If the edema involves the face and larynx, and the patient is experiencing difficulty with respirations, emergency intervention will be required. In that situation, the patient should be transported immediately to an emergency facility.

Management

Epinephrine would most likely be administered in this case. Other medications used would be antihistamines and/or corticosteroids. Prophylactic therapy would include daily antihistamine and possibly corticosteroids as well.

Patient Education

Patient education would include instruction on avoidance of triggers and medication side effects.

CANDIDIASIS

Etiology

Candida is caused by a superficial fungal infection and is commonly found in warm, humid climates. It is not a dermatophyte infection, such as tinea, but it is caused by fungi. Candida is more serious for a host with a compromised immune system, whether metabolic or systemic. The use of broad-spectrum antibiotics may also be a catalyst for the onset of candida. The lesions are most likely to be found in mucosal areas (oral thrush) and intertriginous surfaces, where skin meets skin, such as skin folds of the abdomen, as well as beneath the breasts, groin, and axillae. Other common locations for candida are the genitals (vulvovaginitis and balanitis).

Pathophysiology

On the mucosal surface, the area, such as the tongue, may have a visible white coating, which is friable, and

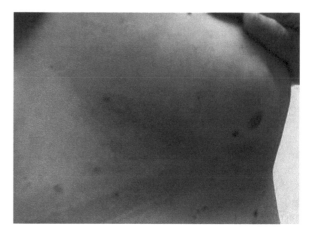
Figure 15.28: Candidiasis

may be removed with a tongue depressor. For cutaneous presentations, the lesions will be erythematous, and the initial papules will coalesce, forming patches, while satellite lesions continue to develop. Vaginal candidiasis will produce severe itching and burning with a thick, white discharge. An intertriginous candida (see Figure 15.28) will present with an erythematous rash that appears wet. Usually, diagnosis is based on history and presentation.

Management

Managing candida is relatively easy unless the infection is long-standing and resistant to treatment. Topical steroids are not a good choice as they will further suppress the reaction of the immune system. Topical antifungal medications are the first line of treatment and should be applied sparingly twice daily for 2 to 4 weeks. These include nystatin, miconazole, and clotrimazole; if oral therapy is required, then itraconazole or fluconazole may be prescribed. If a secondary infection is present, due to mechanical injury or trauma, an oral antibiotic such as a cephalosporin may be added.

Patient Education

Patient education will include keeping the area clean and dry, using a hairdryer on the low or cool setting to dry the area. Also, the patient should change clothes frequently, especially in hot, humid climates and separate skin folds with clean tissue or cotton cloths. The patient should return to the clinic in 2 weeks.

CELLULITIS

Pathophysiology

Acute cellulitis (SSTI, or skin and soft tissue infection) is a bacterial infection involving the deep dermis and

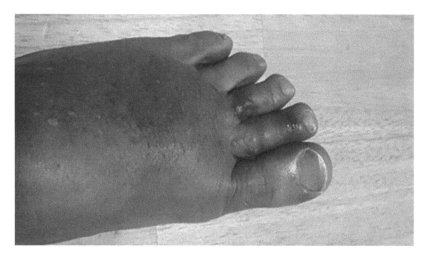

Figure 15.29: Cellulitis

subcutaneous tissues. The presentation includes edema, pain, and erythema and commonly is seen on arms, legs, and at the locations of trauma, abrasions, psoriasis, eczema, or tinea (Figure 15.29). The cause of the infection is usually group A streptococcus, namely *Staphylococcus aureus,* in the adult patient.

Approach to Diagnosis

Diagnosis is usually determined based on history and presentation of symptoms such as warmth, edema, erythema, and localized pain. There may also be systemic associated symptoms such as fever, chills, and general malaise. Blood work may reveal mild leukocytosis with a left shift and an increased sedimentation rate. It is possible to culture the infection; however, the results are more definitive if the patient has an underlying autoimmune disease.

Management

Uncomplicated cellulitis is an infection that is nonpurulent, afebrile, nonimmunosuppressive, and has no exudates or abscess. Treatment would include oral antibiotic therapy with cephalexin, dicloxacillin, clindamycin, or linezolid in order to target beta-hemolytic streptococci. For a complicated cellulitis, one that is purulent, the treatment would focus on cellulitis-associated MRSA (CA-MRSA) and would involve clindamycin, trimethoprim-sulfamethoxazole, doxycycline or minocycline, or linezolid. The patient should elevate the area as much as possible and use cool compresses for pain relief.

Patient Education

Patient education is centered on preventing recurrence of cellulitis. Good personal hygiene should be stressed as well as wound care and keeping the environment clean. The patient should return for follow-up and be referred if the infection is persistent.

CONTACT DERMATITIS (ALLERGIC AND NONALLERGIC)

Etiology

Contact dermatitis is caused by a person's exposure to allergens and/or irritants in the environment. Nonallergic or irritant contact dermatitis (ICD) is common and is the result of exposure to caustic chemicals and irritants, usually found in the work environment. The occupations most likely to suffer from ICD are hairdressers, bakers, beauticians, butchers, painters, dental assistants, machine operators, cleaners, and healthcare workers. Other factors that exacerbate ICD are advancing age, race, gender, fair skin color, and the presence of atopic dermatitis.

Pathophysiology

The patient with ICD may report that they had an immediate reaction to the irritant, describing burning and tenderness at the site of exposure. The lesions may be erythematous patches with accompanying edema and bullae. Chemical burns are the result of exposure to acid and alkaline.

Management

Treatment for ICD would begin with the immediate removal of the offending irritant. Topical steroids are used to control the inflammation. Any secondary infections should be noted and treated as necessary. The patient may have choices to make regarding occupational exposure or perhaps using barrier clothing and equipment to avoid chronicity. Prevention is the key.

Approach to Diagnosis

The patient with allergic contact dermatitis (ACD) may not be aware of the offending allergen. A thorough history will aid the patient in determining the cause of the

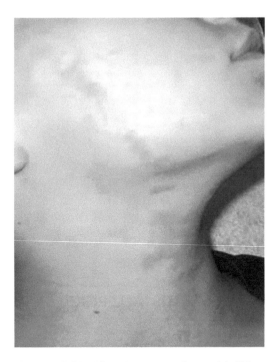

Figure 15.30: Allergic contact dermatitis (Rhus dermatitis from poison ivy)

outbreak. The history should include questions concerning skin-care products, soap, detergent, plants, food, metals, jewelry (common with nickel allergies), and cosmetics. Age does not play a factor in ACD. The infection is a type IV delayed hypersensitivity to a specific allergen. Included in this type of contact dermatitis is Rhus dermatitis caused by poison ivy, poison oak, and poison sumac, the most common form of ACD (Figure 15.30). Urushiol is the resinous sap of these plants and the cause of the allergic response when a person comes in contact with the leaf or the parts of the stem and root. This causes a characteristic linear pattern of the lesions as the plant is drawn across the skin or when the oleoresin is streaked when the patient scratches the lesions.

The patient with ACD will present with an eczematous-like eruption of moist vesicular lesions that are extremely pruritic and accompanied by edema. This may evolve into secondary lesions of scale, crust, and lichenification. Secondary infections might develop as a result of mechanical trauma such as scratching.

Management

Treatment for ACD, as in ICD, begins with avoidance of the offending allergen. Topical steroids are prescribed for clearance and may need to be used for up to 6 weeks. There are over-the-counter medications that directly remove the urushiol in the event of Rhus dermatitis; however, for peak effectiveness, the medication must be used immediately postexposure. Watch for and treat any secondary bacterial infections. The patient should be referred for allergy testing in order to identify any other allergens which may present a problem.

FOLLICULITIS

Etiology

Folliculitis is an infection or inflammation of the hair follicle and may involve the superficial or deep portion of that structure. It is usually caused by an infection, physical injury to the follicle, or by an irritation. Folliculitis may occur anywhere on the body and is not partial to any age, race, or gender. The infection may be caused by fungi, bacteria, yeast, and drug therapy. Bacterial folliculitis is usually caused by *Staphylococcal aureus*.

Approach to Diagnosis

The patient will present with a pustule or pustules in a grouped arrangement and usually without systemic symptoms. Diagnosis may be made by history and presentation alone, or by culturing the pustules. A KOH prep could be used to differentiate between bacterial and fungal infections.

Management

Antibacterial cleansers may be used on the affected area as well as topical antibiotics. If necessary, according to the results of the culture, or if there is lymphadenopathy present, systemic antibiotics may also be needed.

Patient Education

Patient education will involve teaching good personal hygiene to avoid bacterial infections. They should not share personal items with others.

CASE STUDY
HOT TUB FOLLICULITIS

PATIENT HISTORY

A 60-year-old female came to the clinic complaining of a rash on her abdomen. She was seen in a walk-in clinic 2 days ago and was diagnosed with herpes zoster and given an oral antiviral medication. She stated the rash had worsened since then and wanted to be checked again since she was on vacation. She reported that she had spent much of her time in the hotel hot tub. She denied pain but reported that the itching was very intense. She had taken oatmeal baths and used a topical anti-itch cream but did not obtain relief. She denied any other symptoms or exposure. Patient denied fever and chills.

PHYSICAL EXAMINATION

Physical assessment revealed a rash composed of multiple discrete papules and pustules located from her left flank to her abdomen, crossing over the midline and covering the right side of her abdomen as well (Figure 15.31). The lesions did not follow along a dermatomal pattern and did cross the midline of the abdomen. Some of the papules had coalesced into erythematous plaques with many satellite lesions. There were no visible vesicles or pustules, no drainage, no bleeding, and no edema. The area was neither warm nor tender on palpation.

DIAGNOSIS

Due to the presentation of the lesions and the patient's history, this was diagnosed as hot tub folliculitis. Hotel hot tubs frequently host pathogens such as *S. aureus*, *Pseudomonas aeruginosa*, dermatophytes, or candida, especially in a hot and humid climate.

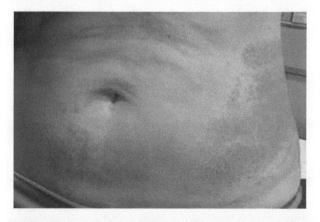

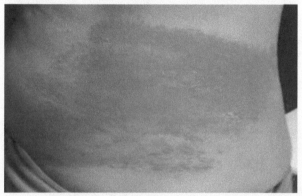

Figure 15.31: Case study–Hot tub folliculitis

TREATMENT

With no lymphadenopathy present, the lesions may be left to resolve spontaneously. The patient should be instructed on how to cleanse the affected area. If the infection is minor, a topical antibiotic may be applied; however, for a severe infection, oral antibiotic treatment would be necessary. This patient was treated with oral cephalexin for 10 days and the rash was resolved within a week. Topical antipruritics may also be applied to relieve itching, as well as oral corticosteroids and/or antihistamines. She was also advised to take warm showers after being in a public hot tub, pool, or spa, using antibacterial soap.

GRANULOMA ANNULARE

Etiology

Granuloma annulare (GA) is relatively common; however, its presentation is easy to confuse with other skin manifestations, such as nummular eczema or tinea. There is some connection between GA (the disseminated type) and the incidence of diabetes. HIV infection is more connected to the generalized type of GA. It is a self-limiting inflammatory condition that affects the dermal layer. It is most common in 30- to 60-year-olds and in women. GA may be the result of trauma, vasculitis, or a skin hypersensitivity.

Pathophysiology

The presentation of GA involves rings of firm papules that may be reddish or flesh-colored. The most common areas of the body for involvement usually are the hands and feet on the lateral and dorsal surfaces. The papular rings may grow from 0.5 to 5 cm in diameter over a period of several months. Most older adults will experience the disseminated type with numerous annular rings of papules. The papules will be concentrated in the areas of greatest sun exposure and the lesions may last for years.

Approach to Diagnosis

Diagnostic testing may involve a punch biopsy with a histologic examination; however, the diagnosis is usually made based on the presentation and characteristics of the lesions.[18]

Management

Because GA is usually self-limited, the lesions are usually left without treatment and may have spontaneous involution. Otherwise, injections of triamcinolone acetonide are given directly into the lesions. Other therapies for disseminated GA are dapsone, isotretinoin, niacinamide, etretinate, narrow-band ultraviolet B therapy, psoralen and ultraviolet A therapy, and hydroxychloroquine.

Patient Education

Because the lesions may be embarrassing and stigmatizing, the patient should be provided adequate support and anticipatory guidance. Education about medication/treatment side effects will be necessary. Treat any secondary infections caused by mechanical trauma or scratching.

HERPES SIMPLEX

There are two types of herpes simplex viruses: HSV-1 and HSV-2. Traditionally HSV-1 has presented as oral lesions (such as cold sores) and HSV-2 has presented as genital lesions. However, that is no longer the case. Frequently, and most likely as a result of sexual contact, HSV-1 may be genital and HSV-2 may be oral. It is a very common infection and approximately 90% of adults in the United States carry the HSV-1 antibodies. The initial phase of the infection involves the virus establishing in a nerve ganglion. The second phase involves a recurrence of the virus at the same location. Many patients do not report symptoms. Modes of transmission may be by respiratory droplets, contact with an active viral lesion, and contact with any fluid, such as saliva or cervical sections that may contain the virus.

Pathophysiology

Within 3 to 7 days after the initial exposure, the patient may experience parathesia or burning at the site of inoculation. Prodromal symptoms may be headache, achiness, tender lymph nodes, or no symptoms at all. The lesions appear as vesicles on an erythematous base, then evolve to pustules with umbilication, and resolving in dry, crusted lesions. Blood tests may reveal an elevated IgG antibody titer.

Management

Treatment usually involves oral antiviral medication, such as acyclovir, valacyclovir, or famciclovir for primary infections. If the patient has recurrent episodes or is immunocompromised, topical antivirals are added.[14]

HERPES ZOSTER

Herpes zoster, more commonly known as shingles, is a viral infection that involves the cutaneous area over a dermatome. While it can happen in all ages, the incidence of infection does increase with age, affecting approximately 10% to 20% of all persons. Immunocompromised persons are also at greater risk for acquiring zoster. The virus responsible for varicella, or chickenpox, is reactivated after remaining dormant in the dorsal root ganglia. Causes of reactivation may be stress, age, fatigue, immunosuppressive medications, trauma, or radiation therapy.

Pathophysiology

The onset of illness begins with the prodromal symptoms of generalized aching and localized itching, burning, or neuralgia at the cutaneous site of reactivation, usually over a single dermatome or over two adjacent dermatomes. Within 4 or 5 days, the lesions erupt, beginning as painful vesicles on an erythematous base. The vesicles may cluster in groups, thus eventually forming a plaque (Figure 15.32). The vesicles evolve into pustules containing purulent fluids, and they may umbilicate as well. The vesicles are not uniform in size or stage of evolution and may continue to erupt for 7 days. Further lesion evolution involves rupture and the lesions form a crust, which may remain for several weeks. A herpes zoster infection may seriously affect the quality of life for the older adult.

One adverse effect of zoster is postherpetic neuralgia (PHN), which is pain at the site of the initial eruption

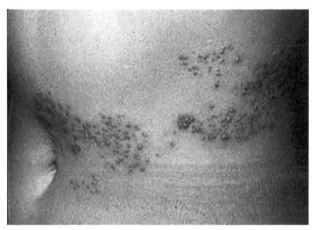

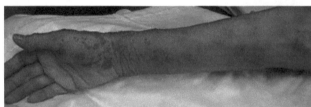

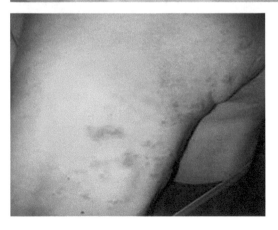

Figure 15.32: Herpes zoster

after the lesions have resolved. This is caused by damage to the peripheral nerves and an increased sensitivity of the central nervous system. This is painful and disrupts the quality of life, especially for the older patient. The herpes zoster vaccine, administered prior to onset of the illness, would reduce the incidence and intensity of PHN.[17]

Another danger of zoster lies in the location of the dermatome. Approximately 10% to 15% of zoster episodes occur on the ophthalmic nerve (herpes zoster ophthalmicus). This may involve the fifth cranial nerve, the trigeminal nerve, which has three branches: the ophthalmic, the maxillary, and the mandibular. Symptoms may include prodromal complaints of nausea, vomiting, and headaches. If vesicles are located on the tip and the side of the nose (or Hutchinson's sign), this may indicate a very severe condition leading to many ocular complications. The pain will persist for several weeks or longer in older patients, even then continuing to increase.

Management

Treatment focuses on pain management and inflammation suppression and includes early administration (within 72 hours after rash onset) of antiviral medications, such as acyclovir, famciclovir, and valacyclovir, especially in patients older than age 50. Treatment is also indicated if a rash is present, the patient experiences pain, the patient is immunocompromised, or if the lesions involve the face or eye. Cool compresses may help to relieve pain and remove crust and dried serum. Pain may be relieved by NSAIDs or acetaminophen.[6]

CASE STUDY
IMPETIGO/ECTHYMA

An 80-year-old male came to the clinic to report a rash on his outer left ankle. He said he first noticed "sores" on his ankle about 4 weeks ago, after walking in the woods with his dog. They were not painful, but very itchy, and he scratched them until they became open and weeping. He stated that a scale or scabs had now developed over the sores. He denied any exposure to chemicals, new detergent or soap, or diet changes but did admit the possibility of insect bites while walking in the woods. He had applied alcohol and antibiotic ointment to the rash with no relief.

PHYSICAL EXAMINATION

Upon inspection, it was noted that on the lateral left ankle, there was a large plaque of multiple papulovesicular and pustular lesions. There were noted erosions and ulcerations, all on an erythematous base. The entire area was covered with a thick, golden crust with visible weeping of fluid beneath the crust. Upon palpation, the area was tender and edematous (Figures 15.33 and 15.34).

DIAGNOSIS

A diagnosis was made of impetigo, and because the infection eroded beyond the epidermal layer, a secondary diagnosis of ecthyma was made. The primary lesions had evolved due to excessive scratching and infection.

TREATMENT

This patient was prescribed oral cephalexin for 10 days and a topical antibacterial ointment applied three times daily until all lesions were cleared. The patient was instructed in good handwashing hygiene with antibacterial soap and to avoid scratching the rash. Gentle washing was recommended to remove the crusting. The lesions were cleared by 12 days.[6,7]

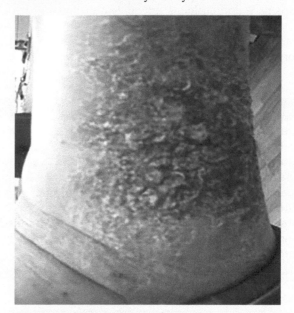

Figure 15.33: Impetigo/ecthyma

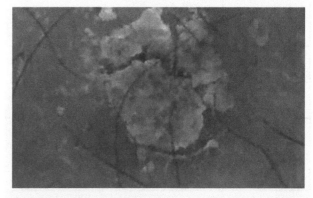

Figure 15.34: Impetigo

PRESSURE ULCERS

Etiology

Pressure ulcers, or decubitus ulcers (also called bed-sores), occur when there is continuous pressure from bony prominences on the skin. This pressure compromises the perfusion of blood to the skin and sores develop, commonly on hips, the sacral area, and the heels of the feet. These sores can be extremely painful, and cause infections, and even death.

Approach to Diagnosis

The size and characteristics of each lesion should be carefully documented and recorded with photos. Inspect for any compromise in the skin integrity and examine for signs of infection (warm, redness, drainage, tenderness). Prevention measures should be in place, such as frequent repositioning of immobilized patients, good skin hygiene, gentle massages to increase circulation to the area, hips pads and cushions, adequate nutrition and hydration, active or passive range of motion exercises, and vigilant observation and documentation. Refer to Box 15.4 for staging criteria for pressure ulcers.

Box 15.4: Staging of Pressure Ulcers

Stage I: The skin is intact, but there is erythema, which persists at least 30 minutes after relief of pressure.
Stage II: The skin is now broken, and there is a visible shallow sore. Drainage may be present.
Stage III: The stores extend past the epidermal layers, into the dermis and subcutaneous layers.
State IV: The wound extends into the layer of muscle and may even extend to the bone. There is usually a large amount of drainage and wound debris.

PSORIASIS

Psoriasis affects approximately 120 million people, mostly adults, worldwide. It is a chronic inflammatory condition of the skin, immune-mediated, which is usually chronic and requires long-term management. It affects males and females equally, usually occurring between 15 to 30 years of age, although it can occur at any age. There is often a first-degree relative who also has a history of psoriasis.[2]

Etiology

Causes may include medications, such as beta-blockers, emotional stress, excessive alcohol intake, smoking, bacterial and viral infections, trauma, or surgery. The presentation of psoriasis can be so severe that it can create a stigmatizing situation for the patient, as well as a loss of quality of life (Figure 15.35). There are six subtypes of psoriasis (Table 15.1).

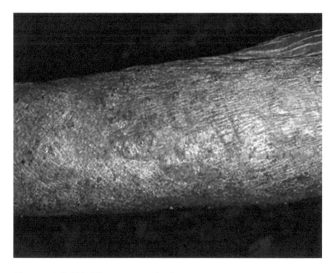

Figure 15.35: Plaque psoriasis

Table 15.1: Psoriasis Subtypes

Subtype	Description
Plaque Psoriasis	Well-demarcated erythematous plaques are thick, red, sometimes with a silvery scale. They are usually found on scalps, knees, and elbows. If the scale is removed there will be bleeding from punctate blood vessels (Auspitz sign). This aids in the diagnosis.
Scalp Psoriasis	Lesions appear on the scale and are thick, silvery, and erythematous. It is accompanied by intense itching and scaling.
Palmoplantar Psoriasis	Lesions appear on the palms of the hands and the soles of the feet. They may appear as erythematous papules or patches, vesicles, and pustules.
Guttate Psoriasis	Lesions are smaller and usually found on the trunk and extremities and may accompany other infections, such as a streptococcal throat or a sinus infection. Lesions are pink with a white scale.
Inverse Psoriasis	May be mistaken for fungus or candida because it is found in the intertriginous areas. Lesions are thin and erythematous without scale. Usually found on flexor surfaces, groins, and axillae.
Erythrodermic Psoriasis	Lesions are generalized over the entire body. More severe form triggered by environmental factors or as a reaction to a medication.

Many patients also have psoriatic nails. The finger- and toenails become thick and yellow. Because of frequent accompanying onycholysis, the condition may be mistaken for a fungal infection. Some patients will also have pitting and/or dystrophy of the nails. Severe psoriasis may also be associated with joint disease and other comorbidities, such as diabetes, hypertension, cardiovascular disease (CVD), and Crohn's disease.

Management

Common pharmacologic treatments for mild to moderate involvement include topical corticosteroids, topical immunomodulators, vitamin A and D analogs, tar preparations, and keratolytic agents. For more severe psoriasis, treatments may include ultraviolet light, retinoids, and methotrexate.

Patient Education

Common nursing measures include education to avoid the triggers known to exacerbate psoriasis, the prevention and management of comorbidities such as CV disease and diabetes, diet and exercise counseling, cancer screenings, psychologic screening and counseling, and avoidance of alcohol and tobacco products. The patient should be educated to avoid hot baths and showers, use only mild soap, and pat the skin dry with a soft towel.[1]

ROSACEA

Rosacea is a very common skin condition affecting more than 16 million people. It is commonly mistaken for sunburns, acne, or contact dermatitis. It is more common in women than men and is not reversible. Contributing factors are believed to be vasodilation with persistent erythema, microbial agents, chronic sun exposure, inflammation, ethnicity, and connective tissue and immune disorders.

Relevant Social Determinants of Health

▪ Rosacea is most common among middle- and older-aged adults and persons of Irish, Scottish, Welsh, and English origin.

Approach to Diagnosis

There are guidelines that aid in the diagnosis of rosacea, which is made primarily based on appearance and history. The primary subtype may include flushing or blushing, which causes persistent erythema, papules, pustules, and telangiectasis. The secondary subtype may include edema, dryness, burning, plaques, and the spreading of initial papules and pustules. The most disfiguring subtype is rhinophyma, or hypertrophy of the nose, accompanied by a thickening of the skin. Finally, ocular symptoms may also develop, such as dry, gritty, and burning eyes, photosensitivity, blurred vision, hordeolum, chalazion, blepharitis, conjunctivitis, and foreign body sensation.

Management

Treatment is aimed toward the prevention of the progression of rosacea. Patient education includes teaching the patient to cleanse the face twice daily with an antibacterial soap, use sunscreen daily, avoid oily facial and hair products, and avoid the use of harsh scrubs or exfoliants on the skin. Avoidance of triggers should also be emphasized; triggers include hot or spicy food and drink, sun exposure, hot baths, hot tubs or saunas, aged food products (cheese, wine), stress, cosmetic irritant, caffeine, smoking, and the avoidance of medication that cause vasodilation.

Medical treatment includes topical metronidazole cream/lotion/gel, topical azelaic acid, and topical sulfacetamide, as well as oral tetracycline, doxycycline, erythromycin, and oral contraceptives. If there is no improvement with 3 months of oral and topical therapy, a referral to a dermatologist should be made. Laser treatment for the removal of telangiectasia has been largely successful.

SCABIES

Etiology

Scabies is a pruritic, communicable rash caused by *Sarcoptes scabiei*, a mite that burrows in the skin. It is almost always passed by close contact with another person who has an infestation of scabies. The mites burrow in areas that are moist and warm, such as axillary folds, the beltline, interdigital spaces, areolae, and genital areas. They may be sexually transmitted. Because these mites have the ability to survive a few days without a human host, they may also be transmitted via clothing or bedding. Human mites are not transmitted by contact with animals. Much like myths surrounding pediculosis, many believe those infected with scabies have poor hygiene. However, this is not the case, although these beliefs may cause embarrassment and stigmatism for those who are infected.

After the transmission of the mite from one person to another, the mite population grows to about 10 to 12 adult mites. The males die after mating. The female then burrows into the epidermal layer of the skin, laying approximately three eggs daily for her lifetime, which is 1 to 2 months. In less than 2 weeks, these eggs have evolved into adult mites.

Pathophysiology

The patient commonly will complain of extreme itching, which may be worse at night and is the result of a reaction to the fecal material left by the mite. The patient may cause excoriation and scaling from scratching the lesions. There will be visible mite burrows, which are gray or skin-colored and may be a few centimeters long. The lesions will be vesicular and filled with fluid;

papules may also be visible and caused by a hypersensitivity reaction (Figure 15.36). A less common variation of the presentation would occur with crusted, or Norwegian, scabies. This variant might occur with older patients and patients who are immunocompromised. The infestation would involve millions of mites and would present with thick crusts and scales with warty growths. Itching is not usually a bothersome symptom with crusted scabies.

Approach to Diagnosis

Diagnosis may be confirmed with a good history and physical examination of the lesions. However, a scraping of the burrow may be seen under microscopic examination. The crusts on crusted scabies may need to be scraped off prior to treatment. Treatment with a topical scabicidal medication, such as permethrin or sulfur, is necessary for killing the live mites. Lindane is now discouraged due to the toxic side effects and has FDA approval only for patients who are intolerant to other treatments. All scabicides may have a more toxic effect on older adults and pregnant or lactating women; therefore, caution must be exercised. For control of the pruritis, antihistamines and topical antipruritics and steroids may be used. If a secondary infection has developed, antibiotic treatment with cephalexin or dicloxacillin would be warranted.[19]

Patient Education

The patient will need education concerning the application and administration of any of the medications, as well as handwashing hygiene and avoidance of scratching the lesions. Clothing and bedding should be laundered in hot water.

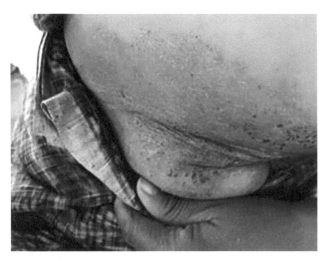

Figure 15.36: Scabies

SEBORRHEIC DERMATITIS

Etiology

Seborrheic dermatitis is a chronic and inflammatory process that affects all ages and may have an intermittent pattern of recurrence. Causes may be related to environmental exposures, yeast, medications, or a genetic component. Causes may also be related to coexisting conditions, such as Parkinson's disease, Down syndrome, stroke, head injury, and psychologic disorders. The lesions are erythematous and wax-like with a yellow scale. Dandruff is a mild form of seborrheic dermatitis.

SD may be caused by an inflammatory response to the yeast *Malassezia*, which inhabits the skin, causing a dysfunction in the skin barrier. Lesions usually appear anywhere on the body, more often on the scalp, forehead and face, ear, and in the peri- and postauricular area. The rash is scaly with erythematous papules that often evolve into plaques. Pruritus is usually a factor. Diagnosis may be made empirically or with a Wood's light.

Management

Current treatment involves medicated shampoos, topical antifungal agents, topical steroids, immunomodulators, and oral antifungals. Patient education would involve information concerning shampooing and body hygiene, and frequent follow-up.

SEBORRHEIC KERATOSIS

Etiology

Seborrheic keratosis (SK) is a common benign neoplasm occurring at any age; however, it occurs more frequently in older adults. The origin is unknown; it is believed to be nonviral, and perhaps to have a genetic connection.

Pathophysiology

The clinical presentation of SK may have either a smooth or a rough surface. The smooth-surfaced lesions are very small, 1 mm, dome-shaped; are embedded in the surface of the skin; and may have black or white specks of keratin. The more common rough-surfaced lesions are flat-domed, oval or round, and easily picked or scraped off (Figure 15.37). They may be misdiagnosed as a melanoma; therefore, it is important to be able to recognize the differing characteristics. SK lesions occur more commonly on the arms, chest, back, and face. Stucco keratosis, also called barnacles, a type of SK, are scaly papules usually found on the legs, ankles, and feet. They may be brown or white, appear to be "stuck on," and are frequently located on sun-exposed areas.

Management

Because the SK lesions are benign, treatment is unnecessary.

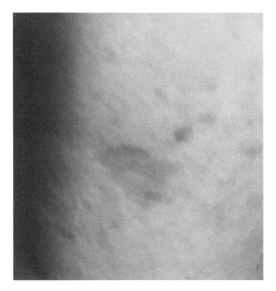

Figure 15.37: Seborrheic keratosis

TINEA

Etiology

Tinea is a fungal infection caused by dermatophytes. Because of their annular presentation, tineas are often called "ringworm," thus necessitating a thorough explanation to the patient that they do not have a worm in their skin. Tinea rubrum is the most common type of tinea infection and causes the majority of outbreaks. Other subtypes are caused by *T. tonurans* and *M. canis*. The fungus is transmitted by direct contact with a host, either human or animal or soil. Dermatophytes have the ability to survive on fomites, or inanimate objects, such as clothing, beddings, brushes and combs, hats, locker room floors, shower tiles, and mats used for wrestling or yoga. It is more common in warm, moist climates, and found often in adults and adolescents. The word "tinea" is often followed by the location of the lesions: tinea capitis (head; Figure 15.23), tinea corporis (body; Figure 15.38), tinea faceii (face), tinea axillaris (axillae; Figure 15.39), tinea barbae (beard), tinea manuum (hand), tinea unguinum (finger/toenails), tinea cruris (groin), and tinea pedis (foot; Figure 15.40). Tinea pedis is more commonly known as athlete's foot, caused by the wearing of sweaty socks and shoes.

Pathophysiology

Tinea lesions erupt about 1 to 2 weeks after contact. They are annular, erythematous, scaly, macular, or popular, with a raised border. There is a clear flatter central area that darkens from red to brown. The border may advance to evolve into a large plaque with asymmetric

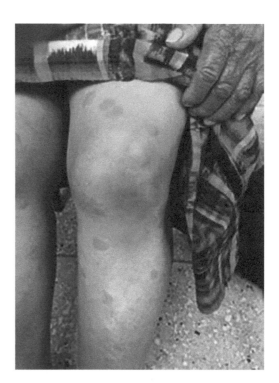

Figure 15.38: Tinea corporis

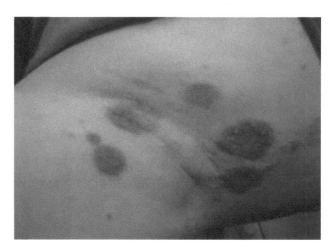

Figure 15.39: Tinea axillaris

edges. Tinea pedis may have a variant presentation with fissures in the interdigital spaces. It is contagious and spreads rapidly and is accompanied by extreme pruritis. Tinea versicolor presents with hypopigmented macules and patches usually seen on sun-exposed areas (Figure 15.42). The skin with the tinea does not tan in the sun; therefore, the rest of the skin appears to be unchanged in color. A KOH prep may be used for diagnosis based on the presence of fungal spores and hyphae.[5]

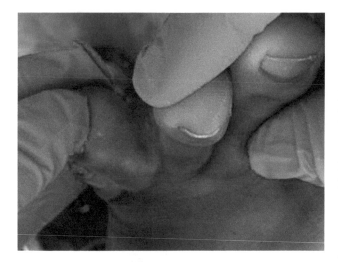

Figure 15.40: Tinea pedis

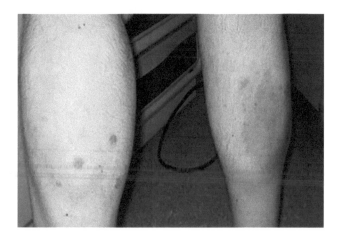

Figure 15.41: Tinea incognito

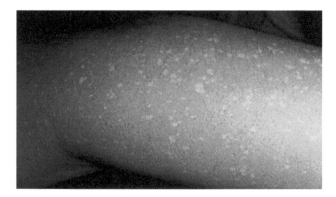

Figure 15.42: Tinea versicolor

Approach to Diagnosis

Diagnosis is based upon history and presentation. However, a Wood's light may be used to determine fluorescence.

Management

Treatment would involve an antifungal cream for any tinea on the body with the exception of tinea capitis, which would require oral griseofulvin. An antifungal shampoo is helpful with tinea versicolor. If the lesions are inappropriately treated with topical steroid creams, the lesions may mutate and become tinea incognito (Figure 15.41).

Patient Education

Patient education would involve careful hygiene and preventive measures.

URTICARIA

Etiology

Urticaria, often referred to as hives or wheals, is an extremely pruritic condition usually caused by mucosal edema from plasma leakage in the superficial dermis. There is a release of mast cell mediators, histamines, eosinophils, and neutrophils. Capillaries dilate and the adjacent tissues are filled with plasma. The reaction may be acute and last a few hours or a few weeks, and it may be intermittent. The reaction may instead be chronic, lasting more than 6 weeks. Older adults have a higher incidence of chronic urticaria. Usually the cause is unknown; it may be a reaction to medication, food, infection, insect bites, mast cell activation, IgE mediation, systemic disease, hormones, or physical stimuli. Angioedema may accompany urticarial, resulting in possible airway obstruction and the need for emergency intervention and care.[20,23]

Pathophysiology

The lesions are circumscribed, erythematous, edematous, pruritic, and usually generalized over the entire body. They begin as edematous papules and evolve into plaques, which vary in shape and size. The central edematous area is called the wheal with the outer red area called the flare (Figure 15.44).

Approach to Diagnosis

A very thorough history is crucial; many times, the offending cause is idiopathic and not identified, especially in chronic cases. If the lesions are painful and nonresolving, a punch biopsy may be performed.[21]

Management

Treatment modalities include antihistamines, H2 receptor antagonists, leukotriene receptor antagonists, anti-itch topicals, and a dermatology referral.

Patient Education

Educate the patient to avoid hot showers, humidity, tight clothing, known allergens or triggers, alcohol, unnecessary medications, spicy foods, stress, infections, and poor

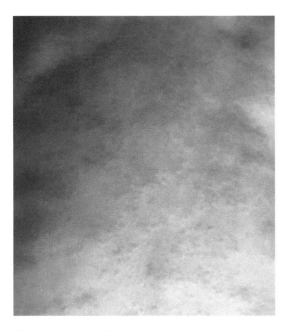

Figure 15.43: Urticaria

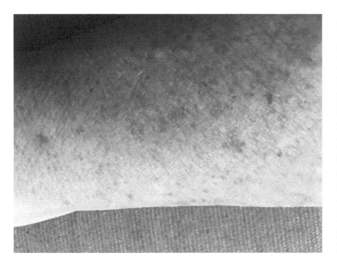

Figure 15.44: Actinic keratosis

sleep. Cool, moist compresses may be helpful to control itching. Counsel the patient to immediately report to an ED or call 911 if they experience shortness of breath, tightness of the throat, swelling of lips, tongue or mouth, nausea, or vomiting.[13]

SUN-INDUCED SKIN DISORDERS

Actinic Keratosis

Actinic keratosis (AK), also called solar keratosis, is a common superficial epidermal precancerous lesion caused by sun exposure and the aging process. Typically, the patient will be fair-skinned with freckles and flat macules and a history of overexposure to the sun (Figure 15.47).

Risk Factors

These lesions must be watched carefully as up to 20% of them may evolve into squamous cell carcinoma. This is caused by trauma to the keratinocytes by ultraviolet radiation. The clinical presentation of the lesions is a rough, erythematous area that develops into scales or crusts, and they are commonly found on sun-exposed areas, such as the face, dorsal surface of the hands, arms, ears, and nose.

Approach to Diagnosis

A biopsy is usually performed to rule out cancer if the AK has not responded to a previous therapy, such as topical immunotherapy or cryotherapy. Typically, a shave biopsy is sufficient for diagnosis.

Management

Management and health promotion will include sun-safety measures and patient education according to risk factors.

Basal Cell Carcinoma

Etiology

Basal cell carcinoma (BCC) is the most commonly reported neoplastic malignancy. The patient may often present with a sore that heals but continues to recur with bleeding and scabbing. Those persons at most risk are fair-skinned, blonde or red-headed, have light eyes, have poor ability to tan, female, with a history of excessive sun exposure, and are middle- to older aged adults. The lesions are most commonly found in the sun-exposed areas, such as the head, face, neck, and back. The most pervasive casual factor is damage to the basal keratinocytes in the epidermis, adnexa, and hair follicles by overexposure to ultraviolent radiation for many years. Tanning beds are a common factor as well as sun exposure.

Pathophysiology

The BCC lesions present as thick and ulcerated sores that appear to heal and then return, often with bleeding. Rarely is there any metastasis to the organs. The lesions may be nodular, which is the most common, with a pink or white pearly dome-shaped papule. Telangiectasia may be present on the surface of the lesions. Another presentation is pigmented with a black, brown, or blue color, with an elevated translucent border. Cystic BCC will have a lesion that is round and smooth and resembles a cyst. There are also BCC lesions (morpheaform), which may be waxy and firm, yellow or white, and firm or mildly elevated. Another subtype is superficial BCC, which is a lesion of the epidermis, presenting as a scaly, pink macule.

Approach to Diagnosis and Treatment

Diagnosis is obtained by a skin biopsy, either by a punch, shave, or curette technique. Treatment depends on the subtype, size, location, and severity of the lesion and may include topical immunotherapy, cryotherapy, electrodesiccation and curettage, radiation therapy, or a surgical excision. Patient education will center on appropriate follow-up, sun-safety measures, and continuing skin cancer screening examinations regularly.

Squamous Cell Carcinoma

Etiology

Squamous cell carcinoma (SCC) is a malignant condition that has doubled in incidence in the past four decades. Sun exposure and UVB exposure have been contributing factors. SCC is found more often in males, older adults, and persons with fair skin who have a history of chronic sun exposure. It occurs more often in African Americans and Asian Indians while BCC occurs more often in those who are Hispanic, Japanese, Chinese, and Caucasian. Cellular DNA has been mutated as a result of trauma to keratinocytes and these cells form tumors in the dermal layer.

Pathophysiology

The lesions of SCC are popular or nodular; many evolve into plaques, occurring in sun-damaged areas of the skin, especially the head, face, and neck.

Approach to Diagnosis and Treatment

Diagnosis is made based on the results of a shave biopsy. Treating SCC may involve surgical excision, Mohs micrographic surgery, immunotherapy, radiation therapy, or a combination of any of these. Patient education requires adequate follow-up and sun safety measures.

Malignant Melanoma

Etiology

The most serious form of skin cancer, and the most deadly, is melanoma, responsible for 75% of all skin cancer-associated deaths (Figure 15.45). In the United States, the incidence doubled between 1982 and 2011. It is the number one cause of deaths from cancer in females aged 25 to 30, the most common cancer in those in their mid- to late 20s, and the second-leading cause of cancer in adolescents to young adults. Melanoma is also very common among older adults, especially those in their mid-50s to late 60s. Those who are most affected are White, fair-skinned, blonde or red-headed, freckled, and blue or green-eyed. They have a history of sunburns, a family or personal history of melanoma, the presence of more than 60 nevi, and perhaps immunosuppression. The most important factor is the overexposure to ultraviolet radiation.

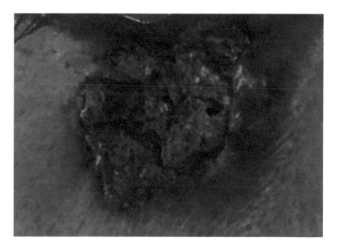

Figure 15.45: Skin cancer—melanoma

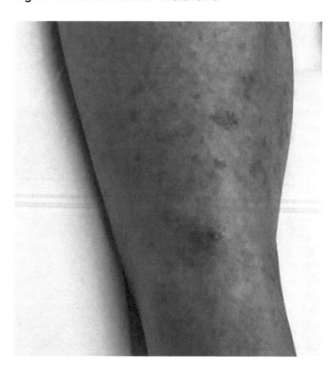

Figure 15.46: Skin cancer—squamous cell carcinoma
Source: Erin Bishop

Pathophysiology

These malignant melanocytes may be in the skin, gastrointestinal tract, ears, eyes, and mucous membranes of the mouth and genitalia. The heart, brain, and other organs may also be malignant from metastasis. The presentation of the lesions varies depending upon the person's skin color; they may be popular, macular, or nodular (Figure 15.46). Usually, the lesions fit somewhere in the *ABCDE* mnemonic used by the American Cancer Society:

■   A—asymmetry

■   B—border irregularity

- C—color variation
- D—diameter greater than 6 mm
- E—enlargement, elevation, or evolution

Approach to Diagnosis and Treatment

A thorough history and physical examination are necessary prior to any diagnostic testing. Diagnosis is made by a biopsy of the primary lesions. Clinical staging is conducted. The most common choice of treatment is surgical excision, if appropriate. Treatment modalities also include nonsurgical therapy, such as imiquimod, cryotherapy, and radiation therapy.

Patient Education

Health education includes frequent follow-up, yearly skin examinations, and sun safety measures.

CONCLUSION

Some skin disorders can be challenging to diagnose and treat in primary care. This chapter provides an overview of the most common skin disorders seen in primary care. There are many circumstances where the nurse practitioner will be able to manage the patient without referral to a dermatologist or another specialist. However, in some circumstances, a referral will be essential to achieve the best outcomes. So having the knowledge and skills to perform a thorough history and physical examination will help inform the treatment and appropriateness of a referral to a dermatologist.[11,12]

REFERENCES

References for this chapter are online and available at https://connect.springerpub.com/content/book/978-0-8261-8414-6/part/part01/toc-part/ch15.

CHAPTER 16

Common Eye, Ear, Nose, and Throat Disorders Encountered in the Primary Care Setting

Laura L. Van Auker

LEARNING OBJECTIVES

At the conclusion of this chapter, the learner will be able to:

➤ Discuss normal anatomy and physiology of the special senses: eyes, ears, nose, mouth, and throat.

➤ Recognize age-related changes of the special senses and disorders due to infection or inflammation.

➤ Summarize the impact of age-related and disease-associated alteration in the special senses and resulting sensory deficits of the eyes, ears, nose, mouth, and throat.

INTRODUCTION

The body systems and organs of the eyes, ears, nose, and oropharynx, including the associated organs of the tongue, salivary glands, teeth, and vestibular system, constitute the special sensory systems of the body. They provide the ability to evaluate and respond to internal and external stimuli, as well as provide crucial processes for survival and homeostasis. While each system articulates within dedicated pathways through the central nervous system, the process of stimuli to decoder pathways provides the normal sensory expression. Age-related alterations in visual acuity (presbyopia) may be easily adapted to with corrective lenses. More serious consequences may occur when age-related changes worsen preexisting conditions or manifest as disorders in response to chronic metabolic conditions such as the microvascular disease of diabetic retinopathy. Alterations in the sensory organs can lead to a reduction in quality of life and social isolation, increasing the risk of secondary disorders, such as depression, cognitive impairment, and dementia. This chapter provides an overview of each of these systems with related physiology and pathophysiology and common disorders and associated symptomology.

OVERVIEW OF THE SYSTEM

The Eye and Vision: Normal Anatomy and Physiology

The eyes are two orbit-shaped structures lying within a protective bony space in the anterior skull. They are composed of three layers that provide function and shape. The white outermost layer, called the sclera, surrounds the globe of the eye with a flexible fibrous sheath with the clear lens of the cornea positioned to the anterior body. Light enters through the cornea and through to the lens regulated by muscles and tendons attached to the sclera. The middle layer of the eye, the choroid, forms the ciliary body with smooth muscle fibers that control the shape of the lens and provide focus on incoming light. The lens is a clear, flexible structure that allows focus on shapes. It sits behind the iris and further divides the globe of the eye into two chambers. The aqueous humor, the watery fluid of the anterior chamber, provides nutrients for the cornea and lens and filters out cellular waste products. Posterior to the lens is the vitreous humor, a clear gelatinous material that provides balanced pressure to provide form to the eye in the posterior chamber.

The melanin-containing choroid layer acts to absorb stray light. The diameter of the pupil, the dark center within the colored iris, opens and closes through reflexive action of smooth muscles within the iris in response to light stimulus. The interior layer of the eye is the retina whose outer surface is pigmented like the choroid, with an inner surface containing photoreceptors and nerve cells. The retina contains two types of photoreceptors, nearly 150 million rods, which provide night vision with low-light sensitivity, and approximately 6 million cones, which serve as receptors for bright light, color vision, and visual acuity. The retina is loosely attached to the choroid layer of the eye, with vulnerability to injury and detachment. At the posterior of the retina, axons from the sensory ganglion gather to form the optic nerve (cranial nerve II). This myelinated optic nerve exits the posterior retina on the nasally located circular area called the optic disc along with retinal arteries and veins. The macula lies lateral to the optic disc with the centrally positioned fovea centralis, which is a concentrated area of cones that provides for visual acuity. As the optic nerve exits the optic disc, it enters the optic chasm and branches into the left and right tracts. Visual images are initially projected upside down on the retina, where image processing begins. The sensory nerve impulses then transmit through the optic nerve to the visual cortex located in the occipital lobe, where the brain provides the final processing of the image (Figure 16.1).

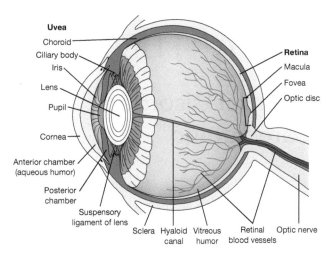

Figure 16.1: The anatomy of the eye and optic nerve

Sourc: Tkacs N, Herrmann L, Johnson R. *Advanced Physiology and Pathophysiology: Essentials for Clinical Practice*, 1st ed. Springer Publishing Company; 2020.

Exterior structures of the eye provide further function and protection. The eyes are covered with a fragile membrane called the conjunctiva, which extends from the inner lining of the upper and lower eyelids and across the exposed portion of the eye. Opening and closing of the eyelids controls the amount of light entering the eye. The eyelashes act as protective brushes through blinking and are lined with exocrine meibomian glands that prevent dehydration of the eye. Tear glands provide lubrication of the conjunctiva and tear ducts and allow excess drainage of tears.

Anatomy of the Eye and Optic Nerve

Light enters the eye through the cornea and travels through the pupil to the lens, which focuses the light rays on the retina. Posterior to the cornea, the outermost layer of the eye is the sclera. The uvea is the next layer, made up of the iris, ciliary body, and choroid. The innermost layer is the retina, the site of photoreceptor cells and other cellular elements. The retina also includes the macula, fovea, and optic disc, which is the point of attachment of the optic nerve and retinal blood vessels.

Evaluation of Visual Changes

Initial evaluation of visual changes and impairment requires a clear history of the pattern of visual loss based on onset, duration, clinical course, and associated or premonitory symptoms, such as pain, scotoma, or floaters, as well as prior history. Classifying the pattern and associated signs and symptoms of visual changes provides insight into the pathophysiology of the condition and should characterize as unilateral, bilateral, transient, persistent, sudden, gradual, painless, or painful (Table 16.1). Further description may include the location of vision

loss as central or peripheral vision loss, night blindness, or blurry or hazy vision. In the primary care office, a minimal eye examination consists of tests for visual acuity, pupil function, and extraocular muscle motility, as well as direct ophthalmoscopy through an undilated pupil.

The American Academy of Ophthalmology recommends that healthy adults without visual problems or symptoms of disease should have a complete eye screening examination once in their 20s and twice in the 30s. At age 40, a comprehensive examination that includes screening for common eye disease is recommended as that is often the time that age-related vision changes begin.[1]

Differential diagnoses can be logically considered based on affected anatomic sites (Table 16.2) and potential causes related to opacities, retinal or optic nerve disease, visual pathway disorders, central nervous system conditions, or functional disorders.

DISORDERS OF THE EYE AND AGE-RELATED CHANGES

Eye diseases and disorders common in aging adults are often identified during a recommended comprehensive eye examination scheduled every 1 to 2 years for the healthy adult older than age 60.[3] Chronic health conditions, such as hypertension and diabetes, require more frequent evaluation to monitor for eye changes requiring intervention to prevent more serious conditions in the eyes such as diabetic or hypertensive retinopathy. Some visual changes such as presbyopia, decreased near vision, are universal and are not considered a disease process. Other normal changes include changes in depth perception (binocularity), peripheral vision, and changes in sensitivity to contrast, color, and glare.[4] These normal changes may alter daily function but rarely are debilitating. Normal vision is considered 20/40 or better on a Snellen chart. Low vision in older adults, called visual impairment, is defined as worse than 20/40 but better than 20/200. Vision equal to or worse than 20/200 is considered legal blindness. Visual field less than or equal to 20 degrees resulting in tunnel vision (associated with conditions such as retinitis pigmentosa or glaucoma) is also considered legally blind and may be life-altering, similar to loss of visual acuity. Beyond conditions resulting in refractory errors, the major causes of vision impairment in older adults include age-related macular degeneration (AMD), cataracts, glaucoma, and diabetic and hypertensive retinopathy.

Presbyopia

Presbyopia is the naturally occurring age-related loss in the eye's ability to focus, resulting in refractive error for near vision. Occurring typically between age 40 to 50 years, it is speculated to be the result of loss in elasticity of the lens. Changes in the curvature of the lens over time with the weakening of the ciliary muscles that would normally

Table 16.1: Causes of Vision Loss

Transient Vision Loss (Less Than 24 hours)
• Amaurosis fugax: Unilateral lasting only minutes • Migraine: Vision loss 10 to 60 minutes • Ocular ischemic syndrome (carotid occlusive disease) • Papilledema: Raised intracranial pressure or malignant hypertension • Retinal detachment • Sudden change in blood pressure: Orthostatic hypotension • Transient acute increase in intraocular pressure: Acute angle–closure glaucoma or retro/peribulbar hemorrhage • Vertebrobasilar artery insufficiency: Vision loss is bilateral and lasts minutes • Vitreous hemorrhage • Vitreous detachment
Vision Loss Greater Than 24 Hours: Sudden, Painless
• Exposure (Welder's flash): Prolonged exposure to intense light/sunlight • Ischemic optic neuropathy: To prevent permanent loss, rule out giant cell temporal arteritis • Other retinal or central nervous system disease: Occipital lobe CVA causing cortical blindness • Optic neuritis • Retinal artery/vein occlusion • Retinal detachment • Vitreous or aqueous hemorrhage (hyphema)
Vision Loss Greater Than 24 Hours: Gradual, Painless
• Cataracts • Cerebral neoplasm • Chronic retinopathy: Age-related macular degeneration, diabetic retinopathy • Chronic corneal disease: Corneal dystrophy • Corneal ulcer • Open-angle glaucoma • Optic neuropathy/atrophy: Compressive lesion, toxic-metabolic cause, radiation • Pseudotumor cerebri • Refractive error • Retinitis pigmentosa
Vision Loss Greater Than 24 Hours: Painful
• Acute angle closure: Glaucoma • Corneal hydrops: Keratoconus • Corneal abrasion/ulcer • Herpes simplex/zoster • Ocular onchocerciasis: River blindness, *Onchocerca volvulus* worm • Optic neuritis • Orbital apex/superior orbital fissure/cavernous sinus syndrome • Uveitis

Source: Gibson CM, ed. Vision loss. https://www.wikidoc.org/index.php/Vision_loss#Functional_disorder

Table 16.2: Differentials for Impaired Vision

Refractive Error
Eyelids
Ptosis
Edema
Blepharospasm
Cornea
Abrasion
Infection
Edema
Degeneration
Anterior Chamber
Iritis
Hyphema
Lens
Cataract
Tumescence (e.g., poorly controlled diabetes)
Vitreous
Hemorrhage
Floaters
Retina
Age-related macular degeneration (ARMD)
Central serous retinopathy
Inflammation
Trauma
Detachment
Diabetes
Hypertension
Vasculature
Retinal artery occlusion
Giant cell (temporal) arteritis
Retinal vein occlusion
Optic Nerve
Atrophy (glaucoma)
Inflammation
Compression
Ischemia
Other (inherited, drugs, toxins, deficiencies)
Psychiatric
Hysteria
Malingering

Source: Reproduced with permission from Goroll AH. *Primary Care Medicine: Office Evaluation and Management of the Adult Patient*. 7th ed. Lippincott Williams & Wilkins; 2014.

bend and straighten the lens may also contribute to presbyopia. Most individuals recognize a loss in the ability to see things up close, such as for reading. Adjusting for the blurry vision requires holding print farther out to focus and using increased light or large-print materials. Presbyopia may result in eye strain, eye fatigue, and headache. Symptoms worsen over time but stop getting worse after age 65.[5]

Presbyopia is not curable and eventually exceeds the eye's ability to accommodate, resulting in blurred vision. An evaluation is provided with a comprehensive eye examination by an eye care professional. Reasonable optical correction may be obtained with the use of glasses or contacts. The use of "monovision" management with a single contact allows the corrected eye to focus upon near vision and the opposite eye to provide farsightedness. Some patients have difficulty tolerating the variance in focus. Surgical options are improving and include corneal inlays, lens replacement, and monovision LASIK or keratoplasty.

Cataracts

Cataracts are characterized by clouding of the lens causing opacity (Table 16.3A) and visual impairment (Table 16.3B). Age is the major risk factor for onset, but the progression and severity are influenced by multifactorial influences of genetics, environment, and socioeconomic and biochemical factors acting synergistically.[6] Cataracts are the most common cause of blindness in the world. In the United States, age-related cataracts affect 70% of White Americans by age 80 compared to 53% for Blacks and 61% for Hispanic Americans.[7] Cataracts may occur congenitally as the result of trauma or due to systemic disease such as diabetes or exposure to medications (steroids, statins) or from excessive sun exposure. The most common, age-related (senile) cataracts are considered a normal part of aging, with two-thirds of cases causing functional impairment after age 70. Cataracts may occur as the result of reduced metabolic efficiency in the lens, leading to progressive insoluble proteins that may impact a portion of or the full lens. Both eyes are typically involved but progress independently and possibly asymmetrically. Symptoms include a gradual loss of visual clarity and may include loss of color perception, especially blues and greens; double vision; and excessive sensitivity to glare. Patients may report fixed spots, halos in vision, and difficulty seeing at night. They may report an increasing need for prescription eyeglass adjustments. On examination, the lens is translucent with yellow discoloration and a dark spot can be visualized on the fundoscopic examination. Treatment is surgical to maintain activities of daily living with intra- or extracapsular extraction of the cataract with lens replacement. Surgical risks are minimal, and the prognosis is excellent restoring vision to 20/20 to 20/40. Social disparities occur in treatment when resources for curative surgical intervention are inadequate. Untreated cataracts

Table 16.3: Eye Disorders

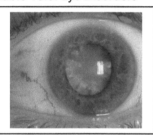	**A: Senile cataract (National Eye Institute, NEI)** *Source:* https://medialibrary.nei.nih.gov/search?keywords=cataract&photographer=&orientation=All&type=1#/media/3539
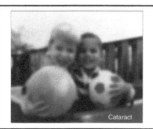	**B: Patient view with cataracts** *Source:* https://medialibrary.nei.nih.gov/search?keywords=cataracts#/media/1811
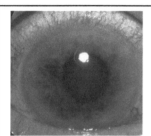	**C: Ciliary flush in acute angle glaucoma** Angle-closure glaucoma is a sudden elevation in intraocular pressure that occurs when the iris blocks the eye's drainage channel—the trabecular meshwork. *Source:* Jonathan Trobe, M.D. The Eyes Have It
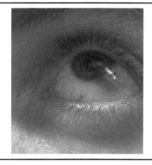	**D: Mild subconjunctival hemorrhage** *Source:* https://upload.wikimedia.org/wikipedia/commons/thumb/e/e8/Subconjunctival_hemorrhage_02.jpg/512px-Subconjunctival_hemorrhage_02.jpg
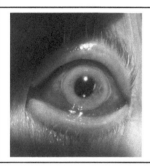	**E: Severe subconjunctival hemorrhage—consistent with trauma** *Source:* James Heilman, MD

(continued)

Table 16.3: Eye Disorders (*continued*)

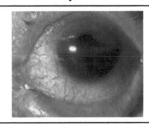	**F: Hyphema: posttrauma blood filling the anterior chamber, causing a horizontal fluid level.** *Source:* By Rakesh Ahuja, MD
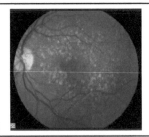	**G: Macular degeneration** *Source:* https://medialibrary.nei.nih.gov/search?keywords=macular%20degeneration#/media/3533
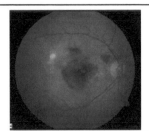	**H: Macular degeneration** *Source:* https://medialibrary.nei.nih.gov/search?keywords=macular%20degeneration#/media/3531
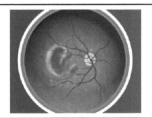	**I: Macular degeneration** *Source:* https://medialibrary.nei.nih.gov/search?keywords=macular%20degeneration#/media/3530
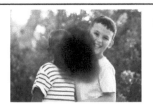	**J: Central vision loss (macular degeneration)** *Source:* https://medialibrary.nei.nih.gov/search?keywords=macular%20degeneration#/media/1203
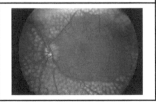	**K: Diabetic retinopathy: fundus showing scatter laser surgery for diabetic retinopathy** *Source:* National Eye Institute, National Institutes of Health https://commons.wikimedia.org/wiki/File:Fundus_photo_showing_scatter_laser_surgery_for_diabetic_retinopathy_EDA09.JPG

(continued)

Table 16.3: Eye Disorders (*continued*)

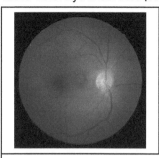

L: Hypertensive retinopathy with AV nicking, silver wire arterioles, and mild vascular tuosity

Source: By Frank Wood

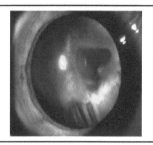

M: Slit lamp view retinal detachment

Source: https://en.wikipedia.org/wiki/Retinal_detachment#References

may increase the risk of secondary glaucoma and may fully occlude visualization of the retina necessary to monitor other retinal disease.

Glaucoma

Glaucoma is a condition defined as increased intraocular pressure (IOP), with the potential to cause optic nerve damage and blindness.[8] The eye depends on continuous fluid production of aqueous humor in the posterior chamber within the ciliary body located above the eye's lens. The secretion of aqueous humor is important to maintain eye shape and normal vision. Pressure in the eye depends on a balanced rate of production and drainage of aqueous humor from the posterior to the anterior chamber through the trabecular meshwork and canal of Schlemm. This drainage system may clog over time and is influenced by the anatomic angle between the iris and the cornea where flow occurs. When a blockage occurs, intraocular pressure increases, exceeding the normal range of 10 to 21 mmHg. Glaucoma presents in four main types and may be acute or chronic.

Open-Angle Glaucoma

Open-angle glaucoma is the most common form with a gradual onset and typically affects people older than age 40. It is frequently associated with a family history of glaucoma or diabetes and occurs more commonly in individuals of African descent.

Normal-Tension Glaucoma

Normal-tension glaucoma (NTG) is a form of open-angle glaucoma presenting with normal IOP measurements, consistently lower than 21 mmHg, but presenting with optic neuropathy, abnormal cup/disc ratios, and greater than expected visual field loss. The etiology of NTG is unclear, and metabolic and other system disorders causing optic neuropathy must be ruled out. NTG has been associated with diffuse cerebral ischemia, autoimmune disorders, migraine headaches, and Raynaud syndrome. Vasospastic events, optic hypoperfusion, nocturnal hypotension, hypercoagulopathy, and increased blood viscosity have been identified as contributing factors. NTG is a diagnosis of exclusion and may require adjunctive lab and diagnostic testing for infectious or inflammatory conditions, carotid artery pathology, and 24-hour blood pressure monitoring in close consultation with the comprehensive ophthalmology consultation.[9]

Primary Congenital Glaucoma

Primary congenital glaucoma (PCG) is a rare genetically determined malfunction within the trabecular meshwork and anterior chamber of the eye resulting in IOP. It is identified early in childhood, with surgical intervention being the primary treatment. Prognosis in the United States is generally adequate to preserve sight, but outcomes worldwide are variable based on early detection of the condition. Lifelong monitoring is required.

While there are no current means to prevent glaucoma, active treatment and management may reduce the risk to the IOP that creates optic nerve pressure, retinal damage, and blindness. Most individuals are well managed with topical eye drops and avoidance of medications and uncontrolled metabolic conditions that may increase eye pressures. Topical agents that can be used to reduce the IOP include prostaglandin analogs, alpha$_2$ agonists, carbonic anhydrase inhibitors, and miotics.

Primary Acute Angle Closure

Primary acute angle closure presents as elevated IOP when occlusion of the anterior chamber outflow mechanism occurs and is considered a medical emergency requiring immediate ophthalmology evaluation to avoid irreversible blindness. Acute angle closure may be due to either pupil block, causing the peripheral iris to move forward, and/or peripheral adhesion of the iris to the drainage channel caused by intraocular inflammation.[10] Factors that may precipitate acute angle closure include dim light and certain drugs (e.g., bronchodilators, cough mixtures, cold and flu medication, antidepressants, antihistamines, and anticonvulsants).

Risk factors for angle closure include female sex, older age, Asian ethnicity, and those with a family history of angle-closure glaucoma, especially in first-degree relatives. The unilateral sudden rapid rise in the IOP is usually associated with eye pain, haloes, and blurring or loss of vision. Associated headache, nausea, vomiting, or diaphoresis are common features. When presenting with abdominal pain, it may be misdiagnosed as gastroenteritis. Physical examination includes a circumlimbal injection (ciliary flush); a fixed, mid-dilated nonreactive pupil; steamy cornea; tearing; and decreased visual acuity. The "bloodshot" appearance of ciliary flush is distinguished from other conjunctival injection by the organized radiation of vessels radiating from the border of the cornea (Table 16.3C). Identifying the most efficient means of accessing ophthalmology consultation may depend upon available community resources, with either direct call to the consulting ophthalmologist for same-day emergency evaluation or to the local ED with on-call specialty services. Rapid pressure control with topical and systemic medications is required to limit optic nerve damage followed by iridotomy to alleviate the pupillary block.

Age-Related Macular Degeneration

AMD (or ARMD) is the leading cause of irreversible central vision loss and blindness in older adults in the Western world. It is a condition more common in the older White population with approximately 14% experiencing some degree of macular degeneration by age 80. In the United States, lower rates seen in the Black population, but increasing identification in Hispanics has prompted projections of nearly a sixfold increase in expected cases between 2010 to 2050. Estimates for total cases in the United States are expected to rise from the current number of 2.07 million to 5.44 million cases by 2050.[7] In addition to age, risk factors for AMD include toxic drugs and effects from chloroquine, hydroxychloroquine, and phenothiazines. Hydroxychloroquine, a malaria drug, is commonly used in rheumatologic conditions; it can cause a highly accelerated form of macular retinopathy and requires at least an annual comprehensive eye examination. Smoking is an independent risk factor for AMD, with a dose-related effect, and smoking cessation is an immediate priority.

AMD is a condition of degenerative and oxidative changes within the eye leading to accumulation of drusen, small, yellowish deposits of cellular debris within the multilayer Bruch membrane of the retina. Bruch's membrane provides interaction between the retinal pigment epitheliums (RPE) for retinal cell nutrition, removal of cellular waste, and blood flow from the choroid layer. Drusen disrupt normal cellular function leading to atrophy (dry macular degeneration) and progressively to neovascular degeneration with retinal hemorrhage and fibrosis (wet or exudative macular degeneration). Early-stage AMD is insidious and asymptomatic, with early diagnosis possible only by age-appropriate screening for AMD prior to the onset of visual changes. Gradual loss of central vision is the chief feature, with metamorphopsia, the phenomenon of experiencing wavy or distorted vision, frequently occurring (Table 16.3J). This can be documented on examination using a special testing tool where the patient is prompted to stare at a standardized Amsler grid. Patient reporting of wavy-line distortion with the Amsler grid closely correlates to the onset of wet macular degeneration from macular neovascularization and hemorrhage (Figure 16.2). The Amsler grid is now available for patient self-evaluation online through the National Eye Institute (NEI), National Institutes of Health (NIH) website, "Age-Related Macular Degeneration, What You Should Know" (www.nei.nih.gov/learn-abouteye-health/resources-for-health-educators/outreachmaterials/age-related-macular-degeneration-what-youshould-know). AMD is rapidly progressive at this point with serous leaks leading to mottling, hemorrhages, macular scarring, and fibrosis notable on retinal examination (Table 16.3G, 16.3H, 16.3I).

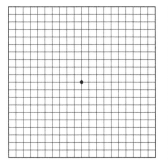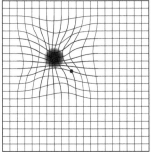

Figure 16.2: Amsler grid
Left shows grid as seen by an individual with normal vision. Right shows grid as seen by an individual with metamorphopsia of age-related macular degeneration.
Source: National Eye Institute, NIH Media.

Without effective treatment or cure available, early detection is critical to managing AMD progression to wet form macular degeneration and significant vision loss. According to the Age-Related Eye Disease Study (AREDS), nutritional therapy with a healthy diet high in antioxidants (vitamin C, vitamin E, lutein, zeaxanthins, zinc, copper) is the treatment for early dry AMD and may slow disease progression by 25% through supporting the macular cells.[45] Wet AMD treatments may include laser photocoagulation therapy to stop vascular leaking or anti-VEGF therapy, intravitreal injections of vascular endothelial growth factor (VEGF) inhibitors. Drawbacks to laser photocoagulation include recurrence of bleeding in up to 50% within 2 years. VEGF, a normal stimulator for healthy epithelial cell renewal in the eye, becomes unhealthy in wet AMD and is targeted with intravitreal injections to disrupt the progression of hypervascularization of new weak blood vessels that leak blood, lipids, and serum into the retinal layers. The goal is to disrupt the progressive scarring and inflammation that kills macular cells, as well as photoreceptor rods and cones.[46] Side effects of intravitreal injections may include serious eye infection with eye pain, light sensitivity, and vision changes; increased eye pressure; retinal detachment; and vitreous floaters.

RETINAL CHANGES OF SYSTEMIC DISEASES

Diabetic Retinopathy

Diabetic retinopathy (DR) results from the medical condition of both type 1 and type 2 diabetes mellitus and typically occurs 10 to 15 years post–diabetic disease onset with steady increases with projections of doubling in the American population from 2010 to 2050 (Figure 16.3). It is the leading cause of blindness in Western countries, affects 93 million people worldwide, and is the leading cause of blindness in people aged 20 to 64. It represents 12% of all new cases of blindness in the United States annually with a prevalence rate of 28.5% for all diabetics over age 40 years.[11] As a systemic condition, the goal of prevention and management is optimal control of blood glucose levels to control diabetic microvascular complications throughout the body, including the vessels of the retina (refer to managing diabetes in Chapter 26). Additional risk factors for progression to diabetic retinopathy include poorly managed hypertension, obesity, and possibly lipid control. In the United States, minorities are disproportionately affected by diabetes; have disparities in access to care, screening, and treatment; and are two to three times more likely to develop significant visual complications including retinopathy.[11] According to projections by the NEI, a national epidemic of diabetic retinopathy will arise as the number of Americans with diabetic retinopathy is expected to nearly double, from 7.7 million to 14.6 million between 2010 to 2050 with Hispanics showing a disproportionate rise in cases[7] (Figure 16.3).

The earliest changes in DR may be asymptomatic and only identified by an ophthalmologist or retinal specialist in a minimally annual comprehensive diabetic eye examination. In response to chronic hyperglycemia, the initial phase of DR is nonproliferative with venous dilation, microaneurysm, retinal hemorrhages, retinal edema, and exudates (Figure 16.4). Exudates are thought to be caused

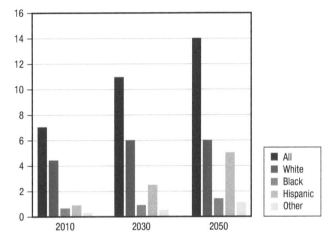

Figure 16.3: Projections for diabetic retinopathy, 2010–2030–2050

From 2010 to 2050, the number of Americans with diabetic retinopathy is expected to nearly double, from 7.7 million to 14.6 million. Hispanic Americans are expected to see the greatest increase in cases, rising more than threefold from 1.2 million to 5.3 million.

Source: National Eye Institute. Diabetic retinopathy data and statistics. Updated November 19, 2020. https://www.nei.nih.gov/learn-about-eye-health/resources-for-health-educators/eye-health-data-and-statistics/diabetic-retinopathy-data-and-statistics

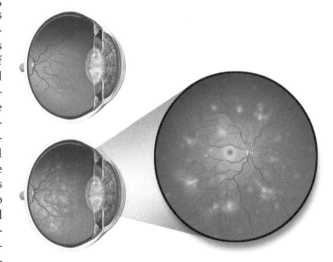

Figure 16.4: Normal retina and diabetic retinopathy
Source: Blausen.com staff. Medical gallery of Blausen medical 2014. *WikiJ Med.* 2014;1(2):1. doi:10.15347/wjm/2014.010

by the deposit of fatty components leaked from weakened blood vessels with hard exudates (yellow spots seen in the retina) and soft exudates (pale yellow or white areas with ill-defined edges) displaying in compact groups. The result is retinal ischemia, neuron dysfunction, retinal basement cell thickening, and a cascade of interconnecting biochemical pathways. In this earliest stage of nonproliferative diabetic retinopathy (NPDR), it may be staged as mild, moderate, or severe. Progression to proliferative diabetic retinopathy (PDR) is more ominous, with neovascularization, vitreous hemorrhage, and increased risk to secondary complications of DR, including diabetic macular edema, diabetic glaucoma, and retinal detachment. The resultant retinal ischemia of PDR prompts fragile vascular proliferation in front of the retina, where the vessels tend to bleed with concomitant fibroblastic activation and inflammation leading to tears and retinal detachment (Table 16.3K).

The primary goal of DR is to prevent progression to PDR with permanent retinal injury. Close monitoring by a retinal specialist is central to care in addition to aggressive primary care management of diabetes, obesity, cardiovascular disease, and behavioral risks, such as smoking, diet, and sedentary lifestyle. A team-based approach engaging the patient in shared decision-making for care decisions and lifestyle modifications is essential. Treatment for DR may include pan-retinal photocoagulation with targeted laser scatter treatment to reduce neovascularization. Later stages of PDR may require intravitreal injection with the anti-VEGF class of drugs (see macular degeneration) and corticosteroids with the goal of reducing proliferative neovascular areas. Anti-VEGF injections require repeat administration as often as monthly, adding significant cost and burden for the patient and the healthcare system, reinforcing the goal of avoiding PDR through glycemic control.

Hypertensive Retinopathy

Hypertensive retinopathy describes the target organ retinal changes secondary to the systemic cardiovascular changes in uncontrolled hypertension (Table 16.1). Patients may present with symptoms of headache with associated double vision, eye swelling, ruptured blood vessel, or reduced vision. Increased risk for vessel damage of the eye is seen in women and people of African and African Caribbean descent. Increased risk is associated with chronic untreated blood pressure, heart disease, diabetes, atherosclerosis, smoking, being overweight, having high cholesterol, drinking alcohol, and eating a diet high in animal fat, trans fats, and sugary and high-sodium foods. In uncontrolled systemic hypertension, arteriolar narrowing and atherosclerotic changes demonstrate disease advancement and are observed on the fundoscopic examination. This is most reliably observed using pupillary dilation. The retinovascular changes are manifestations of chronic hypertension, but acute hypertension can have a significant retinal impact as well. As the singular opportunity in the body to directly observe vascular changes, the retinal examination is considered a strong indicator and predictor of end-organ vascular correlation to hypertension duration and severity. Retinal blood vessels have distinct features, which differentiate them from other blood vessels in that there is an absence of a sympathetic nerve supply, the autoregulation of blood flow, and the presence of a blood-retinal barrier. This uniquely allows the direct response to an increase in blood pressure (BP) to the retinal vessels, which initially constrict. Eventually, an increasing BP overcomes the retinal constrictive response, and endothelial and muscle layer damage ensues. This process has been identified by stages based on the physiologic retinal response and observable changes of the retina on funduscopic examination. In the vasoconstrictive phase, vessels demonstrate retinal arteriole narrowing evidenced by the decrease in the normal arteriole to venule ratio of 2:3. On examination, arteriolar narrowing, arteriovenous (AV) crossing changes (compression of the underlying venules) called "nicking," and increased light reflex of the arterioles may be seen (copper-wire and silver-wire arterioles). With arteriosclerosis in older patients, only focal arteriolar narrowing will develop as affected vessels lack the ability to vasoconstrict. In the sclerotic phase, chronic persistent BP elevations promote vessel wall changes with intimal thickening, hyperplasia, and hyaline degeneration of the arteriolar wall.

The exudative phase of retinal hypertension occurs with severe levels of BP elevation, which disrupts the blood-brain barrier, leaking blood and plasma into the vessel walls and disrupting the autoregulatory mechanisms. Retinal hemorrhage (flame-shaped and dot blot) is evident with hard exudate formation. Eventual necrosis of smooth muscle cells occurs with retinal ischemia recognized by cotton-wool spots. Malignant hypertension, the most severe phase, involves elevated intracranial pressures leading to optic nerve ischemia and edema (papilledema). As the choroidal arterioles necrose, choroidopathy becomes evident with infarction of choriocapillaris. On examination, Elschnig's spots (overlying pigment of the retinal pigmented epithelium that appears yellow), Siegrist's streak (retinal pigmented epithelium [RPE] hyperplasia over infarcts of the choroidal area), rings of exudates around the retina called macular "stars," and neurosensory RPE detachments are evidence of choroidopathy. A loss of visual acuity progresses with increasing macular involvement.

Differentials include retinopathy caused by other conditions, such as diabetic retinopathy and retinopathy associated with autoimmune disorders, anemia, and radiation therapy. Preventing systemic and retinal hypertension is the primary aim, with goals to limit and reverse target organ damage of the retina through lowering of high blood pressure. Treating antihypertensive medications is associated with lower risks to cardiovascular disease and death, as well as destructive changes of the retina. Promoting a healthy diet, exercise, weight management, and avoiding smoking are essential patient lifestyle recommendations for hypertensive disease management.

Retinal Detachment

Retinal detachment occurs in about five in 100,000 persons per year with otherwise normal eyes with a reported lifetime risk of one in 300. This rises to 20 in 100,000 per year in the middle-aged and older adult population. Approximately 67% of all retinal attachments are associated with severe myopia (above 5–6 diopters) when it presents in a younger population. Higher risk is also associated with cataract surgery (5–16/1,000 surgeries), especially in those with severe myopia, where the risk for retinal detachment may persist for years. Retinal detachment may occur as the result of eye trauma or in the presence of choroid tumors. Evidence of trauma, such as bleeding into the anterior chamber of the eye (Table 16.3F) or mild to severe subconjunctival hemorrhage (Table 16.3D, 16.3E), should increase concern for retinal detachment and requires emergent referral to an eye specialist. In proliferative retinopathies of diabetes or sickle cell disease, abnormal cell growth (neovascularization) into the retina and vitreous may cause significant traction on the retina resulting in detachment. Often this is preceded by posterior vitreous detachment.

Patients may present with a sudden loss of partial or full vision, prompting emergent referral to the eye specialist. Unilateral involvement is typical, but bilateral attachment occurs in about 7% of cases. Other symptoms include a sense of heaviness on one eye, "a veil or curtain dropping" effect over the field of vision, brief flashes of light (photopsia) in the extreme peripheral vision, or a sudden significant increase in floaters (age-related fibers of debris floating within the vitreous that cause dark spots or strings in the vision). A loss of central vision is significant as well as a progressive "shadow" moving from the periphery to the center of vision. Straight lines may also appear curved. Without prompt referral and treatment, permanent vision loss will occur. Treatment for detached retina focuses on finding the retinal tear, sealing the break, and relieving the source of present and future vitreoretinal traction (Table 16.3M). Following treatment, a 15% chance of occurrence in the opposite eye remains with an increase to 25% to 30% risk in patients who have undergone bilateral cataract surgery.

Temporal Arteritis

Temporal arteritis, also known as giant cell or Horton's arteritis, is a granulomatous inflammation of the temporal arteries which supplies blood to the scalp from the heart. The arteries become inflamed and swollen, resulting in constriction and reduced blood flow to the head. Thought to be of autoimmune origin, the true etiology is unknown but is associated with another autoimmune disorder, polymyalgia rheumatica (PMR), in about 30% of cases. While relatively rare, it is not uncommon, occurring in about five out of 10,000 people, typically after age 50, with women affected more often than men. The most common presenting symptom is a unilateral or bilateral throbbing headache which may be associated with fatigue, fever, jaw pain worsened by chewing, and localized tenderness of the scalp or temples. Associated symptoms can include muscle aches of the upper torso, lower back, thighs, and buttocks; a loss of appetite; and weight loss. Most concerning are symptoms of broader vasculitis causing vision problems that, if not treated, may result in irreversible vision loss. Symptoms such as double vision, blurry vision, or transient (brief) vision loss are urgent hallmarks of broader vasculitis, which may result in sudden partial or full vision loss. Vasculitis involving the larger blood vessels of the aorta and its branches may damage vessels, resulting in aneurysms, stroke, and transient ischemic attacks. Differentials for temporal arteritis include temporal mandibular joint pain (TMJ), scalp injury, and other causes of altered vision or headaches.

Management of temporal arteritis requires rapid identification and treatment to avoid potential serious sequelae. Suggested clinical diagnosis of temporal arteritis is made by history and physical findings with the patient often demonstrating scalp tenderness and swelling. Headache may be variable in intensity, necessitating careful evaluation locally of the temporal arteries. The temporal arteries should be examined from immediately in front of the tragus of the ear and along the temple. Palpation should be performed bilaterally, with a comparison of pulse strength between the involved and noninvolved arteries as well as notation of a nodular or tender artery. Temporal artery pulse evaluation should always occur in an older patient with headache, unilateral visual changes, and with symptoms suggestive of polymyalgia rheumatica. Rapid diagnosis and treatment are usually successful and focus on reducing vessel inflammation using corticosteroid therapy. Providing resources for individuals with low vision needs is a common approach aside from the clinical diagnosis. The primary care provider provides an important coordination of services with appropriate specialists. Maximizing vision through corrective optical devices, increased contrast and lighting, and the use of low vision assistance devices and assistive technology will promote optimal social engagement and reduce the risk to depression associated with sensory impairments. Environmental modifications in the home and work are necessary to address the high risk of falls associated with low vision, including increased lighting, removing clutter, using enlarged print safety instructions, and maintaining clear exits. Resources to promote autonomy and provide for progressive needs for accommodation are available through a variety of local and national resources for individuals with visual impairment and low vision (Table 16.4).

Table 16.4: Low Vision Educational Resources and Support Services

- American Foundation for the Blind
- American Academy of Ophthalmology
- The American Optometric Association (AOA) Foundation
- National Eye Institute, National Institute of Health (NEI/NIH)
- Help for Students With Visual Disabilities
- American Macular Degeneration Foundation
- Library of Congress
- Lighthouse Guild
- Lions Clubs International
- States Departments of Rehabilitation
- (VA) Blind and Low Vision Rehabilitation Services

DISORDERS OF THE EARS, HEARING, AND VESTIBULAR SYSTEM

Normal Anatomy and Physiology

The human ear provides both the sensory function of hearing as well as the vestibular ability to detect body position and balance. The three divisions of the ear—the outer, middle, and inner ear—innervate with neural pathways to the brain to regulate these functions. The outer ear consists of a cuplike cartilaginous auricle (pinna) that assists in sound capture, directing it into the external ear canal, which terminates at the tympanic membrane. This normally unrestricted passage represents conductive hearing. When transmitted sound reaches the tympanic membrane (eardrum), the vibrations of sound are transmitted by the drum-like tympanic membrane to the inner (middle) ear ossicles. These three small bones—the malleus (hammer), incus (anvil), and the stapes (stirrup)—create chain-like articulations amplifying the vibrations to the membrane of the oval window, the opening to the inner ear. From the membrane of the oval window, vibrations create fluid wave action in the spiral-shaped cochlea, where it travels through the organ of Corti. Within the organ of Corti, the motion of the hairlike neuro hearing receptors (cilia) stimulates dendrite cells at their bases to transmit neuroelectric impulses to the vestibulocochlear nerve (cranial nerve VIII). The sensorineural hearing process that began at the oval window is completed when the impulses are delivered to the temporal lobe of the brain for final decoding in the hearing process.

The vestibular and proprioceptive mechanisms occur in the inner ear, coordinating postural equilibrium and eye movement through innervation with the brain.

Disease or injury within the vestibular system may have an impact on hearing and vision functions in addition to the vestibular mechanism controlling balance and postural equilibrium, leading to dizziness, vertigo, and increased risk of falls.

HEARING LOSS

Hearing loss is defined as impairment of either partial or total ability to hear and may be unilateral or bilateral, temporary or permanent. While some hearing impairment originates in childhood, the most common hearing loss comes with aging. Hearing loss in adults has multiple causes including exposure to noise, infections, trauma, or medication toxicity (Table 16.5). Genetics may play a role in both congenital and age-related hearing loss (ARHL). Approximately half of worldwide hearing loss is thought to be preventable with public health measures of ear protection from noise, immunization against infections impacting hearing, and appropriate management of ear infections.

Hearing loss is initially measured using primary care office-based audiometry and can be categorized by severity, type, and configuration (Figure 16.5). During a hearing test (audiometry), reception of sound is measured for sensitivity to intensity of sound measured in decibels (dB), and the threshold is measured at different frequencies measured in Hertz (Hz). The frequency at which hearing loss occurs may have a significant impact on the severity of disability experienced by an individual. Severity is defined as mild (2–40 dB), moderate (41–55 dB), moderate-severe (56–70 dB), severe (71–90 dB), or profound (greater than 90 dB). Frequency levels for screening audiometry may test in the 250 Hz to 8 kHz range. The recognized frequencies for critical speech recognition lie in the 1 kHz to 4 kHz range. The type of hearing loss is defined by the cause of hearing impairment, with the outer and middle ear producing conductive hearing loss and sensorineural hearing loss occurring within the inner ear. In addition to the two types of hearing loss, conductive and sensorineural, a third category, mixed hearing loss, may include compounded functional or pathophysiologic changes in multiple areas of the ear.

Conductive Hearing Loss

Conductive hearing loss is caused by blocked or impaired transmission of sound from the outer or middle ear to the inner ear and brain. Blockage or obstruction can be caused by conditions in the external canal such as impacted cerumen or exudative debris or canal swelling in otitis externa or from conditions such as persistent middle ear fluid effusion or hereditary osteosclerotic overgrowth of bones in the middle ear (Table 16.5).

Table 16.5: Cause of Hearing Loss: Differential Diagnosis by Location

CONDUCTIVE HEARING LOSS	SENSORINEURAL HEARING LOSS
OUTER EAR CAUSES	INNER EAR CAUSES
Outer ear malformations (surgery or trauma)	Presbycusis (aging)
Otitis externa	Noise exposure
Impacted cerumen	Ménierè's disease
Osteoma	Viral cochleitis
Exostosis	Acoustic neuroma
Foreign object in canal	Ototoxic drugs
MIDDLE EAR CAUSES	Meningitis
Otitis media	Barotrauma
Tympanic membrane perforation	Meningioma
Cholesteatoma	Multiple sclerosis
Otoschlerosis	Vascular disease
Glomustumors	Head trauma
Temporal bone trauma	Viral infection
Paget's disease	Autoimmune inner ear disease
Eustachian tube dysfunction	Hereditary
Residual fluid from colds or allergies	Inner ear malformation

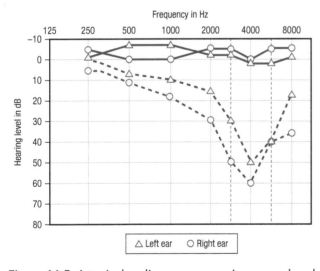

Figure 16.5: A typical audiogram comparing normal and impaired hearing. The dip or notch at 4 kHz, as shown, or at 6 kHz is a symptom of noise-induced hearing loss. *Source:* Trauz B. *Handbook for Acoustic Ecolog.* Cambridge Street Publishing; 1999. https://www.sfu.ca/sonic-studio -webdav/handbook/Audiogram.html

Sensorineural Hearing Loss

Sensorineural hearing loss is the result of damage or impairment of the cochlea in the inner ear or to neural pathways. The most common presentation is the gradual loss in ARHL also called presbycusis. When ARHL occurs, the loss of high-frequency sounds is the most common loss and further impacts the ability to understand words in an environment with strong background noise. While there is a wide range of causes for sensorineural hearing loss throughout adulthood (Table 16.5), acoustic trauma from occupational or recreational noise exposure represents a significant source of damage to the cochlea from sounds exceeding 85 dB (Figure 16.6). Sensorineural hearing loss from noise or ototoxic medication exposure is permanent but largely preventable with cautionary measures of ear protection and pharmacotherapeutic choice and drug-level monitoring. Other causes of sensorineural hearing, such as from Ménierè's disease, trauma, or infection, may result in temporary or permanent hearing impairment.

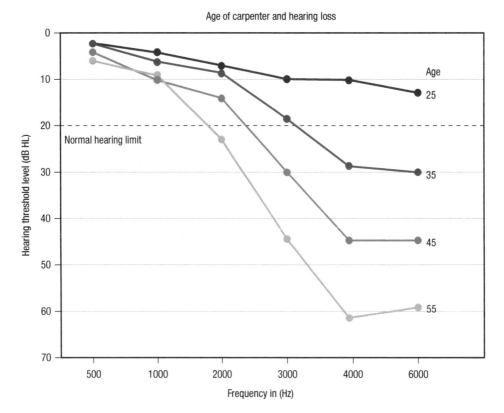

Figure 16.6: Occupational noise-induced hearing loss in carpenters by age
Source: National Institute for Occupational Safety and Health 25 year old carpenter has 50 year old ears - noise: facts and statistics. (https://www.cdc.gov/niosh/topics/noise/factsstatistics/charts/chart-50yrold.html)

AGE-RELATED CENTRAL AUDITORY PROCESSING DISORDER

The development of age-related central auditory processing disorder (CAPD) in older adults is gaining recognition as a silent impairment of the cognitive ear, which is the ability to hear and process as receptive communication. It is defined as a change in the auditory network that disrupts auditory perception and/or speech communication performance.[13] It is frequently coupled with ARHL and is gaining research interest due to the frequent association with the cognitive decline of dementia and the frequent comorbidity of depression, decreased socialization, and isolation.

Evaluation of a complaint of hearing loss in adults requires a careful otoscopic examination, which may reveal the cause of conductive hearing loss due to obstruction, inflammation, or trauma. History and additional evaluation using tympanometry, and the Rinne and Weber tests, may differentiate conductive from sensorineural hearing loss within the primary care setting. Concern for systemic conditions may require appropriate laboratory diagnostics. Comorbidities should be taken into account as sources of vascular, neurologic, or inflammatory etiologies of hearing impairment. Undetermined etiology, sudden loss,

or unresolved hearing loss should be referred for a comprehensive evaluation by an otolaryngologist or audiologist. Advanced hearing evaluation may include auditory brainstem response (ABR), brainstem auditory evoked response (BAER), otoacoustic emissions (OAE), or behavioral audiometry evaluation. For more information about hearing tests and patient self-screening, visit the American Speech-Language-Hearing Association website (www.asha.org/public/hearing/Hearing-Testing).

PRESBYCUSIS, AGE-RELATED HEARING LOSS

One of the most common conditions affecting older and elderly adults presents as a gradual bilateral sensorineural hearing loss. There is no differentiation by race or gender. Between the ages of 65 and 74, approximately one in three people in the United States has some degree of hearing loss. By age 75, nearly half will experience difficulty hearing, especially in the higher frequencies. There is frequently associated bilateral tinnitus, a constant ringing, buzzing, or whistling sound heard by the patient. Genetic predisposition for ARHL has been identified, and the condition is amplified by ototoxic medications or damaging levels of noise exposure. Evaluation, treatment, and rehabilitation of individuals with ARHL requires a multidisciplinary consultation team, which may include specialists in the fields of otolaryngology, audiology, neurology, and psychology. The full range of differentials for sensorineural hearing loss must be considered and may include blood tests for autoimmune-induced hearing loss and CT or MRI to exclude tumors or anatomic abnormalities. Treatment may include amplification devices (hearing aids), lipreading, assistive listening devices for telephones or television, or consideration for cochlear implant. Cochlear implants are considered when the hearing loss is refractory to hearing aids and relatively intact central neural pathways exist in the presence of cochlear changes. While ARHL is not curable, the goal is mitigation of impacts on daily function and socialization. The use of hearing aids is not universally beneficial with only about 10% to 20% experiencing benefit with committed use. Routine follow-up with the otolaryngologist and audiologist is important for the patient's acceptance of amplification devices, monitoring of changing hearing thresholds, and the routine adjustment of devices to optimize benefit and utilization.[14]

NOISE-INDUCED SENSORINEURAL HEARING LOSS

Noise-induced sensorineural hearing loss (NIHL) is the second-most common form of hearing loss in adults following presbycusis and is the direct result of loud, repeated sounds over time that result in damage to the inner ear. The three types of NIHL are impact noise, such as a gun blast or explosion; continuous noise, such as from machinery; or amplified musical devices or loud intermittent noise, such as a loud passing parade. Normal conversation is about 60 dB, and a rock concert is about 120 dB. When sounds exceed 85 dB, there is the risk of causing damage and degeneration to the hair cells and associated nerve fibers of the inner ear. If the noise exposure is persistent, frequent, or extreme without adequate ear protection, the hearing loss may become permanent. Historically, NIHL has been occupationally related but has become increasingly associated with the use of headphones for listening devices at damaging volume in younger individuals. There is a high correlation of NIHL within certain professions due to noise or ototoxic chemical exposure (Figure 16.6, occupational hearing loss). In 1971, the Occupational Safety and Health Administration was formed within the U.S. Department of Labor to address worker health and safety with specific requirements of worker protection from occupational noise-related hearing injury.[44] NIOSH, the National Institute for Occupational Safety and Health, conducts research and monitoring for work-related injury and illness. A 2014 NIOSH report[15] identified about 22 million workers exposed to hazardous noise annually and about 10 million workers with exposure to ototoxic chemicals, solvents, and ototoxic pharmaceuticals.

Initial evaluation of NIHL follows the same measures as any identified hearing impairment. However, it may be necessary to differentiate potential occupational etiology which requires referral to employer-based resources for work injury evaluation and mandatory reporting.

NIHL is entirely preventable and public health campaigns by the NIOSH and the Centers for Disease Control and Prevention (CDC) have promoted a hearing conservation program focused upon hearing loss from both recreational noise-induced loss (www.cdc.gov/media/dpk/injury-violence-safety/noise-induced-hearing-loss/hearing-loss.html) and occupational causes regulated by the U.S. Department of Labor and OSHA (www.osha.gov/noise).

TINNITUS

Tinnitus in its common form is a subjective phantom sound described as ringing, humming, or buzzing in the ears bilaterally and unrelated to a physical source. Objective tinnitus, when an actual sound is produced as the result of a vascular or muscular source in the ear, head, or neck, is relatively rare. Tinnitus in its subjective form is very common, affecting an estimated 10% to 15% (30–40 million) of Americans. It may occur at any age but is more common with aging, occurring in 85% of individuals with sensorineural forms of hearing loss such as ARHL and NIHL.[16] Acute forms may be associated with vestibular symptoms of vertigo and associated nausea and vomiting. More commonly, it presents as a chronic condition, which can have significant negative functional and emotional impacts on the individual. It often is associated with increased levels of anxiety, depression, and greater work absenteeism. A temporary form of vertigo may develop after exposure to an explosive sound or event such as a loud concert. This form of tinnitus should have spontaneous resolution in a few hours. The initial history of tinnitus is critical to identify potentially life-threatening conditions that present with tinnitus and require immediate referral for evaluation. When the patient describes the tinnitus as one-sided or pulsatile, there is concern for the possibility of a cerebellopontine angle (CPA) tumor or glomus tumor of the middle or inner ear. The majority of CPA tumors are benign and include vestibular schwannomas (acoustic neuromas), hemangiomas, vascular malformations, and lipomas. Malignant tumors are rare but surgical interventions and tumor bulk can have a significant residual impact on hearing. When tinnitus presents in a fluctuating pattern or is associated with dizziness and hearing loss, Ménière's disease should be considered.

Pathophysiology

The pathophysiology of tinnitus is complex. Tinnitus associated with sensorineural cochlear damage results in a reduction in stimulus within the middle ear and neural conduction to the brain. The area of damage, called the lesion projection zone (LPZ), responds to the lack of sensory input with subcortical and cortical projections that adjust with efforts at reordering the sensory pathway. This is described as neuroplasticity and is the brain's mechanism for filling gaps in neural messaging, normally rewiring for alternative pathways. In tinnitus, it results in an altered tonotopic organization and the distressing phantom sound heard by the patient. The reduction of regular and organized stimulation leads to an increase in the spontaneous firing rate and an increase in the sound frequency representation in the adjacent neurons bordering the region of sensorineural damage. These areas are described as lesion edge frequencies and provide the neural conduction that results in the tinnitus sound perception by the patient.

Successful treatment for tinnitus is highly variable and often must address the emotional response of the patient in order to facilitate adaptation and tolerance of what can be a highly distressing daily stressor. Antidepressants, cognitive behavioral therapy (CBT), and biofeedback are accepted modalities. CBT as an evidence-based therapy focuses upon the individual's negative response to tinnitus when elimination of the auditory perception cannot be altered. Sound-based therapies fall into four general mechanisms of action using devices to alter sound perception of tinnitus. "Masking" devices expose the patient to an external sound at a loud enough volume to cover the perception of the tinnitus sounds. "Distraction" devices use external sound to divert the patient's attention to provide respite from highly irritating tinnitus sounds. "Habituation" produces a sound stimulus to the brain to assist the brain in reclassifying the tinnitus sound as unimportant or unworthy of conscious recognition as meaningful sound. Using the neural plasticity of the brain, it retrains the brain to ignore the sound frequencies of the tinnitus. "Neuromodulation" uses specialized sound to reduce the neural hyperactivity that occurs in the LPZ that is thought to be the underlying cause of tinnitus. A comprehensive evaluation for modalities of sound therapy is provided by speech and hearing specialists. Cochlear implants for tinnitus, especially associated with sensorineural hearing loss, are becoming a more common approach to refractory cases with a positive reduction in tinnitus handicap.

EUSTACHIAN TUBE DYSFUNCTION

Eustachian tube dysfunction is a common condition affecting the ability of the ear to normalize pressure between the middle ear and the atmosphere. This auditory tube links the posterior pharynx to the middle ear and more recently is referred to as the pharyngotympanic tube. The Eustachian tube serves three main functions, protecting of the middle ear from pathogens and providing middle ear

ventilation. The third function, equalizing air pressure on both sides of the eardrum, allows the drum to vibrate properly for sound conduction and to drain secretions from the middle ear. The length of the Eustachian tube in adults measures approximately 35 mm. Some instances of congenital narrowing of the tube occur with chronic Eustachian tube dysfunction (ETD), leading to significant mucus collection and may impair hearing. Chronic partial or complete Eustachian tube blockage, referred to as "glue ear," is more commonly identified in childhood but may persist into adulthood. The condition can cause ear pain, diminished hearing, ear popping, dizziness, and experiencing increased pressure effects with altitude change. The condition can be identified by direct visualization of the tympanic membrane, which may demonstrate reduced movement with Valsalva or insufflation and may demonstrate a retracted membrane, especially with "glue ear." The presence of a Type C tympanogram may reveal a negative peak pressure associated with Eustachian tube dysfunction or a new or resolving middle ear infection.

When increased middle ear pressure exists while participating in activities requiring pressure normalization such as in scuba diving, hiking at elevation, and in air travel, the added pressure can increase the risk for barotrauma. Barotrauma symptoms can include dizziness, hearing loss, ear pain, ringing in the ears, ear bleeding, and an inability to "clear" the ears. This condition is usually temporary but requires avoidance of the precipitating activity. Resolving Eustachian tube dysfunction and symptoms may benefit from yawning, performing the Valsalva maneuver, swallowing, applying a warm washcloth, and using nasal decongestants or nasal corticosteroids. Conditions unresolved by conservative therapy may require surgical insertion of ventilation (myringotomy tubes), which involves puncturing the eardrum and insertion of a myringotomy tube to allow drainage of fluid, mucus, blood, or pus and creating direct access for normalizing middle ear pressure with atmospheric air pressure. Primary management of Eustachian tube dysfunction focuses on prevention of chronic middle ear congestion that may result from a recent upper respiratory infection or chronic allergic rhinitis with retrograde mucus flow from the nasal pharynx space through the Eustachian tube and into the middle ear. Nasal corticosteroids, antihistamines, and decongestants may be beneficial with increased hydration to maintain mucoid thinning. Initiating multiple "sets" of Valsalva (hold nose and "blow out ears," held for 1 to 2 seconds) at the first signs of decreased middle ear clearing anecdotally may aid in prevention and resolution of Eustachian tube dysfunction.

When ETD becomes chronic, surgical interventions include balloon dilatation of the Eustachian tube, transtubal application of fluids to achieve patency by way of a nasal microendoscope, and Eustachian tubalplasty as alternatives to pressure-equalizing tubes.

VESTIBULAR SYSTEM: CONDITIONS IMPACTING BALANCE

Dizziness in the older adult interferes with everyday activities in up to 30% of persons by age 70.[17] The aging of the vestibular structures within the ear begins in earlier adulthood, with a loss of hair cells that progresses asymptomatically. Disorders of the vestibular or balance mechanism are often multifactorial but aging presents risk factors for symptoms of dizziness which compromise mobility and increase risk to secondary complications of falls and anxiety around fear of falling. The most common causes of dizziness in older age include sensory deficits, vestibular disorders, and central disorders of the central nervous system.[17] Central conditions of balance and gait changes may be further explored in the chapter associated with neurology and fall risks in the older adult. The most common conditions seen in primary care associated with the vestibular system (Table 16.6) include treatable conditions, such as benign paroxysmal positional vertigo (BPPV); self-limiting conditions, such as labyrinthitis; and potentially persistent or intermittent conditions, such as Ménière's disease, which requires treatment and adaptation measures actively supported by the primary care provider in conjunction with a specialist team.[18]

MÉNIÈRE'S DISEASE

Ménière's disease, also called endolymphatic hydrops, does not have a known etiology, but symptoms are attributed to the distension of the endolymphatic compartment of the inner ear.[19] This results in episodes of dizziness or vertigo and typically unilateral hearing loss. The episodes of vertigo may occur without warning and resolve spontaneously within 20 minutes to several hours. The vertigo often precipitates nausea. Rarely, the vertigo may last up to 24 hours. Episodes are recurrent; they may disappear completely for a period of time, recurring without warning. Over time the frequency of episodes may decrease. Treatment is targeted at symptoms of nausea and vertigo with meclizine having some benefit in acute episodes only.[20] The condition is often associated with intermittent sensorineural hearing loss which most often becomes permanent. Hypersensitivity to sound may develop, and tinnitus, the sound perception of buzzing, ringing, whistling, or roaring, may frequently accompany Ménière's disease presenting outside the episodes of vertigo. Patients may experience a sense of pressure (aural fullness) in the affected ear. Differential diagnoses for Ménière's disease include otosclerosis and acute vestibular labyrinthitis or neuronitis, which can mimic the vertigo of Ménierè's attacks as well as other vestibular disorders.

LABYRINTHITIS

Labyrinthitis, also known as vestibular neuritis, neurolabyrinthitis, and acute peripheral vestibulopathy, is a condition associated with an infection or inflammatory condition of the inner ear. Viral infection from an upper respiratory source or postinfection inflammation causes about 50% of cases.[21] Peak age of onset is between 30 to 50 years, with a range up to 88 years. Individuals with autoimmune disorders may be predisposed to the condition.[22] Physical examination findings include unilateral vertical or horizontal nystagmus with the fast phase of the beats away from the affected side. In the *head impulse test*, the examiner rapidly rotates the head to each side, observing the ability of the patient to maintain forward focus. With a positive test, the gaze on the affected side is initially pulled laterally before regaining fixed forward focus. The patient may demonstrate gait instability but maintain the ability to ambulate, with imbalance causing a tilt toward the affected side. Hearing loss may occur in labyrinthitis but is absent when only vestibular neuritis is present. The absence of other significant neurologic changes, such as weakness

Table 16.6: Vestibular Disorders

Common Vestibular Disorders	Less Common Vestibular Disorders	
Benign paroxysmal positional vertigo (BPPV)	Perilymph fistula	Enlarged vestibular aqueduct
Vestibular migraine	Superior semicircular canal dehiscence (SSCD)	Mal de Débarquement
Labyrinthitis or vestibular neuritis	Acoustic neuroma	Autoimmune inner ear disease
Ménière's disease	Bilateral vestibular hypofunction	Secondary endolymphatic hydrops
Age-related dizziness and imbalance	Ototoxicity	Cholesteatoma
Head injury concussion or traumatic brain injury	Neurotoxic vestibulopathy	Persistent postural perceptual dizziness (PPPD)

Source: Adapted from Vestibular Disorders Association. What is vestibular? https://www.vestibular.org

or sensory loss, lessens the likelihood of central nervous system differentials, including cerebellar and brainstem hemorrhages or ischemia presenting as in stroke.[22]

Although usually self-limiting within days to weeks, patients may experience profound disabling symptoms of dizziness, vertigo, nausea, vomiting, temporary loss of hearing, and gait impairment. Treatment is focused on managing symptoms with antiemetics, antihistamines, anticholinergics, and benzodiazepines. Rarely, when symptoms do persist for months or years, a multidisciplinary team of otolaryngology, physical therapy, and mental health support is required with an exploration of other etiology through brain imaging. Treatment includes physical therapists trained in vestibular rehabilitation. Recurrence is uncommon, but the presentation of benign paroxysmal positional vertigo (BPPV) may occur.

BENIGN PAROXYSMAL POSITIONAL VERTIGO

BPPV is one of the most common vestibular disorders with a 2.4% incidence across the life span. The pathophysiology of BPPV is thought to be caused by the displacement of otoconia, the natural calcium stones (canaliths and cupuloliths) that normally stimulate semicircular canal cilia communicating positional sense to the vestibular receptors.[23] It is seen most commonly in the 50- to 70-year-old age group, with an incidence of about 9% by 60 years. Women are affected more than men by about 2:1 and association with a patient history of migraine, Ménière's disease, and low serum vitamin D with the onset of BPPV has been observed.[24] Up to 86% of affected individuals report difficulty in maintaining their activities of daily living and increased absenteeism from work.[18] The hallmark symptom is brief vertigo associated with head movement manifesting observable nystagmus. While the experience of BPPV with head movement may last only seconds, recurrent episodes are common until spontaneous remission in days to weeks, or the patient receives successful treatment with repositioning maneuvers. Other neurologic symptoms or sensory changes are significantly absent, allowing BPPV to be reliably identified by history and physical examination in the office setting. The "Dix-Hallpike maneuver" is performed in the office with a series of rapid positional maneuvers intended to stimulate the onset of vertigo and associated nystagmus. It has a high diagnostic value when accompanied by careful history and physical examination with neurologic focus and hearing screening to rule out medication or central nervous system conditions associated with vertigo and dizziness, such as multiple sclerosis. Rapid recovery from vertigo and nystagmus produced from the provocative Dix-Hallpike procedure strongly suggests the peripheral vestibular etiology of BPPV. Delayed recovery beyond 30 seconds suggests a central nervous system condition that requires further evaluation. Basic lab work, including

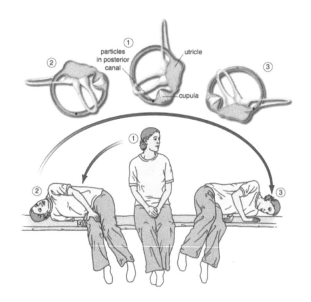

Figure 16.7: Canalith repositioning maneuver

Source: Parnes LS, Agrawal SK, Theriault J. Benign paroxysmal positional vertigo. In: Kountakis SE, ed. *Encyclopedia of Otolaryngology, Head and Neck Surgery*. Springer; 2013. doi:10.1007/978-3-642-23499-6_583

general chemistries, serum evaluation for anemia, and a vitamin D level, aid in excluding systemic conditions as the cause for dizziness and vertigo.

Treatment is evidence-based use of applied positional maneuvers with the goal of passing semicircular canal debris and otolithic stones from the posterior canal to the common crus and then to the vestibule where they naturally exit. There are variants of positional maneuvers with the "Epley's canalith repositioning maneuver" and "Semont's liberatory maneuver" being the most widely known with Level 1 research supported efficacy. Success rates of 90% have been achieved when properly administered with appropriate speed and positioning during the maneuver.[24] These maneuvers for canalith repositioning may be applied within the primary care office setting or can be referred to vestibular-trained physical therapists. There are no contraindications due to age or other neurologic conditions. In some cases, patients may be taught to self-administer the maneuvers at home when BPPV is recurrent or multiple maneuvers are required to resolve the condition. Pharmacologic agents are not routinely required.

DISORDERS OF THE NOSE, SINUSES, MOUTH, AND THROAT

Normal Anatomy and Physiology

The human nose serves two major purposes: as the first organ for the respiratory system and breathing and as the olfactory system providing the sensory mechanism for smell and taste. The nose is a prominent feature of the face and is highly variable in structure and size. As the first component of the upper respiratory system, the nasal epithelium and its mucoid lining provide particulate filtration, warming and moisturizing of air on the way to the lungs. Cilia move the debris containing mucus toward the oropharynx. It is a complex integration of multiple systems involving the nose, sinuses, mouth and throat, esophagus, and larynx (nasopharyngeal system). The pulmonary function is best integrated into disorders of the respiratory system. Disorders of voluntary and involuntary functions of chewing and swallowing are traditionally appropriated to the gastrointestinal system.

The second function of the nose, the olfactory sensory system (cranial nerve I and part of cranial nerve V), is closely associated with the sensory function of taste (cranial nerves VII and IX). Within the olfactory epithelium are receptor cells that recognize seven primary classes of olfactory stimulants: camphoraceous, musky, floral, peppermint, ethereal, pungent, and putrid. In addition to cranial nerves, taste involves multiple nerves located in the tongue, soft palate, uvula, pharynx, and upper esophagus. The five primary sensations of taste—sour, salty, sweet, bitter, and umami—are processed by taste receptors (taste buds) located on specific areas of the tongue. Together the olfactory and taste sensory systems create the perception of flavor.

Olfactory disorders and taste dysfunction (gustation) become more common with aging and may occur separately or together. The loss of olfactory sensory neurons and degradation of cells within the olfactory bulb located in the inferior cerebral hemispheres at the front of the brain may lead to a loss of appetite, malnutrition, and safety concerns when loss of sensitivity to noxious odors occurs. Age-related changes to salivary gland function within the oral cavity may cause drying of mucous membranes resulting in xerostomia (dry mouth), which increases the risk of poor oral health, dental cavities, and edentation (loss of teeth). Additionally, many medications taken by adults and older adults for chronic health conditions have associated side effects of oral and nasal mucosal drying. A history of radiation therapy to the head or neck may also affect one's sensitivity of smell.

DISORDERS OF SMELL AND TASTE

Some loss of taste (hypogeusia) and smell (anosmia) occurs naturally after age 60, becoming more significant by age 70. Other factors may precipitate alteration in taste and smell in adulthood such as nasal and sinus problems related to allergies causing nasal congestion or obstruction by nasal polyps. Certain medications including beta-blockers and angiotensin-converting enzyme (ACE) inhibitors may dull the senses of smell and taste. True taste loss is rare and is associated with alterations in the central nervous system. Most temporary loss is due to nasal congestion and is a function of impaired smell. However, a recent recognition of COVID-19-related symptoms has included temporary changes in loss of taste or smell.[25] The distortion of odors

or taste may result in dysgeusia, a condition in which a burning sensation in the mouth may accompany a foul, salty, rancid, or metallic taste perception. This occurs most commonly in middle-aged and older women, and the precise cause is unknown but may be related to reduced saliva production and dry mouth (xerostomia). A loss of taste and smell can increase health risks for heart disease, diabetes, and stroke as individuals add too much sugar or salt to enhance food flavor.[26] A loss of smell and taste may lead to loss of appetite, undesired weight loss, and undernutrition in the older adults or overeating leading to obesity.[27]

CONDITIONS OF THE MOUTH AND THROAT

Conditions of the mouth and throat may be temporary, such as minor traumas or infections, and are frequently encountered in primary care. Often conditions may be chronic or involve neoplastic changes that have a significant impact upon function, morbidity, and even mortality.

XEROSTOMIA

Xerostomia (dry mouth) may be quite distressing and may have a significant impact on oral health. Assessment requires evaluation of all medications, including over-the-counter (OTC) therapeutics for potential drying effects. Blood work and imaging of the salivary ducts may reveal the cause of dry mouth, and cell biopsy from the salivary glands in the lip may be appropriate to evaluate for Sjogren's syndrome. Treatment will target changes in medications as appropriate and using products containing xylitol to moisturize the mouth, such as Biotene Dry Mouth Oral Rinse or Act Dry Mouth Mouthwash. Prescription products that stimulate saliva production include pilocarpine (Salagen) or cevimeline (Evoxac). Special attention must be paid to oral hygiene with the goal of preventing tooth decay. A dental evaluation may offer protective fluoride trays to wear at night. Chlorhexidine oral rinse once weekly may help control cavities.

ORAL CANDIDIASIS

Oral candidiasis occurrence is increasing in older adults who also have a greater tendency to experience recurrent episodes.[28] Similar to infants, older adults have a greater risk of being immunocompromised. The lesions present as a pseudomembranous lesion with the appearance of white moss that can be scraped off or with eruptions of erythema or mucosal hyperplasia.[28] The use of immunosuppressive drugs, inhaled corticosteroids, antibiotics, poor nutrition or oral hygiene, and use of dentures may contribute to recurrent oral fungal infection. Diabetes, anemia, leukemia, HIV, chemo- or radiation therapy for cancer, and smoking cigarettes may contribute to the risk of oral thrush as well. Older adults are also at greater risk for developing systemic spread leading to systemic candidiasis and sepsis. Treatment with antifungal medication is usually in oral gels or liquids for topical application, although tablets may be used. Prevention should focus on best oral hygiene and addressing conditions, such as poorly controlled diabetes, that may provide a fungal-friendly environment for oral thrush.

ORAL LEUKOPLAKIA

Oral leukoplakia is the presence of clinically visible but often asymptomatic predominantly white plaques on the oral mucosa. These lesions are described as premalignant or potentially malignant lesions that may progress to oral squamous cell carcinoma, most frequently affecting middle-aged and older people.[29] While human papillomavirus plays a significant role in oropharyngeal cancers, it is less often the etiology for oral squamous cell carcinoma. Oral leukoplakia most commonly is associated with smokers without gender preference older than ages 30 to 40 years and may have a malignant transition in 2% to 3% or more at the site of the leukoplakia or elsewhere in the mouth, head, or neck region.

"Erythroplakia" is a red plaque presenting orally that does not resolve and is associated with a high risk of progression to malignancy.[30] It is a diagnosis of exclusion rather than histology and is associated with tobacco use. Surgery with or without additional radiotherapy or chemotherapy offers a 60% survival rate for these cancers.[29]

ORAL CANCERS

Oral cancers may occur at primary sites in the lips, mucosa, gums, tongue, and bony structures supporting teeth. Squamous cell carcinoma is the most common oral cancer originating in the mucosa of the lips and mouth. Tobacco use accounts for 75% of oral cancers, with people of male gender affected twice as often as women. Black and Hispanic males have the highest rates. Alcohol use is an added risk factor. Peak occurrence is between 60 and 70 years with 10.5 adults per 100,000 affected in the United States.[32]

For additional oral health training, the reader is referred to the Smiles for Life (SFL) online training resource, a comprehensive oral health curriculum developed by a national steering committee of physicians and dentists formed within the Society of Teachers of Family Medicine, and specially tailored for primary care clinicians and educators. The online modules are self-paced with excellent resources for oral care across the life span with an integrated approach to preventive oral health and systemic disease prevention. Modules are available without charge (http://www.smilesforlifeoralhealth.org/).

Salivary Glands

The salivary glands produce saliva, which is delivered into the mouth by the salivary ducts. These glands are part of the exocrine system, regulated by feedback loops of the

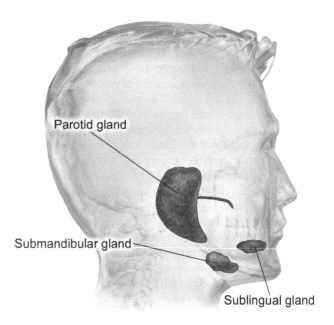

Figure 16.8: Salivary glands
Source: Blausen.com staff. Medical gallery of Blausen Medical 2014. *Wiki J Med*. 2014;1(2):1. doi:10.15347/wjm/2014.010

sympathetic and parasympathetic nervous systems. There are three major glands and ducts—the parotid, submandibular, and sublingual (submental)—that are supported by 800 to 1,000 minor salivary glands in the mucosa or the oral cavity (Figure 16.8). Salivary glands serve a broad range of purposes, producing about 0.5 L to 1.5 L of saliva per day. Initial chemical digestion of food begins with the production of salivary amylase to break down starches in food. Salivary glands moisturizes the oral cavity to help with chewing, swallowing, and speech and facilitates the tongue in experiencing taste. Although mostly water, saliva produces essential antibacterial chemicals that fight bacteria in the mouth and produces proteins and minerals that protect tooth enamel and prevent tooth decay and gum disease. Disorders of the salivary glands may be caused by exocrine dysregulation, as well as inflammatory, infectious, or obstructive processes, that may result in hyposalivation, causing dry mouth (xerostomia). An increased risk of upper respiratory infection has been associated with xerostomia, with speculation that impairment of the oral and airway mucosa reduces its effect as a physical barrier, allowing increased adhesion and colonization of pathologic viruses. A reduction in the presence of antimicrobial proteins and peptides from the saliva further increase the risk of infection.[33]

SIALADENITIS

Sialadenitis is the inflammation of a salivary gland that can occur due to viral, bacterial, inflammatory, or obstructive causes. The most common infectious agents are mumps, HIV, *Staphylococcus aureus*, *Moraxella catarrhalis*, *Streptococcus viridans*, *Pseudomonas*, *Escherichia coli*, and tuberculosis. Sjogren's, an autoimmune disorder, reduces salivary production and may enhance inflammatory processes. Sialolithiasis (salivary stones or salivary calculi) may obstruct the salivary ducts, leading to inflammation and infection resulting in cellulitis or abscess. Salivary stones account for about 50% of all salivary gland disease and are twice as common in men as women; they are typically seen between the ages of 30 and 60 years. The condition is uncommon in children but more common with aging when salivary production may naturally reduce or be exacerbated by dehydration or mediations (e.g., use of phenothiazines) that produce dry mouth.

The most common gland involved is the submandibular gland (also called the Wharton's duct). Typical symptoms include pain and swelling of the affected gland, which worsens with the stimulation of salivation by the sight, smell, or taste of food. These recurrent episodes of blockage have been termed "mealtime syndrome," when a stone may shift within the salivary duct to block the outflow. Inflammation or infection may develop and the presence of pustular drainage at the ductal meatus or a report of bad taste with eating is common. The salivary stone may be palpable when at the mouth of the duct (Figure 16.9). Diagnosis is typically made by history and physical findings and exclusion of other differentials. In complex cases, confirmation by x-ray (80% are visible on x-ray), ultrasound, or sialogram may be used for more significant blockage or infection. The suggestion of larger stones or infection requires a referral to ENT or oral-maxillofacial surgeons for evaluation.

While the stone is a calcified mass, an increase in calcium levels has not been determined to be a cause, and beyond an association with dehydration, chronic infection of the glands, and inflammation, the etiology in most cases remains unknown. Treatment for small stones (2–10 mm in size) can be managed noninvasively with warm packs, hydration, the use of nonsteriodal anti-inflammatory drugs (NSAIDs), and having the patient suck on bitter or sour foods that promote salivation, resulting in spontaneous expulsion of the stone. Lemon-drop hard candies or citrus fruits are easily obtainable for this purpose. Some specialists may massage the stone to expulsion or may engage a minimally invasive procedure of sialendoscopy to directly cannulate the salivary duct and remove the stone (sialectomy). Larger stones will require surgical excision with a small excision at the site of the stone to remove. Rarely, surgical removal of the submandibular gland will be required to resolve recurrent stones or infection. While the stone remains in the duct, antibiotics may help reduce the risk of infection.

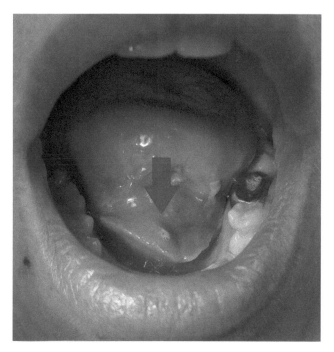

Figure 16.9: Salivary stone: blockage of the submandibular gland by a stone with subsequent infection. Arrow marks pus coming out of the opening of the submandibular gland.
Source: Courtesy of James Heilman, MD

HOARSE VOICE (DYSPHONIA)

Hoarse voice (dysphonia) represents about 1% of all primary care visits and may have a lifetime prevalence of about 30%.[34] Dysphonia describes any change in the sound of the voice characterized by altered voice quality, pitch, loudness, or vocal effort.[35] Although rarely a manifestation of significant medical illness, it may impact upon the ability to communicate and to general quality of life (QOL). In 2% of cases of dysphonia, age-related weakening of muscle tone, irregularity of vocal cord oscillation, or added vocal cord bulk and incomplete closure of the glottis while speaking occur.[34] Dysphonia has many causes with the following distribution of incidence: acute laryngitis (42.1%), chronic laryngitis (9.7%), functional overuse dysphonia (30%), benign tumors (10.7% to 31%), malignant tumors (2.2% to 3.0%), neurogenic factors such as vocal cord dysfunction (2.8% to 8%), and psychogenic factors (2.0 to 2.2%).[34] Men are at greater risk for neck- and larynx-related malignant conditions, which are frequently associated with tobacco use. The most common cause of hoarse voice is acute laryngitis associated with viral infection of the upper respiratory tract. It is self-limited and resolves in 1 to 2 weeks, with efforts made for voice rest. Antibiotics and corticosteroids are not warranted. If symptoms persist, treatment of chronic laryngitis addresses likely etiologic factors of nicotine use, inhaled corticosteroid medicine, inhaled environmental toxins, gastroesophageal reflux with laryngopharyngeal involvement, and all causes stimulating frequent cough.

Table 16.7: Serious Comorbidities of Hoarseness

- History of nicotine and/or alcohol consumption
- Enlarged cervical lymph nodes
- Hoarseness following trauma
- Association with hemoptysis, dysphagia, odynophagia
- Neurologic symptoms
- Unexplained weight loss
- Progression of hoarseness
- Immunosuppression
- Possible bolus aspiration
- Hoarseness after an operative intervention (intubation, neck surgery)

Source: Reiter R, Hoffmann TK, Pickhard A, Brosch S. Hoarseness-causes and treatments. *Deutsches Arzteblatt Int.* 2015;112(19):329–337. doi:10.3238/arztebl.2015.0329

Serious comorbidities require prompt referral for a laryngoscopic examination by an otorhinolaryngologist when associated risks are present (Table 16.7).[34]

Assessment of dysphonia with history and physical examination in most cases will produce a modifiable etiology. Failure to improve or resolve in 4 weeks is suggestive of a more serious cause. Therapy for unresolved benign dysphonia may require surgical evaluation for benign or malignant tumors of the throat and neck, voice therapy, or referral for Botox injections if spastic dysphonia is present.

DENTAL DISORDERS IN AGING: CARIES, PERIODONTITIS, AND EDENTULISM

The rate of edentulism (loss of teeth) in the United States has had a dramatic reduction, with 17% of adults aged 65 or older experiencing tooth loss. This is a 10% drop since 1999 across all sociodemographic groups except non-Hispanic Black adults and current smokers. Rates above average reflect significant social determinants influencing tooth loss with the poor (34%), those with less than high school education (35%), and current smokers (43%) higher compared to those not- poor (11%), those with more than high school education (9%), and those who never smoked (12%).[36] The loss of teeth follows a trend of risk to dental caries that begins in childhood directly related to poor access to dental healthcare.[37] Quality of dental care influences both the incidence of caries, but, more important, the presence of untreated caries that may increase certain health risk factors leading to periodontal disease and loss of teeth. Aging naturally causes structural oral and perioral changes, with a complex interaction among tooth structure, biofluid, and dietary, salivary, and genetic factors.[6] Untreated caries potentiates chronic bacterial infection leading to tissue and bone destruction of the

Caries Prevention and Risk Management Strategies
- Behavioral modification: oral hygiene and diet
- Patients, especially those at high risk of caries development, should be instructed to reduce the amount and frequency of carbohydrate consumption. Patients should limit sugary snacks between meals and eat a healthy diet that limits added sugars and high-acid foods that can affect the mineralization of enamel. Encourage patients to chew sugar-free gum with xylitol, which can promote salivary flow and remineralization, and cannot be metabolized by cariogenic bacteria. All patients should be educated in optimal oral hygiene practices, including brushing with fluoride toothpaste twice a day and cleaning between teeth daily. Although some caries prevention recommendations include using topical antimicrobials (e.g., chlorhexidine rinse) in patients 6 years of age and older who are at high risk of caries, a 2015 *Cochrane Systematic Review* found no trials for the use of antimicrobial chlorhexidine mouth rinses, sprays, gels, or chewing gums to prevent caries in children and adolescents.

supportive gingiva, cementum, alveolar bone, and periodontal ligaments, leading to periodontal disease. Periodontal disease is the cause of tooth loss in developed countries but has also been shown to have an impact on the metabolic status of type 2 diabetics and increased risk of ischemic stroke, acute myocardial infarction, and subacute bacterial endocarditis.[38] This can be addressed through patient education for preventive dental care, policies to improve access to dental care from health disparities, and a concerted integrated public health effort to promote dental health.[37] The American Dental Association has focused guidelines by age, indicating prevention and risk management for adult oral health (Box 16.1).[43]

DISORDERS OF THE NOSE AND SINUSES

Aging brings many physiologic changes that may produce alterations in the function of the nose. These changes may impact neural, histologic, mucosal, and olfactory status, and more than 70% of the older adults report excessive clear rhinorrhea. The mechanism is unclear but appears to be an imbalance of the sympathetic and parasympathetic tone that results in cholinergic hyperactivity and increased secretory nasal secretions. This, paired with reduced overall body water content in aging, lessens the effectiveness of mucociliary clearance, and produces thicker secretions such as postnasal drip, increasing risk to more frequent respiratory infections.[39] Further changes experienced by older adults due to these physiologic and structural changes include dryness, atrophy, or

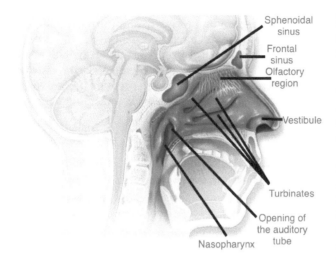

Figure 16.10: Maxillofacial anatomy
Source: https://www.wikidoc.org/index.php/Rhinitis_
pathophysiology

ulceration of the nasal mucosa; more intranasal crusting; and epistaxis, which has multiple etiologies, including mucosal friability as well as digitally induced trauma[40] (Figure 16.10).

RHINITIS

"Rhinitis" is the general term given to any inflammation of the nasal mucosa. There are a wide range of etiologies for nasal inflammation including infectious, allergic, and noninfectious etiologies. Rhinitis is classically associated with nasal membrane edema, congestions, and runny nose. The most common source for infectious rhinitis is a viral upper respiratory infection (URI), labeled the "common cold." Not uncommonly, the extension of infectious source will extend inflammation to the osteomeatal complex of the sinuses and is termed "rhinosinusitis." Noninfectious rhinitis may be divided into two basic types: allergic rhinitis (AR) and the nonallergic rhinitis (NAR), which includes vasomotor rhinitis (VMR) and rhinitis medicamentosa. Recognition of the differences in the rhinitis differentials is important to appropriately target therapy and is best obtained from a thorough past medical history including other atopic type conditions, treatments tried, family history, and occupational and recreational exposures.

Nearly 60 million people in the United States are significantly impacted by nasal congestion, rhinorrhea, sneezing, and itching associated with AR. It has been reported that 35% to 50% of individuals with AR express at least moderate effect on their daily function due to AR symptoms.[39] This presents both a financial burden and an altered QOL for individuals who experience secondary impacts of disturbed sleep, fatigue, daytime somnolence, irritability, attention, and memory deficits in their work and learning environments. AR further burdens society financially with health impacts from associated conditions of asthma, allergic conjunctivitis, and rhinosinusitis.

ALLERGIC RHINITIS

AR is an immunoglobulin E (IgE)-mediated response to environmental antigens such as pollen, molds, dangers, and dust. It may have a seasonal pattern based on antigen stimulus or it may be perennial and chronic. It is frequently associated with other atopic diseases, such as asthma, eczema, and atopic dermatitis, and not uncommonly has an associated positive family history for the same. Symptoms may be confused with the common cold, but there is an absence of fever, and environmental antigens may be seasonably identified. Presenting signs include rhinorrhea (typically clear watery); nasal congestion with pale, boggy, or bluish mucosa; itchy or watery eyes and nose; sneezing; dry cough; and postnasal drip. "Allergic shiners," a bluish halo below the eyes, may be seen as well as an "allergic salute," a crease horizontally across the nose prompted from chronic upward rubbing of the nose. Treatment is focused on avoiding allergens and using antihistamines, intranasal cromolyn sodium antihistamine, or intranasal corticosteroids. While several leukotriene modifiers are used in asthma, only one, montelukast, is approved for use in allergic rhinitis. Oral steroids are not first-line therapy. More severe or recalcitrant cases may be referred for immunotherapy. Simple nasal saline drops can help relieve congestion and can decrease allergic response if used to rinse the nose immediately after antigen exposures, such as pollen.

VASOMOTOR RHINITIS

VMR is a transient condition of nasal congestion and spontaneous clear, watery rhinorrhea not associated with infection or IgE-mediated response. Changes in temperature, especially in cold, dry air; exercise; and exposure to strong odors and tobacco smoke may activate VMR. Hot, spicy foods and alcohol may be additional activators. A common experience is skiing, which involves cold air and exercise. The response can be significant with profuse rhinorrhea. Avoiding irritants when possible is the focus of primary management. While the pathophysiology is not well understood, the benefit from the use of ipratropium bromide or atropine intranasally suggests an enhanced cholinergic glandular secretory hypersensitivity response.[39]

RHINITIS MEDICAMENTOSA

Rhinitis medicamentosa occurs with overuse of decongestant drops or sprays, such as oxymetazoline or xylometazoline, resulting in a "rebound" congestion. This prompts increased use of the decongestant, creating a vicious circle in as early as 3 days of use. Highly effective for providing increased airflow due to the vasoconstric-tive effect and reduced mucosal edema, these alpha-adrenergic agonists are recommended for only short-term and episodic therapy for nasal congestion, with drops applied to alternate nostrils to provide acceptable relief and lower rebound risk. They have no effect on the itching, sneezing, or nasal secretion related to antigen re-sponse, which is better managed by therapies targeted at the etiology of the allergic or nonallergic triggers.

RHINOSINUSITIS

Rhinosinusitis involves inflammation of the ostiome-atal complex and often follows a viral or bacterial URI. It is defined in subtypes based on symptom duration, with acute rhinosinusitis duration less than 4 weeks; subacute, 4 to 12 weeks; and chronic rhinosinusitis lasting greater than 12 weeks.[41] The typical bacteri-al etiology reflects the same organisms found in acute otitis media with *S. pneumoniae, H. influenze,* and, less commonly, *S. aureus* and *M. catarrhalis* as the responsi-ble organisms. Exposure to cigarette smoke, history of trauma, and obstruction of the sinus and paranasal si-nuses due to nasal polyps are risk factors for recurrent acute episodes or chronic unresolved rhinosinusitis (Table 16.8). Acute sinusitis presents with signs and symptoms of nasal congestion, facial pain and pressure,

fever, pain on bending forward, and purulent nasal dis-charge. It may produce referred pain to the upper teeth and purulent postnasal drip, causing an irritative sore throat. Palpation over the affected sinus may be associat-ed with tenderness and increased pressure (Figure 16.11). Decreased light transmission with transillumination of

Table 16.8: Predisposing Factors for Acute Bacterial Rhinosinusitis

> - **Dental infections and procedures**
> - **Iatrogenic Causes:** Sinus surgery, nasogastric tubes, nasal packing, mechanical ventilation
> - **Immunodeficiency:** Human immunodeficiency virus infection, immunoglobulin deficiencies
> - **Impaired Ciliary Motility:** Smoking, cystic fibrosis, Kartagener syndrome, immotile cilia syndrome
> - **Mechanical Obstruction:** Deviated nasal septum, nasal polyps, hypertrophic middle turbinates, tumor, trauma, foreign body, Wegener granulomatosis
> - **Mucosal Edema:** Preceding viral upper respiratory infection, allergic rhinitis, vasomotor rhinitis

Source: Aring AM, Chan MM. Current concepts in adult acute rhinosinusitis. *Am Fam Physician.* 2016;94(2):97–105. https://www.aafp.org/afp/2016/0715/p97.html

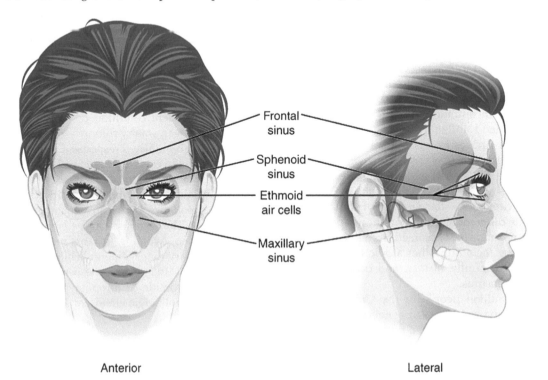

Anterior   Lateral

Figure 16.11: Paranasal sinuses
Source: Betts JG, Young KA, Wise JA, et al. *Anatomy and Physiology.* OpenStax; 2013:Figure 7.18. http://cnx.org/content/col11496/1.6

Table 16.9: Indications for Subspecialist Referral for Acute Bacterial Rhinosinusitis

- Anatomic defects causing obstruction
- Complications, such as orbital cellulitis, subperiosteal abscess, intraorbital abscess, altered mental status, meningitis, cavernous sinus thrombosis, intracranial abscess, Pott puffy tumor (osteomyelitis of frontal bone)
- Evaluation of immunotherapy for allergic rhinitis
- Frequent recurrences (three to four episodes per year)
- Fungal sinusitis, granulomatous disease, or possible neoplasm
- Immunocompromised host
- Nosocomial infection
- Severe infection with persistent fever greater than 102 °F (39 °C)
- Treatment failure after extended antibiotic courses
- Unusual or resistant bacteria

Source: Aring AM, Chan MM. Current concepts in adult acute rhinosinusitis. *Am Fam Physician.* 2016;94(2):97-105. https://www.aafp.org/afp/2016/0715/p97.html

the sinus may be present. Acute sinusitis is a clinical diagnosis and does not initially warrant additional diagnostic studies. Most acute cases are presumed to be viral and will resolve within 2 weeks with watchful waiting and symptom management. When symptoms are more severe in the first 3 to 4 days of illness and worsen and persist 7 days or more beyond initial presentation, with the presence of purulent secretions and rhinorrhea, a bacterial sinusitis may be assumed and treated with appropriate antibiotic therapy.[41,42] Treatment includes pain management with NSAIDs and efforts to reduce membrane congestion with oral and/or nasal decongestants, intranasal corticosteroids, and saline nasal–sinus irrigation and steaming. Cases of rhinosinusitis lasting greater than 4 weeks should be considered for referral to otolaryngology, evaluating for nasal polyps or structural malformations causing obstruction (Table 16.9). At this point, a CT or an MRI may be performed if malignancy or intracranial spread is suspected. Rare life-threatening complications include periorbital cellulitis, intracranial abscess, meningitis, and sinus thrombosis.[41]

RHINITIS IN OLDER ADULTS

Rhinitis in older adults is caused by the same types of items that cause rhinitis in younger adults. Allergic rhinitis remains the most common type with 30% of older adults reporting allergic symptoms and greater than 40% further report their rhinitis symptoms as moderate to severe. Allergic rhinitis is somewhat less frequent in

older adults, but there is an increase in associated ocular symptoms of red, watery, or itching eyes.[39] As older adults have greater concomitant use of medications, drug-induced rhinitis is not infrequent, especially when alpha-1 adrenergic antagonists are used for prostatic hyperplasia. ACE inhibitors, beta-adrenergic inhibitors, and phosphodiesterase inhibitors can induce symptoms of rhinitis.

Caution must be used in the selection of sedating antihistamines in older adults, due to the potential for systemic anticholinergic effects. These agents may induce urinary retention, constipation, delirium, and ocular pressure changes that may have nonreversible consequences.

EPISTAXIS

Epistaxis nosebleeds may occur across the life span, but in adulthood and older adults, the most common causes are trauma (nose picking), nasal dryness, alcohol use, hypertension, or foreign body (including intranasal illicit recreational drug use [i.e., cocaine]; Table 16.10).

Table 16.10: Etiology of Nosebleeds in Adults and Older Adults

Etiology of Nosebleed in Adults and Older Adults
Anterior source: approximately 90% of nosebleeds, usually Kiesselbach's plexus
Nose picking ("epistaxis digitorum")
Trauma
Infection
Nasal foreign body
Dry air
Atmospheric pressure alterations (e.g., increased altitude, lower arterial partial pressure of oxygen [PaO_2])
Allergies
Blood dyscrasias
Malignancy (e.g., leukemia, lymphoma)
Posterior source: approximately 10% of nosebleeds, usually sphenopalatine artery
Iatrogenic coagulopathy (e.g., warfarin, heparin, high-dose aspirin)
Blood dyscrasia
Liver failure
Renal failure
Malignancy
Older age

Source: Mahon BM, Desai BK. Epistaxis control. In: Ganti L, ed. *Atlas of Emergency Medicine Procedures.* Springer; 2016. doi:10.1007/978-1-4939-2507-0_53

Some medications commonly used in adulthood and older adults may increase the likelihood of nasal bleeding and increase the length of time and volume of the nosebleed. These may include over-the-counter medications such as aspirin (ASA) and NSAIDs, as well as certain medications in the following classes: anticoagulants, antiplatelets, antihistamines, anticonvulsants, antibiotics, antifungals, statins, and antidepressants.

Nosebleeds may occur in either the anterior or posterior and typically present unilaterally. The most common bleed originates from the anterior nasal septum (Figure 16.12) in the Little's area, which is also known as Kiesselbach's plexus. This is a highly vascularized region due to the anastomosis of five regional arteries. In the anterior nasal cavity, blood vessels are more superficial and may rupture readily when traumatized. Approximately 90% of nosebleeds occur in the anterior cavity. The balance occurs in the posterior nasal cavity and are prompted by more systemic causes, with poorly managed hypertension and atherosclerosis being the most common causes. Posterior nosebleeds may be more significant and more difficult to manage, leading to greater blood loss, and may be associated with multiple systemic etiologies (Table 16.11). Recurrent or persistent nosebleeds warrant appropriate lab diagnostics evaluating relevant systemic differentials that are more commonly associated with more significant posterior bleeding. While anterior nosebleeds are easily managed by patients themselves or within the primary care setting, posterior bleeds will require referral to the emergency department or otolaryngologist for packing procedures. Due to the high risk of complications, including infection with packing, posterior cavity nosebleed may be referred to inpatient management and monitoring as there is potential for life-threatening arterial hemorrhage.[42]

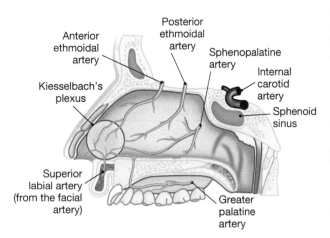

Figure 16.12: Arteries of the nasal sinus region
Source: Mahon BM, Desai BK. Epistaxis control. In: Ganti L, ed. *Atlas of Emergency Medicine Procedures*. Springer; 2016. doi:10.1007/978-1-4939-2507-0_53

Table 16.11: Differential Diagnosis: Nosebleeds

- Trauma, irritation, inflammation, dryness
- Hypertension, atherosclerosis
- Infections such as human immunodeficiency virus (HIV), hepatitis C virus, Epstein–Barr virus, *Helicobacter pylori*, bacterial sepsis with disseminated intravascular coagulation
- Alcohol use disorder
- Nutrient Deficiencies such as vitamin B12, folate, copper
- Primary immune thrombocytopenia
- Posttransfusion purpura
- Myelodysplastic syndromes
- Aplastic anemia

Source: Data from VisualDX. Differential diagnosis & pitfalls. https://www.visualdx.com/visualdx/diagnosis/drug-induced+epistaxis?diagnosisId=55921&moduleId=101#Differential_Diagnosis_And_Pitfalls

 ETHICAL DILEMMAS

Alterations in function of the essential sensory organs for vision, hearing, smell, and taste can create both safety and ethical concerns. The progression in loss of function may occur over time, limiting the individual's ability to accurately assess the limitations that may create hazards. Reduced visual acuity can increase the risk of accidents and falls. A loss of hearing also may increase the risk of accidents as well as of falls if the vestibular dysfunction results in poor balance. Poor oral health and alterations in taste and smell can increase inflammatory processes that potentiate or worsen chronic obstructive pulmonary disease and pneumonia. While direct correlation between oral health and heart disease has not been established, some studies have shown that gum disease increases bacteria levels, resulting in blood infections that may attack heart valves. Poor dentition leading to tooth loss has been associated with more heart disease and diabetics are particularly vulnerable to the potential increased infection risk associated with poor oral hygiene.

There are significant ethical issues related to access to evaluation for disorders of sensory function. In the United States, evaluation for hearing and vision loss is often a function of affordability and insurance coverage. Eyeglasses and hearing aids are costly and are minimally or not covered at all. Hearing aids may run into several thousands of dollars and require replenishment of batteries and maintenance visits. A loss of sensory function and lack of access to evaluation and assistive devices may create significant barriers for individuals in their work, social, and family lives, resulting in reduced income, social isolation, and a loss of psychologic health. While the

American with Disabilities Act provides required accommodations for individuals with sensory system deficits, the support to institute individualized accommodations must include medical providers that the individual is challenged to access to begin with. There are additional societal stigmas associated with hearing and vision loss, which may defer the aging individual from seeking care and use of assistive devices. Cost and a lack of coverage, particularly for dental care and assistive devices such as hearing aids, must be addressed at a higher policy level, but adult-gerontology nurse practitioners can advocate for both the individual through work and school accommodations and for greater population health through increased awareness of the hidden disabilities created with age-related changes in the sensory systems.

CONCLUSION

Disorders of the sensory systems of the body include dysfunction of the eyes, ears, nose, paranasal sinus, and oropharynx as well as the vestibular system that provides balance and sensation of place. The systems are highly complex, and disease or dysfunction has potential for both temporary and permanent impact leading to an inability to respond to internal and external stimuli. Alterations in or loss of vision, hearing, smell, taste, and balance may have a significant impact on the adults and especially older adults, threatening survival and homeostasis. Careful attention to prevention, screening, and appropriate response to early signs and symptoms of dysfunction is the primary responsibility of the clinician in care of this population. Care is optimized by strong clinician–patient relationships establishing common goals of disease prevention and mitigation of genetic, congenital, and behavioral risk factors.[2]

CASE STUDY
A 67-YEAR-OLD FEMALE PRESENTS TO PRIMARY CARE CLINIC

Chief Complaint: "My hearing is getting worse, and I have felt pressure in my right ear for the past week. When I got up from bed this morning, I felt really dizzy."

History of Present Illness: Hearing has been getting worse over the past year; it has become increasingly difficult to hear in busy restaurants. Last week she developed a sense of pressure in her right ear and experienced ear pain when she flew home from her family reunion in Nebraska. This morning she has felt only pressure and decreased hearing on her right side, and she experienced some dizziness upon arising from bed. Occasionally she has high-pitched buzzing in her ears. She has never had hearing evaluation.

Past Medical History: Claims good general health without illness, injuries, hospitalizations, denies chronic conditions except seasonal allergies in spring.

Family History: Father deceased age 79, history of hypertension. Mother 90 years old with Alzheimer's dementia, hypertension, and osteoporosis. No siblings.

Review of Systems: Good general health, no injuries or illnesses, denies fever, chills, weight loss

Eyes: Denies visual changes except reading "cheaters" she buys at dollar store.

Ears: Per history of present illness

Nose: Occasional seasonal allergies, feeling congested during recent stay at family farm

Throat: Denies sore throat except intermittent postnasal drip irritation with allergies.

Cardiovascular: Denies chest pain, palpitations, exercise intolerance, leg pain, history of murmur or blood pressure elevation. Exercises walk/jog about 2 miles three times weekly without difficulty.

Respiratory: Denies shortness of breath, dyspnea, orthopnea, or cough. Never diagnosed with asthma but occasional cough and wheeze with exercise during allergy season.

Gastrointestinal: No bowel changes, denies N/V/D/C, dyspepsia, dysphagia, abdominal pain or bloating, no melena or blood.

Genitourinary: No changes, denies frequency, urgency, dysuria, hematuria.

Neuro: Per HPI + dizziness this morning. Denies history syncope, loss of consciousness, seizures, changes in cognition, gait, sensation, numbness, tingling, tremors, or headaches.

OBJECTIVE

Vital Signs: Temp—97.7; HR—68; BP—122/73; R—14; Wt.—137 lb; SpO$_2$—97% on RA

General: Alert, oriented x4, well nourished, well developed female in no apparent distress.

HEENT: Head: normocephalic, no lesions; Eyes: no redness, injection, discharge, PERRLA; Ears: canals patent, no lesions or swelling, TMS; left normal color, landmarks, light reflex and mobility, right TM dull, pink, poor mobility, does not clear with patient Valsalva.

Rinne: Positive bone conduction heard longer than air conduction

Weber: Does not localize; not reliable due to concurrent acute conductive loss on right due to acute middle ear condition in the potential presence of bilateral age-related sensorineural hearing loss.

Nose: Patent with boggy inflamed red turbinates bilaterally, clear nasal discharge.

Cardiovascular: RRR, no murmurs, gallops, lifts or bruits, carotids without bruit

Respiratory: Chest clear, normal breath sounds, no rales, rhonchi, or wheezes, normal expansion.

Abdomen: Soft, normal BS, nontender, nondistended, no masses, no hepatosplenomegaly, abdominal aorta, normal size, no lifts or bruits.

Neuro: CN II-XII grossly intact, normal gait, no ataxia, DTRs 2+ upper and lower, negative Romberg.

Screening office-based tympanometry and audiogram (Figure 16.13).

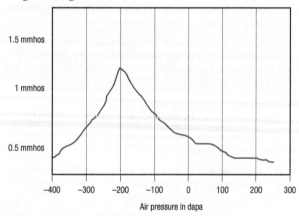

Figure 16.13: Type C tympanogram

Tympanogram: Left ear: Normal peak between +/− 100 daPa, normal compliance 0.3–1.5 mL.

Right ear: Type C tympanogram with shifted peak below −100 daPa as seen in Eustachian tube dysfunction and middle ear effusion, compliance normal at 0.3–1.5 mL.

Screening Audiogram: Moderate hearing loss bilaterally with thresholds exceeding 45(dB) at 1,000–6,000 (Hz), warrants ENT referral for diagnostic puretone audiometry to differentiate conductive loss and level of sensorineural hearing loss.

DIFFERENTIALS/ASSESSMENT AND PLAN

Alteration in hearing

- Left ear, potential moderate age-related sensorineural hearing loss.

- Right ear, likely acute conductive hearing loss associated with middle ear effusion and Eustachian tube dysfunction secondary to allergic rhinitis and airflight-associated barotrauma. Further evaluation required to determine presence of age-related sensorineural hearing loss underlying acute right ear hearing loss and ear pain.

- Eustachian tube dysfunction—Normally recommend Valsalva maneuver holding nose while breath-holding to facilitate clearance of middle ear congestion but must avoid currently due to possible barotrauma from increased middle ear pressure during flight. Increase fluid intake to promote liquefaction and movement of middle ear effusion.

- Barotrauma—avoid increased ear pressure avoiding elevation change till symptoms clear. May try OTC decongestant and antihistamine. Discuss prevention measures.

Allergic Rhinitis: Encourage future early management to avoid secondary middle ear congestion with nonsedating OTC antihistamine and intranasal steroids, avoidance of allergens.

Dizziness: Single episode, etiology unclear but may be associated with middle ear effusion and Eustachian tube dysfunction or barotrauma. Consider otoliths if symptoms persist with referral to PT for Epley maneuver therapy. Observe for other neurologic symptoms.

LAB/DIAGNOSTICS/REFERRALS/FOLLOW-UP

- CBC—evaluate for anemia
- UA—evaluate for infection and hydration
- CMP—evaluate general chemistries and electrolytes
- FBS—evaluate morning glucose
- Referral to ENT for further evaluation of alterations in hearing
- Return to clinic for follow-up if dizziness persists

REFERENCES

References for this chapter are online and available at https://connect.springerpub.com/content/book/978-0-8261-8414-6/part/part01/toc-part/ch16.

CHAPTER 17

Common Neurologic Disorders Encountered in the Primary Care Setting

Vilija Abrute, Tracian Kelly Hershorin, and Debra J. Hain

LEARNING OBJECTIVES

At the conclusion of this chapter, the learner will be able to:

➤ Discuss neurologic anatomy and physiology.
➤ Describe common neurologic health conditions.
➤ Present evidence-based strategies to address common neurologic health problems.

INTRODUCTION

Adolescents through older adults who are seen in primary care can present with chief complaints related to neurologic disorders (e.g., seizure, headache), so the nurse practitioner (NP) must be prepared to address these issues and know when to refer the patient to neurology. This chapter focuses on assessing, diagnosing, and managing common neurologic disorders that NPs may encounter in the primary care setting. These conditions include stroke, seizure disorders/epilepsy, headaches, movement disorders, a brief overview of normal pressure hydrocephalus, and common symptoms, such as dizziness and syncope. Dementia is a common neurologic condition in older adults, but this is not discussed in this chapter (see Chapter 10 for information about dementia).

OVERVIEW OF THE NEUROLOGIC SYSTEM

The neurologic system is composed of two major parts: the central nervous system (CNS), which is made up of the brain and spinal cord, and the peripheral nervous system, which consists of nerves that stem off from the spinal cord and extend to all parts of the body. There are many neurologic diseases, such as neurodegenerative diseases (e.g., Parkinson's disease [PD], Alzheimer's disease), stroke, seizure disorders, cancer, and headaches (see Chapter 10 for information about dementia). A neurologic examination is an important aspect of the approach to diagnosis and management of neurologic conditions. A basic overview of the neurologic examination is presented here; for more information on performing a physical examination, see Chapter 12.

Normal Anatomy and Physiology

The basic units of the nervous system are neurons. Neurons consist of a large cell body and two types of nerve fibers known as axons, which are long, slender nerve fibers that project from a nerve cell and can send messages as electrical impulses to other nerve cells and muscles, and the dendrites, which are made up of branches of nerve cells that receive electrical impulses. The brain and spinal cord also contain support cells called glial cells, which are different from nerve cells and do not produce electrical impulses. There are several types of

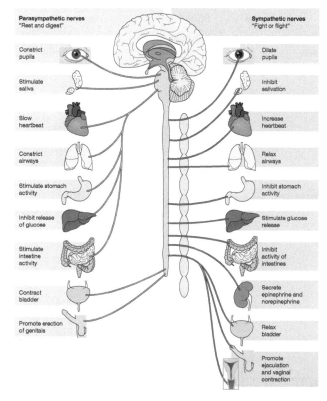

Figure 17.1: The autonomic nervous system

Source: Armitage A, ed. *A Practical Guide to Parkinson's Disease: Diagnosis and Management.* Springer Publishing Company; 2018.

support cells, such as the astrocytes, which provide nutrients and control the chemical components of fluids to and around nerve cells, allowing them to flourish, and ependymal cells, which form along open areas in the brain and spinal cord to create and release CSF that bathes cells of the nervous system. Glial progenitor cells are present throughout the adult brain and can produce new astrocytes and oligodendrocytes to replace those destroyed by injuries or disorders. Microglia cells assist in protecting the brain against damages and assist in eradicating debris from dead cells. These cells can move around in the

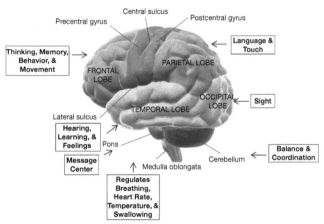

Figure 17.3: Lateral view of the cerebral hemispheres, brainstem, and cerebellum with basic functions

Source: Slota MC, ed. *AACN Core Curriculum for Pediatric High Acuity, Progressive, and Critical Care Nursing.* 3rd ed. Springer Publishing Company; 2018:Figure 4.6.

nervous system and multiply to protect the brain during an injury. Oligodendrocytes form a coating around nerve cell axons and make a specialized membrane called myelin, a fatty substance that insulates nerve axons and speeds the conduction of impulses along nerve fibers.

The brain has several functions based on the various locations within the brain (see Figures 17.2 and 17.3). The blood-brain barrier is a cellular and biochemical structure that is the primary regulator of transporting molecules and cells into and out of the CNS. The neurovascular unit is comprised of endothelial cells, pericytes, immune cells, astrocytes, and basement membrane.

The peripheral nervous system consists of the Schwann cells, which are also known as glial. These cells are like oligodendrocytes and make myelin to insulate axons in the peripheral nervous system. However, the brain and spinal cord consist of gray matter, which has nerve cell bodies, dendrites and axons, glial cells, and capillaries (the smallest of the body's blood vessels), and white matter, which contains relatively very few neurons and consists mainly of axons that are wrapped with many layers of myelin and of the oligodendrocytes that make the myelin. Myelin is what makes the white matter.

Nerve cells routinely increase or decrease the number of connections they have with other nerve cells. This process may partly explain how people learn, adapt, and form memories. However, the brain and spinal cord rarely produce new nerve cells. An exception is the hippocampus, an area of the brain involved in memory formation. The nervous system is an extraordinarily complex communication system that can send and receive voluminous amounts of information simultaneously. The nervous system is vulnerable to diseases and injuries, and the most common conditions are discussed in this chapter.

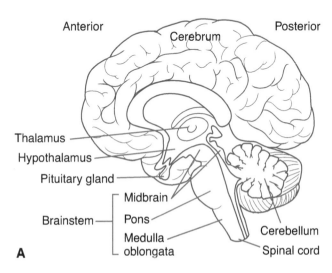

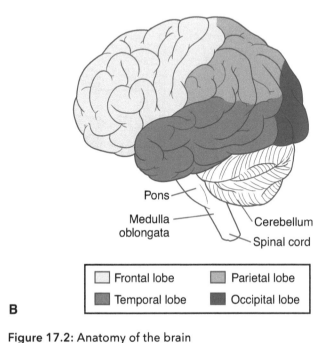

Figure 17.2: Anatomy of the brain

(A) Structures of the brain. (B) Lobes of the brain.

Source: Chiocca EM. Advanced Pediatric Assessment. 3rd ed. Springer Publishing Company; 2020.

NEUROLOGIC EXAMINATION

The following provides an overview of the neurologic examination (see Chapter 12 and refer to your advanced health assessment textbook). When patients present to primary care with complaints such as tremor, headache, numbness or weakness in arms and legs, blurred vision, worsening balance, or cognition, performing a neurologic examination is essential for diagnosing and management of neurologic disorders. The neurologic examination is done when assessing a patient's CNS—brain, spinal cord, and nerves—and the peripheral nervous system. Common CNS disorders include stroke, PD, migraines, meningitis, and brain or spinal cord tumors. If deficits are found during the neurologic examination, ordering neuroimaging can be useful before referral to a specialist, such as a neurologist or neurosurgeon, and helps avoid delays in diagnosis or treatment. If you are uncertain of the neuroimaging

that should be ordered, consulting with a neurologic specialist can be beneficial; it is important to avoid ordering unnecessary diagnostic testing.

The focus of the examination is as follows:

1. Mental Status

   a. **Cognition:** Level of alertness and orientation (person, time, and place) immediate, short-term and long-term (recent and remote), calculation, abstraction

   b. **Language:** Observe how patient speaks, any hesitation, or aphasia (must consider ethnic and racial differences and if English is primary language)

2. **Cranial Nerves** (CN) (see Table 17.1) may not all be evaluated in primary care, but you should be prepared to evaluate all CNs as necessary. Even though evaluating CN might seem like a lot, once

Table 17.1: Assessment of Cranial Nerves

Cranial Nerve	Function	Response
I Olfactory	Smell	Usually not tested; however, it may be a necessary part of the examination, particularly when assessing cognitive function. Have the patient close their eyes and have them identify a scent that is common (i.e., coffee, alcohol, orange, and so on).
II Optic	Vision	Cover one eye and ask how many fingers the patient can see
III Oculomotor	Pupils size/reactivity	Are they equally reactive?
	Extraocular movements (EOM)	Ask the patient to look up, down, and sideways. Is nystagmus present?
IV Trochlea	Eye inward and down	Part of extraocular movement (EOM)
V Trigeminal	Facial sensation	Touch forehead, cheeks, chin
	Jaw movement	Is numbness present?
VI Abducens	Eye side to side	Part of EOM
VII Facial	Facial expression: to show symmetricity	Is smile symmetric? Raise eyebrows Close eyes tightly
VIII Acoustic	Hearing	Can hear equally both ears (Rhine and Weber tests, Whisper test)
IX Glossopharyngeal	Gag/swallow	Usually not tested; however, it is important in those suspected of neurologic disorders that may affect swallowing (i.e., stroke, Parkinson's disease)
X Vagus	Swallow, vocal quality	Voice hoarseness (observe/listen)
XI Spinal accessory	Shoulders, head rotation	Shrugs shoulders Tilts head side to side
XII Hypoglossal	Tongue movement	Ask to stick tongue out, must be straight/midline
	Speech	Articulation (observe/listen)

EOM, extraocular muscle anatomy

you get the routine down, it does not take a long time to perform this very important examination.

3. **Motor Examination**

   a. Pronator Drift: Ask patient to raise an arm up as if holding a pizza tray with eyes closed for 5 seconds; if a lesion exists, one palm will drift inward.

   b. Test Strength in Arms and Legs: Ask patient to push–pull with arms, straighten their leg out, and hold it up against resistance. Ask if they are able to perform activities of daily living (ADLs).

   c. Muscle Tone: Bend arms and legs quickly; note if flaccid, increased tone, or spasticity (significant for upper motor neuron disease).

   d. Involuntary movements

4. **Sensory Examination**

   a. Touch arms and legs and ask if sensation is the same or if there is numbness.

   b. Proprioception: With index fingers, ask to alternate and touch nose and then examiner's finger; movements should be symmetric, without tremor, and accurate.

   c. Reflexes: Very important to note hyperreflexia; it is usually the sign of upper motor neuron disease. Should assess tendon reflexes (biceps, triceps, brachioradialis, knee, ankle) and plantar response (normal response: all toes flex, called a flexor plantar response).

   d. Graphesthesia

   e. Stereognosis

5. **Gait and Coordination**

   a. When the patient ambulates into the examination room, observe gait and balance and how they turn; determine if gait is spastic, magnetic (unable to clear feet off the floor, steady, dropped foot, any use of assistive devices or braces). In older adults, it is essential to assess for fall risk (see Chapter 10).

Obtaining a thorough patient history and performing a neurologic examination supports differential diagnoses and the determination of additional diagnostic studies that may be needed.

"Syncope" is a clinical syndrome for when the patient experiences a transient loss of consciousness (LOC). This is caused by an episode of inadequate cerebral nutrient flow, often due to an abrupt drop in systemic BP. A loss of postural tone occurs with the LOC and the person will collapse. Recovery is usually rapid (seconds), but if it lasts longer, this is not syncope or is not syncope alone (e.g., traumatic head injury [TBI] or another cause). One cause of syncope is reflex syncope, which encompasses vasodilatation and/or bradycardia that leads to systemic hypotension and cerebral hypoperfusion. Causes of reflex syncope are vasovagal, situational syncope, carotid sinus syncope, micturition syncope, and other triggers (e.g., coughing, sneezing, defecation). Orthostatic hypotension, particularly in older adults, can be related to medications (e.g., diuretics, vasodilators, antidepressants), volume depletion (e.g., hemorrhage, gastrointestinal [GI] losses such as vomiting, diarrhea, dehydration due to diminished thirst in older adults), and autonomic failure (e.g., PD, Lewy body dementia, diabetes, spinal cord injury, autoimmune neuropathy). Cardiac causes include tachyarrhythmias, bradyarrhythmia, structural cardiac disease (e.g., severe aortic stenosis, prosthetic valve dysfunction), and cardiopulmonary/vascular (e.g., severe pulmonary hypertension, pulmonary embolus). The initial evaluation is to obtain a complete medical history and perform a physical examination. Based on the history and physical, you will determine next steps, such as diagnostic testing or referral to a neurologist, pulmonologist, and/or cardiologist.

STROKE

Etiology

Each year almost 800,000 people in the United States experience a stroke; 87% are ischemic and about 185,000 are recurrent.[1,2] As secondary stroke prevention strategies have improved, the number of recurrent strokes and transient ischemic attacks (TAI) have decreased. Stroke, or cerebrovascular accident (CVA), historically has been characterized as "a neurological deficit attributed to an acute focal injury of the CNS by a vascular cause, including cerebral infarction, intracerebral hemorrhage (ICH), and subarachnoid infarction (SAH) and is a major cause of disability and death worldwide."[3] The types of strokes include intracerebral hemorrhage (10%), SAH (2%), and ischemic stroke (88%) of all strokes.

Pathophysiology

There are two broad categories of stroke: hemorrhagic and ischemic. These are different conditions; hemorrhagic stroke occurs when too much blood is within the closed cranium, and ischemic stroke is when there is reduced blood resulting in inadequate oxygen and nutrients to the brain. Ischemic stroke is an acute injury to the brain due to thrombosis, embolism, or systemic hypoperfusion. Thrombosis can be the result of an obstruction of the arterial wall from atherosclerosis (most common), dissection, or fibromuscular dysplasia. An embolism occurs when particles of debris starting from somewhere else in the body blocks access to a specific part of the brain. Systemic hypoperfusion is related to general circulatory conditions (e.g., cardiac pump failure due to cardiac arrest or arrhythmia, reduced cardiac output). There are several subtypes of ischemic stroke; see Box 17.1.

Box 17.1: Stroke Subtypes

- Lacunary stroke: lacunar syndrome with normal computed tomography/magnetic resonance imaging (CT/MRI) or subcortical stroke measuring less than 1.5 cm in diameter on CT or MRI. Most, but not all, are related to small-vessel disease.

- Stroke attributable to small-vessel disease: subcortical measuring less than 1.5 cm on CT or MRI without evidence of a concomitant cortical infarct.

- Cardioembolic stroke: attributed to arterial occlusion from an embolus, presumed came from the heart. Imaging is similar to that found on large artery atherosclerosis. Evidence of a TIA or previous stroke greater than 1 vascular territory supports the diagnosis of cardioembolic stroke.

- Cryptogenic stroke: imaging that confirms a stroke with an unknown source after thorough diagnostic assessment was done.

- Stroke caused by large artery atherosclerosis: stroke in the vascular distribution of a major intracranial or extracranial artery with greater than 50% stenosis or occlusion on vascular imaging.

Source: Kleindorger DO, Towfighi A, Chaturvedi S, Cockroft KM, Gutierrez J. 2021 Guideline for the prevention of stroke in patients with stroke and transient ischemic attack: a guideline from the American Heart Association/American Stroke Association. *Stroke.* 2021;52:e1–e104. doi:10.1161/STR.0000000000000375

Hemorrhagic stroke, on the other hand, occurs when there is bleeding directly into the brain parenchyma, forming localized hematoma (spreads along the white matter pathways) and bleeding into the cerebrospinal fluid (CSF) within the subarachnoid space that surrounds the brain. There are two subtypes: intracerebral hemorrhage and SAH.[66]

Intracranial hemorrhage (ICH) usually is from arterioles or small vessels bleeding directly into the brain. Common causes of ICH include the following:

- Hypertension
- Trauma (e.g., fall in older adults, motor vehicle accident)
- Bleeding diatheses
- Amyloid angiopathy
- Illicit drug use (mostly amphetamines and cocaine)
- Vascular malformations

Less frequent causes are bleeding into tumors, aneurysm rupture, and vasculitis.

Major causes of subarachnoid hemorrhage (SAH) are a rupture of an arterial aneurysm and bleeding from vascular malformations. The main causes of an ICH are not common reasons for SAH. For years, healthcare professionals considered TIA to be benign; now, we know this is not true. TIA is no longer defined by neurologic deficits lasting less than 24 hours. People who have a TIA or minor stroke are at risk for recurrent stroke and so require urgent evaluation and treatment. "TIA" is defined as "a transient episode of neurologic dysfunction caused by focal brain, spinal cord, or retinal ischemic, without an acute infarction."[4] There can be permanent brain tissue injury. A minor stroke is when the person has persistent, minor, nondisabling neurologic deficits. Regardless, both are indicative of recurrent ischemic stroke.

Risk Factors

Medical risk factors are hypertension, dyslipidemia, obesity/overweight, obstructive sleep apnea (OSA), diabetes mellitus, atrial fibrillation, coronary heart disease, family history of cardiovascular disease (CVD), previous stroke or TIA, and COVID-19 infection. Lifestyle risk factors are physical inactivity, stress, low educational level, heavy or excessive alcohol use, illicit drug use (e.g., heroin, cocaine), current smoking, and exposure to secondhand smoke. Other risk factors include age older than 50 years, especially those over age 80; African Americans; use of birth control pills or hormone therapies (e.g., estrogen); male gender (after 85 years women have similar or higher risk); and poor nutrition (e.g., regular meat, low green vegetables, added salt at the table, regular sugar).[5]

Approach to Diagnosis

Brain ischemia occurs when there is a stroke; this can last anywhere from seconds to minutes and longer and can also be transient. Ischemic stroke causes a sudden loss of focal brain function. Assessment and treatment must begin as soon as possible because the longer it takes to intervene, the more brain injury will occur. The clinical manifestations of stroke include aphasia, dysarthria, hemianopia, vision changes, and sudden headache (hemorrhagic), often described as the worse headache ever and may be associated with nausea, vomiting, alteration in consciousness, gait disturbance, paralysis (unilateral), facial paresis, and arm drift/weakness. The three most predictive findings in the assessment are facial paresis, arm drift/weakness, and abnormal speech. In older adults, the first presenting symptom can be a sudden fall or acute confusion (delirium).

The first step is obtaining a thorough history and physical. It is important to determine the time of the onset of symptoms because this will provide information about eligibility for treatment with intravenous thrombolysis (less than 4.5 hours from onset of symptoms) and endovascular thrombectomy (less than 24 hours from symptom onset). It is important to consider other differential diagnoses, such as seizures, syncope, migraine, hypoglycemia, hyperglycemia, or drug toxicity. If the patient is unable to provide information, it is critical to ask a family member or a reliable person who would have knowledge about the patient's health condition or if there was recent trauma. The physical examination should include a neurologic assessment. Evaluate the retroorbital regions for vascular bruits and palpate pulses for absence or irregularity of pulses (make sure you assess both sides to determine symmetry). A fundoscopic examination and examination of the head (assess for trauma) should be done. Lungs (abnormal breath sounds, fluid overload, stridor) and heart sounds (assess for arrhythmia, murmur, S3 or S4) should be assessed. A tongue laceration may indicate a seizure. Assess the skin for trauma and signs of endocarditis.

Diagnostics

Urgent brain imaging—CT without contrast—is the fastest and best initial image to confirm a suspected diagnosis and the fastest way to initiate the treatment. Magnetic resonance imaging/magnetic resonance angiography (MRI/MRA) can be ordered later to look at the soft tissues and blood vessels in greater detail and to determine the cause. Imaging is mandatory in patients with sudden neurologic changes (symptoms of acute stroke or neurologic deterioration). In addition, it is important to assess blood glucose using a finger stick and check oxygen saturation. An assessment that can be done as soon as possible in your office (do not delay noncontrast CT if acute stroke is suspected) is the electrocardiogram. If after your assessment you suspect your patient is having a stroke you should call 911 so that they can receive urgent assessment and treatment. Laboratory studies that should be done at the ED are complete blood count (CBC) with platelets, troponin, prothrombin time (PT) and international normalized ratio (INR), activated partial thromboplastin time, and clotting time to determine if the person is a candidate for thrombolytic therapy with alteplase. Other laboratory studies that can be considered are serum electrolytes, liver function tests, toxicology screening, blood alcohol level, and a pregnancy test if in childbearing years and the potential of pregnancy is present. Chest radiography may be done if lung disease is suspected and electroencephalogram if seizures are suspected.

Screening Tools and Tests

Stroke severity is assessed with an impairment-level scale; the most commonly used is the National Institutes of Health Stroke Scale (NIHSS), and for adolescents consider the Pediatric National Institutes of Health Stroke Scale (pedNIHSS). The Canadian Neurologic Scale, European Stroke Scale, and the Scandinavian Stroke Scale have been used in clinical trials. These scales are not useful for making the diagnosis of stroke, only for determining the severity. The NIHSS is a reliable and valid 15-item tool that has become a standard stroke impairment scale for use in clinical trials and clinical care (see www.stroke.nih.gov/documents/NIH_Stroke_Scale_508C.pdf).

Management

The first thing to consider in stroke management is stabilizing the patient. So, if your patient presents with symptoms that are consistent with a stroke, it is important to determine if the situation is emergent or nonemergent by assessing airway, breathing, and circulation along with performing a rapid neurologic evaluation. If the patient has hypoglycemia (which can cause neurofocal deficits), you need to rapidly correct their glucose. Hyperglycemia can also affect the brain and needs to be treated (see Chapter 26 for more information). Patients having an acute stroke have better health outcomes (e.g., reduced morbidity, stroke-related complications) when they receive faster treatment. Antihypertensive medication (reducing blood pressure [BP]) may not be the most beneficial during the initial management of ischemic stroke. There is impaired cerebral autoregulation, the perfusion pressure distal to the obstructed vessel is low, and the distal vessels are dilated and dependent on systemic BP. In addition, you need to consider if the elevated BP is related to the stress of having a stroke or if the patient urgently needs to go to the hospital (this is based on your rapid physical assessment, not just based on BP reading).

The role of primary care NPs in stroke management is first recognizing the patient may be having a stroke (may present to the office or call the office to report concerns). Primary stroke prevention is important in those who are at risk of stroke, so evaluating a person's risk is critical.

Once the person is discharged from the hospital or postacute care, the NP should comanage the patient with other specialists involved in the person's care (e.g., neurologist, cardiologist). Pharmacologic and nonpharmacologic interventions will be necessary. Secondary prevention involves managing health conditions and other risk factors that increase the risk of stroke in adults who have a history of TIA or previous ischemic stroke. You can use a risk calculator that is based on the Framingham Study: https://qxmd.com/calculate/calculator_252/framingham-risk-score-2008.

Pharmacologic

The first-line treatment for acute ischemic stroke is intravenous alteplase within 4.5 hours of the onset of symptoms. Other medications that can be considered include aspirin within 48 hours of the onset of stroke, lipid-lowering medications, and antihypertensive medications (see Chapter 20). Those with intracerebral hemorrhage should have all anticoagulant and antiplatelet medications stopped and reversed right away with IV vitamin K, four-factor prothrombin complex concentration, or fresh frozen plasma. Protamine sulfate can be used for patients with heparin-associated intracerebral hemorrhage. Elevated BP should be treated because it may increase the risk of hematoma expansion, but this should be gradual and not rapid to prevent cerebral ischemia. Patients may need mild sedation to maintain comfort, and the person will need normal saline for hemodynamic stability.

Goals of care in secondary stroke prevention include BP and glycemic control (see Chapter 26). When treating dyslipidemia, consider anticoagulation therapy for those with atrial fibrillation or other arrhythmias that put them at risk (see Chapter 20). For those with chronic nonvalvular atrial fibrillation (AF), you may consider long-term anticoagulation with warfarin or a direct oral anticoagulant (dabigatran, apixaban, rivaroxaban, edoxaban). Antiplatelet therapy with aspirin (50 to 100 mg daily), clopidogrel 75 mg daily, or a combination of aspirin–release dipyridamole (25 mg/200 mg twice daily) may be appropriate. Whenever considering anticoagulant therapy the clinician must assess the benefit versus the risk, paying close attention to bleeding risks.

🏠 Quality and Safety Alert

▨ In older adults at risk of or experiencing recurrent falls, considerations should include the risk of TBI and the use of anticoagulants. The risk of the patient having a subdural hematoma from a fall can be higher than the risk of having a stroke from atrial fibrillation (A-Fib).

((•)) EMERGENCY

▨ Elevate the person's head to manage elevated intracranial pressure (ICP).

▨ Glucocorticoids should never be given to lower ICP.

▨ Seizures can occur with increased ICP.

▨ Dysphagia is common when a person has a stroke, so it is very important to consider risk factors for aspiration pneumonia.

Nonpharmacologic

Primary and secondary prevention of stroke and reducing disability are essential, so it is critical to have the person engage in healthy lifestyle changes before stroke occurs and encourage self-management activities (e.g., taking medications as prescribed, physical activity, eating heart-healthy diet, smoking cessation). The Mediterranean diet has been shown to improve health outcomes in patients with CVD. Once a person experiences a stroke and is stable enough for discharge, consider postacute care in a skilled nursing facility (SNF) or a subacute or rehabilitation center to assist in improving their functional status. Reducing alcohol consumption is very important. Weight reduction in those who are overweight/obese should be one of the areas to address in lifestyle management discussions; the patient will most likely benefit from a consultation with a dietitian. Depression is common after having a stroke, so consider a consultation with a psych/mental health expert after evaluating your patient (see Chapter 18 for more information regarding depression).

Procedures

Patients who have experienced an acute stroke will receive care from another specialist (e.g., neurologist, vascular surgeon, radiologist), and appropriate procedures will be completed to improve survival and reduce disability. Procedures that may be done to restore cerebral blood flow include carotid endarterectomy and mechanical thrombectomy. The discussion of procedures is beyond the scope of this textbook, so reviewing additional resources for further information is recommended.

Patient Education

Individuals should be educated about primary and secondary stroke prevention and the importance of controlling BP, diabetes mellitus, dyslipidemia, hypertension, and other chronic health conditions that may increase risk. In addition, healthy lifestyle management should be reinforced. The Centers for Disease Control and Prevention (CDC) has patient education materials available at https://www.cdc.gov/stroke/materials_for_patients.htm, and the American Heart Association has information at www.stroke.org/en/professionals/stroke-resource-library.

SEIZURES AND EPILEPSY

Etiology

Seizures are common with about 8% to 10% of the population having seizures over a lifetime. Epilepsy affects about 50 million people worldwide, which makes it one of the most common neurologic diseases globally. About 70% of people can live epilepsy-free if diagnosed and receive treatments in a timely manner.[6] Epilepsy is more prevalent in rural areas compared to urban developed countries.[7]

Pathophysiology

A seizure occurs when electrical hypersynchronization of neuronal networks in the cerebral cortex creates a change in behavior. Acute symptomatic seizures can be the result of drug or alcohol withdrawal, metabolic derangements, and acute neurologic disorders (stroke, encephalitis, or TBI). This can be within 1 week of stroke, TBI, anoxic encephalopathy, intracranial surgery, subdural hematoma, encephalopathy due to infection, or within 24 hours of metabolic disturbances. Causes for seizures are noted in Box 17.3. Epilepsy is when at least two unprovoked seizures (unknown etiology) occur 24 hours apart. Seizures are either focal or generalized, which depends if the electrical activity involves a focal area of the brain or both sides of the brain at the same time.

Risk Factors

Risk factors include family history of seizures, abnormal early neurologic development or intellectual disability,

Box 17.2: Steps to Obtain a Patient/Event History

- Description of the event (when started, how long lasted, how did the patient present)
- Timing of the seizure in relationship to sleep
- Ask about LOC
- Postictal period manifestations
- Seizure precipitants or triggers (environmental or physiologic, any triggers immediately preceded the seizure)
- Prior events
- Medications (over the counter)
- Drug use or alcohol intoxication or withdrawal
- Family history
- Risk factors

stroke, Alzheimer's disease, history of intracranial infection, alcohol or drug abuse, immunosuppression, history of cancer, rheumatologic disorders (e.g., systemic lupus erythematosus), and hematologic disorders (sickle cell disease, porphyria, antiphospholipid syndrome).

Approach to Diagnosis

Obtaining a thorough history (see Box 17.2), characterizing the seizure, and ruling out possible causes are essential. Physical history generally does not provide much information in those with epileptic seizures. The physical examination is essential for identifying possible causes of seizure (see Box 17.4). Assessing for trauma-related injury due to a seizure is important. A neurologic examination as discussed earlier is critical. An oropharynx examination is also important to assess for injury to the tongue if the patient has had a recent seizure. If the patient is seen in your office getting rapid point-of-care glucose for those with a first-time seizure, it can help diagnose hypoglycemia. Serum electrolytes and CBC with differential, renal function tests, liver function tests, urinalysis, and toxicology screening can assist in determining causes for seizures. Seizures are considered provoked (acute symptomatic seizures) or unprovoked (epilepsy). Provoked seizures are caused by some triggers (e.g., hypoglycemia, alcohol withdrawal), and once these triggers are removed, the patient is not likely to have another seizure.

Approach to Management

The approach to management depends on if this is a first-time seizure or if the person has a history of epilepsy, type of movement or behavior, frequency, and severity. It is important to identify the cause of the seizure (see Box 17.3). The main goals of management include controlling the seizures, reducing side effects of the treatment, and

Box 17.3: Causes of Seizures

- Acute ischemic or hemorrhagic stroke
- Subdural hematoma
- Subarachnoid hemorrhage
- Traumatic brain injury
- Eclampsia
- Encephalopathy
- Hypoxic-ischemic injury
- Brain abscess
- Meningitis or encephalitis
- Hypoglycemia
- Hyperglycemia
- Hyponatremia
- Hypocalcemia
- Hypomagnesemia
- Uremia (buildup of metabolic toxins in advanced renal failure or acute kidney injury), most often myoclonic
- Withdrawal from drugs, medications (most benzodiazepines), or alcohol
- Drug intoxication, poisoning, or overdose

Box 17.4: Classification of Seizures

Seizures are classified as either being primary generalized or partial. A partial seizure can be followed by a generalized seizure, which results in LOC, which is known as secondary generalization.

Primary Generalized Seizure: There is an irregular electrical discharge that originates from the diencephalic activating system, involves both halves (hemispheres) in the entire cortex, and spreads simultaneously to all areas of the brain. Generalized seizures include the following:

- Absence seizures
- Atonic seizures
- Infantile spasms
- Myoclonic seizures

Partial Seizures: There is a surplus of neuronal discharge that occurs in a focal area of the cerebral cortex, which is located in the temporal lobe, and most often results from structural aberrations. Partial seizures include the following:

- Simple seizures, in which there is no impairment of consciousness
- Complex seizures, in which the activity is reduced but there is no complete LOC

maintaining or restoring quality of life.[8] Referral and co-management with a neurologist should be considered. Classifying a seizure is important; the International

League Against Epilepsy (ILAE) has a classification system of seizure types that is available at www.ilae.org/guidelines/definition-and-classification. If someone witnesses the seizure, it is important to start with early post-seizure management. The seizure may only last about 2 minutes (average time), and so there may be no need for administration of medications at that time; however, IV access may be important for the future administration of medications (if paramedics are present or the person goes to the ED). Determining if the seizure is acute symptomatic (focal) or unprovoked (generalized) is important. Status epilepticus is when a seizure lasts longer than 5 to 10 minutes or there are serial seizures without interictal return to baseline consciousness. Patients should be referred to a neurologist; however, primary care NPs should collaborate with the specialist to assure primary care needs are addressed.

Pharmacologic

A single seizure can occur for many reasons and may not be diagnostic for epilepsy so initiation of antiepileptic drugs (AED) may not be necessary (consultation with a neurologist is important). Adults with a high risk of recurrent seizures should receive AED; initiating therapy after the first seizure reduces the absolute risk by 35% over 2 years. AED therapy is indicated after two unprovoked seizures.[9] For individuals with a low risk who have had a single seizure, delaying the start of an AED is warranted. The choice of AED depends on the type of seizure, the patient's history and presentation, and comorbid conditions. You should weigh the benefits and risks of starting and choosing appropriate medications. Never discontinue AED before assessing the risk of seizure recurrence and the risks and benefits of withdrawal (see Box 17.5 for types of medications to consider).

Box 17.5: Antiepileptic Medications

Types of antiepileptic medications to consider:

- Primary Generalized Seizure: Valproic acid, ethosuximide
  - Lamotrigine, carbamazepine, oxcarbazepine, levetiracetam, and topiramate
- Partial Seizures (Focal Seizures): carbamazepine, lamotrigine
  - Oxcarbazepine, levetiracetam, and valproic acid
- Status Epilepticus (prolong seizures lasting more than 5 minutes, repeated seizures = 3 or more seizures in 1 hour): buccal midazolam
  - Rectal diazepam and lorazepam

Consultation with a neurologist is indicated for evaluation, diagnosis, and treatment of seizures. *See Chapter 13 for more specifics about medication management.*

SPECIAL CONSIDERATIONS FOR ADOLESCENTS TO YOUNG ADULTS

Epilepsy in adolescents is associated with a high risk of experiencing a depressive disorder (about 8%–35%) and may be bidirectional (indicating underlying pathophysiology). (See Chapter 18 for more information about depression in adolescents.) It is important to identify and treat depression because if unrecognized or not treated, the risk of suicide ideation, poor quality of life, and not taking AED as prescribed is high.[10] Adolescents with chronic conditions such as epilepsy may have challenges engaging in day-to-day diseases management. Chapter 11 has information about the care of adolescents living with chronic health conditions.

SPECIAL CONSIDERATIONS FOR OLDER ADULTS

Seizures are common in older adults, and managing seizures can be complex. In older adults (65 and older) the risk of reoccurrence of unprovoked seizure (after experiencing first seizure) is 53% in the first year and a lifetime risk of 80%.[55] A provoked or triggered seizure (acute symptomatic seizures) can be due to stroke, subdural hematoma, hypertensive encephalopathy, TBI, or metabolic disturbances. The most common cause of epilepsy in older adults is cerebrovascular disease. About 10% to 20% of older adults with Alzheimer's type dementia have epilepsy.[11] Manifestations of seizures in older adults include confusion, behavioral changes, unresponsiveness, sudden falls with no warning, and arousal from sleep with confusion. Focal seizures can present with the absence of symptoms that can occur in younger adults.

ⓘ CLINICAL PEARLS

- Start with single monotherapy for AED.
- Titrate gradually to the highest dose that the patient can tolerate and/or leads to seizure freedom (start low and go slow); monitor for side effects.
- If a breakthrough seizure occurs, adding a second medication may be necessary.
- Monitor regularly in the office.
- Establish therapeutic concentration range when the patient is in remission.
- In patients taking phenytoin or other medications that are tightly protein-bound and have low serum albumin levels, it is important to measure free unbound serum levels of phenytoin or drug they are taking.

Nonpharmacologic

Teaching family members or others about how to provide a safe environment during a seizure activity and about AEDs that are prescribed is important. When appropriate, it is essential to monitor therapeutic levels of AEDs. The patient and family should be provided information about safe driving and other activities during which they may be at risk for injury if a seizure were to occur. Alcohol intake in small amounts may not result in a seizure or affect serum levels of antiseizure medications in those with controlled epilepsy, but heavier alcohol intake (three or more drinks per day) increases the risk of having a seizure.

⌂ Quality and Safety Alerts

- Women of childbearing age should be warned about becoming pregnant and the increased risk of major and minor malformations in the fetus when exposed to antiseizure medications.
- Exposure to AEDs can have deleterious effects on cognitive and behavioral outcomes of the child later in life.
- Pregnancy should be planned and close follow-up once the woman is pregnant is essential.
- Folic acid should be prescribed in women of childbearing age who are taking AEDs.
- Enzyme-inducing AEDs can lower the efficacy of hormonal contraceptives, so pregnancy preventive methods should be discussed.

Procedures

Some patients may have drug-resistant epilepsy (failure to adequately control seizures despite two trials of appropriately chosen AED with the patient following the regimen or no improvement after more than 1 year of treatment). It is beyond the scope of primary care NPs to address this issue but being aware of possible interventions can assist you in discussing treatment options with your patient. Options may include epilepsy surgery and vagus nerve stimulation. Referral to a specialized epilepsy center or provider is an option.

PATIENT EDUCATION

Patients and parents of adolescents should be informed about seizure prevention, treatment, and when to contact their healthcare provider. Patient education materials can be found at the following:

- CDC: www.cdc.gov/epilepsy/about/index.htm and www.cdc.gov/healthyschools/npao/epilepsy.htm
- American Association of Neurological Surgeons: www.aans.org/en/Patients/Neurosurgical-Conditions-and-Treatments/Epilepsy
- American Academy of Pediatrics: www.healthychildren.org/English/health-issues/conditions/seizures/Pages/Seizure-Safety-Tips-for-Parents.aspx

Making sure patients have the knowledge and skills to take medication as prescribed because not doing this increases the risk of mortality, hospitalization, and injury. Written instructions on how, when, and why to take the medications and potential adverse events can help the patient take AED as prescribed.

NORMAL PRESSURE HYDROCEPHALUS

Normal pressure hydrocephalus (NPH) syndrome was first described in 1965 by Hakim and Adams as a condition characterized by a triad of progressive disorders: gait disturbance, urinary incontinence, and cognitive impairment in addition to radiologic findings of enlarged cerebral ventricles with normal opening pressure on lumbar puncture.[12,13] Since the initial discovery of NPH, research has tremendously expanded with findings that have supported evidence-based guidelines for management. Interestingly, despite having guidelines and increased clinical information about NPH, it is not always recognized as a possible diagnosis by primary care providers. This is unfortunate because the condition can be effectively treated with the insertion of a ventricular peritoneal shunt (VPS). Studies indicate that 80% of patients improve with insertion of the shunt.[14] It is still an underdiagnosed and undertreated progressive condition causing older adults to progress with dementia and to lose independence. A loss of independence can lead to decreased quality of life, depression, frequent falls, recurrent urinary tract infections, burden on caregivers, and finally admission to a SNF. Therefore, it is important for NPs to recognize NPH in primary care and provide appropriate referral to neurology as early as possible since the condition can be surgically reversible.

Epidemiology

As we witness an increasing global aging population, NPH is an important differential diagnosis for neurodegenerative disorders.[15] Multiple studies reported that the prevalence of idiopathic NPH (iNPH) has been estimated to be 10 per 100,000 to 22 per 100,000 overall, with 1.30% in those aged older than 65 years and 5.9% in those aged older than 80 years.[16] In a prospective Swedish population study, researchers found that the prevalence of iNPH was 3.7% among individuals 65 years and older, and more common in the higher age group, 80 years and older.[6] Studies that included participants with iNPH found that the mean age of onset was 75 years old, and adults in their 40s and 50s being diagnosed with iNPH was extremely uncommon.[17] The difference between men and women was not significant.[6]

Pathophysiology

CSF is a clear colorless liquid that continuously circulates through cavities of the brain and spinal cord that is formed in the choroid plexus of the third, fourth, and each lateral ventricle. CSF circulation occurs from the lateral ventricles to the third ventricle, then passes through the cerebral aqueduct of Sylvius into the fourth ventricles, and finally circulates into the central canal of the spinal cord and into the subarachnoid space. CSF is gradually reabsorbed into the bloodstream via the arachnoid villi in dural venous sinuses. When there is a disruption of CSF flow, an increase in CSF pressure results in ventricular enlargement (see Figure 17.4).

NPH is classified into two groups. Secondary NPH (sNPH) develops due to an impaired absorption of CSF after an antecedent disease, such as SAH, meningitis, radiation-induced trauma or head trauma, while in idiopathic NPH, no obvious or exact underlying cause can be identified.[13] In sNPH, the products of cellular components of intracranial tumors, protein, and cells from SAH or meningitis, adhesions, and fibrosis may lead to CSF viscosity and impairment of CSF reabsorption.[59] There have been many theories and hypotheses proposed regarding the pathophysiology of iNPH, yet none of them has found a unifying concept to explain the disease despite all the known characteristics of CSF flow, cerebrovascular system, and brain environment.[59]

It is important to differentiate that sNPH develops quickly after the initial injury, weeks or months, and may affect any age group, whereas iNPH develops gradually over the years and affects primarily older adults.[59]

Risk Factors

NPH is considered a rare condition compared to other causes of dementia, such as Alzheimer's disease. However, as stated, it is often underdiagnosed so the true incidence and prevalence may not be known. The size of the ventricles increases with aging, so this may be one of the reasons the clinician does not suspect NPH but rather one of the other types of dementia. Because symptoms can improve with shunting, it is important that

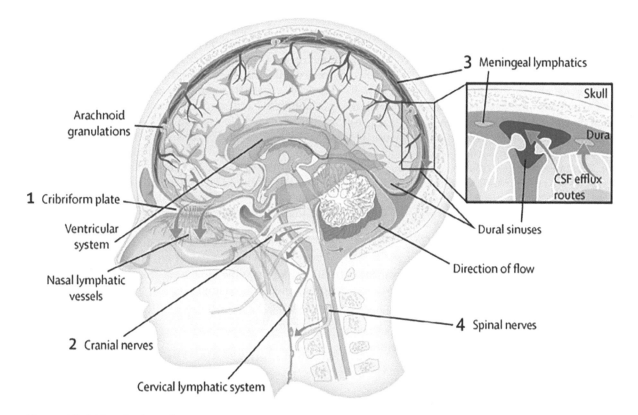

Figure 17.4: Ventricular enlargement

Source: Rasmussen MK, Mestre H, Nedergaard M. The glymphatic pathway in neurological disorders. *Lancet Neurol.* 2018;17(11):1016-1024. doi:10.1016/S1474-4422(18)30318-1

NPs consider this as one of the differential diagnoses when assessing a patient who presents with symptoms of cognitive impairment.

Approach to Diagnosis

Idiopathic NPH patients will present with the triad of cardinal features: gait disturbance, cognitive impairment, and urinary dysfunction. This patient will also have ventriculomegaly, which is the hallmark sign seen on neuroimaging with no obstruction at the level of the third or fourth ventricle.

Gait

It is important to note that gait disturbance is typically the first clinical manifestation of NPH.[59] The gait is characterized as wide-based, short steps, often referred to as "magnetic gait"—the patient is unable to lift their feet adequately off the floor. Frequent falls are also reported. It is important during the assessment to ask the patient to turn—often you will discover that the patient needs to take multiple steps to turn around and might even lose their balance.

Cognitive Impairment

Patients often present with a decline in memory, complaints that they are no longer able to pay bills or make calculations, and decreased attention span or verbal fluency.

Verbal memory and psychomotor speed are likely to respond to shunting.[17]

Urinary Dysfunction

Increased nocturnal urinary frequency and urgency, as well as urinary incontinence, are the most common complaints in outpatient practice. The patient may present with urgency before having incontinence. Characteristics of urinary dysfunction also include a reduction of maximum flow rate, an increase in the residual volume, and a reduction of bladder capacity on a urodynamic test.[17]

Diagnostic Imaging

Oliveira and colleagues,[18] in accordance with International Guidelines, identified key imaging futures in diagnosing NPH (Figure 17.5):

1. Ventricular enlargement with Evans's index greater than 0.3 (Figure 17.5A).
2. Absence of macroscopic obstruction to CSF flow.
3. At least one of these supporting features:
   (a) Enlarged temporal horns of the lateral ventricles not entirely due to hippocampus atrophy;
   (b) Callosal angle of 40 degrees or greater (Figure 17.5B);
   (c) Periventricular signal changes on CT and MRI due to altered brain water content and not entirely attributable to microvascular ischemic changes or demyelination (Figure 17.5C);
   (d) Flow void in the Sylvian aqueduct or fourth ventricle on MRI.

Approach to Diagnosis

Differential diagnosis includes a high number of diseases common in older adults (Table 17.2); therefore, it is important to adequately exclude entities to avoid incorrect diagnosis. When ventriculomegaly is excluded, then NPH symptomatology becomes nonspecific: Dementia occurs in about 35% of people aged 70 years and older, urinary incontinence in 40% of women and 20% of men older than 60, and gait impairment in almost 20% of people aged older than 70.[18]

Diagnostic Procedures

Patients with secondary NPH usually get a shunt placed before discharge from the hospital. For example, patients with TBI or SAH usually have hydrocephalus complications during their hospital stay, so to achieve the best outcomes, the shunt is placed during the index hospitalization.

For those with iNPH, for a definite diagnosis and determining a patient's response to shunting, a short-term continuous lumbar drain (LD) trial is commonly used due to its sensitivity (60% to 100%) and specificity (80% to 100%).[18] Evidence supports that a large volume CSF lumbar puncture test showed a sensitivity of 28% to 62% and a specificity of 33% to 100%.

LD trial is usually performed with patients who are suspected to have iNPH. Various medical centers have their own LD trial protocols, but most commonly, all involve similar practices as follows. Prior to conducting the LD trial, each patient undergoes physical therapy (PT) evaluation. PT utilizes a validated test of functional mobility, the Timed Up and Go (TUG), and Tinetti and the Berg Balance Scale (BBS) tests. A Mini-Mental State Examination (MMSE) is also performed to evaluate cognition; some facilities even add a neuropsychologic examination. On the day of the LD trial, the patient is admitted to the hospital, where an LD is inserted by an interventional radiologist under fluoroscopy guidance. After the procedure, the patient is then admitted to a nursing floor where the nurses monitor the drain by allowing CSF to drain 5 to 10 cc/hr. On the last day of the trial, PT reevaluates the patient, performs the same tests, calculates the scores, and notes if there was an improvement. The final decision and diagnosis of NPH are made by a neurosurgeon, who will be placing and managing the shunt.

Management

There is no pharmacologic treatment for NPH. First-line and standard treatment of iNPH is the insertion of a shunt by a neurosurgeon to divert CSF. Consulting with a neurosurgeon is recommended because the patient will need long-term follow-up. There are two types of shunts. Inserting a ventriculoperitoneal (VP) shunt is a more invasive procedure but with a low failure rate, whereas inserting a lumboperitoneal (LP) shunt is a less invasive procedure.[16]

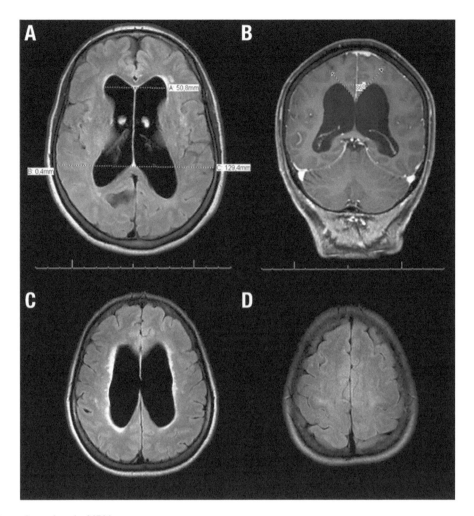

Figure 17.5: Neuroimaging in NPH

NPH, normal pressure hydrocephalus

Source: Oliveira LM, Nitrini R, Román GC. Normal-pressure hydrocephalus: a critical review. *Dement Neuropsychol.*
2019;13(2):133-143. doi:10.1590/1980-57642018dn13-020001. Erratum in: *Dement Neuropsychol.* 2019;13(3):361.

Studies show that gait is one of the most shunt-responsive symptoms, where 60% to 80% of patients report improvement in gait.[16] One group of researchers reviewed all the studies over a 7-year period and concluded that 96% of patients with NPH who received a shunt reported subjective improvement and that, when tested objectively with a timed test, 83% of people showed improvement.[12]

Numerous small studies have reported the rate of complications can be as high as 38%; however, a systematic review of the literature that included 30 studies performed between 2006 and 2020 reported an overall complication rate of 8.2%.[19] Postoperative shunt complications include infection, shunt failure, headache, and subdural hematoma/hygroma due to CSF over drainage. NPH normally affects older adults who already have multiple chronic conditions; therefore, these complications might have a greater impact on this population. Common practice is to use adjustable shunts that can be programmed to drain less fluid to prevent a subdural hematoma. One month after surgery, a CT of the head is performed to confirm stability shunt readjustment based on the patient's symptoms, if needed. The most common complication is shunt overdrainage, in which the patient complains of a headache when they are upright and their symptoms are relieved when lying flat. Symptoms of underdrainage include headaches with increased frequency and more severe upon awakening in the morning. Vomiting and dizziness may also occur. Therefore, it is important for primary care providers to identify these symptoms and direct patients back to the neurosurgeon for evaluation and adjustment of the shunt. It is also important to remember that not every headache or nausea is a sign of shunt failure; careful history must be taken to rule out other potential causes.

Table 17.2: Hydrocephalus Conditions

Vascular Dementias		Other Hydrocephalus Conditions	
Cerebrovascular disease	Binswanger's disease Subcortical infarcts Stroke Multi-infarct dementia Leukoencephalopathy Cerebral autosomal dominant arteriopathy Vertebrobasilar insufficiency	Obstructive hydrocephalus LOVA Arrested hydrocephalus Aqueductal stenosis	
Infectious diseases	Lyme borreliosis Human immunodeficiency virus Progressive multifocal leukoencephalopathy (PML) Floor laxity syphilis	Urologic diseases	Bladder and prostate cancer Benign prostatic hyperplasia Stress incontinence or pelvic urinary tract infection
Neurodegenerative diseases	Alzheimer's disease Parkinson's disease Lewy body disease Frontotemporal dementia Corticobasal degeneration Progressive supranuclear palsy Amyotrophic lateral sclerosis Huntington's disease Spongiform disease Multisystem atrophy	Miscellaneous	Epilepsy Depression B12 deficiency Collagen vascular disorders Spinal stenosis Chronic traumatic brain injury Chiari malformation Wernicke's encephalopathy Carcinomatous meningitis Spinal cord tumor Brain tumor Hyperthyroidism Organ failures Peripheral neuropathy Chronic subdural hematoma

Source: Adapted from Skalický P, Mládek A, Vlasák A, De Lacy P, Beneš V, Bradáč O. Normal pressure hydrocephalus: an overview of pathophysiological mechanisms and diagnostic procedures. *Neurosurg Rev.* 2020;43(6):1451-1464. doi:10.1007/s10143-019-01201-5

🏠 Quality and Safety Alerts

◼ For patients who have a shunt and experience neurologic deterioration, a brain CT scan should be performed to exclude possible subdural hematoma and check catheter position. A shunt series of plain radiography that visualizes the entire shunt system should be considered (checking for obstruction). An abdominal ultrasound may help detect obstruction of the shunt tip.

Patient Education

Most of the shunts that patients with NPH receive are adjustable or programmable valves; therefore, patients will need long-term follow-up by a neurosurgeon. These shunts are MRI compatible; however, due to a strong magnetic field, a shunt may need to be readjusted back to the same pre-MRI settings within 24 hours. Patients can safely travel through the airport security scanners as these will not affect the shunt setting. It is recommended that patients carry a card in their wallet with information about the shunt and the current setting.

MOVEMENT DISORDERS

Movement disorders have been described as neurologic syndromes in which there is either an excess of movement (hyperkinesia) or a paucity of voluntary and automatic movements (hypokinesia), unrelated to weakness

Table 17.3: Classification of Movement Disorders

Hypokinesias	Akinesia/Bradykinesia
	Apraxia
	Blocking (holding) ticks
	Cataplexy and drop attacks
	Catatonia, psychomotor depression, and obsession slowness
	Freezing phenomenon
	Hesitant gates
	Hyperthyroid slowness
	Rigidity
	Stiff muscles
Hyperkinesias	Abdominal dyskinesia
	Akathitic movements
	Ataxia/asynergia/dysmetria
	Athetosis
	Ballism
	Chorea
	Dystonia
	Hemifacial spasm
	Hyperekplexia
	Hypnogenic dyskinesias
	Jumping disorders
	Jumpy stumps
	Moving toes and fingers
	Myoclonus
	Myokymia and synkinesis
	Myorhythmia
	Paroxysmal dyskinesias
	Periodic movements in sleep
	REM sleep behavior disorder
	Restless legs
	Stereotypy
	Tics
	Tremor

Source: Adapted from Fahn S. Classification of movement disorders. *Mov Disord.* 2011;26(6):947-957. doi:10.1002/mds.23759.

or spasticity.[20] In the same paper, Dr. Fahn also described how he and his colleague came up with the term in 1986 when they tried to establish a clinic that would treat hyperkinetic, as well as parkinsonian, disorders at the University of Pennsylvania. In 2011 Fahn and his colleagues classified movement disorders into two groups—hypokinesias and hyperkinesias—and listed the disorders that belong to them (Table 17.3).

Pathophysiology of movement disorders is not clearly understood but it is thought that most of the disorders are accompanied by prominent and characteristic changes in firing rates and patterns in the basal ganglia, thalamus, cortex, cerebellum, and pedunculopontine nucleus, which are all highly significant in these disorders.[21]

"Tardive dyskinesia" is a medication-induced movement disorder associated with dopamine receptor blocking agents such as the first- and second-generation antipsychotic medications. Patients most often present with spontaneous movements of the mouth and tongue. However, arms, legs, trunk, and respiratory muscles may be involved. Less common is dystonia involving a focal area of the body like the neck. The best chance of recovery is early intervention. which is discontinuation of the offending medication. Avoidance of dopamine-receptor blocking agents is the best way to prevent TD. However, some patients will require these medications, so prescribing the lowest dose and for the shortest duration is necessary. The second-generation antipsychotics have a smaller chance of causing TD, so if you have to prescribe these medications consider one of these drugs. Avoid acute drug-induced parkinsonism and akathisia because these are risk factors for future TD. When prescribing antipsychotic medications, it is critical that you monitor patients for TD.

There is a lot to be known about movement disorders (there is a subspecialty within neurology just focused on movement disorders); however, we present the most common movement disorders seen in primary care, starting with PD.

PARKINSON'S DISEASE

"Shaking Palsy" was an essay published in 1817 by James Parkinson that described characteristics of a disease we now call PD.[22] PD is a movement disorder and one of the fastest growing neurologic conditions in the world.

Epidemiology

There are reports that in the industrialized countries the estimated prevalence of PD is 0.3% in the general population, 1.0% in people older than 60 years, and 3.0% in people 80 and older.[11] It was estimated that in 2016, there were 6.1 million individuals in the world with PD, and it grew by 2.4 times since 1990.[25] The sharp increase in cases has been attributed to improved methods in detecting the disease, greater awareness, longer life expectancy, and possibly increased environmental exposure, such as pesticides, solvents, and metals in industrialized countries.[25] More men than women are affected by the disease, with a ratio of 3:2 or ratio of 1.4:1; age of onset is 50 years or older, with most cases reported at age 70, but then incidence declines past 70 years of age.[23,24] Studies also show that 5% to 15% of cases occur in the same family.[23,24] However, it has been also identified that some factors decrease the incidence of PD, such as cigarette smoking, coffee drinking, calcium channel blockers, and statins;[24] more research is needed to identify the true effect of behaviors such as cigarette smoking and coffee intake and medication before we recommend these to our patients.

Pathophysiology

The cause of PD is unknown; however, the main feature is characterized by death of dopaminergic neurons in substantia nigra (subsequently it turns pale) and the presence of Lewy bodies.[24,25] It is estimated that at the time of diagnosis of PD, up to 60% of dopaminergic neurons are already lost.[24] There are multiple theories and hypotheses regarding PD. Armstrong and Okun described the most widely used Braak's hypothesis to explain the pathophysiologic progression of the disease.[25]

Braak's hypothesis suggests that there are four stages of PD. During Stages 1 and 2, PD starts in the medulla and olfactory bulb, presenting with symptoms such as decreased smell and a loss of normal rapid eye movement sleep (or muscle paralysis during this sleep stage); therefore, one will physically act out their dreams while sleeping. Stages 3 and 4 are when the disease progresses to other parts of the midbrain. During these stages, the patient presents with classic motor symptoms (see the following discussion) and is usually the time when PD is diagnosed. Finally, the hypothesis suggests that in the advanced stage, PD progresses to cerebral cortices, and patients may present with cognitive impairment and hallucinations.

Providers must also recognize that some patients might also present with conditions that exhibit PD-like symptoms, called secondary parkinsonism. Secondary parkinsonism is usually abrupt onset, and several other symptoms or antecedent diseases will be present as well. Drug-induced parkinsonism is the most common secondary parkinsonism after PD.[24] The most common drugs used to treat PD are antipsychotics, or mood stabilizers, or antidepressants; calcium channel blockers; antiemetics; medications used to treat seizures; and/or dopamine-depleting drugs. These are discussed next.

Approach to Diagnosis

Cardinal signs of PD are resting tremor (usually unilateral at first), rigidity, postural instability, bradykinesia (slowness of movement), akinesia (loss of movement), and other motor and nonmotor symptoms, such as freezing of gait and abnormal postures.[22,24] Patients can have hypographia and hypophonia as the disease progresses. Constipation and depression are often present before the actual diagnosis and can occur anytime during the progression of the disease. It is important to monitor for signs and symptoms of depression (see Chapter 18 for more information about depression and Chapter 22 for constipation).

There is still no diagnostic test to test for the disease; the gold standard for diagnosing is based on clinical criteria.[22] Tarakad and Jankovic found that diagnostic accuracy performed by movement disorder specialist at the initial assessment was 79.6% and increased to 83.9% at a follow-up visit. PD causes motor and nonmotor symptoms (Table 17.4). Nonmotor symptoms develop gradually and over the years, and patients normally do not discuss them with the provider during the visit because they may feel embarrassed, are unaware that they are part of the disease, or, many times, are never asked because the focus is usually on motor symptoms that are observed. Therefore, most often diagnosis of PD occurs quite late in the diseases, only when the patient presents with motor symptoms.

The International Parkinson and Movement Disorder Society (MDS) propose an official Clinical Diagnostic Criteria for Parkinson's Disease. These criteria were proposed in 2015, and it was intended for use in clinical research as well as to guide clinical diagnosis.[28] Clinical diagnostic criteria for PD require an individual to have bradykinesia and at least two of four supportive criteria: (a) resting tremor, (b) a dramatic improvement with dopaminergic therapy, (c) the presence of levodopa-induced dyskinesias, or (d) olfactory loss or positive myocardial innervation imaging.[63] Great attention must be paid to the absolute exclusion criteria (if present, rule out the disease), and there must be no red flags (Box 17.6 and Box 17.7).

The resting tremor seen in PD usually begins as unilateral, so if a patient presents with an action tremor the diagnosis is most likely essential tremor (ET), the most common neurologic disorder that causes action tremors. The risk increases with age, although it can affect young adults, especially if familial. ET most often affects the hands and arms and can be asymmetric. Less often you can see ET involving the head, voice, trunk, and legs. The evaluation for patients with tremors is a thorough history and physical examination and certain laboratory tests (i.e., thyroid; screening for heavy metal poisoning, such as mercury or arsenic, if an environmental cause is suspected; hypoglycemia). Disorders that can cause tremors are hyperthyroidism, PD, dystonia, Wilson disease, or drugs. Paying attention to the age of onset and evolution of tremor is important. A detailed neurologic examination must be performed to identify clinical manifestations of tremors and what are the activating conditions.

Table 17.4: Parkinson's Disease Symptoms

Parkinson's Disease Symptoms		
Motor	Gait disturbance:	Freezing of gait
		Festination
		Start/target/ obstacle hesitation
	Slowed movements	Bradykinesia
		Akinesia
		Hypokinesia
	Hypomimia	
	Micrographia	
	Alterations in blinking/ eye movement	
	Resting tremor	Tremor not present during movement and temporarily disappears when the limb is held outstretched
	Rigidity	Resistance to passive movement
Nonmotor	Psychiatric symptoms	Depression
		Anxiety
		Apathy
		Hallucinations
		Psychosis
	Genitourinary symptoms	Urinary frequency
		Urgency
		Reduced libido
		Sexual dysfunction
	Cardiovascular symptoms	Blood pressure variations: postural, postprandial, dysrhythmias
	Dementia Cognitive impairment	Initially affecting attention, executive, and visuospatial functions
	Sensory symptoms	Pain
		Visual dysfunction
		Olfactory disturbance
	Sleep	Disturbances
		Wakefulness
		Daytime sleepiness
	Hyposmia	
	Fatigue	
	Hypophonia	
	Gastrointestinal symptoms	
	Trouble swallowing Sialorrhea	

Source: Adapted from Armstrong MJ, Okun MS. Diagnosis and treatment of Parkinson disease: a review. *JAMA*. 2020;323(6):548–560. doi:10.1001/jama.2019.22360; Tarakad A, Jankovic J. Diagnosis and management of Parkinson's disease. *Semin Neurol*. 2017;37(2):118–126. doi:10.1055/s-0037-1601888; Balestrino R, Schapira AHV. Parkinson disease. *Eur J Neurol*. 2020;27(1):27–42. doi:10.1111/ene.14108

Box 17.6: Exclusion Criteria

1. Cerebellar abnormalities (cerebellar gait, limb ataxia, or oculomotor abnormalities)
2. Downward vertical supranuclear gaze palsy
3. Diagnosis of frontotemporal dementia or primary progressive aphasia
4. Parkinsonian features restricted to the lower limbs for more than 3 years
5. Treatment with a dopamine receptor blocker or a dopamine-depleting agent
6. Absence of response to high-dose levodopa
7. Unequivocal cortical sensory loss, clear limb ideomotor apraxia, or progressive aphasia
8. Normal functional neuroimaging of the presynaptic dopaminergic system
9. Documentation of an alternative condition known to produce parkinsonism

Source: Adapted from Postuma RB, Berg D, Stern M, et al. MDS clinical diagnostic criteria for Parkinson's disease. *Mov Disord*. 2015;30(12):1591–1601. doi:10.1002/mds.26424

Box 17.7: Red Flags

1. Rapid progression of gait impairment with regular use of wheelchair within 5 years of onset
2. A complete absence of progression of motor symptoms or signs over 5 or more
3. Early and severe dysphonia, dysarthria, or dysphagia within first 5 years
4. Inspiratory respiratory dysfunction: either diurnal or nocturnal

(continued)

5. Severe autonomic failure in the first 5 years of disease:
   - Orthostatic hypotension
   - Severe urinary retention or urinary incontinence in the first 5 years of disease
6. Recurrent (>1/year) falls because of impaired balance within 3 years of onset
7. Disproportionate dystonia or contractures of hand or feet within the first 10 years
8. Absence of any of the common nonmotor features of disease despite 5-year disease duration.
   - Sleep dysfunction (sleep-maintenance insomnia, excessive daytime somnolence, symptoms of REM sleep behavior disorder)
   - Autonomic dysfunction (constipation, daytime urinary urgency, symptomatic orthostasis)
   - Hyposmia
   - Psychiatric dysfunction (depression, anxiety, or hallucinations)
9. Unexplained spasticity and weakness (lower extremities) or clear pathologic hyperreflexia
10. Bilateral symmetric parkinsonism.

Source: Adapted from Postuma RB, Berg D, Stern M, et al. MDS clinical diagnostic criteria for Parkinson's disease. Mov Disord. 2015;30(12):1591-1601. doi:10.1002/mds.26424

Management

Management of PD is complex, and it must be tailored to the specific needs of the individual as patients experience motor and nonmotor symptoms of various intensities. The International Parkinson and Movement Disorder Society 2018 concluded that to date, there are no interventions to prevent or slow disease progression; however, interventions for treating motor symptoms continue to become available with emerging evidence. There are four major categories of pharmacologic agents that are used in treating PD in addition to other compounds (see Table 17.5). It is beyond the scope of a primary care NP to diagnose and treat patients with PD; however, it is essential that NPs recognize when a patient may have PD and make an appropriate referral to a neurologist (best would be to a movement disorder specialist if available). There are movement disorder centers at which an interprofessional team collaborates about managing patients with PD and providing support for family members.

PD is a complex disorder: There are no therapies available to stop the neurodegeneration, and only symptomatic treatments are available. At the early stages of the disease, pharmacologic treatments work well to help patients with rigidity and tremors, prevent falls, or reduce freezing of gait. As the disease progresses

medications are less effective, and patients are left to face other complications of PD. Other complications include anxiety and depression, difficulty swallowing, sleep disorders, hallucinations, fatigue, pain, BP variability, falls, dysarthria, urinary incontinence, cognitive impairment, and complications associated with long-term pharmacologic treatment. In advanced PD, patients are left to face severe disability, a loss of independence, and significantly reduced quality of life. Caregiver burden may be high, requiring increased supportive services. Taking a person-centered co management with neurologist approach to care is critical because although the symptoms are similar, living with the disease can vary from patient to patient.

Pharmacologic
Levodopa
The gold standard and initial treatment of PD motor symptoms is levodopa. Recent research shows that individuals treated with levodopa had small but persistent mobility benefits 7 years after initiation and improvement in performing ADLs.[63] This study was conducted over a 7-year period, and it was also observed that patients receiving levodopa, especially with higher doses, were more likely to develop dyskinesias. When treating a patient with levodopa, the benefit of medications is "ON" time, and when medications wear off, the "OFF" time manifests as tremor, dyskinesia, and other motor symptoms.[63] Carbidopa-levodopa, long-acting formulation, has been shown to reduce motor fluctuations and dyskinesias while maintaining "on" time.[22] In advanced disease, when the patient may have dysphagia, a combination of levodopa–carbidopa intestinal gel can reduce the motor symptoms without bothersome dyskinesia; however, surgical intervention requires placing a gastrostomy catheter.[11,3] Discussion about placing a gastrostomy tube for nutritional reasons and medications administration should include the patient and family; the benefits, risks, and alternatives are part of the conversation. Levodopa agents also remain the first choice in treating freezing of gait.[4]

Subthalamic Nucleus Deep Brain Stimulation
Subthalamic nucleus deep brain stimulation (STN-DBS) is a surgical option that helps to reduce dyskinesias and optimize levodopa effects.[3] Research shows that STN-DBS is superior to pharmacologic treatment, effective in controlling motor symptoms, motor complications, and some nonmotor symptoms, and its use in long-term patients led to reduced doses of medications.[24] DBS is recommended for those patients when medications reach such high doses that the patient can no longer tolerate the side effects or cannot tolerate the medication event at small doses; in addition, motor symptoms are so severe that patients cannot work or have a good quality of

Table 17.5: Pharmacologic Agents Used for Motor Symptoms in PD

Category (Specific Agent)	Most Common Adverse Effects	Therapeutic Uses: Early Symptomatic, Levodopa Adjunct, Wearing Off, Dyskinesia
Levodopa:		
• Carbidopa-Levodopa IR • Carbidopa-Levodopa CR • Carbidopa-Levodopa ER • Inhaled Levodopa	All preparation causes nausea. Inhaled might also cause upper respiratory tract infections.	Inhaled not used for early use of treatment and dyskinesias
Nonergot Dopamine Agonist:		
• Pramipexole IR or ER • Ropinirole IR or ER • Rotigotine transdermal • Apomorphine injection	Orthostatic hypotension, dizziness, nausea, sleepiness, and might cause site reactions	Injection is used only for wearing off symptoms
Monoamine Oxidase-B Inhibitors		
• Selegiline • Rasagiline • Safinamide • Zonisamide	Nausea, dizziness, orthostatic hypotension; Selegiline might cause insomnia	Zonisamide used only for wearing off
Catechot-O-Methyltransferase Inhibitors		
• Entacapone • Opicapone • Tolcapone	Nausea, diarrhea, falls, insomnia, orthostatic hypotension, GI symptoms, sleep disorders, falls	All agents used only for wearing off or dyskinesias
Other:		
• Antiholinergics	Dizziness, anxiety	Used for early symptoms and as levodopa agent
• Amantadine	Orthostatic hypotension, hallucinations, edema, gastrointestinal symptoms	Not used for wearing off
• Istradefylline	Nausea, hallucinations	Used only for wearing off
• Clozapine	Sleepiness, dizziness, tachycardia, constipation, orthostatic hypotension, sialorrhea	Used only for dyskinesias

CR, controlled release; ER, extended release; IR, immediate release; PD, Parkinson's disease.
Source: Armstrong MJ, Okun MS. Diagnosis and treatment of Parkinson disease: a review. *JAMA*. 2020;323(6):548–560. doi:10.1001/jama.2019.22360

life. Evidence supports that many patients who received DBS have improved quality of life, are able to return to activities they enjoy, and are able to return to work if appropriate. Patients who are interested or referred for DBS must be carefully selected by a multidisciplinary team and meet the following: (a) must respond well to levodopa agents, (b) device may worsen psychiatric symptoms, (c) can worsen cognitive function, and (d) may worsen speech disturbances.[24] Every patient undergoes a lengthy neurocognitive evaluation by a neurologist to make sure that there is no underlying psychiatric or cognitive disease. The neurosurgeon implanting the device also reviews with the patient and sets clear expectations of what the device can do and possible side effects.

Dopamine

Dopamine agonist medications are the first choice in younger patients and only for mild to moderate PD symptoms with the goal to delay levodopa treatment and to avoid dyskinesias.[63] Impulse control disorders, such as gambling, compulsive spending, and abnormal sexual or eating disorders, were associated in 40% of patients receiving a dopamine agonist.[63] Dopamine should also be used with caution in patients with cognitive impairment such as orthostatic hypotension, hallucinations, confusion, somnolence, leg edema, and impulse control disorders.[22]

Monoamine Oxidase-B Inhibitors

Adding monoamine oxidase B (MAO-B) inhibitors helps prolong the benefits of levodopa by blocking enzymes that degrade dopamine.[63] Early treatment with an MAO-B inhibitor delayed the additional dopaminergic therapy; however, the natural course of PD was not modified.[24] Trials have also shown that adding MAO-B inhibitors to the treatment regimen showed a reduction in freezing of gait after 3 months of treatment.[4]

Pharmacologic Treatment for Essential Tremor

The pharmacologic treatment for essential tremor (ET) is beta-blocker propranolol; you may also consider primidone and anticonvulsant agent. Propranolol can be used as monotherapy or in combination with primidone. The initial dose is 60 to 80 mg/day (may choose intermediate-release or extended-release formulation); increase dose as needed based on response and tolerability. The usual dose range is 60 mg to 320 mg/day. There are no renal dose adjustments.

The initial dose of primidone is 50 mg to 62.5 mg once daily, and the dose is increased gradually based on the response and tolerability of the patient. Dose increases are increments of 62.5 mg to 125 mg every 1 to 3 days or by 250 mg every week and administered in two to three divided doses. Lower maintenance doses have been found to be equally or more effective than higher doses, and this can benefit the patient with fewer adverse effects. This medication should be avoided in those with end-stage kidney disease (ESKD) and will require renal dose adjustments for those with chronic kidney disease (CKD). Other second-line medications include topiramate and gabapentin.

Catechol-O-Methyl Transferase (COMT) Inhibitors

Metabolism of levodopa occurs through COMT enzymes; therefore, by inhibiting these enzymes researchers were able to increase the half-life of levodopa.[24] COMT inhibitors used together with levodopa prolong on time and decrease the off time, reducing motor fluctuations altogether.[3,10]

Other Compounds

Anticholinergic drugs have been found to improve some motor symptoms, such as tremors, but unfortunately worsen cognitive deficits.[24] Extended-release amantadine that has an anticholinergic component is able to decrease levodopa-induced dyskinesia symptoms.[24]

Nonpharmacologic

The International Parkinson and Movement Disorder Society in 2018 suggested that dietary supplements or nutritional supplements such as Q10, creatinine, and vitamin D remain popular among people with PD; unfortunately, little research has been done and what has been completed has not demonstrated efficacy.

There are PD rehabilitation programs that have demonstrated effectiveness in helping patients have a better quality of life. One such program is Lee Silverman Voice Treatment (LSVT) and Big and Loud programs (www.lsvtglobal.com). Big is an evidence-based exercise program that teaches the person how to move to their fullest potential, and Loud is a method for treating speech and voice impairments. Support groups can be helpful for patients and families.

Patient Education

Patient/family education is essential. There are many resources available to assist you in educating patients:

- American Parkinson's Disease Association: www.apdaparkinson.org/resources-support
- Parkinson's Foundation: www.parkinson.org/understanding-parkinsons
- Michael J Fox Foundation: www.michaeljfox.org

HEADACHES

Etiology

Headaches are among the most common complaints in primary care. Headaches can be classified into two groups: primary and secondary. Primary headaches, a condition without an underlying disease, are more common in primary care than secondary headaches. Secondary headaches are usually caused by another etiology, such as vascular disease (i.e., stroke or aneurysms), brain trauma, infection, and psychiatric disorder. Paying attention to red flags that may indicate a serious underlying condition is important when assessing for secondary headaches (see Box 17.8). Primary headaches can be classified as migraine, tension-type, and trigeminal autonomic cephalgia (most common are cluster headaches), with the most frequent being episodic tension-type headache. Trigeminal autonomic cephalgia is an uncommon diagnosis in primary care but can lead to significant disability.[29]

The most common primary headaches are migraines, tension headache, and trigeminal autonomic cephalgia (cluster headaches). It is estimated that 90% of patients who present to primary care for evaluation have primary

Box 17.8: Quality and Safety Alerts

Red Flags:
Presenting Symptoms of Headache May Be Secondary to a Serious Underlying Condition

- Fever
- Neoplasm history
- Neurologic deficit
- Onset sudden or abrupt
- Adult older than age 50
- Pattern different from usual headache
- Papilledema and change in mental status
- Positional headache
- Progressive headache and atypical presentation
- Precipitated by sneezing, coughing, or exercising
- Progressive headache and atypical presentations
- Pregnancy or puerperium
- Painful eye with autonomic features
- Posttraumatic onset of headache
- Immune system compromised such as in HIV
- Taking pain medication (overuse) or new medication at onset of headache
- Worst headache of one's life

Source: Do TP, Remmers A, Schytz HW, et al. Red and orange flags for secondary headaches in clinical practice: SNNOOP10 list. Neurology. 2019;92:134. doi:10.1212/WNL.0000000000006697; Rizzoli P, Mullally WJ. Headache. Am J Med. 2018;131(1):17–24. doi:10.1016/j.amjmed.2017.09.005

headache disorders and often undergo unnecessary imaging with total costs of more than $1 billion per year.[29] Headaches affect about 50% of the adult population; about 50% of those have acute tension-type headaches and 10% have migraines.[6] About 3% to 4% of patients with episodic headaches (tension or migraine) become chronic. The cost of chronic migraines ($8,250) is three times the cost of episodic migraines ($2,650) each year.[31] In the United States, it is estimated that due to the migraines, there are 112 million collective workdays lost annually, which estimates to $16 billion productivity loss and $1 billion in medical costs.[33]

Migraines are a major health condition that can lead to many years of lost productivity and can impact daily life for those who have chronic migraines. According to the Global Burden of Disease study 2019, migraines remain the second overall cause of disability in both genders and all ages; however, young women have the highest prevalence of migraines. Migraines are the third-most prevalent disorder in the world.[11]

Pathophysiology

The pathophysiology of headaches depends on the classification. Tension-type headaches (TTH) are the most common types of headaches in the general population. There are three main types: infrequent (less than 1 day a month), frequent episodic (episodes 1–14 days a month), and chronic headaches (15 days or more a month). Precise mechanisms for TTH are not known, but the environment seems to be a major contributor to episodic TTH. The chronic TTH seems to be due to the sensitization of pain pathways in the CNS due to prolonged nociceptive stimuli from pericranial myofascial tissue.[34] Pathophysiology is complex, but in simple terms can be described as genetically induced hypersensitivity of the brain to homeostatic changes that act as headache triggers, subsequently causing complex vascular and nerve activation that is difficult to control and extinguish.[29]

Risk Factors

Key risks for progression to chronic headaches include the following:

- Acute medication use month after month at greater than 2 days per month
- Stress and life events, particularly with unrecognized/untreated anxiety and/or depression
- Obesity
- Caffeine use.[53]

Approach to Diagnosis

Obtaining a comprehensive history is crucial in the diagnosis of headaches (Box 17.9).

Box 17.9: Questions to Ask During the Examination

- Family history of migraine
- Childhood migraine proxy symptoms: carsickness, gastrointestinal complaints
- Age of onset
- Frequency, severity, and tempo over time
- Triggering, aggravating, or alleviating features
- Autonomic features
- Aura features
- Current and prior treatments
- Lifestyle features
- Comorbid conditions

Source: Rizzoli P, Mullally WJ. Headache. Am J Med. 2018;131(1):17–24. doi:10.1016/j.amjmed.2017.09.005

MIGRAINES

Migraines are usually caused by triggers such as stress, menstruation, visual stimuli, weather changes, nitrates, drinking wine, sleep disturbances, and aspartame. Migraines can be disabling, and there are two major types: migraine without auras—a clinical syndrome characterized by headache with specific features and associated symptoms (Table 17.6)—and migraine with aura—primarily characterized by the transient focal neurologic symptoms that usually precede or occasionally accompany the headache.

Migraines are episodic and the most common complaint is a severe headache usually associated with nausea and/or light (photophobia) and sound sensitivity (phonophobia).

Migraines can be described in four phases: prodrome, aura, headache phase, and postdrome.

Prodrome phase may be present in up to 60% of patients, can start hours or days prior to the headache, and consists of multiple symptoms, such as hyperactivity, depression, cravings for a particular food, irritability, repetitive yawning, fatigue, and neck stiffness.[29] During postdrome phase, some feel fatigue and have impaired concentration, whereas others feel refreshed and hyperactive.[29] The POUND mnemonic can be used for the diagnosis of migraine (see Box 17.10).

Box 17.10: POUND Pneumonic for Diagnosis of Migraine Headache

- ■ **P**ulsating or throbbing pain
- ■ **O**ne-day average duration
- ■ **U**nilateral location
- ■ **N**ausea or vomiting
- ■ **D**isabling

Source: Ebell MH. Diagnosis of migraine headache. *Am Fam Physician.* 2006;74(12):2087-2088. https://www.aafp.org/afp/2006/1215/p2087.html

TENSION-TYPE HEADACHES

Patients with TTH may present or complain that the headache is mild to moderate intensity, bilateral, and non-throbbing; many times, the complaint is nonspecific with descriptions such as "dull," "pressure," "head fullness," "feels like a tight cap," or a "heavy weight on my head or shoulders." The pain can be severe, but this is not common. There may be tenderness of pericranial myofascial tissue, and the number of myofascial trigger points is increased. There may be muscle tenderness of the head, neck, or shoulder. It is important to perform manual palpation of the pericranial muscle. Ask the patient about stress and emotional tension that may have precipitated the headache.

TTH diagnosis is based on history and clinical presentation. The International Classification of Headache Disorders, Third Edition (ICHD-3) has diagnostic criteria for TTH, which are in Table 17.7.

Obtaining a headache diary (document date, duration, symptoms, treatment, outcome of each headache episode) can help, but keep in mind that patients may not be

Table 17.6: International Classification of Headache Disorders, Third Edition

International Classification of Headache Disorders (ICHD-3) Third Edition
Migraine Without Aura Diagnostic Criteria
1. Headache attacks lasting 4 to 72 hours (when untreated or unsuccessfully treated) 2. Headache must have two of the following characteristics: • unilateral location • pulsating quality • moderate or severe pain intensity • aggravation by or causing avoidance of routine physical activity (e.g., walking or climbing stairs) 3. During headache at least one of the following: • nausea and/or vomiting • photophobia and phonophobia 4. Not better accounted for by another disease diagnosis.

Source: Adapted from Olla D, Sawyer J, Sommer N, Moore JB 4th. Migraine treatment. *Clin Plast Surg.* 2020;47(2):295-303. doi:10.1016/j.cps.2020.01.003

Table 17.7: Diagnostic Criteria for Tension-Type Headache

Classification of TTH	Criteria
Episodic TTH *Infrequent episodic* TTH is when episodes occur on fewer than 1 day per month on average (fewer than 12 days per year) *Frequent episodic* TTH is when headache episodes occur 1 to 14 days a month on average (12 or greater and 180 or fewer days per year)	At least two of the following: • bilateral location • pressing or tightening (nonpulsating) quality • mild to moderate intensity • not aggravated by routine physical activity such as walking or climbing stairs Both of the following: • no nausea or vomiting • no more than one photophobia or phonophobia

(continued)

Table 17.7: Diagnostic Criteria for Tension-Type Headache (*continued*)

Chronic TTH	A. Headache occurring on 15 or more days per month on average, for more than 3 months (180 days or more) and meeting criteria B through D
	B. Lasting hours to days or unremitting
	C. At least two of the following:
	Bilateral location
	Pressing or tightening (nonpulsating) quality
	Mild to moderate intensity
	Not aggravated by routine physical activity such as walking or climbing stairs
	D. Both of the following
	No more than one photophobia, phonophobia, or mild nausea
	Neither moderate nor severe nausea or vomiting
	E. Not better accounted for by another ICHD-3 diagnosis

Source: Headache Classification Committee of the International Headache Society. The International Classification of Headache Disorders, 3rd edition. *Cephalalgia*. 2018;38(1): 1-211. doi:10.1177/0333102417738202

consistent when completing the diary. When obtaining the history, ask the same questions as in the headache diary along with questions related to the classification of headache. Try to identify the most likely reason for the headache and assess for the underlying condition. If there is the possibility of an underlying serious condition, then perform an urgent assessment and intervene as appropriate. If there is a low probability, then determine if migraine, TTH, or possibly another cause (e.g., cluster headache) is responsible.

TRIGEMINAL AUTONOMIC CEPHALGIA (CLUSTER HEADACHE)

Cluster headache is also known as "suicide headache" because pain is extremely severe unilateral orbital pain associated with increased lacrimation, nasal congestion/ discharge, and partial Horner's; it is more common in men, is episodic, and produces restlessness, characterized by "clusters" with one to eight episodes per day lasting from 2 weeks to 3 months.[29] There are two forms of treatment: acute and preventative.

Diagnostics

Neuroimaging is not recommended in patients with primary headaches unless the person has a nonacute headache and unexplained abnormal finding on neurologic examination or atypical headache or headaches that don't meet diagnostic criteria for TTH or migraine. Another cause of headaches is medication overuse. In addition to red flags (Box 17.10) identified during the history and examination, a CT of the head may be necessary.

Management

Preventative treatment is the best approach for headaches; when there is a need to treat, it is essential to take a person-centered approach. It is essential to listen to the patient, paying attention to possible triggers or other indicators of TTHs or cluster headaches. There are four types: pharmacologic, nonpharmacologic, nonsurgical, and surgical. TTHs are typically not as severe as migraine headaches; however, they are far more common, with a lifetime prevalence in the general population of up to 80%.[29] There are three main types: infrequent (less than 1 day a month), frequent episodic (episodes 1 to 14 days a month), and chronic headaches (15 days or more a month).

Pharmacologic

Migraine Treatment

Pharmacologic treatment of migraines includes prophylactic and abortive medications (Table 17.8). The goal of abortive medications is for them to be used early in the attack for quicker relief and add later preventative medications of poor response. The use of preventative medications is recommended if, during a 1-month period, there are 6 days with headaches, the patient is impaired for 4 days, or complete disability occurs for 3 days.[29]

Treatment for Episodic Tension-Type Headaches

Treatment is only abortive, with nonsteroidal anti-inflammatory drugs (NSAIDs) having been shown to be most effective. Evidence supports that the best pharmacologic option is the combination of ibuprofen 400 mg and acetaminophen 1,000 mg.[11] Shah and Hameed also found that aspirin use was equivalent to placebo and that muscle relaxants had no efficacy in treating episodic TTH.[11]

Treatment for Chronic Tension-Type Headaches

Amitriptyline (tricyclic antidepressant) was found to be the most effective drug; it should be started at very low doses initially, and it takes about 3 to 4 weeks to reach an effect. The medication can be discontinued in 6 months, but if TTH returns, the medication can then be used long term.[11] Patient education plays a very important part when using amitriptyline, as the patient might be impatient and discontinue the drug prematurely or escalate the dose too fast and experience undesired side effects. Side effects include dry mouth, dizziness,

Table 17.8: Pharmacologic, Nonpharmacologic Treatment for Migraines

Prophylactic	Reduce the frequency and severity of the migraine attacks	Antihypertensives: 1. Beta-blockers • Atenolol (Tenormin) • Propranolol • Metoprolol • Nadolol 2. Calcium channel blockers • Diltiazem (Cardizem LA) • Nimodipine (Nimotop) • Verapamil (Isoptin, Calan) 3. Angiotensin-converting enzyme inhibitors • Lisinopril (Prinivil/Zestril) • Candesartan (Atacand) Antidepressants • Paroxetine (Paxil) • Fluoxetine (Prozac) • Sertraline (Zoloft) • Amitriptyline (Elavil) • Nortriptyline (Nortriptyline Hydrochloride, Nortriptyline Hydrochloride Oral Solution, Pamelor) • Imipramine • Doxopin (Silenor) • Protriptyline (Vivactil) Anticonvulsants • Topiramate (Topamax) • Gabapentin (Neurontin) • Divalproex sodium (Depakote) Antihistamines • Benadryl • Claritin Herbals • Feverfew • Butterbur • Coenzyme Q10 (CoQ10) • Magnesium supplements
Abortive	Prevent an individual migraine attack or to stop it once it starts	Triptans • Sumatriptan (Imitrex) • Rizatriptan (Maxalt) • Naratriptan (Amerge)

(continued)

Table 17.8: Pharmacologic, Nonpharmacologic Treatment for Migraines (*continued*)

Abortive	Prevent an individual migraine attack or to stop it once it starts	Triptans
		   • Zolmitriptan (Zomig)
		   • Eletriptan (Relpax)
		   • Almotriptan (Axert)
		   • Frovatriptan (Frova)
		Nonsteroidal anti-inflammatory drugs
		   • Naproxen (Naprosyn, Anaprox, Anaprox DS)
		   • Ibuprofen (Motrin, Advil)
		   • Ketorolac (last resort)
		Combination analgesics
		   • Acetaminophen, caffeine, and aspirin
		Corticosteroids
		   • Dexamethasone
		   • Prednisone
		Narcotics
		   • Butalbital
		   • Tramadol
		   • Codeine
		   • Norco
		   • Oxycodone

Nonsurgical	Prophylactic treatment to prevent migraine headaches or lessen their severity	Botulinum toxin type A(BTX-A) injections
Surgical	Reduction in frequency, severity, or duration or complete elimination	Surgical release of trigger points

urinary retention, cardiac arrhythmias, and glaucoma. Medications that showed no efficacy or very poor response were selective serotonin reuptake inhibitors, serotonin/norepinephrine reuptake inhibitors, and muscle relaxants, and even botulinum toxin type A has varying efficacy.[11]

Nonpharmacology

Nonpharmacologic treatment for migraines consists of behavior modifications, such as avoiding triggers like certain foods or limiting alcohol intake, managing stress, implementing sleep hygiene measures, and avoiding a sedentary lifestyle.

There are multiple nonpharmacologic treatment options for TTH. These include physical therapy (relaxation, posture improvement, exercise), biofeedback, cognitive behavioral therapy, massage, manipulation, acupuncture, and osteopathic manipulative medicine, which have also shown improvement in both acute and chronic presentations, using measures such as increasing range of motion of the head.[11,29]

Medication Overuse Headache

One of the disadvantages of current antimigraine medications is the induction of a headache. "Medication overuse headache" (MOH) is defined as a headache for more than 15 days per month in a person with a preexisting primary headache, developing because of regular overuse of acute or symptomatic headache medication.[35] "Overuse is also defined as 15 or more days per month for nonopioid analgesics and 10 or more days a month for ergotamine, triptans, opioids, and combination of drugs from more than one class."[31] MOH has no specific clinical symptoms and may vary among patients. Usually, the patient may describe insidious onset of increasingly frequent headaches mostly upon awakening or early in the day. Neck pain is common, and autonomic and vasomotor inability are often present. Many patients have sleep disturbances, especially depression, anxiety, and obsessive-compulsive disorders. Diagnosis is based on a thorough history. Therefore, patients should keep not only a diary to record their headaches but also a record of acute treatment as well.

Table 17.9: Treatment for Cluster Headaches

Acute treatment	Oxygen therapy	Effective in less than 10 min No side effects However, mostly not covered by insurance
	Triptans • Sumatriptan (subcutaneous injection) • Zolmitriptan (nasal spray)	An oral medication of any form is not recommended, as the time of onset is often longer than the headache
	Other: • Intranasal lidocaine (with reported 33% response) • Octreotide • Ergotamine	
Preventative treatment	Suboccipital blockade	Adverse events are nonserious such as injection site pain and low-level headache
	Verapamil	Regular ECGs to monitor cardiac function Only C-level evidence
	Other: • Lithium • Oral steroids • Valproic acid • Melatonin • Intranasal capsaicin	
Surgical treatment for drug resistance	Electrical stimulation Vagus nerve stimulation	Stimulations of sphenopalatine ganglion, occipital nerve, and vagus nerve
	Deep brain stimulation	Stimulation of hypothalamus

Source: Kandel SA, Mandiga P. Cluster headache. In: *StatPearls.* StatPearls Publishing; 2021. https://www.ncbi.nlm.nih.gov/books/NBK544241

Patient Education

It is important to discuss preventative strategies and treatment with patients. Websites that can assist with patient education follow:

- NIH: www.ninds.nih.gov/Disorders/All-Disorders/Headache-Information-Page
- National Headache Foundation: https://headaches.org
- American Headache Society: https://americanheadachesociety.org

BRAIN CANCER

Brain tumors, masses or clusters of abnormal cells in the brain, are called primary CNS tumors and are divided into two groups: benign and malignant. Tumors that arise from other cancers in the body are called metastatic tumors. Benign tumors do not invade healthy cells, have clear borders, and grow slowly; examples are meningiomas, pituitary adenoma, schwannoma, and craniopharyngioma, among others.[36] Malignant brain tumors invade healthy cells, and the tumor borders are not clearly visible and grow quickly; examples include glioma, ependymal, or pineal tumors.[36] Further brain tumors are classified by World Health Organization (WHO) standards according to how fast the brain tumors grow, from grade I, the slowest, to grade to II, III, and IV, the fastest growing. Brain tumors are further classified into stages of how fast they spread to nearby cells.[36] Stage 0 means that the tumor is cancerous but has not spread to nearby cells. Stages 1 through 3 mean that cells are cancerous and spread rapidly, while Stage 4 means that cancer spreads throughout the body.

Etiology

The most common brain tumors in adults are meningiomas, gliomas, and intercranial metastasis from systemic cancer; therefore, we discuss them in more detail later. The most common malignant brain tumors, representing 75% of all malignant brain tumors, are gliomas; they arise from glial or precursor cells.[37] Glioblastomas are the most common glioma, making up 15% of all primary brain tumors and 45% of all malignant tumors, with an incidence of 3.2 per 100,000, with a median age at diagnosis of 64 years.[38] Brain metastases comprise the majority of brain tumors, with an incidence 10 times more common than primary tumors, while meningiomas account for 35% of all primary tumors.[38] It is also important to mention that often seen in primary care clinics are the pituitary tumors and cancers that metastasize to the spinal cord: leptomeninges (covering of the spinal cord), conus medullaris, epidural spaces (will cause compressions of the spinal cord), and even individual nerves.[38] The Central Brain Tumor Registry of the United States (CBTRUS) 2020 (https://cbtrus.org/cbtrus-fact-sheet-2020) has data from 2013 to 2017 that have been analyzed indicating that the incidence rate of all brain and other CNS tumors in the United States was 23.79 cases per 100,000, with the rate being higher in women. The data show that the incidence worldwide was 3.5 per 100,000. Incidence rates by sex were 3.9 per 100,000 in males and 3.1 per 100,000 in females. In addition, incidence rates were higher in high-income countries (5.1 per 100,000) than in low-middle (2.2 per 100,000) or low-income countries (1.5 per 100,000). The average annual mortality rate in the United States between 2013 and 2017 was 4.42 per 100,000 population.

Pathophysiology

The main cause of cancer is an uncontrolled growth of cells that occurs when the DNA sequence is altered by mutation and the gene malfunctions due to environment, lifestyle, eating habits, sunlight, and even viruses.[36] There are three categories of genes that are responsible for cancer: (a) tumor suppressors that control the cell death cycle, (b) malfunctioning of repair DNA genes, and (c) proto-oncogenes that fail to control the cell division cycle.[36]

Risk Factors

There have been multiple studies showing that industrial exposures and an association among tobacco, alcohol, or dietary factors may contribute to brain cancer; unfortunately, most of the studies were inconclusive and did not show clear evidence.[39] For a majority of patients with glioblastoma (GBM) brain tumor, less than 5% had critical germline alteration, fewer than 20% had a strong family history of cancer, and very few patients developed GBM after ionizing radiation.[40]

Approach to Diagnosis

Clinical presentation of any tumor is usually related to the functional properties of the brain structure it arises from. See Table 17.10 to review the structures and the functions of the brain to help understand the signs and symptoms

patients may present with. Although primary care NPs will not diagnose and treat brain tumors, it is important to recognize the signs and symptoms to inform the appropriate referral to a neurologist. Some tumors grow very slow, cause no harm to the brain, and are usually incidentally found during a workup after a fall or traumatic accident. Some patients may present with nonspecific signs such as seizure (50%–80% cases), headaches (30% cases), and symptoms of increased ICP (15% of cases; headaches worse at night, morning nausea/vomiting, drowsiness, blurred vision with papilledema, horizontal diplopia).[37]

A brain cancer diagnosis can be invasive or noninvasive. A noninvasive approach is brain scanning with CT and MRI. MRI with contrast is more superior over the CT as a radiologist can identify the tumor in greater detail and it helps for surgical planning as well. The gold standard for brain cancer diagnosis is by obtaining a biopsy.[37]

Management

Glioblastomas

Malignant brain tumors are very difficult to treat due to fast tumor progression and reoccurrence. The European Organization for Research and Treatment of Cancer and the National Cancer Institute of Canada Clinical Trials Group in 2005 published guidelines of postoperative management of glioblastoma called "stupp protocol." Upon diagnosis of glioblastoma, it is imperative that an experienced neurosurgeon safely removes the maximum amount of tumor, followed by "stupp protocol" that entails close monitoring and management by the neurooncologist with chemotherapy in combination with a long course of radiation treatment by a radiation oncologist.[23] Unfortunately, these patients have only a 5-year overall survival.[37,40] Gliomas are further divided into glioblastomas, astrocytoma, oligodendrogliomas, and ependymomas. Meningiomas are tumors of the meninges (covering of the brain) that are often benign and surgically removed.

Meningioma

Treatment of meningioma depends on pathology findings (Table 17.11). No treatment is indicated for benign meningioma with total gross resection. For grades II and III meningioma subtotal resection, radiation is recommended. Chemotherapy in the past was used mostly as salvage therapy due to its limited role; however, recent studies have found novel oncogenic mutations that may respond to therapeutic agents; more research is underway.[37]

Metastatic Tumors

There is no universal standard for how to care for patients with metastatic brain tumor; it usually depends on the type of tumor, and prognosis is poor due to many having advanced systemic disease.[38] Treatments are usually palliative; however, if the patient is young, has excellent performance status, and has a tumor with an estimated

Table 17.10: Signs and Symptoms

Brain Structure	Function	Example of Signs and Symptoms
Frontal lobe	• Higher intellectual functions: consciousness and responsiveness to outside stimuli • Personality • Motor coordination for swallowing, salivation, vocalization, chewing, facial expressions, hand, arm, torso, pelvis, and foot	Patient might present with limb weakness or dysphasia
Parietal lobe	• Visual and touch sensations • Coordinates input from different senses for understanding • Sensory control of the body writing, mathematics, and language • Controls body positions (drawing ability), handling of objects, and verbal and nonverbal memory	Patient might present with numbness, hemineglect (will have no awareness that arm, or leg, is weak or dragging), or spatial disorientation. Visual field deficit.
Occipital lobe	• Seeing: interpreting what is seen and actual visual images. • Reading and writing, finding objects, identifying colors, seeing accurately, recognizing words and drawn objects, and recognizing that object is moving	Visual field deficit, loss of vision, nystagmus, ataxia, and vomiting
Temporal lobe	• Hearing, understanding, organizing, and concentrating on what is seen or heard • Recognition of tones, music sounds, and nonspeech information • Long-term memory • Personality behavior and sexual behavior	Mild personality changes, mood disorders, and short-term memory deficits
Cerebellum	• Balance, posture, and motor coordination, including extremities, and some memory for reflex movements	Patient presents with poor balance, uncoordinated movements (examine walk and finger-to-nose test)
Brainstem	• Basic functions of the body necessary for life: breathing, heart rate, digestion, level of alertness, sleep, and balance. Coordinate movements in the eyeball, swallowing, vomiting, coughing, hiccups, sneezing. Coordinate movements.	Extraocular eye movements are impaired, drooping eyelid, double vision, face becomes asymmetric, trouble swallowing, gagging, limb weakness of one side. Nausea/vomiting.
Pituitary	• Hormones • Growth • Fertility	Visual field deficit, blurry vision, increase in shoe or hand size, exercise intolerance, weight gain, decreased libido, irregular menses

Source: Data from Lapointe S, Perry A, Butowski NA. Primary brain tumours in adults. *Lancet.* 2018;392(10145):432–446. doi:10.1016/S0140-6736(18)30990-5; Tortora GJ, Grabowski SR. *Principles of Anatomy and Physiology.* 10th ed. John Wiley & Sons; 2003.

long survival time, the tumor is recommended to be resected.[38] If the metastatic tumors are caught early while they are still small and fewer than three masses are found, the preference is to perform stereotactic radiosurgery or Gamma Knife.[38] Advances in immunotherapy and the development of agents that cross the blood-brain barrier have been found to be extremely effective in treating metastatic disease; more research is underway.

Patients with a brain tumor are also at risk for multiple complications that primary care providers will address as the NPs comanage the patient with the hematology-oncology group (Table 17.12). Unfortunately, there are limited data on beneficial interventions.

Patient Education

Often when a patient is diagnosed, they start searching for answers as to why this has occurred and did they do something to cause brain cancer. At this point, psychologic and emotional support is needed. There are several

Table 17.11: Treatment for Meningiomas

Grade	Was Gross Total Resection Achieved?	Treatment Plan
Grade I (Benign and most common)	Yes -> No ->	No additional treatment needed, follow up with MRI Frequent MRIs, may need treatment
Grade II (78% survival in 5 years)	Yes -> No ->	Frequent MRI Frequent MRIs and radiation
Grade III (44% survival in 5 years)	Yes -> No ->	Frequent MRIs Frequent MRIs and radiation

Source: Adapted from Lapointe S, Perry A, Butowski NA. Primary brain tumours in adults. *Lancet.* 2018;392(10145):432–446. doi:10.1016/S0140-6736(18)30990-5

Table 17.12: Complications of Metastatic Tumors

Complication	Patient Presentation	Diagnosis	Management
Fatigue		Evaluate medication, depression, sleep disturbance, anemia, nutritional deficiencies, alcohol/substance abuse, endocrine health conditions	• Reported benefit from exercise and corticosteroids • Studies of psychostimulants in patients with brain tumors have yielded mixed results • Antidepressants or mood stabilizers • Wean off steroids • Occupational and cognitive speech therapy
Seizures		Diagnosis is based on patient history and diagnostic evaluation as described in seizure section of the chapter	• Antiseizure medications are usually started upon new diagnosis of gliomas. • For other low-grade tumors, seizure medications are used only postoperatively and restarted later if seizures reoccur.
Mood and other psychiatric disorders including depression	• Psychosis, mania, or irritability due to steroid use • May present with symptoms related to living with brain cancer or due to tumor growth • Can occur after whole radiation or whole-brain radiation		• Steroid weaning • Starting antidepressants or mood stabilizers

(continued)

Table 17.12: Complications of Metastatic Tumors (*continued*)

Complication	Patient Presentation	Diagnosis	Management
Cerebral edema	• Worsening of neurologic deficits arising from culprit brain mass • Edema may cause an increase in ICP and patient may present with confusion, headache, nausea, or vomiting • Can be seen in patients who have brain radiation • Patient can self-report	• Clinical diagnosis: cerebral edema is visible on brain imaging but should be treated based on symptoms	• Corticosteroids, specifically dexamethasone
Endocrinopathies	• Common after brain radiation, particularly those of pituitary or hypothalamus masses	• Standard laboratory testing based on symptoms suggest TSH, cortisol, testosterone, FSH LH, GH	• Hormone replacement based on the laboratory results

FSH LH, follicle stimulating hormone luteinizing hormone; GH, growth hormome; ICP, intracranial pressure; TSH, thyroid stimulating hormone.

Source: McFaline-Figueroa JR, Lee EQ. Brain tumors. *Am J Med.* 2018;131(8):874–882. doi:10.1016/j.amjmed.2017.12.039

resources that can be used to support patients. Providing education and recommending support groups can be beneficial. Family support is also important. It is essential that the patient have advance care plans so their wishes are honored in situations where the person can no longer voice their wishes and preferences for care. If the patient is terminal, hospice care should be discussed. A typical patient education resource is the National Institutes of Health: www.cancer.gov/types/brain.

COMMON SYMPTOMS IN OLDER ADULTS

This section presents a brief overview of some common symptoms or health conditions adults may experience.

HUNTINGTON'S DISEASE

Huntington's disease (HD) is a genetic neurodegenerative condition characterized by choreiform movements, psychiatric disorder, and dementia. The cause is related to a cytosine-adenine-guanine (CAG) trinucleotide repat expansion in the huntingtin (HTT) gene on chromosome 4p, an autosomal-dominate pattern. The worldwide prevalence is about 2.7 cases per 100,000 persons and the incidence is about 0.38 cases per 100,000 per year. Although this is not a disorder primary care NPs will diagnosis, your patient may present with symptoms that require further evaluation and referral to a neurologist. Initially, the symptoms begin insidiously and have a slow persistent decline in cognitive and physical function. The key defining symptom of chorea is characterized by brief, abrupt, involuntary, and unconventional movements involving the face, trunk,

and limbs. Hypotonia with hyperreflexia is seen early in the disease. Abnormal eye movement can be a prominent feature, especially in younger adults. The psychiatric symptoms are irritability, depression, and/or disrupted social relationships that usually occur years before the chorea. Some patients may experience paranoia, delusion, and hallucinations that can occur at any time during the illness. Cognitive decline will occur with HD, and the person can present with executive dysfunction and a decreased ability to make decisions, multitask, and switch from one set of cognitive goals to another. Patients rarely have insight into their deficits. The diagnosis is based on the presentation of typical manifestations of HD, family history (if known), and genetic confirmation. Referral to a neurologist is important for diagnosis and comanagement of the patient.

NEUROPATHIES

Neuropathy is extremely common in clinical practice and presents with varying degrees of sensory and/or motor loss. Patients usually present with complaints of sensory loss, burning or prickling sensation (paresthesia), weakness, and varying degrees of pain. Subsets of neuropathy are polyneuropathy, mononeuropathy, and mononeuropathy multiplex. Polyneuropathy is axonal or demyelination changes in the peripheral nerves, with the patient presenting with a combination of sensory loss, pain, and the motor loss most prominent distally.[41] Mononeuropathy is a lesion in a single nerve that is due to trauma, focal entrapment, ischemia, infection, or tumor, with the patient complaining of symptoms in a single nerve or nerve redistribution.[41] Mononeuropathy multiplex is painful, asymmetrical, multifocal sensory, and motor neuropathy involving at least two separate affected nerve areas. The most common example of mononeuropathy—carpal tunnel disease—and the most common example of polyneuropathy—diabetic neuropathy—seen in primary care are discussed.

CARPAL TUNNEL SYNDROME

The most frequent mononeuropathies encountered in clinical practice are entrapment neuropathies; nerve damage occurs when it passes through narrow, restricted space.[42] These neuropathies are defined as idiopathic as most of the causes are largely unknown; even though only a small portion of nerve is entrapped, it can have substantial physical, psychologic, and economic consequences.[42] The most studied and the most common mononeuropathy worldwide is carpal tunnel syndrome (CTS).[42,43]

Epidemiology

CTS is so common that it is believed that one in 10 people develop CTS at some point in their lives.[43] Other studies suggest that approximately 3% of the general adult population will develop CTS.[43] The prevalence of CTS is similar in men and women, with a ratio of 1 to 1.4; however, the prevalence is almost four times higher than in men at the age of 65 to 74 years old.

Risk Factors

A large study found that forceful hand exertion is the most important factor in the development of CTS in workers. Evidence supports repetitive motions like typing and wrist movement over and over again can lead to CTS. However, association between computer use and carpal tunnel syndrome is still controversial.[42,43] A history of diabetes mellitus, family history, obesity, menopause, arthritis, hypothyroidism, tobacco smoking, pregnancy, and rheumatoid arthritis are additional risk factors for developing CTS.[42,43]

Approach to Diagnosis

The presentation of pain and paresthesia in the distribution of the median nerve are the hallmarks of CTS, which includes the palmar aspect of the thumb, index finger, and middle fingers and radial half of the ring finger.[43] The first symptom a patient may experience is intermittent nocturnal paresthesias and dysesthesias that increase in frequency and occur during waking hours followed by loss of sensation with weakness and finally thenar muscle atrophy.[42] Symptoms can also vary, with some patients complaining of involvement of the wrist and entire hand with radiation to the forearm and entire shoulder.[42,43]

The gold standard in diagnosis is physical assessment and taking accurate history. Tinel's sign and Phalen's maneuver are common diagnostic tests for CTS and widely used, whereas assessing sensory function is not useful unless performed carefully with specific tools.[43] Nerve conduction studies should be obtained to confirm CTS by detecting impaired median nerve conductions across the carpal tunnel; in addition, if the study reveals a severe case, the patient will be less likely to have complete recovery after the surgery.[43]

Differential Diagnosis

The most common disorder confused with CTS is cervical radiculopathy. Cervical radiculopathy is a clinical description of when a nerve root in the cervical spine becomes inflamed or damaged, leading to changes in neurologic function such as numbness, altered reflexes, or weakness that can radiate to the shoulder, arm, hand, or fingers. Therefore, careful assessment and nerve conduction studies may help to distinguish between CTS and other disorders.[43]

Management

Management of CTS depends on the severity of the disease. In mild to moderate cases, splinting is recommended at night as a first-line treatment.[43] There is increasing evidence to support local carpal tunnel corticosteroid injections that may provide patients with symptomatic relief anywhere from 1 month to 10 weeks and sometimes lasting even more than 1 year.[43] The goal of conservative management is to delay the need for surgery. Even though research showed that most of the patients did have surgery by 1 year, a second steroid injection provided symptomatic improvement beyond 12 months, delaying surgery even more.

Patient Education

After carpal tunnel release, surgery patients will be able to return to work in about 2 weeks. However, some patients do report pain up to 1 year. The most common complication of surgery is surgical scar pain or pain near the area of tendon release. Carpal tunnel decompression provides a lasting, good outcome in 70% to 90% of cases.[43] Surgery is the treatment of choice for patients with severe median nerve damage as characterized by permanent sensory or motor loss or ongoing axonal loss or denervation on electrodiagnostic studies.

DIABETIC NEUROPATHY

According to the World Health Organization, as many as 422 million adults globally were living with diabetes in 2014. This number is expected to increase by some estimates [to] as many as 642 million adults worldwide between the ages of 20 and 79. At [a] prevalence rate of 8.8%, [much] of the population may be afflicted [with] diabetes by 2040.[44] The International Diabetes Federation calls diabetes the largest global epidemic of the 21st century.[48] Every single provider, even if not practicing in primary care, will have a patient with diabetes, as it is one of the most common diagnoses in clinical practice. One of the most disabling adverse comorbidities is polyneuropathy, more commonly known as diabetic neuropathy.[43] The most common complaint patients will have is distal symmetric polyneuropathy "stocking and glove distribution," which can lead to sensory disturbances such as diminished protective sense, making patients prone to foot injuries, leading to deterioration in quality of life.[44]

Epidemiology

Diabetic peripheral neuropathy is the most common cause of neuropathy worldwide, and it occurs in upwards of 50% of individuals with diabetes.[44] It is estimated that the annual cost of neuropathy and its complications are more than $10 billion in the United States.[45] The incidence of neuropathy is higher in individuals with type 2 diabetes in comparison to type 1; the prevalence of diabetic neuropathy increases from 8% to 42% in patients with type 2 diabetes over 10-year period.[45]

Risk Factors

Major predictors of diabetic neuropathy are the duration of diabetes and uncontrolled hemoglobin A1c levels. Other risk factors are obesity, hyperglycemia, hypertension, abdominal obesity, low high-density lipoprotein levels, and finally smoking, alcohol abuse, increased height, and older age.[45]

Pathophysiology

The etiology of diabetic neuropathy is not clearly understood; however, there are a few proposed mechanisms. The mechanisms include a derangement of normal metabolic homeostasis, an autoimmune condition, and microvascular disease first affecting the longest axons, such as distal limbs.[44,45]

Approach to Diagnosis

Diagnosis is primarily based on comprehensive history and physical examination with a focus on pain. Approximately 30% to 50% of patients with diabetic neuropathy develop neuropathic pain with the most common complaint of burning pain in the feet as well as paresthesia and nonnoxious stimuli-evoked pain.[45] Clinicians should ask about the onset of symptoms, progression, and what therapies have been attempted. Bedside testing should include a sensory examination: vibration testing (using a 128-Hz tuning fork placed over the dorsum of the distal phalanx of the hallux), pinprick or pain (using monofilament applying to dorsal or plantar aspect of hallux), temperature (mostly cold), proprioception, and light touch. The loss of vibratory sensation is the earliest sign

of underlying neuropathy.[43,44] Clinicians should also evaluate peripheral pulses and examine for swelling, skin temperature changes, erythema, bony deformities, and ulcerations, including deep tendon reflexes (DTR will be diminished).[43] Assessment of gait is important. It is common to see waddling gait, hammertoe deformities, wasting or weakness of muscles of the feet and weakness, and atrophy of the hands in later stages.[43] Nerve conduction studies provide an objective evaluation of neuropathy.

Differential Diagnosis

It is very important to assess for vitamin deficiency, such as vitamins B12 (especially when taking metformin), B6, and B1; alcohol use; thyroid dysfunction; uremia; and heavy metal exposure—as these are also common causes for peripheral neuropathy.[43] Clinicians may also assess for genetic neuropathies, neoplasia, medication-induced neuropathy (therapy and HIV treatment), and amyloidosis.[45]

Management

The main goal of treatment is pain management and prevention of wounds. The consensus of multiple studies is that first- and second-line treatments for painful diabetic neuropathy should include anticonvulsants (lamotrigine, topiramate, oxcarbazepine, carbamazepine), calcium channel ligands (gabapentin, pregabalin), serotonin and noradrenaline reuptake inhibitors (SNRIs; duloxetine, venlafaxine), and tricyclic antidepressants (amitriptyline, nortriptyline, desipramine).[45] If the patient does not achieve the desired outcome with these medications, then a second agent may be needed; for example, if anticonvulsant agents are not effective, then adding a tricyclic antidepressant may be appropriate. Opioid use due to addictive properties and poor response is highly discouraged and not recommended.[44,45]

Patient Education

Treatment of hyperglycemia is the best preventative treatment (see Chapter 26 for more information about diabetes). One study in which patients received a structured exercise program compared to a second group who received only lifestyle counseling found that exercise could prevent nerve injury and promote nerve degeneration; more research is needed.[45]

BELL'S PALSY

Bell's palsy (idiopathic facial nerve palsy or facial nerve palsy if suspected viral etiology) is the most common reason for acute spontaneous peripheral facial paralysis. Most cases are due to the activation of the herpes simplex virus. The facial nerve is a mixed nerve; motor fibers innervate the facial muscles, whereas parasympathetic fibers innervate lacrimal, submandibular, and sublingual salivary glands;

afferent fibers from taste receptors from the anterior two-thirds of the tongue; and somatic afferents from the external auditory canal and pinna (see Figure 17.6).

Epidemiology

About 40,000 people in the United States have Bell's palsy, and each year the incidence is highest in those who are 15 to 45 years old. Most often, the cause of Bell's palsy is not known, but the annual incidence rate is between 13 and 34 cases per 100,000 population. There is no difference in gender, race, or geographic location, but pregnant women have three times the risk, especially during the third trimester or the first week postpartum. Individuals with diabetes account for about 5% to 10% of cases.

Pathophysiology

The mechanism for Bell's palsy is inflammation and possible infectious cause. The most common cause is the herpes simplex virus. Herpes zoster is the next common cause, and other infections include cytomegalovirus, Epstein–Barr virus, adenovirus, rubella virus, mumps, influenza B, and coxsackievirus. Diabetes is a risk factor for microangiopathy that can lead to Bell's palsy via the microcirculatory failure of the vasa nervorum. The risk during pregnancy may be related to fluid retention leading to compression of the nerve or perineural edema.

Risk Factors

Risk factors are pregnancy, preeclampsia, obesity, hypertension, diabetes, and upper respiratory infections.

Approach to Diagnosis

The diagnosis is based on the clinical presentation. Patients typically present with acute unilateral facial weakness. The following criteria are used to diagnose Bell's palsy: The patient presents with a diffuse facial nerve involvement that includes paralysis of the facial muscles with or without loss of taste on the anterior two-thirds aspect of the tone or altered secretion of the lacrimal and salivary glands, and onset is acute over a day or two. The course is progressive, with maximum clinical weakness/paralysis within 3 weeks or less from the first day of visual weakness. Recovery or some degree of function can occur in about 6 months. The physical examination should include a neurologic examination, particularly of the CNs. You should have the patient their close eyes, elevate the brow, frown, show teeth, pucker lips, and tense the soft tissues of the neck to observe for platysma

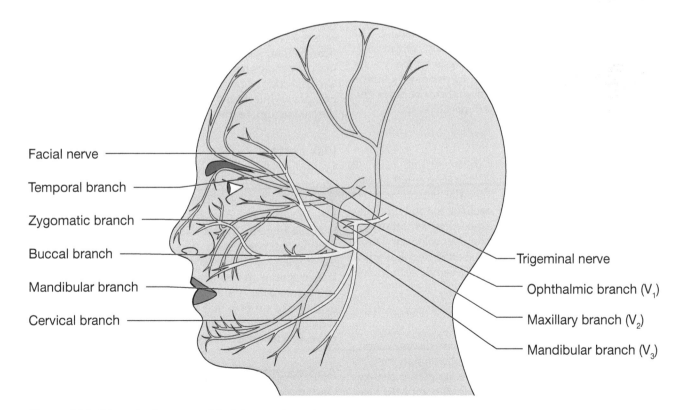

Figure 17.6: Trigeminal nerve and facial nerve branches

Source: Myrick KM, Karosas LM, eds. *Advanced Health Assessment and Differential Diagnosis*. Springer Publishing Company; 2020: Figure 3.5

activation. Facial nerve palsy can be caused by other health conditions and may be confused with Bell's palsy. Some of these are herpes zoster infection, Guillain–Barre syndrome, otitis media, Lyme disease, HIV infection, sarcoidosis, Sjögren syndrome, tumor, or stroke.

Diagnostics

In some cases, you may consider obtaining an electrodiagnostic study such as an electromyography (EMG) and imaging studies (e.g., MRI or CT scan) if signs are atypical and there is a slow progression beyond the usual 3 weeks or if there is no improvement at 4 months. Motor nerve conduction studies can be ordered by the neurologist. Serologic testing for Lyme disease is recommended for adults with acute onset of facial palsy.

Management

Pharmacologic treatment is the main treatment. All patients will require meticulous eye care to prevent corneal dryness and injury until eyelid closure has improved. Most recover in 6 months to 1 year, but about a third will have functional and cosmetic outcomes related to facial weakness and may consider surgical intervention or Botox injections.

Pharmacologic

Short-term oral glucocorticoid treatment is used, in severe cases in combination with antiviral therapy. The best time to start treatment is within 3 days of the onset of symptoms. The recommended dose is typically a 10-day tapering dose starting with 60 mg per day.[46] Caution should be taken with people with diabetes because glucocorticoids increase the risk for hyperglycemia.

Patient Education

It is important to discuss the treatment and possible adverse reactions to notify the NP. It is essential to protect their eye from injury because the person may experience interruption in the eyelid's natural blinking ability, which leaves the eye exposed to irritation and drying. The National Institute of Neurological Disorders and Stroke have patient education material at www.ninds.nih.gov/Disorders/Patient-Caregiver-Education/Fact-Sheets/Bells-Palsy-Fact-Sheet

MULTIPLE SCLEROSIS

Multiple sclerosis (MS) is an autoimmune disease characterized by multifocal regions of demyelination in the CNS with optic nerve involvement and white matter changes having characteristics of Dawson's fingers on MRI head images.[41] MS is thought to be due to the complex interaction between different genetic and environmental factors, with its incidence and prevalence continuing to rise worldwide, especially in North America and Europe.[47] MS is categorized into several clinical subtypes: (a) clinically isolated syndrome (representing the first attack), (b) relapsing-remitting MS (RRMS), (c) secondary progressive MS, and (d) primary progressive MS (PPMS).

Epidemiology

MS usually affects young adults between ages 20 to 40 years old, female-to-male ratio varies between 1.5:1 and 2.5:1. MS is a leading cause of nontraumatic neurologic disability in young adults.[47] Smoking (women are more affected than men when it comes to smoking) has been linked to MS. Recently, more women have been diagnosed with MS compared to men. This is thought to be related to hormones, and women are more inclined to seek medical assistance. In addition, advances in diagnostic MRIs may have resulted in a higher prevalence of MS.[47] Interestingly, minorities in the United States, such as Hispanic Americans and Black Americans, have experienced faster disease progression than do White Americans.[47]

Pathophysiology

"MS is a chronic central nervous system inflammatory disease of autoimmune etiology, mediated by activated T cells with evolving evidence of significant contribution from B cells and cells of the innate immune system."[47] MS causes a variety of motor deficits such as spasticity, weakness, tremor, and ataxia. Specificity is due to disruptions in upper motor neuron networks, and the weakness and loss of dexterity are due to interruption of input to motor neurons, while tremor and ataxia are due to lesions in the cerebellum, brainstem, thalamus, and basal ganglia.[49]

Risk Factors

Multiple risk factors have been identified in MS. Low vitamin D deficiency and cigarette smoking have been identified as the most important environmental risk factors, in addition to diet and obesity in early life.[47,48] There is also a hygiene hypothesis that suggests that multiple infectious exposures in early childhood reduce the risk of developing autoimmune and allergic diseases; however, late infections in young adults, such as Epstein–Barr virus, increase the risk of developing MS.[48] There is no clear evidence to support that MS is an inherited disease, even though there are reports of families that may have two or three affected individuals.[47]

Approach to Diagnosis

Once the primary care NP suspects MS, referral to a neurologist should be made. The diagnosis of MS is usually made after reviewing clinical, imaging (MRI with contrast of brain and spine), and laboratory results. Laboratory findings include a lumbar puncture to obtain CSF to look for inflammatory markers such as OCBs and elevated immunoglobin G (IgG) index; these markers are present in up to 85% of patients with MS.[47] MS is divided into RRMS (85% of cases) and a chronic progressive pattern called PPMS.[49] During RRMS, patients present with symptoms such as trouble seeing, sensitivity to heat, numbness worse in the feet, depression, urinary urgency, trouble with balance, a lack of coordination, weakness, fatigue, and difficulty thinking clearly. Symptoms last at least 24 hours and get progressively worse before full or partial recovery. MS diagnosis is made when two discrete episodes of neurologic dysfunction occur at least 30 days apart in different locations of CNS or a diagnosis can be made in those with one relapse who show evidence of dissemination in time and dissemination in space on MRI (with every relapse MRI shows 5 to 10 times as many lesions).

For every clinical relapse the patient experiences, the MRI shows 5 to 10 times as many lesions.[49] For more information on diagnostic criteria refer to McDonald Criteria at the National MS society webpage at www.nationalmssociety.org.

Management

Pharmacologic treatment is the mainstay of management. Psychosocial support is also very important for patients, particularly when first diagnosed.

Pharmacologic

Studies examining treatment for relapses did not find a difference between oral and IV administration of methylprednisolone (IV-MP); however, if a patient fails to improve, a second course of high dose of IV-MP is recommended, and if the patient has severe deficits and still fails to respond to MP, plasmapheresis may be considered (Table 17.13).[47] With the increasing discovery of disease-modifying treatments, the clinical management of patients has become more complicated. There are two therapeutic approaches in the clinical setting: (a) an escalation strategy, starting treatment with moderately effective medication and escalating to more effective; unfortunately, this approach might be potentially less safe and more expensive; and (b) an induction strategy, starting with highly effective therapy with the aim of obtaining a persistent disease remission; this approach is usually initiated for highly

Table 17.13: Disease-Modifying Therapies

Generic Names	Brand Names	Benefits	Common Side Effects
Interferons	Rebif Betaferon Extavia Plegridy	• Early treatment was associated with a 47% reduction in the hazard ratio for all-cause mortality. • Overall safe medications, safety data collected over 20 years • Single dosing injections every 2 weeks is available	• Very rare liver toxicity
Glatiramer acetate	Copaxone	• Similar safety and efficacy data as with interferons • Can be administered three times weekly	• No side effects reported • No monitoring needed
Dimethyl fumarate	Tecfidera	• Significant reduction in ARR* 49% and disability progression 32%	• Flushing • Gastrointestinal symptoms
Teriflunomide	Aubagio	• Reduction of ARR by 36% and disability progression by 30%	• Hair thinning • Elevation off serum liver enzymes mild leukopenia
Fingolimod	Gilenya	• Reduced the ARR by 52% to 55% and disability progression by 30% • Contraindicated to be used in presence of heart disease	• Careful monitoring is needed for bradycardia, macular edema, and infections
Natalizumab	Tysabri	• Reduced ARR by 68% and disability progression by 42% • Reserved as a last resort of treatment	• High risk of progressive multifocal leukoencephalopathy (PML)

(continued)

Table 17.13: Disease-Modifying Therapies (*continued*)

Generic Names	Brand Names	Benefits	Common Side Effects
Alemtuzumab	Lemtrada	• 45% to 49% production of ARR and 43% reduction off disability progression	• Delayed secondary autoimmune events • Thyroid disease • Immune thrombocytopenia • Rare cases of under glomerular basement membrane disease
Ocrelizumab	Ocrevus	• Production of ARR 46% to 47% and decrease the risks of 24-week confirmed disability progression by 37% to 43%	• Low incidence of serious side effects

*Reduced annualized relapse rate (ARR).[50]

active or rapidly evolving disease.[49] Unfortunately, more effective medications for MS have been associated with serious adverse events, such as alemtuzumab, which can cause severe autoimmune adverse events and infection.[48]

Patient Education

An extensive systemic review completed by Wendebourg and colleagues in 2017[52] identified that fatigue has been a major disabling factor in MS patients. Ten randomized controlled trials on educational interventions for MS-related fatigue were found to be effective in reducing patient-reported fatigue for 1 year. When comparing effectiveness of sports interventions, pharmaceutical treatments, and educational programs, they also found that educational programs had the largest effect in terms of reducing fatigue. It was also discovered that cognitive behavioral therapy seems to be most effective in reducing fatigue compared to other educational programs; it was thought to be due to the individual approaches, closer interaction, and face-to-face time spent with the patient. Patient education can be found at the National MS Society: www.nationalmssociety.org/Chapters/CAN/Services-and-Support/MS-Education.

DIZZINESS

Dizziness is a common complaint of older adults seen in primary care. It can be challenging trying to determine the etiology, and in some cases, the NP may not be able to identify the cause. Other clinical categories are vertigo, unsteadiness, gait instability, lightheadedness, and disequilibrium. Dizziness can be due to a mixed pathology, such as medications and neurologic disorders, as well as otolaryngologic, cardiovascular, and mental health conditions. In adults 70 and older, benign paroxysmal positional vertigo (BPPV; inner ear disorder) is a common reason for dizziness. If after a thorough history and physical examination there is no identifiable cause, then the diagnosis of prebystasis is appropriate; this diagnosis concerns age-related changes often associated with difficulty with ambulation.[50] See Box 17.11 for possible descriptions of the symptoms.

Approach to Diagnosis

Vertigo and dizziness are often used interchangeably by patients seen in primary care, so it is important to obtain a thorough history and physical to assist with diagnosis. Patients who describe the "room as spinning" may be experiencing vertigo. Vertigo is caused by vestibular etiologies. Patients experiencing orthostatic hypotension may report a spinning sensation when they change from sitting to standing, but this usually only lasts for seconds. In other cases, patients may describe a spinning sensation when they have dizziness, so it is important to determine timing, triggers, and associated symptoms.

Box 17.11: Symptoms That May Indicate Cause for Dizziness[50]

- Vertigo: Patient feels the room is spinning and may have nausea, vomiting, unsteadiness, or visual disturbances. Causes can be postviral illness, vestibular neuritis, benign paroxysmal positional vertigo, migraine, CVA (especially if neuro symptoms present), Méniere's disease, or head or neck pain posttrauma
- Presyncope: Sensation of almost fainting
- Disequilibrium: Sense of imbalance. Associated symptoms are hearing loss, chronic lower extremity sensory deficit, poor coordination, and feeling weak
- Lightheadedness: Can be presyncope, or can be due to anxiety

Box 17.12

Orthostatic Hypotension
A diagnosis can be made based on a decrease in systolic BP of 20 mmHg or diastolic BP decrease equal to or greater than 10 mmHg within 3 minutes if standing. An increase in heart rate greater than 30 beats per minute after rising from a supine position may indicate autonomic disturbances, such as postural orthostatic syndrome.

Source: Dix-Hallpike test. https://dizziness-and-balance.com/disorders/bppv/dix%20hallpike.htm

Consider medications as a potential cause, particularly in older adults with polypharmacy. Your physical examination will be based on the history. It is always important to check for orthostatic hypotension (see Box 17.12). If you identify orthostatic hypotension, it is essential to identify the cause, which could be dehydration, cardiac dysfunction, autonomic failure, or medication adverse effect.[51]

Positive torsional nystagmus (the superior pole of the eye beats toward the affected side) is diagnostic for BPPV. Even if the patient complains of dizziness during the maneuver, if there is no torsional nystagmus, the test is negative for BPPV. Your neurologic examination, as described earlier and in Chapter 10, can provide further information to support a diagnosis. An abnormal gait may indicate neuropathy, and a positive Romberg's test is suggestive of the involvement of proprioceptor receptors and their pathways. There is a limited role for routine laboratory testing in adults with dizziness. If your patient has diabetes, you should obtain a finger-stick for glucose. If you suspect cardiac involvement, referral to a cardiologist is important. A CT should be considered if you suspect a stroke, brain tumor, or there has been head trauma. A cardiac Doppler could be ordered if you suspect a vascular cause.[51]

Management

Treatment is based on your assessment findings. If BPPV is the diagnosis, you can use a particle repositioning maneuver (PRM). The Epley maneuver is the treatment for posterior semicircular canal BPPV (most common variant). Pharmacologic treatment with antiemetics and benzodiazepines could be considered for acute and brief episodes (caution with benzodiazepines in older adults). Avoid these medications in patients with BPPV because of the increased risk of falls.[51] Consider Meniere's disease as a differential diagnosis for those with ringing in their ears (see Chapter 16 for more information).

CASE STUDY
84-YEAR-OLD WITH PARKINSON'S DISEASE AND OTHER CONDITIONS

Jerry is an 84-year-old Caucasian male who has been in an SNF for cardiac rehabilitation after being hospitalized for an acute anterior myocardial infarction 2 months ago. His hospitalization was somewhat prolonged because of his PD and other comorbid conditions. He has been in the SNF for 5 weeks but now has several additional problems that seemed to have worsened over the past few weeks, which is why a care conference is being called today.

His wife is very worried that he is not eating very well as, according to her, he has always had a good appetite. She thinks he has lost weight and is not acting like himself. She reports that he is staying in bed a lot because he is afraid of falling. He has trouble feeding himself because of his tremor; she thinks it is worse. She wants to be to be able to take him home, but is afraid that she could not care for him in his current condition.

The physical therapist thinks he has made progress and is able to sit and then stand from the bed with one person assist and walk 100 feet. He thinks Jerry could improve more if he would only put forth more effort, but Jerry is disinterested and has declined therapy with increasing frequency over the past few days. PT is also concerned that he has had some freezing when he walks and that there is increased rigidity, and the PT therapist thinks Jerry is experiencing increased weakness. PT wants to discharge Jerry because he is not making progress with therapy.

The dietitian reports that Jerry is eating less than 50% of his meals and more recently less than 25%; he is on a mechanical soft diet with meats cut up. His current weight is 164 lb, and his weight on admission was 185 lb, which is his usual weight. She knows that his weight loss is putting him at greater risk and wants to change his diet.

His admission diagnoses are ACS 2 months ago, dyslipidemia, CAD, hypertension (HTN), GERD, BPH, PD diagnosed at age 75.

Medications

- Aspirin 81 mg daily
- Metoprolol 100 mg daily
- Atorvastatin 20 mg daily
- HCTZ 25 mg daily
- Levodopa/carbidopa ER 25/100 mg each night
- Levodopa/carbidopa IR 25/100 one by mouth every 8 hours

(cont.)

- Entacapone 200 mg one by mouth with each dose of levodopa/carbidopa
- Omeprazole 20 mg every day 69 minutes prior to breakfast
- Multivitamin
- Saw palmetto for BPH

Allergies: NKDA

ROS pertinent to PD (obtained from staff and family):

GI: Occasional c/o bloating and gas, increased constipation, is receiving Colace and Miralax

Urinary: occasional incontinence of urine

MS: seems weaker with difficulty in standing up and walking. Gait instability

Neurologic: many problems related to PD

Psychiatric: outbursts of anger, frustration with staff alternating with periods of crying. Is withdrawn from other residents. Only wants to see family, keeps door closed to his room

Vital signs and weights: T = 39 °C, HR = 74, R = 20, BP = 140/80 mmHg. Oxygen saturation on room air is 94%. Height is 74 in. Weekly weights (lbs) in chart: Admit: 185, Wk 1–183m Wk 2–180, Wk 3–178, Wk 4–172, Wk 5: 164

Case Study Questions

1. What is the significance of this weight loss in someone with PD?

2. His posture is stooped, and he leans slightly to his right even while sitting. He mostly stared straight ahead without blinking during the examination. What does this have to do with PD?

3. What are his diagnoses related to his current problems (not PMH)? What stage of PD is he in? List three positive findings used to determine the stage.

4. What is the most appropriate plan of care?

Answers

1. He is close to losing 10% of his body weight and is now on a downward trajectory. This unintentional weight loss can lead to muscle wasting and immunocompromise. Weight loss has put him at higher risk for infection, depression, and death. Conditions associated with unintentional weight loss are depression, cancer, cardiac disorders, and some GI conditions. Polypharmacy may also contribute to his weight loss. Studies have shown an increased risk of death associated with loss of 10% of body weight, and the standard guidelines in nursing homes are that 5% weight loss in 1 month is associated with increased mortality.

2. These symptoms are consistent with akinesia and postural disturbance, two of the hallmarks of PD. With the loss of dopamine in the neostriatum secondary to loss of pigmented dopaminergic neurons in the substantia nigra pars compacta of the midbrain comes a significant impairment of overall motor function. The constellation of symptoms related to akinesia includes slowness, reduced amplitude, fatigue, and interruptions in ongoing movements. On examination, we view this as lack of facial expression (masked) and reduced blinking ("reptilian stare"), soft monotonous speech (hypophonia, impaired swallowing resulting in drooling [sialorrhea]), and handwriting that starts small and proceeds to get smaller with each new word (micrographia). It is also the cause of the shuffling gait, reduced arm swing, and difficulty arising from a low chair. Postural disturbances are related to decreased proprioception and an inability to correct one's balance. This significantly increases his risk for falling and should be addressed with the interprofessional team.

3. advanced PD—stage 4, limited ability to walk straight or stand independently, slowing of physical movement, inability to feed himself

- dysphagia
- weight loss
- fall risk
- depression
- constipation
- urinary incontinence
- cognitive impairment

4. Consultation with neurologist and pharmacist about optimizing his medication regiment; discuss the consideration of the use of MAO inhibitors (selegiline or rasagiline) or dopamine agonist (pramipexole, rotigotine, or ropinirole)

- Dysphagia: discontinue current diet and start a dysphagia diet that includes thicken liquids
- Weight loss: discuss with dietitian how you can increase calories, ask family what foods he likes and if they can be present at meals, and encourage his wife to bring foods in from home that fit within the dysphagia diet. Offer nutritional supplements between meals and at bedtime. Continue weekly weights
- Fall Risk: institute fall precautions, provide 24-hour sitter until his condition improves
- Depression: consider adding an antidepressant to his regimen. Depression is the commonly overlooked issue in patients with PD. In PD, the frontal lobe, which regulates mood, is underactive.

(cont.)

Serotonin production can also be affected; therefore, SSRIs are often used to treat depression (see Chapter 18 for more information about treating depression). His appetite changes could be related to his depression, so treating depression may also help with his appetite.

- Urinary incontinence: may be associated with high doses of levodopa and worsened by bradykinesia and difficulty getting out of bed to go to the bathroom. Institute a coordinated fluid intake and toileting regimen in which he is taken to the bathroom every 2 to 4 hours and at bedtime and any time he awakens at night. Avoid fluid for 2 to 3 hours before he goes to sleep.

- Constipation: occurs in more than 50% of patients with PD and is a common early finding. The abdominal examination may yield findings consistent with constipation and there can be distention, diffuse tenderness to palpation without guarding, and rebound tenderness. A rectal examination may reveal hard, impacted stool in the rectal vault. The pathophysiology of GI symptoms is not well understood, but some postulate dopaminergic etiology. Increase fiber in diet, and increase fluid intake. Consume a regular regimen of stool softeners and laxatives as needed. Monitor for distention and/or abdominal pain.

- Cognitive impairment: the prevalence of dementia in persons with PD ranges from 20% to 40%. This is typically a late finding; see Chapter 10 for more information about dementia. Consider referral to a neuropsychologist or memory disorder clinic for evaluation of his cognitive status.

CONCLUSION

The neurologic system is very complex. When patients present to a primary care office with complaints or symptoms of possible neurologic conditions, it is critical to obtain a thorough history and perform a neurologic examination. The management of the patient will depend on the findings of the history and physical. It is important to appropriately refer to a neurologist or other specialist to comanage your patient.

REFERENCES

References for this chapter are online and available at https://connect.springerpub.com/content/book/978-0-8261-8414-6/part/part01/toc-part/ch17.

CHAPTER 18

Common Mental Health Disorders Encountered in the Primary Care Setting

Beth M. King and Diane Esposito

LEARNING OBJECTIVES

At the conclusion of this chapter, the learner will be able to:

➤ Describe the assessment of most common mental health disorders, with a focus on symptomatology and screening tools.

➤ Review pharmacologic treatment for mental health disorders.

➤ Discuss complementary and alternative therapies for persons with mental health disorders.

➤ Discuss ethical dilemmas in mental health.

➤ Review cultural assessment specific to mental health.

INTRODUCTION

Statistics offer a forboding picture of the impact of mental illness in the United States and worldwide. According to the World Health Organization (WHO), 14% of the burden of disease worldwide is due to mental, neurologic, and substance abuse disorders.[1] In the United States, as of 2019, approximately 51.5 million adults, 18 years and older, experience mental illness, and 13.1 million or 5.2% were diagnosed with a serious mental illness in the past year, not including substance or drug use disorder.[2] Education and early prevention and treatment can improve these statistics and the lives of persons with mental health disorders.

This chapter discusses the most common mental health disorders among adolescents and older adults: attention deficit hyperactivity disorder (ADHD), anxiety disorders, eating disorders, depressive disorders, bipolar disorders, neurodevelopment disorders (autism spectrum disorders [ASD]), thought disorders, substance use disorders, trauma, and stressor-related disorders, such as adjustment disorders. Assessments specific to mental health disorders are discussed, in particular the mental status examination (MSE), psychiatric review of systems, and screening tools. Evidence-based, pharmacologic, psychotherapeutic, psychosocial, and complementary and alternative treatments are also presented. A review of the following concepts assists in the treatment of mental health disorders: brain development, neuroplasticity, epigenetics, neurotransmitters, psychologic development, resilience, and recovery. Assessment is crucial to understanding the mental health disorders of clients. Fundamental to assessment is the relationship between you and your client and the development of trust and caring communication skills. These basic skills enable you to gather the necessary information for formulating a diagnosis and treatment plan.

As a nurse practitioner (NP), you are familiar with assessing the client's description of the current problem or chief complaint, medical history, review of systems, and laboratory and x-ray reports. Clients with a mental health disorder need further assessment, which includes the following:

■ **Past Psychiatric History:** Identify hospitalizations or treatment for psychiatric issues, history of psychotropic medications, history of self-harm and/or violence.

■ **Family History:** Identify any family history of psychiatric issues; history of psychiatric illness in family and past generations, and family history of suicidal attempts and/or success, history of violence in the family. Construct a genogram to assist in visualizing the family history.

■ **Development History:** Review the prenatal, perinatal, and postnatal history of the person and any significant factors and delays in development, learning disabilities, and psycho-educational testing.

• **Individual Developmental Stage:** Identify a person's stage of development according to Erickson.

• **Family Developmental Stage:** Identify any recent changes in family systems.

■ **Trauma History**: Review person's experience of traumatic events, such as divorce, violence, war, bullying, and accidents.

■ **Substance Use History:** Review the person's history of nicotine usage, alcohol, cannabis, illicit drugs, and caffeine.

• Age of first use of nicotine, alcohol, cannabis, prescription drugs, street drugs

• Usual pattern of use for substances

• Date, time, and amount of last use

- **Risk Assessment:** Assess for any suicidal thoughts and behaviors, plan and access, homicidal ideation, other harm to self and others, cutting or other self-mutilation, or any other harm to self and others, including cruelty to animals and fire-setting.
- **Legal History:** Review any legal history, which can contribute to stress and anxiety.
- **Environment:** Identify a person's living situation, the safety of the environment, who the persons living with, and availability of running water and refrigeration.
- **Social History:** Discuss the person's social activities, interests, and activities.
- **Educational History:** Review the person's educational background, psycho-educational testing, and any learning disabilities.
- **Occupational and Military History:** Discuss the person's occupation, both past and current positions. Review military history and experiences in combat.
- **Culture:** Review with the person's cultural background and identification.
- **Stressors:** Identify current stressors in life and past and current coping skills. Discuss success in coping with stressors.
- **Strengths:** Identify a person's strengths, both self-identified and evident from the interview.
- **Support System:** Identify the support system of the person, family, friends, animals, and others; availability of support system and frequency of interaction.

MENTAL STATUS EXAMINATION

The MSE is the most useful tool for the NP. The MSE will provide a picture of the person's mental changes and behaviors related to mental disorders. The following categories are included in the examination:

- **General Description:** This includes an account of the person's appearance, behavior, psychomotor activity, and speech.
- **Mood and Affect:** Both adolescents and older adults are at a higher risk for suicide. Both affect and mood must be assessed, along with direct questions related to thoughts of suicide or intent.
- **Thought Content and Process:** Assess for thought disorders demonstrated by a flight of ideas, blocking, and word salad. In addition, evaluate thought content for preoccupations, fears, phobias, and obsessions. A loss of abstract thinking may indicate early dementia.[4]
- **Perceptions:** Hallucinations in the older adult may indicate a need for further diagnostic tests, as "brain tumors and other focal pathology"[4] may be related to the perceptual disturbance.
- **Sensorium and Cognition:** Assessment of the cranial nerves relate to sensorium and cognition or information processing may be assessed through conversation and screening tools.
- **Memory:** Assessment of immediate, recent, and remote memory can indicate cognitive disorders, with loss of recent memory one of the first indicators.
- **Judgment/Insight:** A common question, "What would you do if you smelled smoke in a movie theater?" is used to assess a person's judgment.
- **Intelligence:** When assessing a person's intelligence, the educational level, language, and life experiences must be considered as influencing factors.

Psychiatric Review of Systems

The psychiatric review of systems provides further information in order to obtain a comprehensive assessment of the person. The psychiatric review of systems includes the following:

- **Change in Appetite:** Increase or decrease
- **Sleep Disturbance:** Increase or decrease, early morning awakenings, disturbance of sleep cycle
- **Eating Patterns:** Change in type of food, timing of eating
- **Neuro-Vegetative Symptoms:** Altered concentration and anhedonia
- **Libido Levels:** Altered libido, interest in sex
- **Somatic Symptoms:** Physical symptoms, such as headaches, gastrointestinal (GI) complaints
- **Energy Level:** Alteration in energy, decrease or increase
- **Depression:** Symptoms of depression
- **Anxiety:** Symptoms/behaviors of anxiety
- **Mania:** Symptoms/behaviors of mania
- **Gastrointestinal:** Symptoms suggestive of medication side effects

Suicidal Assessment

Suicidal assessment is necessary for all clients. Reports of loneliness, recent losses, and illness are key indicators to pursue suicidal thoughts/intentions. "Have you ever thought about hurting yourself?" is a necessary component of all psychiatric assessments. The adolescent and older adult population are at increased risk for suicide, and it is imperative that this question be asked and a plan for treatment implemented.

Screening Tools

Screening tools provide additional information for your assessment. The Substance Abuse and Mental Health Services Administration–Health Resources and Services Administration (SAMHSA–HRSA) Center of Excellence for Integrated Health website provides numerous screening tools and resources (www.thenationalcouncil.org/integrated-health-coe).

SPECIFIC ASSESSMENT FOR ADOLESCENT AND GERIATRIC POPULATIONS

Adolescent Review of Systems

- **General:** chronic fatigue, mood, weight changes, increased or decreased need for sleep, drug or alcohol use, sexual activity
- **Integument:** dry skin cuts, burns, bruises, excoriation, severe acne, lanugo
- **HEENT:** chronic headaches, microcephaly, frequent ear infections, snoring, tooth decay or erosion, dry mouth
- **Cardiac:** chest pains, hypo- or hypertension, palpitations
- **Respiratory:** chronic cough, dyspnea, sob
- **GI:** diarrhea, constipation, vomiting, peptic ulcer or heartburn, abdominal pain
- **Endocrine:** obesity, excessive sweating, precocious puberty, intolerance to heat or cold
- **Genitourinary (GU):** enuresis, encopresis, pregnancy, abortions, irregular menses
- **Musculoskeletal:** involuntary movements, multiple fractures
- **Neurologic:** tics, tremor, seizures, memory loss

CHILD AND ADOLESCENT: MENTAL HEALTH DISORDERS

The following mental health disorders are frequently identified in children and adolescents: ADHD, ASD, disruptive mood dysregulation disorder (DMDD), adjustment disorders, separation anxiety disorder, and eating disorders.

ATTENTION DEFICIT HYPERACTIVE DISORDER

ADHD is a neurodevelopmental disorder that usually presents in early childhood as problems with inattention and/or hyperactivity. ADHD was previously referred to as hyperkinesia or hyperkinetic disorder, as hyperactive behavior was generally thought to be the hallmark symptom, although greater acceptance of the inability to focus or concentrate is now equally recognized.

Prevalence

The prevalence of ADHD is not clear. The incidence of ADHD is reported as 5% of children and 2.5% of adults in the *Diagnostic and Statistical Manual of Mental Disorders (DSM-5)*;[6] however, the Centers for Disease Control and Prevention (CDC)[7] report rates of 11% of children in the United States diagnosed with ADHD as of 2011.

According to Visser et al.,[8] the National Survey of Children's Health also indicated parental reports of the prevalence of ADHD diagnosis in children in the United States were 11%. They report that most were being diagnosed by pediatricians utilizing a behavioral checklist, and the median age at diagnosis was 7 years.[8] Another national survey from 2016 reported that the prevalence of ADHD in children ages 2 to 17 was 9.4%, and almost a quarter of them never received treatment for ADHD.[9]

A meta-analysis of the epidemiology of ADHD recently calculated worldwide pooled prevalence of 7.2%.[10] ADHD occurs greater in males than in females 2:1. Persons with ADHD are more likely to also experience other mental disorders, such as depression, anxiety, substance use disorders, or other learning disorders than the general population.[8]

Risk Factors

Like most mental disorders, the etiology of ADHD is often unknown, although there may be a genetic predisposition, as the occurrence is often familial. There are several risk factors that have been identified, largely exposures that occur in utero, such as cigarette smoking, alcohol, or drug use during pregnancy, and exposure to environmental toxins, such as lead, during pregnancy or at a young age; a low birth weight; and brain injuries.

ADHD is thought to be a disorder of executive function, and so behavioral therapy that focuses on organizational skills with the use of external motivation sources can be helpful. Schedules and checklists, with frequent reinforcement, can assist an individual with ADHD using behavior modification. Parenting strategies that apply these approaches, called parental training in behavioral management (PTBM), are also beneficial and are recommended as a first line of treatment for preschool children up to age 6. PTBM is especially effective when combined with medication management for older children.[11]

Approach to Diagnosis

Table 18.1 provides a summary of the *DSM-5* diagnostic criterion for ADHD. Symptoms of inattention or behavioral activation can occur as a result of many other causes, and so diagnosis of the disorder must consider other organic, as well as psychologic, factors. This is especially true when considering a new diagnosis of ADHD in an adult, as according to the diagnostic criteria, symptoms must have been present before the age of 12. Sleep disorders, especially obstructive sleep apnea (OSA), are often misdiagnosed as ADHD, and ADHD symptoms frequently improve after treatment of OSA.[12] It is also important to consider medication-induced symptoms as medications such as those used to treat asthma can cause these symptoms.

Table 18.1: *DSM-5* Diagnostic Criteria for ADHD

- A pattern of inattention and/or hyperactivity that interferes with functioning greater than 6 months, characterized by six or more symptoms of inattention and/or six or more symptoms of hyperactivity and impulsivity
- Frequently interrupts or is intrusive with others
- Symptoms were present before 12 years old
- Symptoms are present in two or more settings (school/work/home)
- Symptoms interfere with social, academic, or occupational functioning
- Symptoms do not occur with diagnosis of a psychotic disorder or are not better explained by another mental disorder.
- *Specify if predominantly inattentive, hyperactive/impulsive, or combined presentation. *Specify if mild, moderate, or severe.

Source: Data from American Psychiatric Association. *Diagnostic and Statistical Manual of Mental Disorders, DSM-5.* 5th ed. American Psychiatric Publishing; 2013:69-60.

The following mental disorders should also be considered in the differential diagnosis process: oppositional defiant disorder (ODD), specific learning disorders, intellectual disability, ASD, reactive attachment disorder, anxiety disorders, depressive disorders, bipolar disorder, DMDD, or substance use disorders. The American Academy of Pediatrics updated the Clinical Practice Guideline for the Diagnosis, Evaluation, and Treatment of Attention-Deficit/Hyperactivity Disorder in Children and Adolescents with a major key action statement recommending healthcare providers screen patients with ADHD for those other commonly occurring comorbid disorders.[11] These guidelines also continue to recommend referrals for parental behavioral management training as well as screening and evaluating for symptoms in at least two settings, which can include requesting behavioral rating scale completion from parents and teachers as well as healthcare providers.[11]

Assessment Tools

- Child Behavior Checklist[13]
- Conner's Rating Scale-Revised (CRS-R)[14]
- NICHQ Vanderbilt Assessment Scales[15]

NEURODEVELOPMENTAL DISORDERS: AUTISM SPECTRUM DISORDER

The characteristics of ASD involve impairment in social communications or repetitive or restricted patterns of behavior. The symptoms are present from early childhood and impact the level of functioning of the individual from mildly to severe. The level of this impairment does vary for each individual, may be dependent on their environment, and may not become obvious until greater demands are placed on the individual. This wide range in impact leads to the recent change in nomenclature from autism to ASD. ASD now encompasses disorders previously referred to as infantile autism, pervasive developmental disorders, Reye's syndrome, or Asperger's disorder.

Prevalence

There has been a marked increase in the incidence of ASD over the last two decades. The CDC has a surveillance program—the Metropolitan Atlanta Developmental Disabilities Surveillance Program first estimated ASD prevalence among children aged 3 to 10 in 1996 to be 3.4 per 1,000; the most current report shows a prevalence of 14.7 per 1,000 children in 2012.[16] This marked increase will contribute to greater numbers of adults with ASD in the future, with consideration for the healthcare needs of this population being more imperative.

Risk Factors

The cause of ASD is unknown, although it is genetic in nature. There is an increased risk of siblings with ASD. Older parents have an increased risk of having a child diagnosed with ASD. The increased rates of ASD are currently being studied, and risk factors including genetic, environmental, pregnancy, and behavioral factors are all being explored. Males are diagnosed 4.5 times more frequently than females.

Approach to Diagnosis

Table 18.2 provides a review of the *DSM-5* diagnostic criteria for ASD. Early diagnosis is important because intervention from birth to 3 years old, with physical, occupational, and speech therapy, can promote verbal, social, and other developmental skills. Early identification of developmental delays is important, and most states have an early intervention system in place. NPs can be instrumental in providing this access to care. Developmental delays, such as not meeting these milestones, can be early symptoms and warrant evaluation by a behavioral specialist. Additional therapies include applied behavior analysis, sensory integration therapy, speech therapy, occupational therapy, and a picture exchange communication system. While there is no one medication indicated for ASD, medication may be used for symptom management, for example, psychostimulants for hyperactivity, selective serotonin reuptake inhibitors (SSRI) for obsessive or compulsive behaviors, atypical antipsychotic for poor reality testing, and others.

Table 18.2: *DSM-5* Diagnostic Criteria for Autism Spectrum Disorder

- Persistent deficits in social communication and interaction across multiple contexts, as manifested by all of the following:
  - Deficits in social-emotional reciprocity, reduced sharing of interests or emotions, or failure to initiate or respond to social interactions
  - Deficits in nonverbal communicative behaviors used for social interaction
  - Deficits in developing, maintaining, and understanding relationships
- Restricted, repetitive patterns of behavior, interests, or activities, as manifested by at least two of the following:
  - Repetitive motor movements or use of objects
  - Insistence on sameness, inflexible routines
  - Highly restricted, fixated interests that are abnormal in intensity
  - Hyper- or hyporeactivity to sensory input
- Symptoms must be present in the early developmental period (but may not become fully manifest until social demands exceed limited capacities or may be masked by learned strategies in later life).
- Symptoms cause clinically significant impairment in social, occupational, or other important areas of current functioning.
- These disturbances are not better explained by intellectual disability disorder.

Source: Data from American Psychiatric Association. *Diagnostic and Statistical Manual of Mental Disorders, DSM-5.* 5th ed. American Psychiatric Publishing; 2013:50-51.

Assessment Tools

- Autism Behavior Checklist (ABC)[17]
- Autism Spectrum Screening Questionnaire (ASSQ)[18]
- Autism Spectrum Quotient (AQ)[19]
- Checklist for Autism in Toddlers (CHAT)[20]
- Childhood Autism Rating Scale, Second Edition (CARS 2)[21]
- Early Screening for Autistic Traits (ESAT)[22]
- Gilliam Autism Rating Scale–2nd Edition (GARS-2)[23]

DISRUPTIVE MOOD DYSREGULATION DISORDER

DMDD is one of the newest additions to the *DSM-5*. It was intended to prevent the inappropriate use of bipolar disorder or oppositional defiant disorder in children who present with disruptive behaviors.

Prevalence

As a new diagnosis added to the *DSM-5* in 2013, DMDD's prevalence is difficult to ascertain. There is a paucity of empirical data on the incidence of the disorder, and as a new disorder, it is considered controversial. If a child meets the criteria for both DMDD and ODD, they are only to be assigned DMDD (Table 18.3). The disorder cannot be diagnosed before the age of 6.

Risk Factors

Parental mental health disorders may be a risk factor, as a higher rate of DMDD has been identified in children whose parents have been diagnosed with a mental disorder, specifically substance use disorders. The experience of other mental health disorders may also be risk factors for DMDD, as 92.8% of youth diagnosed with DMDD met the criteria for another mental disorder (Table 18.5), including mood disorders, conduct disorder, ODD, ADHD, and substance abuse, and the majority had already received treatment for comorbid disorders.[24]

Table 18.3: *DSM-5* Diagnostic Criteria for Disruptive Mood Dysregulation Disorder

- Severe, recurrent **temper** outbursts that are grossly out of proportion to the situation/provocation
- Inconsistent with the developmental level
- Occur three or more times/week
- Mood between temper outbursts is persistently **irritable or angry**
- Duration is 12 or more months, without symptom-free interval of 3 or more consecutive months
- Symptoms are present in at least two of three settings (home, school, peers) and are severe in at least one setting
- **Age** at onset is **before 10 years**
- Diagnosis not made for the first time before age 6 years or after 18 years
- Full criteria for manic/hypomanic episode have never been met
- Behaviors do not occur exclusively during an episode of major depressive disorder and are not better explained by other disorders like dysthymia, ASD, posttraumatic stress disorder, and separation anxiety disorder.
- Diagnosis cannot coexist with bipolar disorder, intermittent explosive disorder, and ODD.

Source: Data from American Psychiatric Association. *Diagnostic and Statistical Manual of Mental Disorders, DSM-5.* 5th ed. American Psychiatric Publishing; 2013:156.

Approach to Diagnosis

Just like the name denotes, DMDD is in the category of depressive disorders, yet it is exhibited by disruptive or irritable behaviors, typical of childhood depression, in addition to problems regulating the mood, or mood swings. It is also a disorder of childhood in that the onset of symptoms must occur before age 10, with a diagnosis before age 18. Treatment includes treating the comorbidities and may include the use of antidepressants, cognitive behavioral therapy, family therapy, or behavioral parent training. There is not a specific assessment tool since the diagnosis is so new, but the Child Behavior Checklist: Dysregulation Profile has been used.

Assessment Tool

■   Child Behavior Checklist—Dysregulation Profile[25]

ANXIETY DISORDERS

Anxiety is an emotion that is experienced by most people in today's busy societies. Anxiety can be an emotion of fear or worry and can contribute to increased physical activity. Anxiety disorders are the most frequently occurring of all mental disorders and can include a generalized anxiety disorder (GAD), specific phobia, separation anxiety disorder, or panic disorder with or without agoraphobia. Anxiety disorders that develop in childhood may persist into adulthood. Significant levels of anxiety can impact the autonomic nervous system, associated with the flight-or-fight system, and cause a cascade of physiologic responses that are then experienced by the individual as physical symptoms and can be mistaken for medical causes.

An anxiety disorder frequently experienced in childhood may be separation anxiety disorder, a specific phobia, or social anxiety. In social anxiety disorder or social phobia, the individual is fearful or anxious about social interactions, resulting in avoidance of these settings. This may include social interactions such as meeting new people or situations involving eating or drinking in front of others. The individual fears being negatively evaluated by others through being embarrassed, humiliated, or rejected or may even fear offending others.

Specific phobias frequently experienced in children and adolescents include fear of animals, bugs, the dark, water, and medical procedures, among many others. Individuals with a first-degree relative experiencing a specific phobia are more likely to experience it as well. Separation anxiety is essentially excessive fear or anxiety about separation from home or attachment figures. It may be manifested as fears about the harm or death of their loved one in their absence, thus interfering with their ability to separate.

Table 18.4: *DSM-5* Diagnostic Criteria for Separation Anxiety Disorder

- Developmentally inappropriate and excessive fear or anxiety concerning separation from those to whom the individual is attached—meets at least three symptom criteria (see list).
- The fear, anxiety, or avoidance lasts at least 4 weeks in children and adolescents and 6 months or more in adults.
- The disturbance causes clinically significant distress or impairment in home, work, or school settings.
- The disturbance is not better explained by another mental disorder.

Source: Data from American Psychiatric Association. *Diagnostic and Statistical Manual of Mental Disorders, DSM-5.* 5th ed. American Psychiatric Publishing; 2013:190-191.

Prevalence

Separation anxiety is more prevalent in children, with prevalence being 4% in that age group, 1.9% in adolescents, and 1.6% in adults as reported in the *DSM-5*.[6]

Risk Factors

Risk factors for the experience of an anxiety disorder can include the experience of a situational stressor, parental overprotectiveness, trauma, abuse, or loss. Having a first-degree relative with an anxiety disorder also increases the likelihood of experiencing one. Individual temperament, specifically inhibition or negative affectivity, is associated with an increased development of anxiety disorder as well.

Approach to Diagnosis

Diagnostic criteria for separation anxiety disorder are listed in Table 18.4. The best approach for treating anxiety disorders in children and adolescents includes cognitive behavioral therapy, systematic desensitization therapy, exposure therapy, and family therapy. Pharmacotherapy with Prozac (fluoxetine), one of the only SSRI medications that is approved by the Food and Drug Administration for use in children, may be helpful as well. Engaging in the use of technology may be instrumental as well, such as the use of the SmartCAT app.[26]

Assessment Tools

■   Children's Separation Anxiety Scale (CSAS)[27]
■   Screen for Child Anxiety Related Emotional Disorders Adult version (SCARED-A)[28]

TRAUMA AND STRESS-RELATED DISORDERS

The reorganization of the *DSM-5* combined the attachment disorders of childhood, commonly seen in situations of abuse or neglect, with posttraumatic stress disorder

(PTSD) and adjustment disorders, providing a separate and distinct category, Trauma and Stressor-Related Disorders. This took PTSD out of its familiar place with anxiety disorders, but the psychologic underpinnings and connections of these disorders make this a reasonable change.

When infants or children do not receive appropriate care or face stressful situations outside of their ability to cope, they are prone to the development of trauma and stressor-related disorders. Reactive attachment disorder and disinhibited social engagement disorder are often seen in cases of neglect, and the symptoms may carry over after neglect has been rectified. In reactive attachment disorder, the child does not seek out interaction or attention from a caregiver, which can lead to failure to thrive. In disinhibited social engagement disorder, the child may indiscriminately seek out attention from unfamiliar adults or in inappropriate ways, thus placing them at risk for additional abuse or harm.

According to a very large retrospective study of a large health maintenance organization by Felitti et al.,[29] children who had adverse childhood experiences (ACEs) such as various forms of physical or emotional abuse or neglect as well as household dysfunction or traumatic losses correlated with poor mental and physical outcomes in adolescence and adulthood. ACEs were relatively common, in that about 50% of the sample of 9,508 reported at least one. Those who experienced four or more had a significant risk of developing serious problems, such as substance use disorders, depression, or suicide attempts.[29]

Early identification of children who encounter ACEs with access to proper mental health treatment could mitigate some of these later outcomes, although access to mental health professionals remains limited in many communities.

ADJUSTMENT DISORDER

Adjustment disorders are commonly occurring in all age groups and consist of the presence of emotional or behavioral symptoms in response to a specific stressor. The stressor may be something as common as the termination of a romantic relationship, or something unique to the individual. Stressors may affect the specific individual, their family, or a larger group or community. Some stressors may accompany specific developmental stages, such as changes in family development, or may follow the death of a loved one when the intensity, quality, or persistence of grief reactions exceeds what normally might be expected. The increased prevalence of incivility or bullying in schools and social media can contribute to this problem. Adjustment disorders are potential triggering events that may increase the risk of suicide.[6]

Prevalence

Adjustment disorders are common and the percentage of patients in an outpatient mental health center with a principal diagnosis of an adjustment disorder can range from 5% to 20% and up to 50% of psychiatric consultations in the inpatient setting, as reported in the *DSM-5*.[6]

Risk Factors

Individuals from lower socioeconomic backgrounds or other disadvantaged circumstances are more likely to be exposed to multiple stressors, causing an increased risk for the development of an adjustment disorder. Individual resiliency traits can be protective factors, and instruction in stress management, problem-solving, and coping skills should be provided to these groups.

Approach to Diagnosis

It is important to differentiate a normal stress response from the diagnosis of an adjustment disorder. To be considered a disorder, it must cause impairment in the individual's functioning, and their response is considered out of proportion to the stressor. It is very normal to be upset when difficult things happen, but when it interferes with the functioning of an individual who does not meet the criteria for a personality disorder; the individual may be experiencing an adjustment disorder (Table 18.5). Supportive, brief insight-oriented psychotherapy; cognitive behavioral therapy; and group or family therapy are the best approaches to treating adjustment disorders, and treatment may take place in the outpatient setting, but in extreme situations, inpatient treatment may be warranted.

Table 18.5: *DSM-5* Diagnostic Criteria for Adjustment Disorders

• The development of emotional or behavioral symptoms in response to a significant stressor that occurs within 3 months of the event.
• These symptoms or behaviors cause distress that is out of proportion to the severity of the stressor, considering the external context and the cultural factors that might influence the symptom, and causes impairment in social, occupational, or other important areas of functioning.
• The stress-related disturbance does not meet the criteria for another mental disorder or indicative of a preexisting mental disorder.
• The symptoms are not those associated with a typical bereavement.
• After removal of the stressor, the symptoms do not persist for more than an additional 6 months, as this would be an acute stress disorder.
Specify whether with depressed mood, or anxiety, or both (mixed). Specify acute (<6 months) or chronic (>6 months)

Source: Data from American Psychiatric Association. *Diagnostic and Statistical Manual of Mental Disorders, DSM-5.* 5th ed. American Psychiatric Publishing; 2013:286–287.

Assessment Tools

- Diagnostic Interview Adjustment Disorder (DIAD)[30]
- Kessler Psychological Distress Scale[31]
- WHODAS II[32]

POSTTRAUMATIC STRESS DISORDER

PTSD was first coined in 1980 by the American Psychiatric Association to describe the emotional reactions to intense trauma. Wars have been a prime cause of this problem in soldiers, and during World War I and II, it was called "shell shock" or "battle fatigue." Although all individuals react differently to exposure to traumatic events, the basic feature of PTSD is a certain set of symptoms following a traumatic event that are outside the range of usual experience. Some believe that the name should exclude the word "disorder" as it may prevent some individuals from seeking treatment due to stigma, while others believe the need to maintain it as a disorder to encourage access to various treatments to help treat this condition.

Prevalence

Mulvihill[33] conducted an integrative review of the literature regarding childhood trauma between 1997 and 2003 and found that 30% of children exposed to trauma develop PTSD, compared to a statistic of 5% to 10% of adults. Due to the prevalence of exposure to trauma, it is reported that PTSD is the fourth-most common psychiatric disorder and that there is a lifetime prevalence of 7% to 12% in the general population and a higher incidence in women (10%–12%) than in men (5%–6%).

Women are more likely to be exposed to interpersonal violence, and men have greater exposure to violence or military combat. Older adults are more likely to experience sub-threshold symptoms of PTSD that can cause significant impairment.[6]

The National Center for PTSD reports the prevalence of PTSD among adolescents based on data from the National Survey of Adolescents to be estimated at 3.7% for boys and 6.3% for girls.[34] A study using the National Comorbidity Survey Replication (NCS-R) estimated the lifetime prevalence of PTSD among adult Americans to be 6.8% and a lifetime prevalence of PTSD among men was 3.6% and among women was 9.7%.[35]

Risk Factors

Resiliency factors are often considered as preventative for developing PTSD and research regarding resiliency building is ongoing. Mulvihill[33] identified that supportive adult relationships and increased social supports were strong resiliency factors, as children who had these available were less likely to develop PTSD following a traumatic experience. Conversely, deficits in social supports are risk factors for developing PTSD.

Approach to Diagnosis

The main symptoms of PTSD are described as reexperiencing, avoidance, negative alterations in cognitions and mood, and alterations in arousal and reactivity (Table 18.6). These symptoms may manifest in patients' lives in many ways, such as recurrent dreams, flashbacks, distress caused by triggers, or physiologic reactions to memories of the event(s). Clinical practice guidelines recommend the use of cognitive behavioral therapy, dialectical behavioral therapy, exposure therapy, mindfulness-based stress reduction (MBSR), eye movement desensitization and reprocessing (EMDR), hypnotherapy, and SSRI or SNRI medications as evidence-based approaches to treat PTSD.[36,37]

Assessment Tools

Assessment tools can be accessed through the U.S. Department of Veteran Affairs website: www.ptsd.va.gov/professional/assessment/overview/index.asp.

Table 18.6: *DSM-5 Diagnostic Criteria for Posttraumatic Stress Disorder*

- Exposure to actual or threatened death, serious injury, or sexual violence in one of the following ways: (a) directly experiencing the traumatic event; (b) witnessing, in person; or (c) learning that the traumatic event occurred to a close family member or close friend.

- Presence of **intrusion** symptoms associated with the traumatic event, beginning after the traumatic event occurred, such as recurrent intrusive and distressing memories, dreams, or flashbacks.

- Persistent **avoidance** of people, places, or things that trigger memories, thoughts, or external reminders of the traumatic event.

- **Negative cognitions** or changes in mood and/or thoughts associated with the traumatic event resulting in an inability to remember important aspects of the traumatic event; exaggerated negative beliefs or expectations about oneself, others, or the world; or distorted thoughts about the cause or consequences of the traumatic event that lead the individual to blame themselves or others.

- Changes in arousal and reactivity associated with the traumatic event, resulting in **hypervigilance**, irritable behavior and angry outbursts, reckless or self-destructive behavior, exaggerated startle reflex, and trouble concentrating or initiating sleep.

- The disturbance lasts more than 1 month and causes significant distress or impairment in functioning.

Source: Data from American Psychiatric Association. *Diagnostic and Statistical Manual of Mental Disorders, DSM-5.* 5th ed. American Psychiatric Publishing; 2013:271-274.

Posttraumatic Stress Disorder Tools:

- Primary Care PTSD Screen (PC-PTSD)
- PTSD Checklist (PCL)

Adult Self Report:

- Davidson Trauma Scale (DTS)
- Distressing Event Questionnaire (DEQ)
- Impact of Event Scale–Revised (IES-R), Los Angeles Symptom Checklist (LASC)
- PTSD Checklist (PCL)—Civilian, Military
- Specific Trauma, Screen for Posttraumatic Stress Symptoms (SPTSS)
- Trauma Symptom Checklist–40 (TSC-40)
- Trauma Symptom Inventory (TSI)

Adult Clinician-Administered Interviews:

- Clinician-Administered PTSD Scale (CAPS) (gold standard)
- PTSD Symptom Scale–Interview Version (PSS-I)
- Structured Clinical Interview for *DSM-IV* PTSD Module (SCID)
- Structured Interview for PTSD (SI-PTSD)

Child Clinician-Administered Interview:

- Child PTSD Reaction Index (CPTS-RI)
- Children's Impact of Traumatic Events Scale–Revised (CITES-2)
- Children's Posttraumatic Stress Disorder Inventory (CPTSDI)
- Clinician-Administered PTSD Scale for Children & Adolescents (CAPSCA)
- Trauma Symptom Checklist for Children (TSCC)
- Traumatic Events Screening Inventory (TESI)
- Dimensions of Stressful Events (DOSE)

Child: Self or Parent Report:

- Child PTSD Symptom Scale (CPSS)
- Parent Report of Child's Reaction to Stress
- Trauma Symptom Checklist for Young Children (TSCYC)
- UCLA Child/Adolescent PTSD Reaction Index for *DSM-5*
- When Bad Things Happen Scale (WBTH)
- My Worst Experiences Survey

EATING DISORDERS

Eating disorders are officially classified as feeding and eating disorders in the *DSM-5* and are described as persistent disturbances in eating behaviors that result in alterations in the consumption or absorption of nutrition that impairs the physical or psychologic functioning. These disorders include pica, rumination disorder, anorexia nervosa, bulimia nervosa, and binge-eating disorder, as well as avoidant/restrictive food intake disorders associated with infancy or early childhood. Three of the most commonly occurring eating disorders, anorexia nervosa, bulimia nervosa, and binge eating disorder, are discussed. Binge-eating disorder is a new addition to the *DSM-5*.

Prevalence

According to the *DSM-5*,[6] anorexia nervosa and bulimia nervosa are both more common in females than males, at a 10:1 ratio. The prevalence of anorexia nervosa among females was reported to be 0.4%, while bulimia nervosa is reported to be more prevalent, at 1% to 1.5% of females. Binge eating disorder is more prevalent than anorexia or bulimia and is also more common in females, although the ratio is much lower, with prevalence estimated at 1.6% of females and 0.8% of males in the United States. Eating disorders are considered to be culture-bound syndromes; these disorders occur in similar frequencies in most industrialized countries and are rare in other nations, where food and fashion have entirely different values.

Risk Factors

All three of these eating disorders appear to run in families, which may reflect genetic influences. In addition, individuals with obsessional traits or anxiety disorders in childhood, or participants in activities that encourage a thin appearance, such as dance, modeling, and some athletics, also are associated with increased risk of anorexia nervosa. Also, the experience of weight concerns, low self-esteem, depressive symptoms, social anxiety disorder, and overanxious disorder of childhood are associated with increased risk for the development of bulimia nervosa.

Approach to Diagnosis

The diagnosis of an eating disorder is based upon the elements of distorted self-image or sense of self-worth, and restriction of intake or loss of control over intake, with feelings of distress; these are outlined in Tables 18.7 to 18.9. A number of physical symptoms of starvation

Table 18.7: *DSM-5* Diagnostic Criteria for Anorexia Nervosa

- Restriction of intake, leading to a significantly low body weight
- Intense fear of gaining weight or of becoming fat
- Disturbance in the way in which one's body weight or shape is perceived

Specify restricting or binge eating/purging type.

Source: Data from American Psychiatric Association. *Diagnostic and Statistical Manual of Mental Disorders, DSM-5.* 5th ed. American Psychiatric Publishing; 2013:338–339.

Table 18.8: *DSM-5* Diagnostic Criteria for Bulimia Nervosa

- Recurrent episodes of binge-eating: eating an amount of food that is larger than what most individuals would eat in a similar time frame, and
- A sense of lack of control over eating during the episode, and
- Recurrent compensatory behaviors to prevent weight gain, such as self-induced vomiting; misuse of laxatives, diuretics, or other medications; fasting; or excessive exercise.
- Binge/purge behaviors occur at least once a week for 3 months.
- Self-worth is focused on body shape and weight.
- Behaviors are not better correlated with anorexia nervosa.

Specify mild, moderate, severe, or extreme based on number of episodes.

Source: Data from American Psychiatric Association. *Diagnostic and Statistical Manual of Mental Disorders, DSM-5.* 5th ed. American Psychiatric Publishing; 2013:345.

Table 18.9: *DSM-5* Diagnostic Criteria for Binge Eating Disorder

- Recurrent episodes of binge eating: eating an amount of food that is larger than what most individuals would eat in a similar time frame
- A sense of lack of control over eating during the episode
- Three of the following:
  - Eating more rapidly than normal
  - Eating until feeling uncomfortably full
  - Eating large amounts of food when not hungry
  - Eating alone due to embarrassment from quantity of food eaten
  - Feeling depressed or very guilty after eating
  - Distress regarding binge-eating
- The binge eating occurs at least once a week for 3 months
- Not due to anorexia or bulimia nervosa

Specify mild, moderate, severe, or extreme based on number of episodes.

Source: Data from American Psychiatric Association. *Diagnostic and Statistical Manual of Mental Disorders, DSM-5.* 5th ed. American Psychiatric Publishing; 2013:350.

may accompany anorexia nervosa, with emaciation, hypothermia, hypotension, and bradycardia, which can be life-threatening. Treating eating disorders will usually combine family and behavioral therapy and often requires inpatient treatment for stabilization of the physical status. Long-term residential treatment of 2 to 4 weeks is also common, especially when the disorder has gone on in secrecy for a long term, as time is needed for behavioral change. Most individuals will continue to participate in individual or group outpatient therapy on a continuous basis as well.

Assessment Tools

- The Eating Attitudes Test (EAT-26)[39]
- The SCOFF Questionnaire[40]

OLDER ADULT: MENTAL HEALTH DISORDERS

The following mental health disorders are frequently identified in older adults: mood disorders, generalized anxiety disorder (GAD), schizophrenia, substance abuse, and somatic symptom disorder. For other mental health disorders, the *DSM-5* provides descriptions and symptomatologies to guide your diagnoses.

MOOD DISORDERS: MAJOR DEPRESSIVE DISORDER

Prevalence

According to the *DSM-5*,[6] 7% of the population suffers from major depressive disorder (MDD) at some point in a 12-month period, and in 2018, intentional self-harm (suicide) was the 10th-leading cause of death in the United States.[41] Suicide was the second-leading cause of death for persons between the ages of 10 and 34, the fourth-leading cause of death for persons between the ages 35 and 54, and the eighth-leading cause of death for persons between the ages 55 and 64 in 2018.[42] Suicide is highest among American Indian and non-Hispanic males and females, followed by White, non-Hispanic males and females.[42] Sadock et al.[4] report the majority of persons with depression have suicidal ideation, and 10% to 15% commit suicide. In addition, persons living in nursing homes who suffer from depression are at an increased risk for death the first year of admittance.[6]

Risk Factors

The following factors place the person at risk for depressive symptomatology: female gender, chronic physical disorder, first-degree family members with a diagnosis of MDD, *social isolation, disability, and stressful life events.*[43]

Approach to Diagnosis

Table 18.10 provides an overview of symptomatology for a diagnosis of MDD according to the *DSM-5*.

Table 18.10: *DSM-5* Diagnostic Criteria for Major Depressive Disorder[6]

- Depressed mood
- Loss of interest or pleasure
- Weight loss or weight increase
- Insomnia or hypersomnia
- Psychomotor agitation or retardation
- Feeling of worthlessness or guilt
- Decreased ability to think clearly or make decisions
- Fatigue, tiredness
- Thoughts of death, suicidal ideation

Source: Data from American Psychiatric Association. *Diagnostic and Statistical Manual of Mental Disorders, DSM-5.* 5th ed. American Psychiatric Publishing; 2013:160–162.

Older adults often present with physical symptoms that need further assessment. One of the essential features of the diagnosis relates to time; a *depressed mood must be present for at least 2 weeks, nearly every day with a loss of interest or pleasure.*[6] In addition, at least five of the following symptom in Table 18.10 must be evident.

BIPOLAR I AND BIPOLAR II

Prevalence

The prevalence in the United States for Bipolar I is 0.6% with the suicide rate estimated to be *15 times* higher than among the general population.[6] Bipolar II prevalence is 0.8% in the United States.[6]

Risk Factors

The primary risk factor associated with bipolar disorders is genetic inheritance, with a 10-fold increased risk with relatives with the same diagnosis. Persons from high-income countries are at an increased risk, as well as those who are separated, divorced, or widowed.[6]

Approach to Diagnosis of Bipolar I

Table 18.11 provides an overview of symptoms associated with a diagnosis of Bipolar I. In order to have a diagnosis of Bipolar I, the person must experience a manic episode, which is defined as "a distinct period of abnormally and persistently elevated, expansive, or irritable mood and abnormally and persistently increased goal-directed activity or energy, *lasting at least 1 week* and present most of the day, nearly every day."[6] At least *three* of the symptoms in Table 18.11 must also be present.

Table 18.11: *DSM-5* Diagnostic Criteria for Bipolar I[6]

- Grandiose behavior or increased self-esteem, confidence
- Decreased sleep requirement
- Talkative and pressured speech
- Racing thoughts and flight of ideas
- Difficulty focusing and easily distracted
- Agitation or increased goal-directed activity
- Engagement in activities such as gambling, spending sprees, sexual activities
- Marked impairment of social or occupational functioning

Source: Data from American Psychiatric Association. *Diagnostic and Statistical Manual of Mental Disorders, DSM-5.* 5th ed. American Psychiatric Publishing; 2013:124.

Approach to Diagnosis of Bipolar II

Table 18.12 provides an overview of symptoms related to a diagnosis of Bipolar II. The main distinguishing factor for this diagnosis is an episode of current or past hypomanic behavior for *4 days* and current or past major depression for a *2-week period but does not impair social or occupational activity or require hospitalization.*[6]

Assessment Tools

A variety of tools are available to assess depression and mania. The most common tools are discussed in the following, including clinician rating tools and self-reported tools.

Table 18.12: *DSM-5* Diagnostic Criteria for Bipolar II[6]

- Hypomanic episode
  - Grandiose behavior or increased self-esteem, confidence
  - Decreased sleep requirement
  - Talkative and pressured speech
  - Racing thoughts and flight of ideas
  - Difficulty focusing and easily distracted
  - Agitation or goal-directed activity
  - Engagement in activities such as gambling, spending sprees, sexual activities
  - Change in functioning recognized by others
- Major depressive episode
  - See Table 18.10

Source: Data from American Psychiatric Association. *Diagnostic and Statistical Manual of Mental Disorders, DSM-5.* 5th ed. American Psychiatric Publishing; 2013:132–133.

- **The Geriatric Depression Scale (GDS):** The GDS originally developed with 30 questions but was revised to a 15-item scale; it was designed for the geriatric population. Suicidality is not assessed in this tool.[44]
- **Beck Depression Inventory (BDI):** The BDI developed in 1961 by Aron Beck is a 21-item self-report questionnaire, measuring attitudes and depressive symptoms.[45]
- **Hamilton Rating Scale for Depression (HAMD):** The HAMD tool developed in 1960 is used to measure the severity of depression for an inpatient population by a clinician.[46]
- **Patient Health Questionnaire (PHQ-9):** The PHQ-9 is a tool to measure the severity of depression, a self-reporting instrument consisting of nine questions based on the *DSM-IV* criteria for major depression. Patients rate themselves on the frequency of experiencing symptoms of depression during the last 2 weeks, from 0 (*not at all*) to 3 (*nearly every day*). Total scores ranging from 5 to 9 indicate mild depression, 10 to 14 moderate depression, 15 to 19 moderately severe depression, and 20 to 27 severe depression.[47]
- **Zung Self-Rated Depression Scale (SDS):** The SDS self-report scale, developed in 1965, consists of 20 items (half positively worded and half negatively worded) used to screen for depression.[46]
- **Center for Epidemiologic Studies Depression Scale (CES-D):** The CES-D tool was developed in 1977 by Radioff and consists of 20 items related to symptoms of depression.[48]
- **Mood Disorder Questionnaire (MDQ):** The MDQ is a screening tool used to assess for bipolar disorders. The tool consists of 13 items related to symptoms of mania and asks for a yes-or-no response to the symptom.[49]

ANXIETY: GENERALIZED ANXIETY DISORDER

Anxiety disorders are the most commonly occurring mental disorder in the United States. This is both related to the high-paced lifestyle, as well as genetic predisposition and other modifiable risk factors.

Prevalence

The prevalence of GAD is 2.9% for adults in the United States, with a higher rate of incidence among females.[6] Anxiety can be debilitating for older adults, leading to isolation, loneliness, and severe psychosocial impairment.

Risk Factors

Several risk factors are associated with GAD, specifically genetic inheritance, negative thinking and affect, and harm avoidance.[6]

Table 18.13: *DSM-5* Diagnostic Criteria for General Anxiety Disorder[6]

- Disproportionate anxiety and worry
- Inability to control the worry
- Restlessness, shakiness
- Tired, fatigued easily
- Irritable
- Muscle tension
- Difficulty with sleep

Source: Data from American Psychiatric Association. *Diagnostic and Statistical Manual of Mental Disorders, DSM-5.* 5th ed. American Psychiatric Publishing; 2013:122.

Approach to Diagnosis

Table 18.13 lists the most frequent symptoms associated with GAD. Disproportionate worry and anxiety for *more than 6 months* is the primary symptom of GAD; worry about own health, children, monies, and friends consumes their everyday life and begins to interfere with their psychosocial functioning. In addition, three or more of the symptoms in Table 18.13 *must be present for 6 months.*[6]

Assessment Tools

The two most common tools used to assess anxiety are the Hamilton Anxiety Rating Scale (HAM-A) and the State Trait Anxiety Inventory (STAI).

- **HAM-A:** The HAM-A, developed in 1959, is a tool utilized by a clinician to assess both cognitive and somatic symptoms of anxiety. Fourteen criteria are scored from 0 to 4, with 0 indicating the symptom is not present to 4 indicating the symptom is severe.[4]
- **STAI:** The STAI is a self-report tool, measuring both state (current feeling of anxiety) and trait anxiety (propensity for anxiety). The tool contains 40 items, 20 questions related to the State Anxiety subscale and 20 to the Trait Anxiety subscale.[6]

SCHIZOPHRENIA

Although the incidence of schizophrenia is less than 1%, it is the mental disorder that causes the greatest disease burden, due to the significant impairment that it causes.

Prevalence

Reports of the prevalence of schizophrenia range from 0.3 to 0.7%[6] to 1%.[4] The ratio of male to female is equal, but the onset of symptoms is earlier in men.[4]

Risk Factor

The major risk factor associated with schizophrenia is genetic loading. Persons are at an increased risk if a first-order relative has schizophrenia. Additional risk factors include prenatal exposure to influenza, gestational complications, and maternal starvation during pregnancy.[4]

Approach to Diagnosis

Table 18.14 presents the most common symptoms associated with schizophrenia. At least one of the symptoms of delusions, hallucinations, or disorganized speech must be present for *at least a month*, along with another criterion, and impairment of functioning at work, in relationships, or in care of self must be evident for at *least 6 months*.[6] Persons diagnosed with schizophrenia must also be closely monitored for suicide intent as 10% commit suicide and 20% to 40% attempt suicide.[50] In addition, the risk for metabolic syndrome is increased for persons on antipsychotic medication, thus requiring monitoring for obesity, diabetes, and cardiac disease.

Assessment Tools

■ **Brief Psychiatric Rating Scale (BPRS):** The BPRS is a 20-item scale used to assess psychiatric symptoms, which include somatic concerns, anxiety, emotional withdrawal, conceptual disorganization, guilt feelings, tension, mannerisms and posturing, grandiosity, depressive mood, hostility, suspiciousness, hallucinatory behavior, motor retardation, uncooperativeness, unusual thought content, blunted affect, excitement, disorientation, severity of illness, and global improvement. The tool is recommended for use for persons with "significant impairment."[4]

■ **Positive and Negative Syndrome Scale (PANSS):** The PANSS is a clinician rating tool used to assess the positive and negative symptoms associated with schizophrenia.[51]

Table 18.14: *DSM-5* Diagnostic Criteria for Schizophrenia[6]

- Altered perceptions: delusions, hallucinations
- Speech: loose associations, word salad, incoherent
- Behavior: catatonic, avolition, impaired impulse control
- Cognition: impaired memory, executive functioning, poor insight
- Negative symptoms: anhedonia, flat affect

Source: Data from American Psychiatric Association. *Diagnostic and Statistical Manual of Mental Disorders, DSM-5.* 5th ed. American Psychiatric Publishing; 2013:99.

SUBSTANCE ABUSE: SUBSTANCE USE DISORDERS

The *DSM-5* revised the nomenclature for problems with addiction from terminology of a particular substance abuse, dependence, or withdrawal to the classification-specific substance "use disorder," for example, alcohol use disorder. The substances can involve alcohol, nicotine, prescription, or other illicit substances.[6]

Prevalence

Substance use disorders, specifically alcohol use, are identified as a "growing public health problem" with older adults.[52] The prevalence of alcohol use disorder in persons age 65 and older vary and range from 0.24% to 15.4%.[52]

Risk Factors

Risk factors associated with substance use disorders relate to genetic loading, access to substances, and the presence of other psychiatric disorders.

Approach to Diagnosis

A diagnosis of substance use disorder (Table 18.15) is a "cluster of cognitive, behavioral, and physiologic symptoms indicating that the individual continues using the substance despite significant substance-related problems."[6] Substances associated with substance use disorder include alcohol, caffeine, cannabis, hallucinogens, inhalants, opioids, sedatives, hypnotics, anxiolytics, stimulants, and tobacco.

Assessment Tools

■ CAGE: The CAGE questionnaire is most frequently used to assess alcohol usage and consists of four questions: "Have you ever **C**ut down on your drinking? Have people **A**nnoyed you by criticizing your drinking?

Table 18.15: *DSM-5* Diagnostic Criteria for Substance Use Disorder[6]

- Impaired Control: inability to control use of substance, increased use, craving substance
- Social Impairment: use of substance impacting role at work, home, and school
- Risky Use: use of substance despite physical and/or psychologic results
- Pharmacologic: symptoms of tolerance and withdrawal

Source: Data from American Psychiatric Association. *Diagnostic and Statistical Manual of Mental Disorders, DSM-5.* 5th ed. American Psychiatric Publishing; 2013:483.

Have you ever felt bad about your drinking or Guilty about your drinking? Have you ever had a drink the first thing in the morning, as an Eye-opener, to steady your nerves or get rid of a hangover?"[4] Responses are scored 0 or 1, with a score of 2 or higher indicating clinical significance.

■ Michigan Alcohol Screening Test (MAST): The MAST is a 25-item, self-rated tool used to assess alcohol use disorder.[53]

SOMATIC SYMPTOM DISORDER

The *DSM-5* replaced somatoform disorder with somatic symptom disorder. Somatic symptom disorder involves a person having an excessive focus on physical symptoms that causes changes in behaviors or emotions.

Prevalence

Persons with somatic symptom disorder frequently present themselves to a medical provider before a mental health provider; thus, the prevalence of the disorder is difficult to determine. The prevalence has been reported to range from 5% to 7%[6] to as high as 15%[4] and is diagnosed more in females than in males.

Risk Factors

Risk factors associated with somatic symptom disorder include negative affectivity, symptoms of anxiety, and depression. In addition, low socioeconomic status and educational level, female gender, age, unemployment status, and health issues have been identified as risk factors.[6]

Approach to Diagnosis

The diagnosis of somatic symptom disorder is often made after a complete medical evaluation for the symptoms presented by the person, and no organic cause is found

Table 18.16: *DSM-5* Diagnostic Criteria for Somatic Symptom Disorder[6]

- Somatic symptom: one or more symptoms that are distressing or interfering with daily life

- Excessive thoughts, feelings, behavior related to symptoms: disproportionate or persistent thoughts, high level of anxiety, excessive time and energy related to symptoms

- Length of time: a symptom may not be consistently present, the state of being symptomatic is persistent and usually more than 6 months

Source: Data from American Psychiatric Association. *Diagnostic and Statistical Manual of Mental Disorders, DSM-5.* 5th ed. American Psychiatric Publishing; 2013:311.

to support the amount of focus on the symptoms. The critical component is the focus on the symptoms being at the point of interfering with their daily functioning. It is not appropriate to diagnose a patient with a mental disorder when a medical cause is found for a symptom they are experiencing but rather only when this situation interferes with their functioning (Table 18.16). Treatment generally consists of using psychotherapy, including family, cognitive, or behavioral therapies.

Assessment Tool

PHQ-15: The tool is self-administered and consists of 15 items.[54]

APPROACHES TO TREATMENT

Pharmacologic

Several practice guidelines based on evidence-based research are available to guide the practitioner to determine which pharmacologic agent to prescribe for mental health disorders (Table 18.17). In addition, genetic screening is available to assist with identifying which medication might work best with the client based on genetic makeup. The Beers Criteria should be reviewed prior to prescribing medication to older adults.

Metabolism of psychotropic medications is impacted by the hepatic cytochrome P450 enzymes (1A2, 2D6, 2C9, 2C19, 3A4), which induce or inhibit the metabolism of other pharmacologic agents and may require dosage adjustments. Common medications that act as inhibitors include SSRIs, bupropion, clomipramine, cimetidine, clarithromycin, fluoroquinolones, grapefruit (including juice), ketoconazole, and nefazodone. Medications that act as inducers include carbamazepine, hypericum (St. John's wort), phenytoin, phenobarbital, and tobacco.[55]

Antidepressants

Antidepressants are medications used in the treatment of affective disorders. Symptom improvement is usually noted within 3 to 6 weeks after initiation of treatment and is considered a response when at least 50% of the symptoms improve.[55] Depressed mood, suicidal ideation, and psychomotor retardation respond well to antidepressants, whereas insomnia, fatigue, concentration level, and a lack of motivation may not be as responsive.[55] Serotonin syndrome is a potentially lethal adverse reaction associated with "therapeutic medication use, inadvertent interactions between drugs, and intentional self-poisoning."[56] Antidepressants have a black-box warning for increased risk of suicidality in children and young adults.[57] Table 18.17 lists the most common antidepressants and significant issues related to the medication.

Antipsychotics

Antipsychotics are used in the treatment of schizophrenia and other psychosis, bipolar disorders, and

Table 18.17: Medications to Treat Major Depressive Disorder

- **Selective Serotonin Reuptake Inhibitors (SSRI)**
  - *Fluoxetine* (Prozac) is an SSRI with 5HT2C antagonistic action, which leads to an activating response and is used with caution with persons experiencing agitation, anxiety, or insomnia. Half-life: 2–3 days.
  - *Sertraline* (Zoloft) is an SSRI with dopamine reuptake inhibition and sigma-1 receptor binding which can produce improvement in hypersomnia, energy levels, and mood.
  - *Paroxetine* (Paxil) is an SSRI with muscarinic anticholinergic and norepinephrine reuptake inhibitor actions, which can produce increased sedation and calmness. Abrupt discontinuance can produce symptoms of akathisia, restlessness, gastrointestinal (GI) distress, and dizziness.
  - *Fluvoxamine* (Luvox) is an SSRI with sigma-1 receptor binding and is frequently used to treat obsessive-compulsive disorders and anxiety.
  - *Citalopram* (Celexa) is an SSRI, which at higher doses can increase the risk of QT prolongation.
  - *Escitalopram* (Lexapro) is an SSRI, which has few side effects and is well tolerated.
  - *Side Effects*: The most common side effects of SSRIs include GI distress, headaches, and sexual dysfunction.

- **Serotonin-norepinephrine reuptake inhibitors (SNRI)**
  - *Venlafaxine* (Effexor) is an SNRI, available in extended-release form, used for both mood disorders and anxiety disorders. Notable side effects are increased blood pressure and sweating.
  - *Desvenlafaxine* (Pristiq) is an SNRI, which is used for the treatment of mood disorders, but aids in the relief of vasomotor symptoms related to perimenopause.
  - *Duloxetine* (Cymbalta) is an SNRI which "relieves depression in the absence of pain and pain in the absence of depression."
  - *Mirtazapine* (Remeron) was approved by the Food and Drug Administration (FDA) for depression; notable side effects are weight gain and sedation.

- **Norepinephrine-dopamine reuptake inhibitors (NDRI)**
  - *Bupropion* is an NDRI, which is activating, the sexual dysfunction side effect is not as prevalent; also used to treat nicotine addiction.

- **Tricyclics (TCAs)**
  - Tricyclics were the first generation of antidepressants; were known for their efficacy, but their side effects were also notable: sedation, weight gain, anticholinergic symptoms, constipation, orthostatic hypotension, dizziness, cardiac arrhythmias, and seizures.[55(p344-345)]
  - Medications: clomipramine, imipramine, amitriptyline, nortriptyline, protriptyline, maprotiline, amoxapine, doxepin, desipramine, trimipramine, dothiepin, lofepamine, and tianeptine[55(p342)]

- **Monoamine Oxidase Inhibitors (MAOIs)**
  - Prescribing MAOIs requires knowledge related to dietary restrictions and drug interactions. Dietary restrictions relate to a tyramine restricted diet, which limits aged cheeses; dried, aged, smoked meats; tap and unpasteurized beer; sauerkraut; kimchee; soy products; and banana peels. The potential effect of not avoiding tyramine products is a hypertensive crisis.[55(p331)]
  - The drug interactions related to MAOIs are medications, which have sympathomimetic actions and can cause hypertensive crisis, and serotonin reuptake inhibitors that can cause serotonin syndrome. Caution is used with persons needing surgery and stopping the MAOI for 10 days prior to surgery is recommended. Stahl's provides an overview of drugs to avoid if prescribing MAOIs; most important are avoidance of SSRIs, SNRIs, clomipramine, St. John's wort, meperidine, tramadol, methadone, and fentanyl. A washout period is needed when switching from another antidepressant and prior to starting MAOIs, typically *5 to 7 days* and *5 weeks* if the person was on fluoxetine.
  - Medications: tranylcypromine sulfate (Parnate), selegiline transdermal (ENSAM), phenelzine (Nardil)[58(p579,661,735)]

Sources: Stahl SM. Stahl's *Essential Psychopharmacology: Neuroscientific Basis and Practical Applications.* 4th ed. Cambridge University Press; 2013; Stahl SM. *Stahl's Essential Psychopharmacology: Prescribers Guide.* 6th ed. Cambridge University Press; 2017.

Table 18.18: Antipsychotics: Medications for Thought Disorders

First Generation, Conventional, Typical: This category of antipsychotics includes D_2 antagonists in all areas of the brain; blockage in the mesolimbic pathway reduces positive symptoms of psychosis and blocks the reward mechanism; blockage in the dorsal striatum is associated with extrapyramidal side effects (EPS) and tardive dyskinesia; blockage in the pituitary is associated with hyperprolactinemia; blockage in the mesocortical DA pathway is related to worsening of cognitive and negative symptoms. In addition, blockage of M_1-cholinergic receptors is related to the anticholinergic side effects, and blockage of H1 receptors is related to weight gain and sedation.

Medications: chlorpromazine (Thorazine), haloperidol (Haldol), loxapine (Loxitane), fluphenazine (Prolixin), pimozide (Orap)

Second Generation, Atypical: These antipsychotics are $5HT_{2A}$ and D_2 antagonists, serotonin-dopamine antagonists. Their clinical profile is "equal positive symptom antipsychotic actions, but low extrapyramidal symptoms and less hyperprolactinemia compared to conventional antipsychotics." Monitoring for metabolic syndrome (diabetes, cardiovascular disease, and stroke) is required for atypical antipsychotics.

- *Clozapine* (Clozaril): The first atypical antipsychotic is "the only antipsychotic that has been documented to reduce the risk of suicide in schizophrenia." Enrollment in risk evaluation and management strategy programs (clozapine REMS program) for the risk of agranulocytosis is required and includes protocols for labs.
- *Olanzapine* (Zyprexa): Olanzapine is associated with significant weight gain and increased risk for diabetes and dyslipidemia.
- *Quetiapine* (Seroquel): Quetiapine does not cause "EPS at any dose, nor prolactin elevation . . . preferred atypical antipsychotic for patients with Parkinson disease who require treatment for psychosis." Assess for cataract development.
- *Asenapine* (Saphris): Asenapine is only given sublingually due to high first-pass metabolism and no food or drink for 10 minutes following dose.
- *Risperidone* (Risperdal): Risperidone is associated with increased prolactin levels, weight gain, and EPS depending on dose.
- *Paliperidone* (Invega): Active metabolite of risperidone, less sedating, fewer EPS and less orthostatic hypotension than risperidone.
- *Ziprasidone* (Geodon): Ziprasidone must be given with food for absorption, associated with limited weight gain, dyslipidemia, or fasting triglyceride elevation side effects. Monitor for QT prolongation.
- *Iloperidone* (Fanapt): High half-life of 18 to 33 hours, increased risk for orthostatic hypotension and sedation related to alpha 1 antagonism.
- *Lurasidone* (Latuda): Must be taken with food to increase absorption, associated with limited weight gain or dyslipidemia.
- *Aripiprazole* (Ability): Limited weight gain, dyslipidemia, elevation of fasting triglycerides, or insulin resistance.

Sources: Stahl SM. *Stahl's Essential Psychopharmacology: Neuroscientific Basis and Practical Applications.* 4th ed. Cambridge University Press; 2013; Stahl SM. *Stahl's Essential Psychopharmacology: Prescribers Guide.* 5th ed. Cambridge University Press; 2014; Stahl SM. *Stahl's Essential Psychopharmacology: Prescribers Guide.* 6th ed. Cambridge University Press; 2017.

treatment-resistant depression and "off-label" uses.[55] The use of antipsychotics with the adolescent and geriatric population requires close monitoring for side effects, including extrapyramidal symptoms, metabolic syndrome, QT prolongation, and neuroleptic malignant syndrome (NMS). Antipsychotics have a black-box warning of an "increased risk of mortality in elderly patients treated for dementia-related psychosis."[57] The American Psychiatric Association[60] has new practice guidelines for the treatment of persons with schizophrenia, including guidance for medication and psychosocial interventions. Table 18.18 lists the most common antipsychotics.

MEDICATION USE IN ADOLESCENTS

The safety and efficacy of the use of antidepressants in children and adolescents have been well documented in peer-reviewed medical and nursing journals, yet the formal diagnosis and treatment of depression as a mental health disorder is often overlooked. Very often, the focus remains on the behavioral symptoms or social issues, which are also very important, yet the possibility of an underlying or comorbid depression or other mood disorder should be considered.

The biologic basis for depression has also been long established, and failure to complete a full psychiatric evaluation with consideration of the use of medication may be a missed opportunity to stabilize the youth's mood and prevent long-term adverse outcomes. Too often, when delinquent or antisocial behavior or substance use is involved, the absence of a full psychiatric evaluation may be a missed critical opportunity to preserve normal development of the child or adolescent.

According to Stahl,[55] the monoamine hypothesis is the underlying principle for the treatment of psychiatric

Table 18.19: Mood Stabilizers: Medications for Mood Disorders

- Mood stabilizers are medications used to treat bipolar disorders, targeting symptoms of mania and depression to prevent relapse and reoccurrence. Only the most common mood stabilizers will be discussed. The CANMAT guidelines are an excellent resource for treatment of bipolar disorders.
- *Lithium:* Lithium is considered the "gold standard" for mood stabilization treatment related to mania and, to a lesser degree, depression. The major side effects of lithium are gastrointestinal (GI) distress (nausea/vomiting/diarrhea), weight gain, fine tremors, and incoordination. The mediation requires close monitoring, as the therapeutic range is narrow and toxicity can develop. Prior to treatment, assessment of kidney function, thyroid function, and an EKG is recommended for persons over 50 years.
- *Valproic acid:* Valproic acid is effective in the treatment of the acute phase of mania and is used long term to prevent the reoccurrence of mania.
- *Carbamazepine* (Tegretol): Carbamazepine is also effective in the treatment of mania but is also an inducer of the CYP450 enzyme 3A4 and can be very sedating.
- *Lamotrigine:* Lamotrigine is approved for maintenance treatment of bipolar I disorder. An adverse effect is the development of a rash related to the Stevens-Johnson syndrome.

Sources: Stahl SM. *Stahl's Essential Psychopharmacology: Neuroscientific Basis and Practical Applications.* 4th ed. Cambridge University Press; 2013; Stahl SM. *Stahl's Essential Psychopharmacology: Prescribers Guide.* 6th ed. Cambridge University Press; 2017; Yatham LN, Kennedy SH, Parikh SV, et al. Canadian Network for Mood and Anxiety Treatments (CANMAT) and International Society for Bipolar Disorder (ISBD) collaborative update of CANMAT guidelines for the management of patients with bipolar disorder: Update 2013. *Bipolar Disord.* 2013;15:1-44. doi:10.1111/bdi.12025

disorders, in which the depletion of neurotransmitters, such as norepinephrine, dopamine, and serotonin, contributes to the symptomatology of depression, irritability, psychosis, inattention, or other related mood disorders (Tables 18.19-18.21).

The neurotransmitter receptor theory posits that there is an abnormality with the receptors for these key monoamine neurotransmitters or a problem with the signal transduction from the receptors and associated with intracellular transcription factors that control gene regulation.

The numbers of medications with FDA approval for use in children and adolescents are limited due to a lack of clinical trials with this vulnerable population. There are some studies that document dosage and efficacy with this population, and when there is literature to support its use, practitioners will often use these medications "off label."

Nonpharmacologic Treatment

There are several evidence-based psychotherapeutic interventions that are recommended for the treatment of mental health disorders in adolescents and the geriatric population. The following are the most common approaches.

Motivational Interviewing (MI): MI, commonly used today by all healthcare practitioners, is an approach that assists a person in behavioral changes. Miller and Rollnick[62] describe MI as a "style of being with people, an integration of particular clinical skills to foster motivation for change." The communication skills utilized in MI are "asking open ended questions, affirming, reflecting, summarizing, and providing information, and advice with permission."[62]

Cognitive Behavior Therapy (CBT): CBT developed by Aron Beck in 1976 is an evidence-based approach to

therapy that proposes that "by changing one's thoughts, emotions and behaviors can also be changed."[63] CBT has been found to be effective for numerous mental health disorders, such as depression, anxiety, obsessive-compulsive disorders, and borderline personality disorders.[63]

Dialectical Behavior Therapy (DBT): DBT, based on cognitive behavior therapy, was developed by Marsha Linehan. The approach focuses on behavioral change using persuasive dialogue.[63] This form of treatment has been found to be effective in the treatment of borderline personality disorder and PTSD.[64]

Eye Movement Desensitization Reprocessing: EMDR developed by Francine Shapiro[65] in which the therapist "guides the patient in processing affective, cognitive, and somatic material with procedures and protocols that include some form of bilateral stimulation (BLS) during a session."[63] Wheeler[63] provides a synthesis of multiple research articles, which provide evidence of efficacy of EMDR.

Individual Therapy: Individual therapy can be based on several theoretical frameworks, for example, interpersonal therapy, solution-focused psychotherapy, and humanistic-existential approach. Each is distinct, but all are relationship-centered and used to treat the majority of mental health disorders.

Group Therapy: Group therapy may utilize a variety of approaches, but the principles are universal: instillation of hope, universality, imparting information, altruism, corrective recapitulation of the primary family group, development of socializing techniques, imitative behavior, interpersonal learning, group cohesiveness, catharsis, and existential factors.[63]

Table 18.20: Anxiolytics/Antianxiety: Medications for Anxiety Disorders

Pharmacologic treatment for anxiety disorders requires careful monitoring (due to abuse potential) and dosing titration. Choice of medication is dependent on the diagnosis and severity of symptomatology. The following are anxiety disorders and Stahl's[55(p388-419)] recommended pharmacologic treatment.

- *Generalized Anxiety Disorder:* SSRIs, SNRIs, benzodiazepines, buspirone, and pregabalin and gabapentin.[55(p416)] Benzodiazepines are recommended for short-term use while waiting for the SSRIs and SNRIs to take effect.
- *Social Anxiety Disorder:* SSRIs, SNRIs, pregabalin, and gabapentin. Beta-blockers, MAOIs, and benzodiazepines are considered second-line treatments.
- *Posttraumatic Stress Disorder:* SSRIs and SNRIs
- *Panic Disorder:* SSRIs, SNRIs, benzodiazepines, and pregabalin and gabapentin

Source: Stahl SM. *Stahl's Essential Psychopharmacology: Neuroscientific Basis and Practical Applications.* 4th ed. Cambridge University Press; 2013.

Psychosocial Therapies: Recreational therapy, music therapy, and art therapy are all additional forms of therapy utilized to foster a person's sense of well-being.

Complementary Alternative Therapy: Yoga, Heart Math®, massage, relaxation exercises, meditation, hypnosis, guided imagery, aromatherapy, acupressure, reflexology, biofeedback, and organizational coaching are all forms of complementary therapies used to treat a person experiencing a variety of mental health disorders. Herbal therapies and supplements are also used, but caution is needed due to the drug interactions with psychotropic medications. For example, Sam-e, used for depression, may produce serotonin syndrome, hypomania, or hyperactive muscle movement.[50] Tryptophan used with depression may increase the risk of serotonin syndrome if the person is on an antidepressant that acts on serotonin.[50] St. John's wort accelerates the metabolism of many drugs, which can interfere with treatment.

SPECIFIC TREATMENT FOR ADOLESCENT AND GERIATRIC POPULATIONS

Adolescent

Individual Therapy

It is important to engage an adolescent client and to establish rapport with both the adolescent and the parents. It is helpful if the youth can see the provider as their advocate. It is necessary to first get parental consent in order to treat a minor, although many states do provide

Table 18.21: Psychostimulants: Medications for the Treatment of ADHD

Pharmacologic treatment of ADHD should only be initiated for those who meet the *DSM-5* criteria for ADHD. According to the American Pediatric guidelines, psychostimulant medication is effective for most children in reducing symptoms of ADHD but should only be considered if the child has not responded to parent training in behavior management and in children ages 6 and older. Additional evidence-based pharmacologic treatments include atomoxetine, extended-release guanfacine, and extended-release clonidine. Common adverse effects of stimulants are a decrease in appetite, somatic symptoms, such as headache or stomachache, or sleep disruption.[11(p13)] Prior to administration of a stimulant medication, a cardiac assessment, including family history, should be obtained.[11(p13)] The following are common medications.

Stimulants

- Methylphenidate (Ritalin), dextroamphetamine (Dexedrine), lisdexamfetamine dimesylate (Vyvanse), methylphenidate (Focalin), dextroamphetamine (Adderall), methylphenidate (Concerta), methylphenidate transdermal patch (Daytrana)

Alpha Agonists

- Clonidine (Catapres), Kapvay (clonidine extended-release), guanfacine (Tenex, Intuniv)

Nonstimulants/SNRIs

- Atomoxetine (Strattera)

ADHD, attention deficit hyperactivity disorder.

Source: Wolraich ML, Hagan JF, Allan C, et al; Subcommittee on Children and Adolescents with Attention-Deficit/Hyperactive Disorder. Clinical practice guideline for the diagnosis, evaluation, and treatment of attention-deficit/hyperactive disorder in children and adolescents. *Pediatrics.* 2019;144(4):e20192528. doi:10.1542/peds.2019-2528

laws to allow for the provision of mental health services to a youth without parental consent. It is also important to consider the youth in terms of receiving informed consent, as the adolescent and parents must receive informed consent regarding the use of psychotropic medications, reviewing the risks and benefits as well as alternative treatment options. Best practice calls for receiving consent from all parties and then allowing the identified patient, or the young person, to make decisions whenever appropriate; that is, ask youth whether they would like to be seen alone first or together with parents first. It is also important to spend time seeing the parents or guardian alone also, after making a connection with the youth first.

Family Therapy

Family therapy is often a necessary approach in treating children and adolescents. Family systems theory considers that symptomatic youth may be indicative of problems in family dynamics (e.g., identified patient, relationships may be out of balance in hierarchy, marital strain, detached or with enmeshed boundaries, etc.). Treating the youth alone will not address these issues and so may not be as effective. NPs who are trained in family systems approaches may work with the whole family or, if providing psychiatric evaluation and medication management only, will refer to a licensed family therapist, who may be a psychologist or social worker for follow-up as well.

Group Therapy

Group therapy is very effective with children and adolescents, as due to the developmental stage, youth identify with their peers, and this prevents them from feeling isolated. Group therapy to deal with specific clinical problems, such as sexual trauma, ASD, ADHD, social skills, divorce, grief, and loss, are often available for children and adolescents in the community. There are a number of self-help groups available as well, such as Alateen, or Narateen when there are specific issues related to drug or alcohol use affecting the family system.

Inpatient Psychiatric Hospitalization

It is necessary to provide care for children and their families in the least restrictive environments. Separating a child from their caretakers can be traumatic in and of itself. When the behavior is considered a risk of danger to self or others, considering things like suicidal ideation or actions, sexually acting out, run away behaviors, substance use, and physical or verbal threats or actual incidents of harming others, inpatient treatment in a crisis stabilization unit may be required. These settings are locked psychiatric inpatient units, and most states require separate programs specific to minors. Admission to these programs may be voluntary or may be court-ordered. Treatment is provided in a multidisciplinary treatment team, consisting of a psychiatrist, psychologists, NPs, social workers, other therapists, recreational or occupational therapists, registered nurses, and mental health assistants. An initial psychiatric evaluation is provided, and treatment may include medication management; individual, group, and family therapy; and behavioral therapy, such as the use of a level system or token economy. The length of stay varies greatly depending on patient acuity as well as disposition planning needs for follow-up, which may involve the need for longer term placement, but average length of stay is 4 to 7 days.

Residential Treatment Centers

After several inpatient admissions to a crisis stabilization unit, without improvement in the behavioral symptoms, longer term treatment in a residential treatment center may be needed. These programs also provide treatment from the multidisciplinary treatment team, but the programs are designed to house individuals in more of a homelike atmosphere, for an average of 1 to 6 months, depending on the problem. There are RTCs to treat individuals with specific problems such as substance use disorders or eating disorders, as well as many programs that treat any mental health disorders. These programs also include educational specialists, and the youth continue with their education while in attendance.

Geriatric

The geriatric population responds well to pharmacologic intervention, individual therapy, and psychosocial therapies.

Pharmacologic Therapy

Pharmacologic treatment of older adults must take into consideration comorbid medical conditions and pharmacologic interactions with psychotropic medications. The NP must also consider the side effects and black-box warnings related to psychotropic medication. Consulting the Beers Criteria prior to prescribing medication is recommended.

Individual Therapy

MI, CBT, and individual therapy are all considered to be effective interventions when working with the geriatric population.

Psychosocial Therapies

Therapies that include socialization, communication, and relationship building with others all facilitate the well-being of the person.

CLINICAL PEARLS

Children and Adolescents

When treating children and adolescents, it is helpful to think in terms of treating the whole family system. It is not uncommon for there to be relationship conflict or communication challenges in a family system, and so an awareness of the family dynamic is imperative to any assessment of a young person, as family intervention is often necessary. As minors, there are usually limitations to their capacity to consent to treatment, which is determined state by state. It is imperative that APRNs are familiar with their state laws. Most often, the minor will present with their legal guardians for treatment, but this is not always the case. Some states do allow minors limited capacity to consent for some types of services, such as mental health services, although usually over the age of 14, if they are capable of understanding the nature of the treatment. Confidentiality is of the utmost importance when treating adolescents, and establishing a trusting therapeutic relationship is the first goal of treatment. Even so, whenever there are issues concerning the potential for harm to self or others, confidentiality is limited, so that the appropriate authorities can be made aware. When prescribing medications for minors it is important to complete the medication education, including informed consent risk–benefit analysis, with both the individual and the guardian/caregivers.

NPs must strive to be open and honest about healthcare information provided, as well as aware of the vulnerable status of children and adolescents. Adolescence is a time of risk-taking behaviors, and it may seem appropriate to the healthcare provider to approach the issue from a fear-based approach, emphasizing the potential harms from a certain behavior. These approaches are usually not effective and may even have more negative consequences by jeopardizing the therapeutic relationship, which must be based upon openness and genuineness. It is, of course, important to provide information regarding the negative consequences of behaviors, such as sexual activity or substance use, but the individual's thoughts and feelings must be discussed and validated as well.

High-Risk Behaviors

Adolescence is a period during which the individual is focused on identify versus role confusion according to Erickson's stages of development, and seeking approval from peers is an important component. The sense of identity sought at this time is sexual or occupation-related, and encountering problems during this stage can lead to role confusion. Participation in social media, such as Facebook, Instagram, Snapchat, Twitter and others, is a way for an individual to express their forming identity, and these self-expressions may be positive but may also be negative. Some adolescents become addicted to the instant gratification of contact with peers through these forums.

Access to media through videos on Netflix, YouTube, or other internet websites also may have negative consequences, depending on the content. Some videos may include inappropriate content or discussions and challenges for risk-taking behaviors. Some adolescents can become addicted to the attention received on these sites and engage in videotaping risky behaviors themselves in an attempt to gain internet fame. Other adolescents can become addicted to video games, and this lack of direct interaction with others or physical activity can lead to problems such as social anxiety, or the development of obesity, further straining the self-image.

Potential risky behaviors include substance use, sexual experimentations such as "sexting," or nonsuicidal self-injury (NSSI) that usually presents as self-inflicted lacerations, known as cutting. Youth may be more at risk of cyberbullying due to the potential anonymity of internet behavior. Online exposure to content regarding high-risk activities may even normalize them and in some ways can encourage the behaviors, especially with vulnerable individuals, who are experiencing poor social supports. It is important for nurses to discuss the amount and types of internet usage with their adolescent patients, and especially their parents, to provide education and, when needed, interventions targeting these behaviors.[66] Discussions about sexuality, with recommendations regarding testing for sexually transmitted diseases, are also important for this population.

The U.S. Preventative Services Task Force recommends screening and behavioral counseling interventions for adults, in the primary care setting and for adolescents aged 12 to 18.[67] The SAMHSA recommends the use of the Screening, and Brief Intervention, Referral for Treatment (S-BIRT)[68] for screening individuals, including adolescents, for the use of alcohol or other substance use.[5] A number of screening tools are available for drug and alcohol use.[5] The National Institute on Alcohol Abuse and Alcoholism recommends a two-question screening as part of an annual examination or an acute care visit for youth, using two age-specific screening questions. For younger adolescents, it is recommended to first ask if they have any friends who drank beer, wine, or alcohol in the past year and then to ask if they have ever drunk alcohol. In high school–aged youth, it is recommended to first ask about their own use, in an open-ended format, such as "In the past year, how many days have you had a drink containing alcohol?" and then inquire about having any friends that binge drink. If the screen is positive for drinking alcohol, a risk algorithm is provided with an intervention recommendation according to the level of risk, with the treatment being brief advice for low risk, use of motivational interviewing for moderate risk, with the addition of a referral for treatment for those at high risk.[69] The CRAFFT Screening Interview can also be used to assess substance use in this age group, and the mnemonic acronym refers to the key words in the first six screening items, regarding driving in a car with someone using drugs or alcohol, using themselves to relax, if they ever used alone, or gotten into trouble with friends or family due to the use.[70]

Adolescents also have an increased risk for suicide, and it is the third leading cause of death for this age group, following homicide and accidents. Warning signs of suicidal behavior can include talking or posting online about wanting to die, talking about feeling hopeless, feeling trapped or experiencing unbearable pain, feeling like a burden to others, increased reckless behavior such as increased alcohol or drug use, and isolation. The Suicide Assessment Five-Step Evaluation and Triage (SAFE-T)[71] approach was developed for healthcare providers to identify the risk and protective factors regarding suicide and determine the risk level, with appropriate recommendations for intervention and follow-up.

CASE STUDY
ADOLESCENT WITH NONSUICIDAL SELF-INJURY DISORDER

Ashley is a 15-year-old female who attends 10th grade at her public high school. She resides with her mother and two younger siblings. Her parents divorced last year, after several years of parental discord. She found out that her father was cheating on her mother with another woman he met online. She has had infrequent contact with her father since the divorce. Her grades have decreased; where she previously was an A–B student, she is now getting Cs and Ds. Her mother states that she understands that Ashley is going through a lot right now and has made allowances for the change in academic performance. Ashley's mother works two jobs to make ends meet, and so Ashley frequently has to babysit her younger siblings. Since the divorce, her family's finances have been difficult, and she does not have money to spend on stylish clothing, so she has taken to wearing T-shirts and jeans. She has been feeling very irritable and angry about the situation. Her mother is always working and seems depressed herself since the divorce, so Ashley does not want to talk to her about her feelings, but she has strong emotions and just does not know how to express them. Her previous best friend is now hanging out with the popular crowd and pretends that Ashley does not exist. This group has posted a number of critical remarks about Ashley on social media, some of which were distressing and not true. She met a girl in her study hall, who is a "goth" and dresses in black, seems like she has it all together, and has befriended Ashley. She has shared that she cuts herself as a way to relieve the pain from this life, shows Ashley a number of scars on her arms, and explains the meaning behind each one and how it helped her through rough times. She tells Ashley that she cannot depend on anyone, that life does not have any meaning, and people will disappoint you, but she found a way to control the pain through cutting. Ashley decides to try cutting herself. The first few times she almost faints from the pain, is afraid about the bleeding, and is worried that her mother will find out. The laceration on her arm becomes bright red and acutely painful after a couple of days, and she develops a fever and flu-like symptoms. She tells her mother, who brings her in immediately to be evaluated by an NP at the local urgent care center.

Considerations

Ashley has a number of risk factors and may be experiencing an adjustment disorder with depressed mood or even a mdajor depressive disorder. She is experiencing a potentially traumatic loss due to the circumstances related to the divorce. The bullying experienced on social media is another precipitating factor, and these experiences are possible risk factors for suicide. A complete suicide evaluation, with consideration of protective factors and the development of a safety plan, is imperative, along with the evaluation of the infected laceration. A referral for counseling with a behavioral specialist is imperative, as the development of a trusting therapeutic relationship is needed, as Ashley is at risk for continued maladaptive behaviors. It is important for the NP treating Ashley to make a connection with Ashley, and one way she can do this is to see her privately first. The NP should obtain informed consent about any of her treatment recommendations from both Ashley and her mother. The NP uses the S-BIRT approach during her one-to-one with Ashley, and Ashley denies any drugs or alcohol use. The NP uses the SAFE-T suicide evaluation with C-SSRS and then provides a brief intervention regarding the self-mutilation, with a referral to counseling. Ashley agrees to journal her feelings whenever having thoughts of self-harm and agrees to let her mother know when she is upset. The NP determines that Ashley does not have an active suicidal plan and is a low risk at this time. The NP has a brief discussion with Ashley and her mom about the recent stressors and the need for counseling. The provider prescribes a topical antibiotic cream, as well as a 10-day course of Keflex to treat the infection. The NP meets with both Ashley and her mother together and schedules an appointment to see Ashley again in 1 week to assure that she has followed through with the counseling appointment, and that the wound is healing appropriately.

Case Study Questions

1. In this case, Ashley's mother was aware of the self-mutilation, but if the parent was not aware, what is the nurse's responsibility of informing the parent of a minor about this type of behavior?
2. How can the NP establish a trusting relationship, and maintain the confidentiality of adolescents in cases of self-harm?

Geriatrics

The care of older adults requires skilled assessment, patience, and a supportive presence. Developmentally, the older adult is experiencing many changes. Loss becomes a major issue; loss of friends, spouses, and significant others; retirement; and physical and psychologic changes are all factors that can impact a person psychologically.

Understanding the person's history and cultural background can provide information to support the individual during this time of change. Encouraging social engagement, physical activity, and supportive friends and family is essential to the integrity of the person's psychologic well-being.

In addition, older adults may experience health challenges that can impact their mental health. Chronic health conditions often coincide with anxiety, depression, and other mental health disorders. Some older adults are reluctant to seek assistance with mental health professionals but are willing to talk with their primary care providers. Understanding the complexity of psychosocial treatment along with medical treatment can be challenging. Screening for mental health issues can become an important part of preventative healthcare. The U.S. Preventative Task Force[72] recommends screening for depression in the adult population with "adequate systems in place to ensure accurate diagnosis, effective treatment, and appropriate follow-up."

CASE STUDY
OLDER ADULT WITH TYPE 2 DIABETES AND MAJOR DEPRESSION

Client: Mrs. C, first visit

Subjective: CC: "I'm so sad; my kids are gone and never call me. I've cared for them all my life and now they don't care what happens to me. I need something to help me get out of this funk." HPI: 62 y/o black female c/o sadness and loneliness, which has increased to a daily feeling over the last 2 months. Reports having difficulty sleeping and waking up early, feeling tired all the time, has no interest in anything or going out with other people. Gained 10 pounds last month, reports too tired to exercise. Reports she has not been able to go to work for the last week because she received a negative yearly evaluation because she was unable to complete tasks and make decisions. No family history of depression or suicide, denies suicidal ideation or attempt. Oriented x 4. PHQ-9 score is 16. Children have moved out of state and are busy with their own lives. Social History: Divorced 2 years ago after 35 years of marriage. Two married daughters living out of state. Remains in contact with siblings and has a brother that lives nearby. Works as a secretary at a law office for the last 2 years, prior to that worked in her ex-husband's office. Parents are both deceased. Reports that she had been active in her church, but recently has stopped attending. Unable to report activities that give her pleasure. Substance Use: Denies use of drugs, drinks wine one to three times per week. Denies history of any family substance abuse.

Mental Status Examination: Appearance: Dressed in mismatched pants and shirt, hair combed but roots evident and in need of color. Orientation: Oriented x4. Speech: Slow, soft, difficult to understand. Mood/Affect: Sad affect, depressed mood. Teary-eyed. Thought Process: No delusions or psychotic thoughts; slow in delivery of thoughts. Perceptual abnormalities: No AVH. Memory/Attention: Both short-term memory and long-term memory intact, able to follow direction. Abstraction: Able to decipher proverbs with insight. Fund of knowledge: Appears average. Insight and Judgment: Has insight as to sadness, sound judgment evident.

PMH: Medical: Reports diagnosed with type 2 diabetes 5 years ago; well controlled with diet and exercise but reports that she is going to the bathroom more frequently and her vision is blurry sometimes. Reports daily blood sugar range between 80–100 mg/dL. No history of hypertension, cancer, or cardiovascular disease. Only hospitalization was birth of children. Former smoker (1 PPD for 10 years but stopped with birth of children). Surgical: Denies surgeries. OBGYN: Not sure of date of last examination, several years ago. Psychiatric: Denies hospitalizations or seeing a therapist. Denies history of depression or suicide. Medications: Metformin 850 mg bid. Over-the-counter (OTC): None reported. Allergies: NKDA. Tobacco: Currently a nonsmoker, but smoked 1 PPD x 10 years, quit over 30 years ago. Alcohol/Drugs: Socially, one to three glasses per week with dinner. FH: Reports mother had diabetes, type 2. Denies family history of cancer, cardiovascular disease or mental health problems in the family. SH: Works as a secretary for a law office for 2 years. Review of systems (ROS): Denies palpitations, HA, edema, or change in bowel or bladder habits.

Objective Data

VS: Blood pressure (BP) 134/80, T 98.6, heart rate (HR) 78, RR 18, Wt.: 152, Ht: 5'2, body mass index (BMI) 27.8 (overweight)

Labs: A1C 7.2%, Blood Sugar: 110 mg/dL, thyroid-stimulating hormone (TSH): 3 uU/mL, total T4: 6.0, Free t4: .8, T3: 100 WNL, CBC WNL, PE: WNL.

DSM-5 Diagnosis

Major Depression Disorder Moderate

Recommended Therapy

Cognitive behavior therapy twice a week for 3 weeks, then once a week until return to feelings of pleasure and able to function at work. *Monitoring*: Monitor for thoughts of suicide at therapy sessions and inform client of 211 phone system for assistance if unavailable. Administer PHQ-9 scale monthly. *Prescribed Medications*: Fluoxetine 20 mg daily. *Education*: Inform of nonsteroidal anti-inflammatory drugs (NSAIDs) interaction, reconfirm no history of seizures

Diagnosis

DSM-5 Differential Diagnosis: Depressive Disorder Due to Another Medical Condition

Rationale: Evidence from history that mood disorder may be related to medical condition of Type 2 diabetes. Client is experiencing increased urination, blurred vision, fatigue, and weight gain. Past A1C value WNL. *Recommended Therapy*: Order FBS, A1C. Lipid profile and UA, based on results increase metformin to 900 mg bid; Vision screening for blurred vision. *Monitor*: Continue to monitor for unstable glucose control or hypoglycemia due to fluoxetine which together with metformin may increase risk of hypoglycemia. Encourage monitoring of blood glucose throughout day. Encourage increase in exercise and monitoring of dietary intake. Monitor weight and abdomen circumference at monthly visits.

Case Study Questions

3. In this case, what symptoms would indicate the need for a medication adjustment for Mrs. C?
4. What other evidence-based or nonpharmacologic interventions might the NP consider in the treatment of Mrs. C?

QUALITY AND SAFETY ALERT

Several quality and safety issues/terms related to mental health are discussed in the following:

- *Black-Box Warnings:* The U.S. FDA declares that "boxed warnings, commonly known as black box warnings" are placed on prescription drugs that have significant serious or life-threatening risks.[73] Two black-box warnings to be aware of are the following: (a) Antidepressants: In 2004, the FDA issued the warning for antidepressant medications of an increased risk of suicidality in children and adolescents. In 2007, the FDA added to the warning that there was "increased risks of suicidal thinking and behavior, known as suicidality, in young adults ages 18 to 24 during initial treatment (generally the first one to two months)".[74] (b) Antipsychotics: In 2008, the FDA placed the warning of "an increased risk of mortality in elderly patients treated for dementia-related psychosis"[57] for both conventional and atypical antipsychotics.
- *Amber Alert*: Initiated in 1996 in Texas in response to a kidnapped child, the Amber Alert is the nationwide broadcast alert for abducted children, age 17 and younger. AMBER is America's Missing: Broadcast Emergency Response.[75]
- *Silver Alerts:* Since 2006, state laws have been written to assist in the location of missing vulnerable persons with cognitive impairment, such as Alzheimer's disease or related disorders, through a public broadcasting system.[76]
- *Verbal De-Escalation Techniques*: The current approach to the care of agitated persons is to utilize verbal de-escalation techniques versus restraints and medication. Richmond et al.[77] describe evidence-based practice approaches to de-escalation by "empowering the patient to stay in control while building trust with the caregivers."
- *Involuntary/Civil Commitment:* Involuntary or civil commitment is a legal process whereby a person is admitted to a treatment facility against their will for evaluation and treatment. Each state has its own commitment laws, including standards and procedures. An historical overview of involuntary civil commitment in the United States and ethical guidelines for civil commitment are presented in the Substance Abuse and Mental Health Services Administration (SAMSHA) publication *Civil Commitment and the Mental Health Care Continuum: Historical Trends and Principles for Law and Practice*.[78]
- *SAFE-T Suicide Assessment*: A suicide assessment mobile app for healthcare providers to assess and evaluate a person's risk and protective factors and determine interventions and a treatment plan. It is recommended for use with the Columbia Suicide Severity Rating Scale (C-SSRS). The SAFE-T is available from the SAMHSA.[79]
- *Recovery:* A paradigm shift is occurring in the treatment of mental health illness to a recovery-oriented model of care. SAMSHA defines "recovery" as a "process of change through which individuals improve their health and wellness, live self-directed lives, and strive to reach their full potential."[80] Four major dimensions—health, home, purpose, and community—are part of the recovery model of care.

ETHICAL DILEMMAS

The *Guide to the Code of Ethics for Nurses*[81] assists NPs in their practice. Several ethical principles are important to the care of persons with mental illness: the right to be included in decision-making, the right to treatment in the least restrictive environment, and the right to refuse treatment unless treatment has been court-ordered.[50] Understanding these rights can lead to ethical dilemmas that are discussed next.

- *Informed Consent:* An informed consent includes information for a person to make an informed decision regarding their care and treatment. The type of treatment, risks and benefits of the treatment, risks and benefits of no treatment, alternative treatments, and the diagnosis and prognosis should be included in informed consent. The NP must ensure that the person is cognitively able to provide informed consent.

- *Confidentiality and Duty to Warn:* The right to confidentiality is well established by legislation and ethical standards. There is an exception: The NP has the responsibility to protect others if a person has expressed an intent of harming an identified third party, which was established by the legal case *Tarasoff v. Regents of University of California*, 1976.[82]

- *Prescription Drug Abuse:* The NP must consider the effect of long-term treatment using opioids and benzodiazepines. The opioid crisis in the United States requires that as prescribers, thoughtful assessment and evaluation of treatment be considered with continued use of opioids.

CULTURAL ASSESSMENT

Sadock et al.[4] define "culture" as "a set of meanings, norms, beliefs, values and behavior patterns shared by a group of people." The cultural competence of NPs is an expected competency today. The *DSM-5* provides an outline for a cultural formulation to assist in understanding our client's vulnerability, distress, psychosocial stressors, and resilience and guide the treatment. There are five areas included in the cultural formulation interview (CFI): "(1) cultural identity of the individual; (2) cultural conceptualization of distress; (3) psychosocial stressors and cultural features of vulnerability and resilience; (4) cultural features of the relationship between the individual and the clinician; and (5) overall cultural assessment for diagnosis and care."[6] The CFI includes 16 questions that guide the practitioner. Other cultural assessments are available, but the CFI format offers a comprehensive format within the context of mental health.

CONCLUSION

The geriatric NP has a vital role in the care of the mental health needs of all of their patients. As a primary care provider, a comprehensive assessment, and knowledge of mental health diagnoses and treatment can impact the outcome of the client's well-being. This chapter has provided basic knowledge related to the needs of a person with mental disorders because an integrative approach with a psychiatric mental health practitioner can be beneficial for both the patient and the practitioner. Nonpharmacologic treatment is often the beginning treatment approach with many mental health disorders, which can take time, patience, and practice. An integrative approach to treatment, with early identification of mental health problems and referral to treatment, can provide the patient with the best possible outcome.

REFERENCES

References for this chapter are online and available at https://connect.springerpub.com/content/book/978-0-8261-8414-6/part/part01/toc-part/ch18.

CHAPTER 19

Common Pulmonary Disorders Encountered in the Primary Care Setting

Nancy Harris

LEARNING OBJECTIVES

At the conclusion of this chapter, the learner will be able to:

➤ Distinguish normal and abnormal pulmonary anatomy and physiology.

➤ Present the most common pulmonary health disorders in primary care.

➤ Describe pharmacologic and nonpharmacologic treatment of pulmonary disorders.

INTRODUCTION

This chapter discusses the structure and function of the respiratory system and common disorders of the lungs. Two of the most common causes of severe disease and death to be covered are asthma and chronic obstructive pulmonary disease (COPD). Infectious processes, including acute bronchitis and community-acquired pneumonia (CAP), as well as pleural lung diseases and pulmonary vascular diseases, are examined. Current diagnostics and treatment options for each disorder are presented.

OVERVIEW OF THE SYSTEM

Normal Anatomy and Physiology

The respiratory system is composed of the upper and lower airways, with the boundary between the two demarcated by the glottis. All subglottic structures are considered to be the lower respiratory tract. In this section, we are concerned with the subglottic structures, including the trachea, bronchi, and lungs (Figure 19.1).

The lungs are composed of the tracheobronchial tree, alveoli, connective tissue, vascular structures, lymphatics, and nerves all rooted in an elastic connective tissue substance and bound by pleural membranes. The pulmonary pleurae are a pair of serous membrane sacs that line the inner thoracic wall and envelope the lungs. The outer layer (parietal pleura) clings to the inner chest wall. The inner layer (visceral pleura) covers the surface of the lung and adjoining structures. A potential space exists between the parietal and visceral pleura known as the pleural cavity that contains a thin film of lubricating fluid (pleural fluid). Pleural fluid provides cushion and reduces friction between the two pleural membranes.

The trachea is composed of epithelium and C-shaped cartilaginous structures that maintain its shape and prevent it from collapsing as air flows in and out of the lower respiratory tract. The epiglottis is a flap of tissue that covers the trachea during the act of swallowing. The trachea bifurcates at the carina to form the left and right mainstem or primary bronchi. The right and left primary bronchi then subdivide into three and two secondary or lobar bronchi, respectively. Each lobar bronchus feeds a lobe of each lung. The right lung is composed of three lobes (upper, middle, lower lobes), and the left lung is composed of two lobes (upper and lower lobes). The secondary (or lobar) bronchi continue to further branch into tertiary (or segmental) bronchi that supplies a particular bronchopulmonary segment. Terminal bronchioles further subdivide into respiratory bronchioles.

These respiratory bronchioles branch multiple times into smaller subdivisions that ultimately become microscopic structures that terminate in clusters of tiny air sacs known as alveoli. The alveoli are composed of a single layer of simple squamous epithelial cells that allow for rapid diffusion of gases between the two compartments. The alveoli account for the majority of the volume of the lung.

The right and left main pulmonary arteries arise from the pulmonary trunk that receives right heart cardiac output. The pulmonary arteries carry deoxygenated blood returned to the right atrium by the superior and inferior venae cavae. The pulmonary arteries closely follow the branching subdivisions of the airways to give rise to a dense capillary network that encircles the alveoli to form the respiratory membrane (gas exchange structures). The pulmonary capillaries combine to form pulmonary veins that carry oxygenated blood to the left atrium. The pulmonary interstitium is the supportive connective tissue framework of the lung that encloses the airways, lymphatics, and vasculature of the lung, as well as approximates the gas exchange structures of the lung.

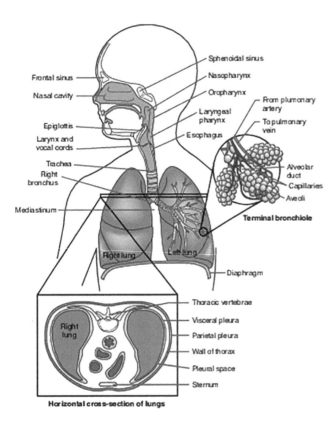

Figure 19.1: The respiratory system

Source: Chiocca EM. *Advanced Pediatric Assessment.* 3rd ed. Springer Publishing Company; 2020.

The lymphatics of the lung are derived from a superficial and deep plexus. The superficial plexus is found beneath the pleura. The deep plexus follows the branching pulmonary vascular network and the expansions of the bronchi. The lymphatics course within the bronchial walls and outside the bronchial walls. There are no lymphatics at the alveolar level. The pulmonary lymphatics act as a conduit for carrying filtered tissue fluid away from the lung and back to venous circulation. Pulmonary lymphatics are also intimately involved in immune surveillance and response.

Brainstem structures, including the pons and medulla, comprise the respiratory control centers. The pons is the pacemaker of breathing. We obviously have conscious control over the rate and depth of breathing. However, these centers receive feedback from mechanoreceptors in the thorax and respiratory muscles and central and peripheral chemoreceptors, as well as vagal afferent receptors in the lung that unconsciously impact the pattern of breathing. Autonomic sympathetic and parasympathetic fibers mediate bronchial diameter, mucus gland secretion, and pulmonary blood flow.

Respiratory rate and the volume of each breath comprise alveolar ventilation which constitutes the amount of air movement into and out of the alveoli. In lung disease, efficient gas exchange is impaired due to alterations in ventilation and/or perfusion that increase the work of breathing. The work of breathing is affected by the compliance of the lung and chest wall, airway resistance, surfactant forces, and the inertia of the respiratory system, which is negligible.

CYSTIC FIBROSIS

Etiology

Cystic fibrosis (CF) is an autosomal recessive inherited disease that results from defective epithelial chloride ion transport. CF is one of the most common genetically inherited diseases of Caucasians.

Pathophysiology

CF is a multisystem disease that affects the respiratory, digestive, and reproductive systems. Mutations in the CF transmembrane conductance regulator (CFTR) gene result in abnormal chloride secretion in epithelial cells leading to decreased hydration of mucus. Chronic respiratory infections and pancreatic insufficiency are common. Pulmonary disease usually develops in infancy or early childhood. Respiratory tract manifestations are due to mucus plugging, airway obstruction, chronic inflammation, and bacterial colonization with damage and remodeling of the airways. Common early symptoms are chronic cough, sputum production, and wheezing. Potential complications of progressive disease include hemoptysis, pneumothorax, and cor pulmonale due to pulmonary hypertension. This is a brief overview. Consider reviewing a pathophysiology textbook for a more comprehensive overview of CF.

Risk Factors

Significant advances in managing CF had resulted in changes in which CF, although a serious condition, is no longer considered the most common life-threatening inherited disorder in the Caucasian population. The incidence is about 1/4,000 in U.S.-born babies.[1] The prognosis has improved over the past decade. CF was considered a disease of children, but now with evidence-based disease management, many adolescents will transition to adult care. In 2018, there were about 55% of patients with CF who were older than age 18.[1] An individual is at higher risk if one or both parents are carriers of a mutated *CFTC* gene or has CF. There is a higher risk if a sibling, half-sibling, or first cousin has CF. More than 10 million Americans are carriers of a *CFTR* gene mutation, and many are unaware. Individuals of Northern European ancestry have the highest risk; it is less common in Hispanics and African Americans, and it is relatively uncommon in Asian Americans.

Approach to Diagnosis

The diagnosis is based on clinical findings that are linked to biochemical or genetic confirmation. Differential diagnoses include immunologic abnormalities, primary ciliary dyskinesis, or Schwachman-Diamond syndrome.

Diagnostics

CF is diagnosed by genetic testing or by a positive sweat chloride test along with one typical manifestation. The sweat chloride test measures the chloride content of sweat. Elevated sweat chloride values are pathognomonic of CF. Advancements in diagnosis and treatment have increased survival and the number of adults with CF now exceeds the number of children.

Screening Tools and Tests

Genetic testing to see if the person has a *CFTR* gene mutation can be done as appropriate. Siblings with CF should be tested whether they have symptoms or not. Other relatives, such as first cousins and half-siblings, may be tested if they have symptoms or the family is concerned that the person may have CF. If the screening is positive, further evaluation is needed to confirm the diagnosis. Families planning to have children may want to be tested, and those already pregnant who have a spouse with CF should consider testing.

Management

Treatment in adult populations involves an interprofessional approach in managing pulmonary and extrapulmonary involvement. Because people are living longer, there is more evidence of gastrointestinal (GI) disturbances ranging from gastroesophageal reflux disease (GERD) and constipation to more complex conditions such as liver disease. Liver involvement is common in CF, with about 30% to 50% of individuals having some type of liver-related disease. Portal hypertension and cirrhosis often present in early childhood. Pancreatic insufficiency, one of the most common GI complications of CF, affects about 85% of patients sometime in their lifetime. Pancreatic duct obstruction during the mother's pregnancy (about the second trimester) leads to pancreatic insufficiency. Patients are at risk for steatorrhea, malnutrition, and fat-soluble deficiencies. CF-related diabetes may develop due to insulin deficiency secondary to pancreatic islet destruction. Nurse practitioners (NPs) should partner with pulmonology and endocrinology specialists to comanage the patient.

Pharmacologic

As the disease progresses, *Pseudomonas aeruginosa* becomes the most common isolated pathogen. Inhaled antibiotics (tobramycin, aztreonam) are the mainstays of pharmacotherapy. Mucolytics (dornase alfa) and hypertonic saline are used as adjunct therapy as well as aerosolized corticosteroids. Oral corticosteroids have been shown to slow the decline in lung function, but their use is limited due to long-term complications. CFTR modulator therapies have revolutionized the treatment of adults and children, correcting the defective protein and moving treatment from therapies directed toward the restoration of lung function and end-organ damage to therapies directed toward the restoration of the function of the CFTR. These medications (ivacaftor, lumacaftor/ivacaftor, tezacaftor/ivacaftor, elexacaftor/tezacaftor/ivacaftor) address the underlying cause of the disease in CF patients identified with *CFTR* genetic mutations.[2]

Nonpharmacologic

Adolescents with CF often have growth failure due to malabsorption, increased energy needs, and reduced appetite. Consulting with a dietitian can be beneficial to evaluate, monitor, and treat nutritional issues. Each person should have an individualized meal plan that meets their nutritional needs as well as includes foods they enjoy eating. Vitamin D deficiency is common and should be evaluated and treated as appropriate. Adolescents may require nutritional and behavioral counseling that focuses on the physical and psychologic aspects of living with CF (see Chapter 11 for more information).

Treatments

Airway clearance therapy (ACT) such as chest physiotherapy, positive expiratory pressure, high-frequency chest wall oscillation, and postural drainage with percussion improves mucous transport and reduces the bacterial load. Aerosolized bronchodilators are no longer recommended for chronic use as evidence of benefit in chronic treatment is low. Organism-specific antimicrobial therapy is an essential part of therapy. *Staphylococcus aureus* is the most common pathogen isolated from the sputum early in the course of the disease. Routine evaluation of patients with stable disease should include posterior/anterior and lateral chest x-rays every 2 to 4 years, with more frequent imaging with symptoms of increased pulmonary exacerbation.

Patient Education

Patients, typically diagnosed in childhood, need to understand the implications of this inherited, long-term multi-organ disease. Proper procedures for postural drainage and percussion should be reinforced with caregivers regularly. Patients should be counseled to avoid infections by frequent handwashing, avoiding crowds, and obtaining a yearly influenza vaccine. Relatives should also be advised as they have a higher risk than average of being carriers of a *CFTR* mutation. Siblings in the family of a person diagnosed with CF should be tested for the *CFTR* gene irrespective of whether they have symptoms or not to identify if they are carriers or have a latent form of the disease itself. Consider genetic

---

Box 19.1: Patient Education: When to Contact a Nurse Practitioner

As this is a multi-organ disease, patients and caregivers should be advised to contact their healthcare provider for the following:

- any symptoms getting worse or new symptoms
- gastrointestinal manifestations such as severe diarrhea, abdominal pain, vomiting, anorexia, or discolored sputum
- new-onset chest pain or tightness
- shortness of breath or wheeze
- fever
- fatigue or inability to maintain normal activities

---

counseling to help individuals understand and cope with outcomes of genetic testing. Patients and their families should be educated about when to contact their healthcare provider (see Box 19.1). The Cystic Fibrosis Foundation (www.cff.org) and National Institutes of Health (NIH; www.nhlbi.nih.gov/health-topics/cystic-fibrosis) should be recommended for patients and families for additional education.

ASTHMA

Etiology

Asthma refers to a heterogeneous group of respiratory diseases with distinct phenotypes relating to individual genetic and environmental factors. Asthma may be categorized as extrinsic or allergic versus intrinsic or nonallergic. Understanding the immunopathology of asthma is important to improve patient outcomes when managing the disease.

Pathophysiology

All forms of asthma are characterized by reversible airway obstruction, bronchial hyperresponsiveness, and airway inflammation resulting in wheeze, cough, dyspnea, and chest tightness. Asthma severity correlates with the degree of airway obstruction, the frequency of symptoms, and subsequently with the frequency of short-acting beta-agonist (SABA) usage. Characteristically, nocturnal symptoms of airway obstruction are more prominent.

Risk Factors

A positive family history of asthma increases risk in atopic families. Research has identified more than 100 associated genes; however, phenotypic expression of asthma appears to be augmented by environmental factors. Indoor allergen exposure (e.g., dust mites, indoor fungi, cockroach allergen, indoor animals, farm animals) plays

an important role in the development of asthma. Exposure to maternal cigarette smoking is strongly linked to childhood asthma. Breastfeeding is associated with a lower incidence of wheezing during the first 2 years of life but does not reduce the risk of wheezing later in childhood. If seen later in childhood, it is most likely atopic asthma. There is a greater incidence of asthma in males. Typical provocative causes for nonallergic asthma include medications, variability in air temperature and weather, exercise, stress, specific aromas, smoke, chemicals, hormones, and variable occupational exposures.

Approach to Diagnosis

The testing for asthma is primarily focused on pulmonary function testing, but other tests, such as chest radiography, blood tests, and tests for allergy, may be appropriate for diagnosis. Patients presenting with signs and symptoms that are consistent with asthma (e.g., cough, wheeze, shortness of breath, chest tightness) should be assessed for other possible causes such as the following:

- **Wheeze:** COPD, goiter in adults and in adolescents, tonsillar hypertrophy, postnasal drip syndrome
- **Cough:** Rhinitis or rhinosinusitis, GERD, bronchitis, angiotensin-converting-enzyme inhibitors, smoker
- **Dyspnea:** Heart failure, COPD, pulmonary embolism, and sarcoidosis

In adolescents and young to middle-aged adults, consider asthma if the person has recurrent episodes of bronchitis and GERD, panic disorder, or sarcoidosis. In older adults, always evaluate if they are/were a smoker, and consider COPD, left-ventricular heart failure, interstitial lung disease, and recurrent oropharyngeal aspiration (especially if the person has a neurologic disorder, dementia, or has had a stroke). There are certain conditions that coexist with asthma that can make the course of the condition worse.

Allergic rhinitis often coexists with allergic asthma and postnasal drip can worsen symptoms. Dyspnea in people who are obese or have COPD may make them appear to have asthma even though they may not have this disease. However, when these diseases coexist with asthma the patient may present with more severe dyspnea. The National Heart, Lung, and Blood Institute of the NIH updated asthma guidelines in 2020, and these can be found at www.nhlbi.nih.gov/health-topics/asthma-management-guidelines-2020-updates.[3]

Diagnostics

Atopy (produces exaggerated immunoglobulin [IgE] immune response to otherwise harmless substances in the environment) is frequently associated with asthma; therefore, a thorough history, as well as family history, is essential. Spirometry with postbronchodilator response is utilized as an important baseline study to support or confirm the diagnosis of asthma. An improvement in forced expiratory volume in 1 second (FEV1) of 12% or more than 200 mL is considered diagnostic of asthma. Asthma is classified as mild intermittent, mild persistent, moderate persistent, or severe persistent depending on symptoms (see Exhibit 19.1).

Screening Tools and Tests

Consider asthma in those with a cigarette smoking history, who are obese, or who have an allergy history. At this time there are no screening guidelines for exercise-induced asthma for athletes; however, some sporting organizations are beginning to establish screening programs for internationally competitive athletes.

Management

Achieving optimal outcomes for those with asthma involves an interprofessional team and implementation of evidence-based strategies with pharmacologic and nonpharmacologic approaches. Consider the Healthy People 2030 objectives when developing a plan of care. These objectives include

- reducing asthma deaths,
- reducing asthma attacks, and
- reducing ED visits for people over the age of 5 years.

NPs focused on controlling asthma should consider two things: (a) reducing impairment, the frequency and intensity of symptoms, and the current or recent functional limitations experienced by the patient and (b) reducing risk, the likelihood of future asthma attacks, progressive decline in lung function, or medication adverse effects. Managing asthma involves medications, evaluating environmental factors that may trigger an attack and worsening of symptoms, and educating and assisting the patient to engage in self-management activities to promote health and well-being.

Exhibit 19.1: Classifying Asthma Severity and Initiating Treatment in Youths 12 Years of Age or Older and Adults

Assessing severity and initiating treatment for patients who are not currently taking long-term control medications.

Components of Severity		Classification of Asthma Severity 12 Years of Age or Older			
			Persistent		
		Intermittent	Mild	Moderate	Severe
Impairment Normal FEV_1/FVC: 8-19 yr 85% 20-39 yr 80% 40-59 yr 75% 60-80 yr 70%	Symptoms	≤2 days/week	>2 days/week but not daily	Daily	Throughout the day
	Nighttime awakenings	≤2 x/month	3-4 x/month	>1x/week but not nightly	Often 7x/week
	Short-acting beta agonist use for symptom control (not prevention of EIB)	≤2 days/week	>2 days/week but not daily, and not more than 1x on any day	Daily	Several times per day
	Interference with normal activity	None	Minor limitation	Some limitation	Extremely limited
	Lung function	•Normal FEV_1 between exacerbations •FEV_1 > 80% predicted •FEV_1 > FVC normal	•FEV_1 > 80% predicted •FEV_1 > FVC normal	•FEV_1 > 60% but <80% predicted •FEV_1 > FVC reduced 5%	•FEV_1 > 60% but predicted •FEV_1 > FVC reduced >5%
Risk	Exacerbations requiring oral systemic corticosteroids	0-1/year	>2/year		
		Consider severity and interval since last exacerbation. Frequency and severity may fluctuate over time for patients in any severity category. Relative annual risk of exacerbations may be related to FEV_1.			
Recommended Step for Initiating Treatment		Step 1	Step 2	Step 3 Step 4 of 5 and consider short course of oral systemic corticosteroids	
		In 2-6 weeks, evaluate level of asthma control that is achieved and adjust therapy accordingly.			

FEV_1 - forced expiratory volume in one second; FVC - forced vital capacity.

Source: National Heart, Lung, and Blood Institute (US). National Asthma Education and Prevention Program, Third Expert Panel on the Diagnosis and Management of Asthma. *Expert Panel* Report 3: *Guidelines for the Diagnosis and Management of Asthma.* Figure 4-5, Stepwise Approach for managing asthma in youths ≥12 years of age and adults; 2007. https://www.ncbi.nlm.nih.gov/books/NBK7222/figure/A2212/

Exhibit 19.2: Asthma Treatment Strategy for Adolescents (12 Years and Older)

Assess lungs and symptoms (characteristics and frequency of symptoms); review interventions that helped treat symptoms, tolerability of medications, side effects of medications, exacerbations, hospitalizations, and patient understanding of how to treat asthma, as well as when to notify the NP. Identify risk factors and comorbid conditions.

Once there is confirmation of a diagnosis, then consider evidence-based treatment strategies that are person-centered and consider the adolescent's lifestyle and wishes. It is important to include a parent(s) while making sure the adolescent's voice is heard.

Plan of Care Pharmacologic interventions include evaluating current therapy and modifying the treatment as indicated. The plan of care should include nonpharmacologic interventions. It is important to develop a person-centered plan of care that includes patient education. In newly diagnosed patients, evaluating the use of an inhaler, how to take other medications, and when to contact their NP is essential.

Medications
- Take a stepwise approach to prescribing medications based on the patient's symptoms, efficiency of medications, tolerability, and presence of adverse events.
- Patients may require an inhaled corticosteroid, long-acting beta₂-agonist, long-acting muscarinic antagonist, leukotriene receptor antagonist, oral corticosteroid, and/or short-acting beta-agonist.

For more details on prescribing medications, see the Global Initiative for Asthma (GINA) 2021 report[4]

Source: Global Initiative for Asthma. *Global Strategy for Asthma Management and Prevention.* Author; 2021. https://ginasthma.org/wp-content/uploads/2021/05/GINA-Main-Report-2021-V2-WMS.pdf

Pharmacologic

A stepwise approach to pharmacologic therapy is utilized in the treatment of asthma, with an inhaled corticosteroid (ICS) as the cornerstone. Using a short-acting beta-agonist alone for mild asthma is no longer recommended. Additional classifications of other medications, such as combination inhalers, leukotriene modifiers, anticholinergic agents, oral and intravenous corticosteroids, and biologics, are indicated based on asthma severity and therapeutic response. Biologic medications, such as omalizumab, mepolizumab, reslizumab, benralizumab, and dupilumab, are typically reserved for poorly controlled moderate to severe asthma. These injectable medications downregulate allergic inflammatory pathways and reduce asthma exacerbations and the need for rescue medications and ED visits.

Nonpharmacologic

It is important for patients to avoid triggers that may exacerbate asthma and engage in smoking cessation behaviors if they continue to smoke. Avoiding secondhand smoke is important. They should receive an annual influenza vaccine to prevent influenza-induced exacerbation; the pneumonia vaccine is recommended. Emotional stress can precipitate or exacerbate asthma. Despite the lack of rigorous studies, relaxation techniques for the treatment of asthma may be one way to help the patient.

Patient Education

Patients should be advised that asthma is a chronic disease-causing airway inflammation and the best way to prevent symptoms is to avoid triggers and take prescribed medications as directed. Self-monitoring instructions should be provided including proper use of a peak flow meter. All patients with asthma regardless of symptom frequency should be counseled regarding the importance of having a SABA for acute symptoms with them at all times. Patients and their family (if appropriate) should be educated about how to use inhalers, peak flow meter, spaces, and an asthma action plan. Discussions about the importance of participating in the treatment plan should be done, particularly with adolescents (Exhibit 19.2) who may experience peer pressure. Education should include red flags when to contact the healthcare provider and what is considered an emergency (see Box 19.3). Patients can also find information at www.aafa.org/asthma-diagnosis.

🔊 EMERGENCIES

Asthma is a chronic disease often triggered by environmental factors. Patients should be advised to contact their healthcare provider for
- shortness of breath not relieved by rescue medication or severe wheezing,
- peak flow readings less than 50% of personal best, and
- cyanosis of fingernails or lips.
- Shortness of breath interfering with normal activities

💡 CLINICAL PEARLS

- Dry powdered inhalers, such as Advair Diskus, have been noted in clinical trials to promote the development of localized infections of the mouth and pharynx with *Candida albicans*. Advise patients to rinse their mouth with water without swallowing following inhalation to help reduce the risk of oropharyngeal candidiasis. When such an infection develops, it should be treated with appropriate local or systemic (i.e., oral) antifungal therapy while treatment with the dry powdered inhaler continues, but at times, therapy may need to be interrupted.

▪ When assessing medication compliance with twice-a-day dosing of asthma medications, be sure to ascertain if your patient is indeed using their medication twice a day. Often patients will "skip" the evening dose to reduce medication costs. Patients need to understand using these medications in this manner leaves them with no treatment for 12 hours, at night, when asthma symptoms often intensify.

RELEVANT SOCIAL DETERMINANTS OF HEALTH

Asthma disproportionately affects individuals of color as well as those of low socioeconomic status.[3] Studies indicate racial disparities in asthma are not related to race-based biologic differences but are due to generations of structural racism, leading to socioeconomic hardship. Increases in housing code violations and poor home quality found in the economically disadvantaged are believed to result in exposure to mold and cockroaches, which exacerbate asthma. This leads to increased ED visits and healthcare costs in this disadvantaged population.

CHRONIC OBSTRUCTIVE PULMONARY DISEASE

Etiology

COPD is a disease of both the airways and parenchyma of the lung and is recognized as a heterogeneous group of diseases with distinct clinical phenotypes. Patients typically present with a fixed pulmonary obstructive deficit with little or no postbronchodilator reversibility. It is a leading cause of global morbidity and mortality and the fourth-leading cause of death in the United States. The most common cause of COPD is cigarette smoking. Other causes include passive smoke and biomass fuel. The amount and duration of smoking are linked to the severity of the disease.

Pathophysiology

COPD and subtypes (emphysema, chronic bronchitis, chronic obstructive asthma) are closely related disorders that cause airflow limitations. Adults with COPD typically manifest symptoms of both emphysema and chronic bronchitis. Chronic obstructive asthma is related to chronic inflammation with airway responsiveness that leads to wheezing, breathlessness, coughing at night or early morning, and chest tightness. Chronic bronchitis is defined as the presence of chronic cough for 3 months of the year for 2 consecutive years. The pathologic features of chronic bronchitis are inflammation, particularly involving the small

airways with bronchial mucosal thickening and edema; smooth muscle hypertrophy and hyperresponsiveness; and mucus hypersecretion with plugging. Hence, common signs and symptoms, including frequent cough productive of mucopurulent sputum, wheeze, coarse rhonchi, breathlessness even at rest, and obesity may be seen. Emphysema is characterized by damage to components of the respiratory acinus with loss of alveolar-capillary surface area and a loss of elastic recoil of the small airways with fixed enlargement of the alveolar airspace. The three cardinal symptoms of COPD are dyspnea, cough, and sputum production, and an early symptom is exertional dyspnea. Less common symptoms are wheezing and chest tightness.

Risk Factors

Tobacco abuse is responsible for the large majority of cases, including studies investigating outbreaks of lung disease associated with e-cigarette vaping devices. More than 70% of all adults with COPD are current or former smokers. Generally, COPD is preventable. Genetic and environmental factors, including abnormal lung development, accelerated aging, and air pollution, are less often contributors. Occupational exposure to toxins, dusts, or industrial chemicals contributes to about 15% of adults with COPD. Nonmodifiable risk factors include a history of childhood asthma or childhood respiratory infections and α1-antitrypsin deficiency.

Approach to Diagnosis

The patient's history is extremely important in the diagnosis. Asking about lifestyle, such as smoking history or passive exposure to cigarette smoke, is essential, and engagement in physical activity and symptoms such as cough, sputum production, and dyspnea are important. Questions about cigarette smoking should include age when started, age of quitting (if no longer smoking), and how much they smoked. Patients who present with increased episodes of cough, purulent sputum, wheezing, fatigue, and dyspnea that occurs episodically with or without a fever may have other health conditions than exacerbation of COPD. These include heart failure, bronchiectasis, and bronchiolitis. When the patient has persistent airflow limitations or pulmonary function test and radiographic findings indicate no heart failure or interstitial lung disease, then COPD is most likely.

Diagnostics

Auscultatory findings in emphysema typically reveal very diminished breath sounds and occasional wheeze. There is little to no cough or sputum expectoration with emphysema. Oftentimes, patients with emphysema appear frail, cachectic, and barrel-chested. Patients often manifest features of both chronic bronchitis and emphysema with small airway inflammation and emphysematous destruction of gas-exchange tissues. In some cases, the emphysematous features dominate the clinical presentation or vice versa. Diagnosis is based on a thorough review of smoking history, exhaustive review of systems, physical examination, and pulmonary function testing (see Box 19.3). Spirometry reveals decreased expiratory flow rates across all lung volumes with a reduction in FEV_1/FVC ratio. Lung volume measurements demonstrate evidence of air trapping with increased residual volume (RV) and functional residual capacity (FRC). Total lung capacity (TLC) is often elevated, especially in emphysema indicative of hyperinflation. Lung diffusion capacity testing is decreased in emphysema due to loss of alveolar-capillary surface area. Chest radiography is mainly used to exclude alternative diagnosis; evaluate for other comorbid conditions, such as lung cancer with airway obstruction, pleural disease, interstitial lung disease, heart failure, or bronchiectasis; or to evaluate for complications of COPD. CT scan has greater sensitivity and specificity than chest radiography for detecting emphysema.[4]

The Global Initiative for COPD (GOLD) works with healthcare professionals and public health officials around the world to increase awareness and prevention of COPD and provide nonbiased current assessment and treatment recommendations for healthcare clinicians. You can find information regarding the latest recommendation at https://goldcopd.org/about-us. NPs can download an app for the GOLD Reports and tools for COPD at https://goldcopd.org/2021-gold-reports and a GOLD pocket guide at https://goldcopd.org/wp-content/uploads/2020/11/GOLD-REPORT-2021-v1.1-25Nov20_WMV.pdf.[7]

Diagnostics

- spirometry sowing airflow limitations (i.e., FEV_1/FVC ratio less than 0.7 or less than the lower limit of normal that is incompletely reversible after administration of an inhaled bronchodilator
- absence of alternative explanation for the symptoms and airflow limitation

The GOLD guidelines recommend repeating the spirometry on a separate occasion to show persistent airflow limitation.[5]

Screening Tools and Tests

More than 16 million Americans have been diagnosed with COPD, and many are unaware they have COPD. The U.S. Preventative Services Task Force does not recommend screening for those without symptoms. However, if your patient is concerned they may be at risk of COPD or have symptoms such as dyspnea or chronic cough, they should be screened. Early detection before symptoms are present does not alter the course of the disease or improve patient outcomes. Screening tests in primary care involve risk assessment via a formal prescreening

questionnaire and, if positive, follow-up with diagnostic spirometry administered without a bronchodilator and, if positive, follow-up with diagnostic spirometry testing.

Management

Managing COPD is aimed at smoking cessation and the use of inhaled and oral medications to stabilize symptoms, reduce exacerbations and hospitalizations, and preserve lung function. The GOLD guidelines, which are a collaborative undertaking among the World Health Organization and the NIH,[5] are the most widely accepted method for classification and management of COPD (see GOLD recommendations https://goldcopd.org/about-us).

Healthy People 2030 Objectives:
- Reduce deaths from COPD in adults.
- Reduce emergency department visits for COPD.
- Reduce hospitalizations for COPD.

Pharmacologic

Pharmacotherapy is started based on the patients' symptoms, the severity of disease, and the risk of exacerbations and adjusted based on the person's response to treatment. The goal of therapy is to improve symptoms, decrease exacerbations, and improve function and quality of life. Pharmacologic triple therapy targets the causes of airflow limitation, which includes anti-inflammatories (inhaled and oral corticosteroids) and medications to induce airway smooth muscle relaxation (inhaled beta-adrenergic agonists), and to reduce mucus hypersecretion (inhaled muscarinic antagonists). A novel class of oral anti-inflammatory medication called Roflumilast, a phosphodiesterase-4 enzyme inhibitor, was developed to reduce exacerbations and hospitalizations in patients with advanced COPD and chronic bronchitis. Unfortunately, the role of this medication is limited to a small subpopulation of patients with COPD. For more complete information regarding managing COPD, staging, and the distinct phenotypes, consult the most current GOLD guidelines.

Nonpharmacologic

Pulmonary rehabilitation with supervised endurance training, interval training, and resistance/strength training of the upper and lower limbs, as well as walking, has been shown to facilitate physical functionality and reduce the psychologic impact of COPD. Studies have indicated vitamin D supplementation reduced exacerbation rates in patients with low baseline vitamin D levels. More research is needed on the role of vitamin D and exacerbations of COPD. Supplemental oxygen may be needed in those who have stable, severe COPD and have chronic hypoxemia. Discussions about goals of care and advance care planning are important.

Patient Education

It is vital for patients with COPD to understand the nature of the disease, risk factors leading to progression, and their role in self-management to obtain optimal health outcomes. The most important element of a COPD treatment plan is smoking cessation; patients should be advised this will slow the progression of the disease. The NP should review inhaler techniques to assure proper usage as there are different types of inhaler devices and nebulizers with slightly different inhalation methods. Respiratory infections trigger COPD exacerbations, and patients should be advised to maintain frequent handwashing and avoid crowds. Patients should receive all recommended vaccines including pneumococcal vaccines, the influenza vaccine, and the pertussis vaccine (booster recommended). Encourage patients to eat a healthy diet and, if overweight or obese, to engage in a weight-reduction diet (consider consulting with a dietitian). For patient education resources, see Box 19.2.

Box 19.2: Resources

- USPSTF recommendations: www.uspreventiveservicestaskforce.org
- American Lung Association: www.lung.org/-health-diseases/ling-disease-lookup/copdliving-with-org
- National Institutes of Health: www.nhlbi.nih.gov/files/docs/public/lung/copd-patient.pdf
- Lung Disease including Asthma and Adult Vaccination: www.cdc.gov/vaccines/adults/rec-vac/health-conditions/lung-disease.html

USPSTF, U.S. Preventive Services Task Force.

EMERGENCIES

COPD is a chronic progressive disease often triggered by respiratory infections. Patients should be advised to contact their healthcare provider for the following:

- shortness of breath not relieved by rescue medication or severe wheezing
- cyanosis of fingernails or lips
- shortness of breath interfering with activities of daily life, confusion, or excessive sleepiness
- fever
- new onset of productive discolored sputum

CLINICAL PEARLS

ALPHA-1 ANTITRYPSIN DEFICIENCY

- GOLD guidelines recommend that all individuals with COPD, regardless of age or ethnicity, should be tested for alpha-1 antitrypsin (ATT) deficiency. The ATT protein is made in the liver and released into serum and ultimately serves to protect the lungs from inflammation. Mutations in the *ATT* gene results in a hepatic buildup of abnormal ATT protein, with ensuing liver disease, and lessened inflammatory protection in the lungs and ultimately pulmonary disease.[5]

- Persons with ATT deficiency, as well as asymptomatic genetic carriers, may be more vulnerable to carcinogen-containing tobacco smoke and COPD. Genetic testing is readily available to identify ATT deficiency, and although there is no cure, treatment including AAT augmentation therapies is available. Identifying ATT deficiency calls for a risk assessment in first- and second-degree family members to identify, protect, and treat these individuals.[6]

ACUTE BRONCHITIS

Etiology

Acute bronchitis is an inflammatory disease of the trachea and major bronchi that affects about 5% of the U.S. population.[7] Viruses are the most common cause, and these include influenza A or B, parainfluenza, respiratory syncytial virus (RSV), coronavirus types 1 to 3, rhinoviruses, and adenovirus. RSV is common in homes with children and nursing homes. In some cases, bacteria or even exposure to noxious inhalants (smoke, volatile chemical fumes, other airborne pollutants) can cause acute bronchitis. Acute bronchitis is commonly seen in primary care practice, accounting for about 10% of visits.

Pathophysiology

Cough is the predominant sign, and this is related to edematous changes in the tracheobronchial tree. Damage to the epithelium causes the release of proinflammatory mediators, which leads to an increase in secretion. The bronchial epithelium becomes damaged, and there is a loss of ciliary function. About 40% of healthy adults will experience transient airflow obstruction and bronchial hyperresponsiveness, which usually resolves in about 6 weeks.[8]

Risk Factors

History of smoking or exposure to pollution are risk factors for acute bronchitis, as well as living in a multigenerational household. Individuals with asthma and allergies also have an increased risk.

Approach to Diagnosis

Cough and sputum production are the hallmark symptoms; in most patients, the cough persists for 1 to 3 weeks. Acute bronchitis is a diagnosis of exclusion that can be distinguished from other significant ailments based on the severity of accompanying symptoms, physical examination, and host risk factors such as age, comorbidities, and lifestyle.

Diagnostics

No specific diagnostic tests are indicated unless more serious etiology is suspected based on a thorough examination. Although cough is the primary symptom, cough itself is also a common manifestation of a more serious illness. Fever and hemoptysis or cough lasting more than 3 weeks should be evaluated with chest radiography. Chest radiographs are either normal or findings are nonspecific; there may be a subtle change consistent with the thickening of the bronchial walls in the lower lobes. A chest radiography may be necessary, particularly in older adults because of the risk of community-acquired pneumonia.

Management

Management is supportive and focused on symptom alleviation, and antimicrobial therapy is typically not indicated unless symptoms are severe or there is underlying chronic lung disease. Antitussive and mucolytic agents are only occasionally useful. Inhaled bronchodilators are of little value unless wheezing is present. The goal of treatment is symptom management. Most individuals will improve without a specific treatment.

Pharmacologic

Some patients will require prescribed medications, but most will be over-the-counter aimed at symptom control. Dextromethorphan or guaifenesin are recommended, but it is important to consider comorbid conditions and possible drug–drug interactions. Because acute bronchitis is most commonly caused by a virus, antimicrobial theory is not indicated. Antimicrobial therapy may be considered in those in which a specific pathogen has been identified or the patient has a high risk for complications. It is very important to be cautious when prescribing antimicrobial therapy because it is important to avoid antibiotic use.[9]

Nonpharmacologic

For those with a bothersome cough, you can suggest throat lozenges and hot tea with honey. Discussing the importance of smoking cessation and/or avoiding secondhand smoke and other environmental irritants is important.

Patient Education

Patient satisfaction with care for acute bronchitis depends most on provider–patient communication rather than on antibiotic treatment. It may be helpful to refer to acute bronchitis as a "chest cold." The NP should discuss

Box 19.3: Quality and Safety ALERT

Selective serotonin reuptake inhibitors may enhance the serotonergic effect of dextromethorphan (e.g., precipitate serotonin syndrome; see Chapters 13 and 18 for more information).[12]

Source: Ding H, Shi C, Xu X, Yu L. Drug-induced chronic cough and the possible mechanism of action. Ann Palliat Med. 2020;9(5):3562. doi:10.21037/apm-20-81

realistic expectations about the clinical course and advise the patient to expect to have a cough for 10 to 14 days after the visit. Providers should reinforce that antibiotics are probably not going to be beneficial and are associated with significant risks and side effects. If the patient cannot sleep due to cough, antitussive therapy such as codeine, dextromethorphan, and benzonatate may be helpful.

 EMERGENCIES

Any worsening symptoms should be evaluated with a chest x-ray.

- Productive cough and fever should be evaluated for secondary pneumonia.
- Pulmonary emboli could be implicated in a patient with cough and shortness of breath.
- Aggressive coughing can result in spontaneous pneumothorax.

OTHER PARENCHYMAL LUNG DISEASE IN BRIEF

Etiology

Parenchymal lung diseases or more commonly interstitial lung diseases (ILDs) are complex diseases of multiple origins that involve the supportive connective tissue framework of the lung that encloses the airways, lymphatics, and vasculature of the lung. A common method of classification is based on known causes such as specific exposures, medications, infections, malignancy, and other underlying primary processes, such as autoimmune connective tissue disorders and granulomatous diseases. Unknown or idiopathic causes are grouped separately based on the natural history of the disease, radiographic features, and histopathologic patterns. Any patient with suspected interstitial lung disease should be referred to a pulmonary specialist, particularly in the case of idiopathic forms due to their progressive course.

Idiopathic pulmonary fibrosis (IPF) is an example of parenchymal lung disease with an estimated 50,000 new cases diagnosed in the United States each year, primarily affecting individuals aged between 50 and 70. The etiology of PF is poorly understood; however, this is a progressive and ultimately fatal fibrosing interstitial lung disease.[10]

Pathophysiology

ILDs occur following some type of injury to the lungs (e.g., infection, radiation, environmental exposures), which results in damage to the epithelial or endothelial layers and the associated basement membrane. The fibrosis may be the way the body is trying to heal and repair. The scarring causes the lungs to be stiff, making it more difficult to breathe. This damage to the lungs is often irreversible and is progressive. Abnormal tissue damage and repair leads to irreversible fibrosis, which results in impairment of gas exchange and a reduction in oxygenation of blood. There are six main categories of identifiable causes: drug-induced, radiation-induced, environmental, autoimmune, occupational, and idiopathic. The most common types identified in the United States are environmental (exposure to mold, animals, or other triggers) and autoimmune (connective tissue disease-related). A history of tobacco abuse is considered to be an independent risk factor, although the exact relationship between smoking and survival in pulmonary fibrosis is not clear. In some situations, like idiopathic pulmonary fibrosis, the cause is not known.

Risk Factors

There are many risks for IDLs such as genetic, certain medications, or medical treatments (e.g., chemotherapy, radiation). Exposure to asbestosis and hypersensitivity pneumonitis have been linked to IDLs. Adults with autoimmune disorders (e.g., sarcoidosis, rheumatoid arthritis) are also at risk.

Approach to Diagnosis

The most important aspect of diagnosis is the history. Paying attention to the onset and duration of symptoms is necessary to help with the diagnosis (acute or subacute). Patients will present with dyspnea, dry cough, fatigue, and unexplained weight loss. Fingertip clubbing could also be noted depending on the progression of the disease. Individuals with history of connective tissue, inflammatory bowel disease, or malignancy may have IDLs. Some medications prescribed to treat cardiovascular disease have been associated with IDLs (e.g., amiodarone). Inquire about smoking, occupation, and environmental exposure, as well as family history. Any patient with symptoms of interstitial lung disease should be referred to pulmonology.

Diagnostics

Routine laboratory testing includes biochemical tests to evaluate hepatic and kidney function (see Chapters 22 and 23). Hematologic testing to evaluate for anemia, polycythemia, leukocytosis, eosinophilia, and urinary issues should be done. Serologic tests are obtained to assess for subclinical rheumatic disease and other autoimmune diseases; this is beyond the scope of a primary care adult-gerontology nurse practitioner (AGNP), so the patients should be referred to a pulmonologist for further evaluation beyond basic laboratory studies. Chest radiography may show a reticular, nodular, or mixed pattern. Although the chest radiograph may be suggestive of IDL, the link between this and histopathologic issues is usually poor. Only honeycombing (small cystic spaces) correlates with pathologic findings (the presence is consistent with a poor prognosis). Most IDLs are restrictive so there are reductions in TLC, FRC, and RV. FVC and FEV_1 are decreased and worsen with progressive disease.

Management

If there is a high suspicion of IDLs it is important to refer the patient to a pulmonologist to establish a diagnosis because misdiagnosis can lead to inappropriate treatment (see Box 19.4).

Pharmacologic

New antifibrotic drugs such as nintedanib, a receptor blocker for multiple tyrosine kinases that causes elaboration of fibrogenic growth factor, and pirfenidone, can slow the progression of certain IPF phenotypes.

Nonpharmacologic

Supportive care includes prescribing supplemental oxygen as needed, patient education, and pulmonary rehabilitation. Psychologic support may be necessary as the individual learns to live with a debilitating disease.

Treatment

Treatment includes oxygen therapy and pulmonary rehabilitation programs. The only effective treatment is lung transplantation. Death is typically within 2 to 5 years after diagnosis.

Patient Education

Patients should be educated about what IDL is and what the risk factors are. Discussing the need to refer them to a pulmonologist and the importance of smoking cessation

---

Box 19.4: Quality and Safety Alert

Even though it is beyond the scope of primary care AGNPs, you may be caring for a patient who has been prescribed pirfenidone, so it is important to be aware of safety issues.

- Drug-induced liver injury that is transient with clinically silent elevations in transaminases has been reported with the use of pirfenidone.

- Perform liver function tests (ALT, AST, and bilirubin) before starting treatment and monthly for the first 6 months and then every 3 months.

Caution with those who have severe hepatic impairment or end-stage kidney disease (ESKD).

is very important. Flu and pneumonia vaccines should be strongly recommended. If pulmonary rehab is needed, helping the patient in understanding the process can help emphasize the importance. Discussing medications and possible adverse events should be included in the education. Being prepared to discuss lung transplant may help you answer questions the patient and family may have.

Educational resources can be found at the following:

- American Lung Association www.lung-health -diseases/lung-disease-lookup/ontersitial-lung.org
- Mayo Clinic www.mayoclinic.org[11]

⦿ CLINICAL PEARLS

- Bilateral fine crackles are often auscultated in patients with pulmonary fibrosis. These crackles have a distinct "Velcro-like" sound during middle to late inspiration as fibrotic lung tissue is stretched.
- IPF is strongly associated with GERD.[12] Although the relationship is not totally understood, one theory is microaspirations may promote or exacerbate IPF. Proton pump inhibitors have been found to slow the progression of this fatal disease. Routine screening for GERD, which many patients believe is a benign condition, should be an element of routine primary care visits to reduce potential IPF risk.

COMMUNITY-ACQUIRED PNEUMONIA

Etiology

CAP refers to acute infection of the pulmonary parenchyma acquired in the community, not in the hospital. It is a leading cause of morbidity and mortality. CAP accounts for more than 4.5 million ED visits each year. Over 650 adults are hospitalized for CAP each year, and about 9% will be hospitalized at least once in the same year. The most common pathogens are *Streptococcus pneumoniae* (*S. pneumoniae*) and respiratory viruses. Common causes can be grouped into three categories: typical bacteria, atypical bacteria, and respiratory viruses (see Box 19.5).

Pathophysiology

CAP, defined as a lower bronchial tree infection acquired outside the hospital, is a common and serious lung disease that can potentially be life-threatening. Individuals with pneumonia manifest signs and symptoms such as cough, purulent sputum production, fever, dyspnea, and hypoxemia related to alveolar spaces filling with inflammatory cellular debris and exudative fluid. Although there are many possible pathogens, the

Box 19.5: Common Pathogens Causing Community-Acquired Pneumonia

Typical Bacteria

- *S. pneumoniae*
- *Haemophilus influenzae*
- *Moraxella catarrhalis*
- *Staphylococcus aureus*
- *Group A streptococci*
- *Aerobic gram-negative bacteria*
- Microaerophilic bacteria

Atypical Bacteria

- *Legionella spp*
- *Mycoplasma pneumoniae*
- *Chlamydia pneumoniae*
- *Chlamydia psittaci*
- *Coxiella burnetii*

Respiratory Viruses

- Influenza A and B
- Severe acute respiratory syndrome coronavirus 2 (SARS-CoV2)
- Other coronaviruses
- Rhinovirus
- Parainfluenza viruses
- Adenoviruses
- RSV

Source: Ramirez JA. Overview of community-acquired pneumonia in adults. In: File TM Jr, ed. *UpToDate*. UpTodate; 2021. https://www.uptodate.com/contents/overview-of-community-acquired-pneumonia-in-adults

emergence of innovative diagnostic methodologies, such as polymerase chain reaction (PCR) assays, which have the sensitivity to detect viral nucleic acid from a nasopharyngeal specimen, are now more routinely able to isolate the causative pathogens. CAP is an infection of the lung parenchyma, in which respiratory pathogens are transmitted from person to person via droplets or less commonly via aerosol inhalation. The pathogen colonizes the nasopharynx and, eventually through microaspiration, reaches the lung alveoli. When the inoculum size is sufficient to cause disease or the host immune response results in inflammation and there is injury to the lung, CAP occurs. In some patients, the local inflammatory response is enough to control the disease, but in others, a systemic response is needed to control the infection and prevent complications (e.g., bacteremia, sepsis). Others may become septic, have acute respiratory syndrome, and/or experience multi-organ failure, which increases their mortality risk.

CAP in older adults with advanced age is associated with a higher incidence and greater disease severity. Among younger adults, CAP is usually due to atypical microorganisms. CAP can be distinguished as "typical" versus "atypical" based on symptomatology, radiographic findings, and other diagnostics.

Risk Factors

Individuals older than age 65 are at increased risk of acquiring CAP, as well as those with a history of smoking, those who are immunocompromised, or those who are malnourished. CAP, COPD, asthma, and treatment with gastric acid–suppressive drugs were also identified as risk factors.

Approach to Diagnostics

The diagnosis is based on the patient's presentation that makes the AGNP suspect CAP. Infiltrates on chest imaging and symptoms consistent with CAP (e.g., fever, dyspnea, cough, sputum production) confirm the diagnosis. Respiratory illnesses that can have a similar presentation as CAP or coexist with CAP include acute exacerbations of COPD, influenza or other viral respiratory infections, acute bronchitis, and asthma exacerbation.

Diagnostics

To make the diagnosis and assist with clinical decision-making, it is important to obtain the following:

- Posteroanterior and lateral chest radiographs, findings of lobar consolidations, interstitial infiltrates, and/or cavitation are consistent with CAP.

- In those patients for whom the chest radiograph is negative but have clinical manifestations of CAP, a CT scan of the chest is appropriate. Adults who are immunocompromised and don't mount a strong immune response and those with exposures to pathogens such as Legionella may have a negative chest radiograph but still have CAP.

- It is important in patients who present with signs and symptoms of pneumonia to consider cardiopulmonary disorders as a possible cause, particularly in those with underlying cardiac disorders.

Screening Tools and Tests

Acute cough is one of the most common reasons a patient may present to your primary care office. The most important thing is determining your patients at risk and implementing preventative strategies such as good hand hygiene, influenza and pneumonia vaccines, and avoiding others with symptoms of respiratory disease.

🏠 Quality and Safety Alert

The presence of three of the following warrant ICU admission:

- Altered mental status (acute confusion)
- Hypotension requiring fluid support
- Temperature (low or high)
- Respirations 30 breaths/minute or
- Arterial oxygen tension to fraction of inspired oxygen (PaO2/FiO2) ratio 250 or less
- Blood urea nitrogen 20 mg/dL or greater
- Leukocyte count <4,000 cells/microL
- Platelet count <100,000/mL
- Multilobar infiltrates[13]

Management

Common causative organisms of typical pneumonia include S. pneumoniae, Hemophilus influenzae, and Moraxella catarrhalis. Patients with atypical pneumonia may exhibit more muted pulmonary symptoms with myriad extrapulmonary manifestations, such as rash and diarrhea, that overshadow the respiratory complaints. Moreover, as opposed to typical pneumonia whose radiographic appearance is consolidative and lobar, infiltrates on chest x-ray in atypical pneumonia are oftentimes nonconsolidated, nonlobar with a patchy interstitial pattern. Keep in mind, these radiographic findings are only generalizations and not absolutes. The causative organism for CAP is seldom identified. Generally in a primary care setting, microbiologic testing is not needed. Hence, empiric treatment is used based on symptom severity, host factors such as comorbidities, age, drug allergies, and, most recently, antimicrobial therapy. Pneumonia severity scoring tools such as the Pneumonia Severity Index (PSI; www.mdcalc.com/psi-port-score-pneumonia-severity-index-cap) and CURB-65 (www.mdcalc.com/curb-65-score-pneumonia-severity) may prove clinically useful regarding risk stratification and the selection of appropriate initial choice of antimicrobial therapy.

Pharmacologic

Empiric treatment with antimicrobial therapy is based on the severity of illness, local epidemiology, patient risk factors for infection with drug-resistant organisms, and status of smoking. In the outpatient setting oral antibiotics are best while considering if the patient has recently been prescribed antibiotics or has a history of structural lung disease. In most adults 65 and older (if they have not recently had antibiotics and are not allergic to PCN), amoxicillin (1 g three times a day) or macrolide (azithromycin, clarithromycin, doxycycline) may be the best choice. For those patients who cannot have amoxicillin, consider cephalosporins or respiratory fluoroquinolone (see Chapter 13 for more information on medication management).

Nonpharmacologic

Adults may experience psychologic distress over concerns of worsening symptoms, particularly if they have other comorbidities that increase the risk of hospitalization or death. Recommending mindfulness or other complementary therapies can assist patients in addressing any anxiety they may experience. In addition, providing education about treatment and prevention strategies is important.

(((•))) EMERGENCIES

Patients with CAP who are treated on an outpatient basis should be closely monitored as treatment failure is common. Acute respiratory failure and acute respiratory distress syndrome (ARDS) are complications often leading to mortality. Patients should be advised to contact their healthcare provider for the following:

- symptoms are not improving, are getting worse, or fever returns
- decreased urination
- experience chest pain with a deep breath
- new onset of hemoptysis
- cyanosis of fingernails or lips
- excessive sleepiness or confusion
- special populations

ADOLESCENTS

CAP in children can be a very serious infection that often results in hospitalization. Most adolescents can be treated as an outpatient. Macrolide antibiotics are recommended for initial therapy for suspected atypical CAP. In those who present with typical CAP and *S. pneumoniae* is suspected as the causative agent, amoxicillin is recommended. The symptoms should resolve in less than 1 month in health children. In those who have atypical CAP it may take a little longer for the cough to abate. Follow-up chest radiographs are not necessary in asymptomatic adolescents with uncomplicated CAP.

OLDER ADULTS

Pneumonia in older adults residing in a nursing home is considered a healthcare-acquired pneumonia and can be challenging to diagnose and treat. Therefore, pneumococcal and influenza immunizations are strongly recommended to decrease the risk of pneumonia.[14] Older adults may not have the typical presentation of pneumonia; however, they may have at least one respiratory sign. The first presenting sign commonly is acute confusion. A low pulse oximetry can be indicated if pneumonia is suspected, but a chest radiograph must be obtained to

confirm. Treatment should be based on the resident's overall prognosis. Oral antibiotics can be used for residents of nursing homes, but if hospitalized, IV antibiotics are the best option. Residents should be treated for a total of 5 to 8 days unless they have a *Pseudomonas aeruginosa* infection, are medically unstable, or demonstrate an inadequate response to the antibiotic therapy.[15]

Aspiration pneumonia can be defined as adverse respiratory consequences as the result of the entry of gastric or oropharyngeal fluids that contain bacteria and/or low pH or other exogenous substances into the lower airways. At-risk patients include those with reduced consciousness level, dysphagia from neurologic disorders (e.g., stroke, dementia, Parkinson's disease), disorders of upper GI tract, mechanical disruption of the glottic closure or lower esophageal sphincter (e.g., tracheostomy, endotracheal intubation, tube feeding), poor dental hygiene, advanced age, and cardiac arrest. The most common presentation in older adults is altered mental status. It is important to consider aspiration pneumonia in your differential diagnosis when caring for older adults at risk.

Patient Education

It is important that patients are educated about preventive measures, such as influenza and pneumonia vaccines. Smoking cessation should be strongly encouraged. Providing resources to help patients stop is important (see www.cdc.gov/tobacco/basic_information/for-health-care-providers/patient-resources/index.html).

ⓘ CLINICAL PEARL

- Two vaccines are currently available to prevent invasive pneumococcal disease: 23-valent pneumococcal polysaccharide vaccine (PPSV 23) and a 13-valent pneumococcal conjugate vaccine (PCV 13). The Centers for Disease Control and Prevention (CDC) recommends all adults 65 years old and older who do not have an immunocompromising condition, cerebrospinal fluid leak, or cochlear implant should receive PPSV23. Once a dose of PPSV23 is given at age 65 years or older, no additional doses of PPSV23 should be administered. Adults 65 years old and older who are potentially at increased risk to PCV13 serotypes (chronic heart, lung, or liver disease; diabetes mellitus; alcoholism; tobacco abuse) should receive the PCV13 vaccine at least 1 year after the PPSV23 vaccine. Further information can be found on the CDC website.

PULMONARY HYPERTENSION

Etiology

Adults that present with symptoms that may be consistent with pulmonary hypertension (PH) will need to undergo extensive diagnostic testing to confirm the diagnosis and identify the underlying cause in order to determine the best treatment. PH is classified into five groups depending on etiology (see Box 19.6).

Pathophysiology

PH is a complex and variable pathophysiologic process associated with multiple disease states and caused by genetic, acquired, or idiopathic means. By definition, PH is the elevation in mean pulmonary artery pressure above 25 mmHg at rest and 30 mmHg with exercise. More simply, PH is due to abnormally high pressure in the pulmonary circulation. PH has been classified into five main groups, with further subdivisions based on etiology, pathophysiologic mechanisms, hemodynamic features, and as a means to delineate therapies. PH is a common complication of cardiovascular and pulmonary diseases and is less often found in other primary disorders, such as venous thromboembolic disease and pulmonary embolism, hemoglobinopathies, metabolic disorders, and other systemic diseases. For this reason, the term "secondary PH" may be seen as a descriptor. Group 3 PH is due to chronic lung disease that causes increased pulmonary vascular resistance due to remodeling of the pulmonary vasculature after years of airway and parenchymal inflammation, fibrosis, and hypoxic pulmonary vasoconstriction as a means to redirect flow with alterations in gas exchange. Chronic lung disease is the second-leading cause of PH behind left heart disease. Group 2 PH owing to left-sided heart disease is due to an elevation in left-heart pressure with an alteration in the forward flow, resulting in a subsequent increase in pulmonary venous pressure (pulmonary venous hypertension) and thus a passive increase in pulmonary artery pressure.

Risk Factors

PH can occur at any age, but the incidence increases with age and is more common among women, non-Hispanic Black people, and adults aged 75 and older. Environmental factors, family history, and genetics also present a risk.

Box 19.6: Clinical Classification of PH

- Group 1: pulmonary arterial hypertension (PAH)
- Group 2: PH due to left heart disease
- Group 3: PH due to lung disease and/or hypoxia
- Group 4: due to pulmonary artery obstruction
- Group 5: PH with unclear and/or multifactorial mechanisms

Approach to Diagnostics

Manifestations of PH include exertional dyspnea, fatigue, presyncope, elevated jugular venous pulse, passive congestion of the liver, lower extremity edema, prominent second heart sound, tricuspid murmur, or diastolic murmur of the pulmonic valve. Over time, PH can progress to chronic right heart failure due to long-standing abnormal cardiac workload related to exaggerated pulmonary vascular pressures in a typically low-pressure circuit. Differential diagnoses for those with signs and symptoms of right ventricular failure include left-sided heart failure, myocardial ischemia due to CAD, liver disease, or Budd-Chiari syndrome (thromboses of the hepatic veins and/or the intrahepatic or suprahepatic inferior vena cava). Based on the severity of symptoms, it has been divided into four functional classes ranging from no symptoms with ordinary activity (class 1) to an inability to perform even minimal physical tasks without symptoms (class 4).

Diagnostics

Pulmonary hypertension is difficult to diagnose and is often not identified in a routine physical examination. The patient history often presents symptoms that mimic other cardiac and pulmonary conditions. Any patient suspected to have PH should be referred to a tertiary care center to coordinate management among cardiologists, pulmonologists, and internists.

Two-dimensional transthoracic echocardiogram is the primary tool used to estimate right-heart hemodynamics if there is suspicion of pulmonary hypertension based on a thorough history, comorbidities, and physical examination. Echocardiography also allows assessment for secondary causes related to left-heart disease. Right-heart catheterization is used to more accurately assess right-heart pressure, exclude other etiologies, and assess vasoreactivity to predict medication responses. If secondary pulmonary hypertension is suspected, workup and management of the PH are directed toward the underlying disease process. For instance, if COPD is the suspected underlying cause, a PFT should be performed for further risk stratification, assessment of disease severity, and to help guide pharmacologic therapy with an appropriate COPD maintenance regimen with or without supplemental oxygen.

Management

Signs and symptoms of PH are nonspecific, but as stated earlier, patients most often present with exertional dyspnea and fatigue that progresses. Over time, the PH becomes severe, and the patient presents with right ventricular failure. Many times, there is a delay in the diagnosis because the signs and symptoms are attributed to age, decondition, or a coexisting health condition. Evidence suggests that about 20% of patients with PH have had it longer than 2 years before being diagnosed; it is more common in those younger than 36 years or those with preexisting health conditions.

Pharmacology

The treatment and diagnosis are beyond the scope of an AGNP; however, it is important for primary care NPs to collaborate with specialists to comanage patients with PH. Pulmonary vasodilators are reserved for group 1 pulmonary hypertension with a few exceptions. There are three main classes of medications: phosphodiesterase type 5 (PDE-5) inhibitors, endothelin receptor antagonists (ERAs), and prostacyclin analogs with calcium channel blockers used in a small subset of patients who demonstrate a positive response to vasoreactivity testing. Depending on etiology, patients may also be placed on anticoagulants and/or diuretics. In group 2, optimization of left-heart diseases is the goal of medications and other treatments. In group 3, the treatment is based on the severity of the associated PH and the severity of right ventricular failure (e.g., elevated right atrial pressure and low cardiac index) and findings of the echocardiography.[16]

Nonpharmacologic

Adults should be encouraged to obtain adequate sleep and engage in physical activity as much as possible, even if this means walking in the house or short distances. The use of supplemental oxygen may be needed. Adequate healthy nutrition is important, so consider having the patient meet with a dietitian if possible.

Patient Education

In the primary care setting, the NP should assure patients have an understanding of medications prescribed by the medical team, evaluate the ability to take medications as prescribed, and discuss the potential side effects and contraindications. Again, depending on etiology, patients may be asked to limit sodium and may require dietary instruction. Smoking cessation is essential for smokers, and alcohol should be limited. Patients should be advised to discuss any exercise program with their medical team prior to initiation; however, exercise as tolerated should be encouraged. Patients should discuss any travel plans with the medical team, and travel to high altitudes may be discouraged. Those with end-stage PH lung transplant or heart/lung transplant (if heart disease is extensive) may be an option. Patients and families can go to the CDC website for more information: www.cdc.gov/heartdisease/pulmonary_hypertension.htm.

ⓘ CLINICAL PEARL

- ■ Patients with PH should receive supportive measures, including avoiding pregnancy, receiving influenza and pneumococcal vaccines, receiving psychosocial support, performing supervised exercise, undergoing in-flight oxygen therapy, and receiving recommendations to avoid general anesthesia if possible (use epidural instead).

PULMONARY EMBOLISM

Etiology

As testing has become more available (D-dimer testing and CT pulmonary angiography), there has been an increase in the number of pulmonary embolisms (PEs). The incidence is about 112 cases per 100,000, with men having a higher incidence compared to women. In the United States, PE accounts for about 100,000 deaths each year. Mortality is high, with African Americans having the highest risk followed by White Americans.

Pathophysiology

PE is the obstruction of a branch or multiple branches of the pulmonary arteries by a thrombus (clot) or thrombi most commonly arising from the deep veins of the lower extremity. However, venous thrombosis may also occur in the upper extremities or the central vasculature and right side of the heart due to intravascular catheters or wires. Once a thrombi lodges in the lung, other pathophysiologic events occur. Some things that can occur are a pulmonary infarction or abnormal gas exchange related to mechanical and functional obstruction of the vascular bed that alters the ventilation-to-perfusion ratio. Atelectasis can occur along with inflammation that stimulates respiratory drive. The patient may then experience hypocapnia and respiratory alkalosis. Hypercapnia and acidosis don't usually occur unless the patient is experiencing shock. Patients may experience hypotension due to diminished stroke volume and cardiac output.

Risk Factors

Risk factors, collectively termed Virchow's triad after a German physician, include venous stasis, vascular endothelial injury, and hypercoagulable states induced by blood clotting disorders, malignancy, nephrotic syndrome, medications, and a multitude of other etiologies. Patients on oral contraceptives or hormone replacement therapy are at risk. Increased rates of blood clots and inflammation have been observed among COVID-19 patients affecting multiple organs, increasing morbidity and mortality.

Approach to Diagnosis

A thorough physical examination and history help to guide and narrow the differential diagnosis. Patients can present with no symptoms, but the most common symptoms are dyspnea followed by chest pleuritic pain, cough, and symptoms of deep vein thrombosis (DVT). Symptoms vary greatly and may be as nonspecific as tachypnea and tachycardia and, less often, hemoptysis and cough. A larger clot burden may manifest with hypotension, syncope, or sudden death. Among older adults, the first symptoms may be altered mental status. Patients with small emboli may be asymptomatic.

Diagnosis

Clinical prediction scoring tools such as the Pulmonary Embolism Severity Index (PESI) and simplified PESI are widely validated tools for risk assessment. Wells Scoring System and Pulmonary Embolism Rule-out Criteria (PERC) help guide diagnosis and critical thinking, and eliminate unnecessary testing. More confirmatory imaging studies include a CT pulmonary angiogram or nuclear medicine ventilation/perfusion scan. Typical findings on plain chest radiography are that of a normal film. Lower extremity venous duplex ultrasound is also commonly performed to confirm the presence of lower extremity thrombi. ECG, cardiac marker testing, and arterial blood gas (ABG) are nonspecific and may strengthen suspicion for PE or support an alternative diagnosis. D-dimer, a fibrin degradation product, is an excellent marker for excluding PE. A normal D-dimer strongly argues against PE.

Management

PE should be considered if your patient presents with acute symptoms of dyspnea at rest or with exertion, pleuritic pain, cough, orthopnea, calf or shin pain, and/or swelling or wheezing. The onset of dyspnea is usually rapid (sometimes this is not the case). The first thing to consider is whether your patient is hemodynamically unstable; if so, 911 should be called and the patient should be transported to the ED. The majority of patients present as hemodynamically stable, allowing time for sufficient evaluation for PE. Differential diagnosis should include dyspnea due to exacerbation of underlying lung and acute chest pain, which may be pneumonia, pericarditis, pleuritis, or rib fracture. Heart failure can cause dyspnea and leg swelling, but unilateral leg swelling is a key feature of a DVT. Chest pain and dyspnea may be due to pneumothorax; this can be differentiated with chest imaging. Acute chest wall pain can be due to musculoskeletal pain, so obtaining a thorough history can help differentiate.

Pharmacologic

Management includes anticoagulation with heparinoids as an initial choice with a transition to an oral anticoagulant unless contraindicated. In the event of hemodynamic instability or impending cardiopulmonary compromise, fibrinolytic therapy with tissue plasminogen activator (tPA) or a similar agent may be indicated unless contraindicated. Embolectomy, either open surgical or catheter-guided, is an alternative therapy for massive PE. With the advent of novel oral anticoagulants such as Factor Xa inhibitors (Xarleto, Eliquis) and direct thrombin inhibitor (Pradaxa), the use of warfarin is losing favor. Additionally, the clinician can immediately initiate a Factor Xa inhibitor, such as Xarleto, without prior anticoagulation with a parenteral anticoagulant. Inferior vena cava (IVC) filters are reserved for those in whom anticoagulation is an absolute contraindication. The American Society of Hematology (ASH)[20] 2020 guidelines[17] recommend that select patients with PE with a low risk for complications should be offered home treatment over hospital treatment. The first dose of anticoagulant therapy should be administered in the hospital or urgent care center. This does not apply to patients who have other conditions that would require hospitalization, have limited or no support at home, cannot afford medications, or have a poor medication adherence history. Although outpatient treatment for uncomplicated PE has been determined safe, this practice is uncommon. (See Chapter 13 for more information regarding medication management.)

Nonpharmacologic

During the acute phase of PE, patients will need supportive care such as analgesia and IV fluids, but once hospitalized AGNPs should discuss with the hospital healthcare team to determine the plan of care for prevention and health promotion. Things that may be recommended include ambulation to promote recovery and prevention, compression stockings, and assuring that the person takes their medications as prescribed, as well as follow-up as recommended.

Patient Education

Providing information about what is a PE and why blood clots are so dangerous is important. Helping them understand the symptoms of PE and DVT and how the diagnosis is determined is important. Preventative measures if the person has a long flight include (a) standing up and walking around every 1 to 2 hours; (b) not smoking just before the trip; (c) wearing loose-fitting, comfortable clothes; (d) moving the legs on a regular basis; (e) if possible, wearing knee-high compression stockings; and (f) avoiding alcohol and medications that make you sleepy (these may impair one's ability to move around).

((•)) EMERGENCIES

At-risk patients should be advised to contact their healthcare provider for the following:

- pain, swelling, or redness in the arm, leg, or any other area of the body
- chest pain or trouble breathing
- fast heartbeat
- excessive sweating
- syncope or near syncope

OBSTRUCTIVE SLEEP APNEA

Etiology

Adults with obstructive sleep apnea (OSA) have obstructive apneas, hypopneas, and/or respiratory effort–related arousals that are caused by repeated collapse of the upper airway during sleep. OSA is the most common sleep-related disorder in the United States, particularly in older males; however, adolescents and women can also have OSA. OSA is the most common disorder that causes daytime sleepiness and is associated with an overall increased risk of two to three times for motor vehicle accidents.[18] OSA is more prevalent in African Americans who are younger than 35 years as compared to non-Hispanic Whites in the same age group. The prevalence is increasing, which may be related to the rising in obesity rates in the United States. Untreated OSA in adolescents can lead to behavior and learning problems. In severe cases, it can result in impaired growth and CV complications (e.g., right and left ventricular dysfunction, hypertension).

Pathophysiology

Sleep apnea can be obstructive when there is a compromised, or completely closed, extrathoracic upper airway (UA); a marked reduction or cessation of brainstem respiratory motor output (central); or a combination of both (mixed). This section is focused on OSA that occurs when there are recurrent episodes of UA obstruction that are "associated with a reduction in ventilation resulting in repeated arousals and episodic oxyhemoglobin desaturations during sleep."[19] OSA is linked to hypertension, and risk of stroke, CAD, heart failure, and atrial fibrillation.

Risk Factors

Risk factors associated with OSA include older age (increases from young adult until the person reaches their 60s and 70s, then plateaus); male gender until a woman is peri- and postmenopausal, when the risk is similar between men and women; obesity; and craniofacial and upper airway abnormalities.[20] Other less common risks are cigarette smoking, a family history of snoring or OSA, and those with nasal congestion. Individuals with heart failure, atrial fibrillation, pulmonary hypertension, hypertension, end-stage kidney disease, chronic lung disease, stroke, Parkinson's disease, and pregnant women have risks for OSA.

Approach to Diagnosis

Patients may present with complaints of excessive daytime sleepiness; however, patients may not report this to the full extent because of the insidious onset and chronicity. So they may instead report fatigue, tiredness, low energy, or a decreased ability to focus. Interestingly fatigue is a common complaint of many older adults, so it is important to consider other possible causes. One of the symptoms of depression is a decreased ability to concentrate, so pay attention to this as a possible reason for the expressed concern regarding a change in concentration level. Questioning the patient and their loved one (or partner) often reveals that the person feels sleepy a lot or falls asleep in passive, boring, and monotonous situations. Common features of OSA include snoring or resuscitative gasping, witnessed apneic periods (episodes of silence followed by loud snoring), and restlessness. Snoring has a sensitivity of 80% to 90% for diagnosis of OSA, but specificity is lower than 50%. Snoring does not have a predictive value for OSA, but if the person does not snore, it decreases the likelihood of OSA, particularly in those with BMI lower than 26. About 10% to 30% of patients present with morning headaches, usually bifrontal and squeezing in quality. Patients may present with other symptoms such as sleep maintenance insomnia (about 30% have this vs. daytime sleepiness), symptoms related to associated conditions (neuropsychiatric symptoms, nocturnal CV events), and increased nocturia (they are awake so have the urge to urinate). Physical findings may be obesity, airway narrowing, a large neck and/or waist circumference, and signs of associated conditions (hypertension, heart failure).[20] Patients should be assessed for OSA whenever there is excessive daytime sleepiness on most days and the presence of at least two of the following: habitual loud snoring, witnessed apnea or gasping or choking during sleep, and diagnosed with hypertension. This is particularly true in the presence of other risk factors. Referral to a sleep medicine specialist for evaluation is important.

Adolescents with suspected OSA should be referred to a specialist in sleep medicine or otolaryngology. Adolescents may require surgical intervention (adenotonsillectomy) or, if mild or moderate OSA (apnea–hypopnea index [AHI] >1 and <10), a watchful waiting for up to 6 months and supportive care may be done.[21]

Diagnostics

Laboratory polysomnography (PSG) is the "gold standard" to assess AHI, which is the hourly rate of apneas and hypopneas averaged over the total sleep time. Classification of severity OSA, based on the AHI, is mild, moderate, and severe.

Mild OSA is an AHI of 5 to 14 events per hour; most people are relatively asymptomatic, but some report daytime sleepiness becoming more noticeable once the person is not stimulated. The daytime sleepiness usually does not impair daily life, but others may notice it. Mild is associated with an increased risk of hypertension, particularly in younger adults.

Moderate OSA (see Box 19.7) is AHI of 15 to 30 events per hour, with patients often being aware of excessive daytime sleepiness and taking steps to avoid falling asleep during the day or sleeping at inappropriate times. Sleep fragmentation in moderate OSA is often observed, hypertension may coexist, and they may experience an increase in motor vehicle accidents.

Severe OSA is AHI of more than 30 events per hour; daytime sleepiness interferes with patients' daily activities, they tend to fall asleep often, are at risk for accidental injury and for CV morbidities such as hypertension and CAD, and have a higher mortality risk.[20]

Screening Tools

There are several instruments that can be used to screen for OSA (see Table 19.1). The U.S. Preventive Services Task Force reports that there is insufficient evidence to make a recommendation on the use of screening tools for OSA in asymptomatic community-residing adults.

Box 19.7: CMS Guidelines for Reimbursement of Positive Airway Pressure Therapy

- AHI is equal to or greater than 14 events per hour, or between 5 and 14 events per hour and associated with excessive daytime sleepiness, impaired neurocognitive function, mood disorder, insomnia, CVD (e.g., hypertension, ischemic heart disease), or a history of stroke.

The CMS will reimburse for an obstructive respiratory disturbance index that is abnormal; this is the number of apneas and hypopneas per hour of recording.

AHI, apnea-hypopnea; CMS, Centers for Medicare and Medicaid Services; CVD, cardiovascular disease.

Source: Centers for Medicare and Medicaid Services. Continuous positive airway pressure (CPAP) therapy for obstructive sleep apnea (OSA) https://www.cms.gov/medicare-coverage-database/view/ncacal-decision-memo.aspx?proposed=N&NCAId=204

Management

The goals of OSA management are to improve sleep quality and normalize the AHI and oxyhemoglobin levels. OSA generally takes an interprofessional approach to achieve the best health outcomes for the patient. Treatment of OSA may lead to less daytime sleepiness, reduced health costs through decreased health utilization, and possibly decreased CV morbidity and mortality. The first step in management is behavior modification and other nonpharmacologic therapies (see the following sections).

Pharmacologic

At this time, there are no medications that warrant replacing nonpharmacologic treatments. Some medications that have been used to replace the burdensome nonpharmacologic therapies are medications that stimulate respiratory drive directly (e.g., theophylline) or indirectly (e.g., acetazolamide) or medications that reduce UA collapsibility (e.g., desipramine), antimuscarinics (e.g., oxybutynin), and nonnoradrenergic agents (e.g., atomoxetine).[22] It is important to avoid prescribing medications that have an inhibitory effect on the central nervous system (particularly benzodiazepine). Some of these medications include antiepileptic drugs, sedating antidepressants, antihistamines, and opiates. If you need to prescribe these medications, it is essential that the patient be closely monitored and that the doses are slowly titrated while paying attention to response and possible adverse events.

Nonpharmacologic

Lifestyle behavior modification includes weight loss (can lead to improved airway patency) and avoiding alcohol (alcohol worsens OSA). Physical activity may not have a direct effect on OSA but engaging in physical activity as part of a weight reduction program can be beneficial. Changing position during sleep to a nonsupine position can enhance airway patency. Continuous positive airway pressure counteracts collapsing forces in UA. Bilevel

Table 19.1: Instruments to Measure Symptomatic Patients for Obstructive Sleep Apnea

Instrument	Purpose
STOP-Bang www.stopbang.ca/osa/screening.php	Eight-item survey on **s**noring, **t**iredness, **o**bserved apneas, blood **p**ressure, **b**ody mass index, **a**ge, **n**eck circumference, and **g**ender; it has a sensitivity of 84% and specificity of 54% for the diagnosis of OSA using AHI threshold of 5 to 14 events.
Sleep apnea clinical score (SACS) www.serenitymedicalservices.com/wp-content/uploads/2020/01/CEREVES_SACS_ENG.pdf	Four-item questionnaire with variables of neck circumference, hypertension, habitual snoring, and nocturnal gasping or choking (score is 0–100). Scores greater than 15 indicate a probability of OSA (defined as AHI greater than 10 events per hour).
Berlin Questionnaire www.sleepapnea.org/wp-content/uploads/2017/02/berlin-questionnaire.pdf	10 items related to snoring and nonrestorative sleep. Sleepiness while driving, apneas during sleep, hypertension, and body mass index. It has a sensitivity of 80% and specificity of 46% with OSA (AHI 5–14 events per hour) and 91% and 37%, respectively, when OSA is defined as AHI greater than 15 events per hour.

AHI, apnea-hypopnea index; OSA, obstructive sleep apnea.

positive airway pressure end-expiratory pressure stents open the airway; inspiratory pressure enhances minute ventilation or decreases hypopneas. Inspire stimulates the UA muscles during sleep, leading to increased airway patience. Another UA stimulator is the autotitrating positive (AP) airway pressure, which uses feedback algorithms to adjust the pressure in response to airway conditions to provide airway patency with minimal mean pressure. Oral appliances that enhance airway patency by stabilizing lateral pharyngeal walls and enhancing AP airway dimensions at the velopharyngeal level include mandibular position devices and tongue retention devices. Some patients will be candidates for surgical interventions that enhance airway patency by reconfiguring soft tissue and/or skeletal structures (palatal surgeries and maxillomandibular advancement).[23]

Patient Education

Patients should be educated about what OSA is, what the symptoms are, testing, and treatment for OSA. In addition, gaining an understanding of the importance of weight loss, adjusting sleep position, and avoiding alcohol or other sedatives is essential. Stressing the critical importance of consistently following treatment recommendations should be completed if OSA is diagnosed. Educational materials can be found at American Thoracic Society,[24] www.thoracic.org/patients/patient-resources/resources/obstructive-sleep-apnea-in-adults.pdf, and the American Lung Association, www.lung.org/lung-health-diseases/lung-disease-lookup/sleep-apnea.

PLEURAL EFFUSION AND PLEURISY

Etiology

Although chest pain is a common complaint seen in primary care (about 1% of all primary care visits), it can be challenging for NPs because of the wide array of possible etiologies. When your patient presents with chest pain, it is critical to determine if it is life-threatening or not by evaluating your patient. In some cases, chest pain is related to pleural effusion or pleurisy, an inflammation of the lung pleura. Causes of pleural effusion include atelectasis, cirrhosis, heart failure (most common cause), drug-induced, endocrine dysfunction, esophageal perforation, infectious parasitic and fungal disease, malignant disease, pancreatic disease, nephrotic syndrome, pneumonia, pulmonary embolism, rheumatoid arthritis, sarcoidosis, systemic lupus erythematosus, tuberculosis, radiotherapy, and viral illness (e.g., HIV/AIDs).[1]

Pathophysiology

A pleural effusion is the abnormal accumulation of fluid within the potential space between the visceral and parietal pleura due to excess production or reduced absorption by lymphatics. The complication of pleural effusion is seen across the life span from an infant with congenital heart disease to the older adult smoker with a primary lung malignancy. Pleural effusions are commonly divided into transudates versus exudates based on the mechanism of fluid accumulation. Transudates are due to an alteration between hydrostatic and oncotic forces (altered Starling forces) while exudates are due to inflammation of the pleura and subsequent alterations in vascular permeability, pleural integrity, and lymphatic drainage. Transudative effusions are a typical complication seen in hypoalbuminemic states, such as cirrhotic liver disease and nephrotic syndrome, and congestive heart failure (pulmonary venous hypertension) whether from alterations of cardiac contractility, preload, or afterload. Transudative effusions are usually bilateral and painless. A less common cause of transudative effusions is atelectasis or translocation of fluid from the peritoneal space into the pleural space through diaphragmatic fenestrations. Exudative effusions are oftentimes unilateral and may be painful. Exudative effusions may be caused by malignancy, parapneumonic process, pulmonary embolism, autoimmune disease, chylothorax, pancreatitis, or another inflammatory, infectious, or malignant subdiaphragmatic process. There is a myriad of other causes for both transudates and exudates, the aforementioned examples being the more common etiologies.

The visceral pleura does not contain pain receptors; however, the parietal pleura, covering the inside of the thoracic wall, is innervated by the somatic nervous system. Trauma or inflammation can result in the affected visceral pleura, extending into the pleural space and stimulating pain receptors in the parietal pleura resulting in localized discomfort. Pleurisy refers to this painful inflammation of the pleura marked by chest pain during respiratory motion that is usually caused by infections, particularly of viral origin, but may be a symptom of a more insidious process such as a complication of pneumonia, an underlying inflammatory syndrome such as rheumatoid arthritis, pulmonary embolism, chest injury, malignancy, pneumothorax, and numerous other conditions.

Risk Factors

There are numerous causes of pleural effusions, but the most common causes of pleural effusions are heart failure, pneumonia, and cancer. Pleurisy is rarely caused by a malignancy; however, pleural effusion may be the result of malignant carcinoma. Age-related changes can increase the risk for pleural effusion.

Approach to Diagnosis

Diagnosis is based on a thorough history and physical. With pleural effusion, many patients are asymptomatic but when symptoms are present, they are usually a nonproductive cough and dyspnea. Auscultation over the affected lung zone reveals muted or absent breath sounds depending on the size of the effusion. A pleural friction rub may be present.[25] It is important to perform a physical examination to identify other possible causes for presentation, such as heart failure neoplasms or trauma.

With pleurisy, the patient may present with chest pain when breathing that worsens when taking a deep breath along with stabbing or shooting chest pain. Pain is usually localized but may radiate to the shoulder. The most comfortable position is usually lying on the affected side. Pleuritic pain is at the site of inflammation, and there is a tenderness that increases with deep palpation. A pleural friction rub may be present but the absence of a friction rub does not exclude the diagnosis of pleurisy. In some patients, there is an underlying disease process, such as pneumonia, pneumothorax, tuberculosis, or pulmonary embolism.

Diagnostics

With pleural effusion, the first step in diagnosis is obtaining the patient's history, paying attention to drugs (nitrofurantoin, amiodarone, ovarian stimulation therapy, or medications that can cause lupus-like syndrome), occupational exposures (asbestos), risk factors for pulmonary embolism, tuberculosis, or other comorbid conditions. Abnormal percussion notes and tactile fremitus are also found with sizable effusions. Imaging with plain chest x-ray, CT scanning, or ultrasonography are the most useful tests to confirm the presence of an effusion. Smaller effusions may be missed on a plain radiograph. Thoracentesis may be done by a pulmonologist to obtain a pleural fluid analysis. Diagnostic and therapeutic thoracentesis is often performed to differentiate transudates from exudates based on pleural fluid chemistries (pleural fluid pH, LDH, protein, glucose), cell count, cultures, and cytology and to relieve symptoms of dyspnea.

With pleurisy, laboratory tests help identify the underlying cause. A complete blood count may reveal an elevated leukocyte count with a shift to the left, which is suggestive of a bacterial infection (e.g., pneumonia). If the diagnosis of pleurisy is not clear, then consider obtaining a CT scan of the chest and tests to evaluate for pulmonary embolism, and consider referral to a pulmonary expert for further diagnostic evaluation.[1]

Management

Ultimately, treatment targeting the primary cause is pursued. Typically, management is supportive and aimed at alleviation of discomfort and treatment of the underlying pathology. Other conditions can have a similar presentation as pleurisy, pneumonia, rib fracture, costochondritis, vertebral fractures, and nerve root pain from herpes zoster infection. Pleurisy is often caused by viral infection, rheumatic disease, and sarcoidosis.

Pleural effusion is caused by pneumonia, tuberculosis, lupus pleuritis, and postcardiac injury syndrome. Treatment is based on the cause of the effusion as is the need for a particular specialist. For example, if there are suspected malignant effusions, then an oncologist and pulmonologist are recommended. Individuals with no underlying respiratory condition or comorbid condition that increases their risk of complications often can be treated in your practice. Those with respiratory distress or who are compromised should be admitted to the hospital.

Pharmacologic

The pain and inflammation of pleurisy are typically treated with nonsteroidal anti-inflammatory drugs (NSAIDs), and occasionally oral steroids.

Nonpharmacologic

Making the patient with pleurisy and/or pleural effusions as comfortable as possible by being authentically present and engaging in shared decision-making is important.

Patient Education

It is important to educate the patient and family about the causes and treatment of pleural effusion and/or pleurisy. Helping them understand the underlying disease process that may have been the cause so they are prepared to engage in health promotion behaviors is an essential aspect of care.[26]

🔆 CLINICAL PEARL

- The normal smooth surfaces of the parietal and visceral pleurae become rough with inflammation. As these surfaces rub together, a rough scratching sound or friction rub can be heard on auscultation. The friction rub is a classic finding in pleurisy.

CASE STUDY
36-YEAR-OLD FEMALE WITH A COUGH OF 3 WEEKS

A 36-year-old female presents to your office complaining of a cough with "green" sputum for almost 2 weeks. She states a cold has been "going around" at home. She had a low-grade fever and sore throat the first few days, which has now resolved except for the cough, which is making sleeping difficult at night. She denies pain apart from a "sore chest" from coughing. Past medical history is noncontributory including no history of asthma or other lung disease.

(cont.)

She denies allergies and takes no medications other than a multivitamin. There is no smoking history. On examination T 98.2 °F, blood pressure 126/70 mmHg, pulse 88, respiratory rate 18 breaths/min, oxygen saturation 99% on room air. Your physical examination is negative, lungs clear to auscultation and there is no lymphadenopathy.

Case Study Questions

1. What is the most likely diagnosis for this patient?
2. What is your management plan that includes a patient-centered approach?

Case Study Answers

1. The most likely diagnosis is acute bronchitis. The patient presents with a report of 3 weeks of cough post–upper respiratory infection, a history negative for lung disease and cigarette smoking, and a negative physical examination. Acute bronchitis is a diagnosis of exclusion; other common causes for prolonged cough, including cough variant asthma, eosinophilic bronchitis, GERD-related cough, atopic cough, and medication-induced cough, should be ruled out. Patients who present with comorbid conditions that contribute to cough, such as atopy or GERD, will most likely present with a multifactorial cough and should be treated for ALL comorbid cough-inducing factors to improve patient outcomes.

2. There is limited evidence of clinical benefit to support the use of antibiotics in acute bronchitis, irrespective of whether the origin is bacterial or viral. Acute bronchitis refers to inflammation of the tracheobronchial tree. Patients should be provided symptom management with antitussives and expectorants. Nasal saline or nasal steroid sprays may improve symptoms if postnasal drip is a cough trigger. Viruses are responsible for more than 90% of acute bronchitis infections and cough with prurient sputum is frequently the presenting symptom. The myth held by patients that green or yellow sputum corresponds with a bacterial origin requiring antibiotics is frequently seen in the primary care office, and education should be provided to dispel this misunderstanding. The color of sputum is not diagnostic. Antibiotic stewardship is vital to reduce antibiotic resistance, now a major health threat, as well as to prevent unnecessary adverse outcomes such as secondary infection with bacteria such as Clostridium difficile. Communicating with patients to explain the potential of antibiotic resistance, as well as the risk of adverse events secondary to the use of unnecessary antibiotics, can create a successful partnership between provider and patient, and promote positive patient outcomes.

CASE STUDY
40-YEAR-OLD MALE WITH PROGRESSING FEVER AND COUGH WITH HEMOPTYSIS

A 40-year-old male presents to your office with nasal congestion, mild sore throat, productive cough, and low-grade fever with malaise for 4 days. Today his fever has increased to 101 °F, and he noticed "specks of blood" in his sputum. He teaches at the local high school, is married with two teenage children, and has a 10 pack-year history of cigarettes. His past medical history is negative. Medications reported are NSAIDs for occasional muscle ache. On examination, he looks ill, with continuing cough and chills. Body temperature is 101.2 °F, pulse 110, respiratory rate 20, oxygen saturation 95% on room air. There is mild erythema of the mucosa of the nose and posterior oropharynx. Ronchi are auscultated in the lungs, with decreased breath sounds. There is dullness to percussion in bilateral lung basis.

Case Study Questions

1. What is your most likely diagnosis?
2. What is your next diagnostic step?
3. What is your treatment plan?

Case Study Answers

1. The most likely diagnosis is CAP. This patient presents with a relatively acute onset of fever, malaise and productive cough with hemoptysis, with progressing symptoms. The 10 pack-year smoking history increases pneumonia risk, as well as exposure to pathogens as a high school teacher and a parent of two teens. CAP can be viral or bacterial. The most common bacterial causes are Streptococcus pneumoniae, Hemophilus influenzae, Chlamydia pneumoniae, and Mycoplasma pneumonia. Viral causes are coronaviruses (primarily SARS-CoV-2), respiratory syncytial virus (RSV), adenoviruses, influenza viruses, metapneumovirus, and Parainfluenza viruses.

2. The gold standard for diagnosis of pneumonia is the presence of infiltrate on chest x-ray (posteroanterior and lateral views). New guidelines recommend all patients with CAP be treated empirically for bacterial infection as frequently patients with CAP caused by a virus also present with a bacterial co-infection. The updated guidelines do not recommend routine collection of sputum Gram stain and culture or blood cultures in CAP patients being treated in the outpatient setting.

3. Guidelines include considering local epidemiology and risk factors to determine the need for drug-resistant pathogens such as methicillin-resistant S. aureus (MRSA) and Pseudomonas aeruginosa. Patients without comorbid conditions or risk factors for drug-resistant pathogens should do well on monotherapy such as amoxicillin, doxycycline, or a macrolide (azithromycin or clarithromycin). Macrolides are now not recommended if there is a possibility of local antibiotic resistance. Patients with comorbidities should receive a broader spectrum antibiotic such as a respiratory fluoroquinolone (levofloxacin, moxifloxacin, gemifloxacin) or a combination therapy with amoxicillin-clavulanate or a cephalosporin plus a macrolide or doxycycline.

CONCLUSION

The respiratory system is responsible for the exchange of oxygen and carbon dioxide in body cells. Stimulated by nerve impulses, the process of respiration occurs every 3 to 5 seconds to promote ventilation to move air in and out of the lungs and facilitate respiration. Disruption of this process secondary to pathologic processes is a leading cause of morbidity and mortality around the world. Timely diagnosis and treatment are essential to maintain homeostasis and promote optimal patient outcomes.

REFERENCES

References for this chapter are online and available at https://connect.springerpub.com/content/book/978-0-8261-8414-6/part/part01/toc-part/ch19.

CHAPTER 20

Common Cardiovascular Disorders Encountered in the Primary Care Setting

Natalie Murphy and Debra J. Hain

LEARNING OBJECTIVES

At the conclusion of this chapter, the learner will be able to:

➤ Review assessment of common conditions affecting the cardiovascular system.

➤ Explore appropriate diagnostic testing for cardiovascular conditions.

➤ Analyze evidence-based treatment options.

➤ Examine alternative, holistic methods of treatment for cardiovascular conditions.

➤ Summarize how culture, ethnicity, and race play a unique role in the pathophysiology and treatment of cardiovascular conditions.

INTRODUCTION

This chapter provides an overview of the anatomy, physiology, and pathophysiology of the cardiovascular system, common health conditions that adult-gerontology nurse practitioners (AGNPs) may see in primary care, and evidence-based strategies to promote health and well-being among adolescents to older adults. In addition, the unique role culture, race, and ethnicity play in the pathophysiology and treatment of cardiovascular conditions is presented. Pharmacologic and nonpharmacologic treatments are discussed. It is important to know the common terms used in cardiology (see Table 20.1) as you review the chapter.

Table 20.1: Glossary of Terms

Ablation: Removing, isolating, or destroying cardiac conduction pathways implicated in arrhythmias
Arrhythmia: An abnormal heart rhythm
Direct current cardioversion: Delivery of a low electrical current to terminate an atrial or ventricular tachyarrhythmia
Ejection fraction: A measurement of the cardiac output with a single heartbeat
Event monitor: Continuous recording of an electrocardiogram (ECG), usually over 10 to 30 days, to diagnose ECG changes
Implantable cardioverter defibrillator (ICD): An implanted device used to treat abnormal tachyarrhythmia by cardioversion, defibrillation, or pacing
Ischemia: Decreased perfusion usually due to reduced blood flow from vessel occlusion or blockage
Holter monitoring: Continuous recording of an ECG, usually over 24 to 48 hours, to diagnose ECG changes
Left ventricular assist device: A surgically implanted pump that helps the left ventricle pump more effectively and improves cardiac output
Left ventricular dysfunction: A heart condition in which cardiac output is reduced because of a deficiency in the left ventricle
Poikilothermia: The inability to regulate core body temperature
Pulses alternans: A condition in which the arterial pulse waveform shows alternating strong and then weak beats
Revascularization: Medical or surgical procedures which restore perfusion when a vessel is blocked. Examples include angioplasty or cardiac bypass surgery.
Syncope: Fainting or transient loss of consciousness which may be related to a cardiac arrhythmia
Wall motion abnormalities: Poor movement of the heart muscle seen on imaging that may reflect underlying ischemia or damage
Xanthomas: Cholesterol deposits on the skin

OVERVIEW OF THE SYSTEM

Cardiovascular disease (CVD) is common in the U.S. population with the majority of individuals with CVD being 60 years of age and older. CVD includes four major areas:

- **Coronary heart disease (CHD):** myocardial infarction (MI), angina pectoris, heart failure (HF), and coronary death
- **Cerebrovascular disease:** stroke and transient ischemic attacks (see Chapter 17)
- **Peripheral artery disease (PAD):** intermittent claudication
- Aortic atherosclerosis and thoracic or abdominal aortic aneurysm

CHD accounts for about a third to half of CHD patients with CVD. Many risk factors for CVD are modifiable through implementing lifestyle behaviors and preventative treatments. CVD is a leading cause of death in the United States and is rapidly increasing in resource-limited countries. The risk for CVD should be considered when engaging in discussions about atherosclerotic cardiovascular disease (ACVD) risks (see Box 20.1). Primary prevention for ACVD is essential (see Figure 20.1). In those diagnosed with CVD, hypertension, dyslipidemia, or other cardiac-related health conditions, health promotion and prevention of comorbid conditions and related complications are critical aspects of the goals of care.

Normal Anatomy and Physiology

The heart is comprised of two "conjoined pumps moving blood through two separate circulatory systems."[1] Structures on the right pump blood through the pulmonary circulation and those on the left through systemic circulation. Arteries branch off to arterioles, becoming smaller vessels (capillaries) that carry blood from the heart to the rest of the body. Venules become veins that carry blood back to the heart. The plasma component of the blood passes through the walls of the capillaries into the interstitial space. The lymphatic system (an important component of the immune system; see Chapter 28) carries lymph back to the cardiovascular system. The heart wall has three structures: myocardium (inner layer), epicardium (outer layer), and pericardium (a double-walled membranous sac that encloses the heart). There are four chambers of the heart: the right atrium, the left atrium, the right ventricle, and the left ventricle. The right heart is a low-pressure system pumping blood through the lungs and the left heart is a high-pressure system pumping blood through the rest of the body. The valves of the heart are atrioventricular valves (tricuspid and mitral valves) and the semilunar valves (pulmonic and aortic valves).

Electrical impulses start with the sinoatrial node (SA), which is located at the junction of the right atrium and the superior vena cava, just above the tricuspid valve

Box 20.1: Risk-Enhancing Factor for Clinician-Patient Risk Discussion

- Family history of premature ACVD (males younger than 55 years and females younger than 65 years)
- Primary hypercholesterolemia (LDL-C 160–180 mg/dL; non-HDL-C 190–219 mg/dL)
- Metabolic syndrome (increased waist circumference, elevated triglycerides (greater than 150 mg/dL, nonfasting), elevated blood pressure (BP), elevated glucose, and low HDL-C (40 mg/dL or lower in men, lower than 50 mg/dL in women) are factors; total of 3 is diagnostic
- Chronic kidney disease (eGFR 15–59 mL/min/1.73 m²) with or without albuminuria, not treated with dialysis or kidney transplantation
- Chronic inflammatory conditions such as psoriasis, Rheumatoid arthritis, lupus, or HIV/AIDS
- History of premature menopause (before age 40) and history of pregnancy-associated conditions that increase later ACVD risk, such as preeclampsia
- High-risk race/ethnicity (e.g., South Asian ancestry)
- Lipids/biomarkers: associated with increased ACVD risk
- Persistently elevated primary hypertriglyceridemia (equal or greater than 175 mg/d, nonfasting)
- If measured, elevated high-sensitivity C-reactive protein (greater than 3.0 mg/dL)

ACVD, atherosclerotic cardiovascular disease; eGFR, estimaged glomerular filtration rate; HDL-C, high-density lipoprotein cholesterol; LDL-C, low-density lipoprotein cholesterol; RA, rheumatoid arthritis.
Source: Arnett DK, Blumenthal RS, Albert MA, et al. 2019 ACC/AHA Guideline on the Primary Prevention of Cardiovascular Disease: Executive Summary: A Report of the American College of Cardiology/American Heart Association Task Force on Clinical Practice Guidelines [published correction appears in *Circulation.* 2019 Sep 10;140(11):e647-e648] [published correction appears in *Circulation.* 2020 Jan 28;141(4):e59] [published correction appears in *Circulation.* 2020 Apr 21;141(16):e773]. *Circulation.* 2019;140(11):e563-e595. doi:10.1161/CIR.0000000000000677

(see Figure 20.1). The action potential moves toward the atrioventricular node (AV node) causing the two atria to contract and begin systole. The AV node located in the intra-atrial septum conducts the action potentials toward the ventricles. Conducting fibers from the AV node

Box 20.2: Healthy People 2030 Objectives

Heart Disease: General
- Improve cardiovascular health in adults.
- Reduce coronary heart disease deaths.

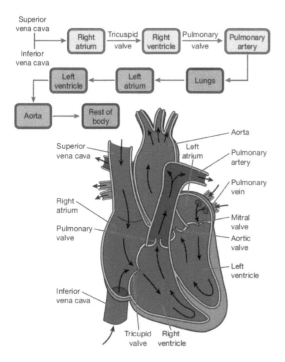

Figure 20.1A: Cardiac circulatory pathway

Circulation of blood through the cardiopulmonary system—tracing the flow of deoxygenated blood from the vena cavae through the right side of the heart and into the lungs, where it is oxygenated and returned to the left side of the heart and pumped to the aorta and the rest of the body.

Source: Myrick KM, Karosas LM, eds. *Advanced Health Assessment and Differential Diagnosis.* Springer Publishing Company; 2021:Figure 6.4.

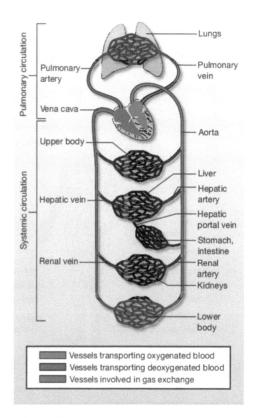

Figure 20.1B: The circulatory system, differentiating systemic and pulmonary circulation

Source: Tkacs NC, Herrmann LL, Johnson RL. *Advanced Physiology and Pathophysiology: Essentials for Clinical Practice.* Springer Publishing Company; 2021:Figure 9.1

converge to become the bundle of His (AV bundle) that then becomes the right and left bundle branches.[1] Even though it is very important to have knowledge of anatomy, physiology, and pathophysiology of the cardiovascular and circulatory system to understand CV health conditions, it is beyond the scope of this chapter to discuss the conduction system of the heart. Consequently, it is important to review an anatomy and physiology or pathophysiology textbook as needed.

PRIMARY (ESSENTIAL) HYPERTENSION

Etiology

Primary (essential) hypertension is the most common cardiovascular disease in the United States, affecting approximately 90% to 95% of patients with elevated BP. Secondary hypertension is less common. Primary hypertension is the most common reason for primary care office visits. The prevalence is higher in men than women, in older adults compared to younger adults, and in non-Hispanic Black adults compared to non-Hispanic White adults. Cardiovascular disease is a primary cause of death in the United States, and hypertension is a major risk factor for CV. In secondary hypertension (no underlying cause is identified), a number of medical conditions or medications can contribute to poor BP control (see the section about risk factors).[2] Many patients have coexisting primary hypertension with secondary hypertension, which can present challenges when trying to achieve adequate BP control.

Pathophysiology

Primary hypertension is the result of alterations in heart rate, stroke volume, total peripheral resistance, kidney function, and the sympathetic nervous system. According to the Eighth Joint National Committee (JNC-8) guidelines, optimal BP for adults should be targeted below 140/90 mmHg and BP of adults older than age 60 should be targeted at 150/90 mmHg or less.

BP is regulated by baroreceptors located in the carotid arteries and aortic arch; endothelial factors, such as nitric oxide; the renin–angiotensin–aldosterone system of the

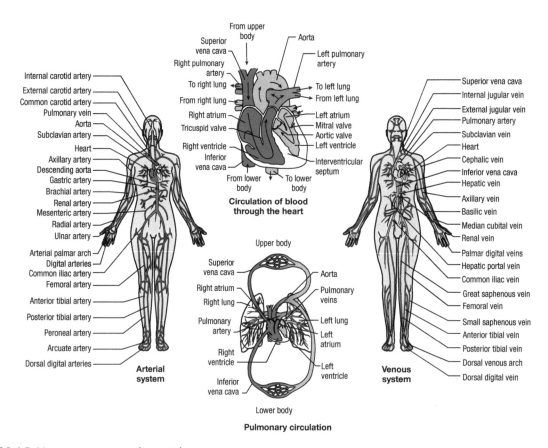

Figure 20.1C: Venous system and arterial system

kidneys; and genetic influences. Obesity, increased sodium intake, stress, and alcohol all contribute to the development of high BP. Untreated hypertension can lead to increased cardiovascular risks (stroke, HF, MI) and end-stage kidney disease (ESKD).

Risk Factors

There are modifiable and nonmodifiable risk factors for primary hypertension. Modifiable risk factors include an unhealthy diet (excessive sodium intake, high in saturated fat and trans-fat, low intake of vegetables and fruit), physical inactivity, tobacco smoking, alcohol, and being overweight or obese. "Nonmodifiable risk factors [are] a family history of hypertension, age [older] than 65 years, and coexisting disease, such as diabetes and chronic kidney disease."[3]

Race is also a nonmodifiable risk factor. In Black adults, primary hypertension tends be more common and severe and occurs earlier in life. This population also seems to have hypertension associated with greater target-organ damage.

Secondary hypertension risk factors include oral contraceptives, nonsteroidal anti-inflammatory drugs (NSAIDs), antidepressants (e.g., serotonin reuptake inhibitors, tricyclic antidepressants, monoamine oxidase inhibitors), corticosteroids, sodium-containing antacids, erythropoietin, stimulants and atypical antipsychotics, illicit drug use, CKD, primary aldosteronism, renovascular hypertension, obstructive sleep apnea, pheochromocytoma, Cushing syndrome, hypothyroidism, hyperthyroidism, and hyperparathyroidism.

Approach to Diagnosis

The American College of Cardiology/American Heart Association (ACC/AHA) states that it is critical to obtain an accurate BP measurement when diagnosing hypertension. It is also important to obtain repeated BP readings. Normal BP systolic is less than 120 mmHg and diastolic less than 80 mmHg; elevated BP is systolic 120 to 129 mmHg and diastolic less than 80 mmHg. Hypertension stage 1 is systolic blood pressure (SBP) less than 130 to 139 mmHg or diastolic blood pressure (DBP) 80 to 89 mmHg, and stage 2 is SBP at least 140 mmHg or DBP at least 90 mmHg. If there is a disparity in category between systolic and diastolic, the higher value determines the stage. The 2020 International Society of Hypertension (ISH) Practice Guidelines recommend hypertension be diagnosed when a person's SBP in the office is 140 mmHg or greater and DBP is 90 mmHg or greater with repeated examination. Isolated hypertension is SBP 140 mmHg or greater and DBP 90 mmHg or less. Whenever possible, the diagnosis should not be made on a single office visit but rather two to three office visits at 1- to 4-week intervals (depends on BP reading). If the BP is 180/110 mmHg or greater and there is evidence of cardiovascular disease, the diagnosis can be made on a single visit. If possible, the diagnosis of hypertension should be confirmed by out-of-office BP[4] (see Box 20.3 for more ISH recommendations). It is important to consider white coat hypertension or masked hypertension as one of the differential diagnoses.

White coat hypertension is used to describe those who only have elevated BP in the medical office/setting but have nonelevated ambulatory or home BP. This type of hypertension is found in approximately 20% to 30% of individuals seen in the office. The diagnosis requires confirmation with repeated office and out-of-office BP measurement. If their total CV risk is low and there is no hypertension-mediate organ damage, medication may not be needed, but they should be encouraged to engage in lifestyle modification and be prescribed antihypertensives if sustained elevated BP is noted. Masked hypertension presents as a normal reading within the office setting but with an elevated ambulatory and home BP. Those with masked hypertension have similar CV risk factors as those with sustained hypertension; the diagnosis requires in-office and out-of-office BP measurements.[40]

Diagnostics

BP should be taken after the patient is seated and relaxed for at least 5 minutes. Home BP logs can also be used to monitor readings, but ensure the manometer used is correctly calibrated. Also, confirm the correct size cuff has been selected based on patient arm circumference.

Once diagnosed, a thorough patient history should be completed. Focus on family history of cardiovascular disease; any current medical risk factors for cardiovascular disease, including diabetes mellitus or dyslipidemia; and review of lifestyle factors that increase risk. Ask about alcohol use (how much and how often), smoking history, current dietary intake of sodium and caffeine, level of stress, current medications, and exercise history. Inquire about any possible signs and symptoms of elevated BP, such as headaches or neck/shoulder pain, although most patients with essential hypertension are asymptomatic.

Physical examination should focus on the vasculature. Eyes should be examined for any signs of retinopathy. Listen for carotid bruits. Carefully auscultate the heart and listen for extra heart sounds or murmurs. While examining the abdomen, evaluate for abdominal or renal bruits. Examine peripheral pulses. Obtain an accurate body mass index (BMI).

A 12-lead ECG should be ordered and examined for signs of left ventricular hypertrophy and/or ischemic changes. Basic fasting serum testing should be completed to identify metabolic and/or renal dysfunction including blood glucose level, hematocrit, potassium level, creatinine and eGFR, calcium level, a lipid profile, and inflammatory markers, such as high-sensitivity C-reactive protein (hs-CRP) and homocysteine levels. A urinalysis with micro-albumin should also be obtained.

Screening Tools

The U.S. Preventative Services Task Force (USPSTF)[2] recommends screening for hypertension in adults 18 years and older with office blood pressure measurement (OBPM). The USPSTF recommends obtaining BP measurements outside of the clinical setting for diagnostic confirmation before starting treatment. Ways to measure BP outside the clinical setting include the following:

▪ **ABPM:** Patients wear a programmed portable device that automatically takes BP measurements, typically

---

Box 20.3: ISH Practice Guideline Recommendations.

Hypertension Diagnosis: Office BP Measurement

▪ **Initial evaluation:** measure BP in both arms, preferred if can do at the same time. If there is a consistent difference between arms of more than 10 mmHg in repeated measurements, use the arm with the higher BP; if the difference is greater than 20 mmHg, consider further investigation.

▪ **Standing BP:** measure in people who are being treated for hypertension after 1 minute and again after 3 minutes when there are symptoms suggesting postural hypotension and at the first visit for older adults and people with diabetes.

▪ **Unattended office BP:** multiple automated BP measurements taken while the patient remains alone in the office provide a more standardized evaluation but also lower BP level than usual office measurements with an uncertain threshold for hypertension diagnosis. Confirmation of out-of-office BP reading is needed for most treatment decisions.

Hypertension Diagnosis: Out-of-Office BP Measurement

▪ Out-of-office BP measurements (by patients at home or with 24-hour ambulatory BP monitoring [ABPM]) are more reproducible than office measurements, more closely associated with hypertension-induced organ damage and the risk of CV events, and identify the white coat and masked hypertension phenomena.

▪ Out-of-office BP is often necessary for the accurate diagnosis of hypertension and for treatment decisions. In untreated or treated individuals with office BP classified as high-normal BP or grade 1 hypertension (SBP 130–159 mmHg and/or DBP 85–99 mmHg), the BP level needs to be confirmed using home or ambulatory BP monitoring.

BP, blood pressure; ISH, International Society of Hypertension.
Source: Unger T, Borghi C, Charchar F, et al. 2020 International Society of Hypertension global hypertension practice guidelines. *Hypertension.* 2020;75(6):1334–1357. doi:10.1161/HYPERTENSIONAHA.120.15026

in 20- to 30-minute intervals (this is set by the health-care provider) over 12 to 24 hours while the person goes about their normal activities and while sleeping. Usually, the patient maintains a diary to help identify activity that may be correlated with elevations in BP.

■ **Out-of-office BP monitoring**: Patients are asked to measure their BP at home with an automated device. Measurements are taken much less frequently than with ABPM (e.g., 1–2 times a day or week, although they can be spread out over more time). BP measurements should be taken at the brachial artery with a validated and accurate device in a seated position after 5 minutes of rest.

Screening should be done every year in adults 40 years and older and in adults at increased risk for hypertension (e.g., those who are obese or overweight, Black adults). Screening can be done less frequently (i.e., every 3–5 years) in adults aged 18 to 39 years who are not at increased risk for hypertension and with a prior normal BP reading.[5]

Specific Assessment for Adolescents, Older Adult Patients, and African American Patients

The prevalence of essential hypertension in the adolescent population is rising. The primary cause of this is the current epidemic of childhood obesity and subsequently the earlier development of atherosclerosis. An obese adolescent with a family history of hypertension is at the greatest risk of developing the condition. African American adolescents may be at greater genetic risk than adolescents of other races. Carefully question patients about the use of stimulant drugs, smoking, and alcohol intake as these also increase risk. Assess the level of stress and the current level of physical activity. Also carefully consider any possible secondary cause, especially kidney or endocrine disease.

With age, atherosclerosis worsens, and subsequently, the prevalence of hypertension increases. Older adults are more likely to develop elevated systolic pressure, widening pulse pressure, and orthostatic hypotension. When assessing BP in older adults, ensure that BP is checked both while sitting and then standing. If diastolic pressure is too low, the heart itself receives less blood flow and oxygen.[6]

Management

Treating hypertension to goal is essential to prevent adverse cardiovascular and nephrology outcomes. Hypertension is the second leading cause of CKD (see Chapter 23 for more information about kidney disease). Cardiovascular complications due to hypertension include left ventricular hypertrophy (LVH), HF, both reduced ejection fraction (systolic) and preserved ejection fraction (diastolic), ischemic stroke (see Chapter 17 for more information), intracerebral hemorrhage, and ischemic heart disease.

Pharmacologic

According to JNC-8 guidelines, hypertension treatment is guided by BP readings,[7] patient age, race, and presence of comorbidities. Patients older than age 60 should have a BP target of less than 150/90 mmHg. Patients less than 60 years of age should have a BP target of less than 140/90 mmHg. Patients of any age who have diabetes mellitus or chronic kidney disease should have a BP target of less than 140/90 mmHg. Race and comorbidities guide the selection of antihypertensive agents.

Drug therapy should be selected with individual patient needs in mind; taking a person-centered approach can result in optimal health outcomes (see Chapter 2 for more information about person-centered care). If the BP is less than 159/90–99 mmHg, the patient can be started on therapy with a single agent. Thiazide diuretics are preferred over other agents in the Black population, but an angiotensin-converting-enzyme inhibitor (ACEI), angiotensin II receptor blocker (ARB), calcium channel blockers, or beta-blockers can also be selected. If the BP is greater than 160/100 mmHg, then therapy should begin with a combination of two antihypertensive agents. In all cases, begin with the lowest dose and titrate upward monthly based on BP response.

When selecting medications, the nurse practitioner (NP) should consider cost and individual patient needs. Cost greatly impacts adherence to therapy. Always consider lower cost, generic agents first. Adherence to the regimen is also enhanced if long-acting and/or combination medications are selected. Fewer pills less often equal better compliance. Match drugs selected to patient need. For example, a Black patient with mild lower extremity edema would likely do well on a thiazide diuretic, which will reduce BP readings and edema. Patients with diabetes or chronic kidney disease may benefit from the renal protection an ACEI or ARB can provide. Patients with coexisting atrial fibrillation can be treated with a beta-blocker or a calcium channel blocker. Also, carefully consider the possible adverse effects of each antihypertensive class. For example, a patient with a history of lower extremity edema is unlikely to tolerate a calcium channel blocker as this may worsen the edema (see Chapter 13 for medication management).

Nonpharmacologic

All patients diagnosed with essential hypertension should be counseled about healthy lifestyle modifications and these should be initiated before pharmacologic treatment. Weight loss to achieve desired BMI should be encouraged by adopting a heart-healthy diet and implementing aerobic activity for at least 30 minutes most days of the week. The DASH diet (Dietary Approaches to Stop Hypertension) should be thoroughly explained; it is important to consider kidney function when recommending a diet. This diet focuses on a whole-food dietary approach heavy in fruits, vegetables, greens, and lean meats and low in saturated fat, cholesterol, and processed foods. Sodium intake should be restricted to no more than 2,400 mg daily. Smoking cessation should be strongly encouraged, and alcohol intake should be reduced or eliminated. The recommended limit of ethanol is 1 ounce per day for men and 0.5 ounce per day for women.

Management Specific to Adolescents and Older Adults

Many adolescents are unaware that hypertension can occur in their age group and incorrectly assume it only happens with advancing age. Family history of hypertension is strongly linked to the diagnosis in young people. Patient education about lifestyle modifications is very important because weight loss, daily exercise, smoking cessation, a low sodium diet, the elimination of stimulant drugs and alcohol, and stress reduction can reverse the hypertensive process. Untreated adolescent hypertension can lead to earlier development of coronary artery disease and kidney disease.

Older adults with hypertension have unique clinical circumstances and needs. Many older adults may have isolated systolic hypertension, which is an SBP above 160mmHg with a DBP below 90 mmHg. This widened pulse pressure (systolic rises and diastolic falls) is mainly due to diminished arterial compliance. However, it can also be related to anemia, hyperthyroidism, aortic insufficiency, arteriovenous fistula, or Paget disease of the bone. Reducing SBP without lowering diastolic pressure too low is often tricky. Lowering DBP below 65 mmHg is associated with an increased risk of CV events. Medication selection should be guided by individual patient characteristics and comorbid conditions. Start at the lowest dose and titrate slowly while closely monitoring BP and possible adverse effects (they may need only half the dose a younger person requires). Older adults may have sluggish baroreceptors and sympathetic neural responses as well as impaired cerebral autoregulation. So, unless it is an emergency, lowering the BP gradually over a period of 3 to 6 months and not hours to days to reduce the risk of ischemic symptoms is important. Be particularly cautious in older adults with orthostatic hypotension (see Box 20.4). An even more cautious approach should be taken in those with advanced age and particularly with adults who are considered frail.

Box 20.4: Orthostatic Hypotension

Orthostatic hypotension is diagnosed when, within 2 minutes of quick standing, one or more of the following is present:

- at least 20 mmHg fall in SBP
- at least 10 mmHg fall in DBP
- symptoms of cerebral hypoperfusion (e.g., dizziness)

Patient Education

Patients should be thoroughly educated about the possible side effects of medications ordered. Many side effects are transient and resolve as the individual adjusts to the lowering of the BP. Collaborate with the patient to help them understand that BP control often takes weeks of trial and error and titration to achieve goals. Encourage them to be patient during this adjustment time. Keep in mind that most patients will require two or more antihypertensive agents to reach goal BP. Estrogen therapy is not recommended in patients with hypertension as it adds to the risk of adverse cardiac events. Lifestyle modifications as discussed previously are key to achieving the goals of BP control. Teaching older adults to slowly change position from sitting to standing to prevent orthostatic hypotension is important.

🏠 Quality and Safety Alerts

- With adolescents and adult females of reproductive age, cautiously consider treatment with an ACEI or ARB because of the possible adverse risks to a fetus.
- Females with hypertension should not be prescribed oral birth control agents that contain estrogen as this increases the likelihood of adverse cardiac/thrombotic events.
- Older adults are sensitive to volume depletion, autonomic insufficiency, and dysregulation of baroreceptors. Consequently, they are more likely than their younger counterparts to develop symptomatic orthostatic hypotension. This leads to an increased incidence of falls, fractures, and increased mortality rates.

💡 CLINICAL PEARLS

- Most patients require more than one medication to meet BP goals.
- The medication plan must be individualized. The NP must consider age, race/ethnicity, cost, and comorbidities when developing a plan of care.

📡 EMERGENCIES

- Severe hypertension (SBP over 180 mmHg and/or DBP above 120 mmHg) with evidence of acute end-organ damage (e.g., encephalopathy, stroke, retinal hemorrhages, papilledema, acute kidney injury) is a hypertensive emergency.
- This can be life-threatening and requires immediate treatment, which most often occurs in a hospital where the patient can receive parenteral medications and be monitored.
- BP pressure should be gradually reduced to reduce the risk of CV events.

In patients that have SBP 180 mmHg or higher and/ or DBP above 120 mmHg and are asymptomatic, there is no proven benefit to sending the patient urgently to the hospital.

Hypertension urgency often can be managed in your office with BP reduction over days. Most often, the cause is related to the patient not taking medications as prescribed. Once beginning treatment, it is essential to have close follow-up over the next few days. If you give the patient medication in your office or other primary care settings, it is important to monitor their response over several hours before sending the patient home.

Box 20.5: Healthy People 2030 Objectives

- Reduce the proportion of adults with high BP.
- Increase BP control in adults through heathier eating, weight loss, and increased physical activity.

Relevant Social Determinants of Health

- Assess for patient's difficulties obtaining medications due to financial constraints and transportation issues.
- Evaluate challenges obtaining recommended foods by determining if there are financial constraints, food insecurity, or a food desert in the community.

EVOLVING CASE STUDY

Stephen, a 75-year-old Black overweight male, presents to the office for a routine visit. He has a past medical history of diabetes mellitus, which has been fairly well controlled. His last hemoglobin A1C obtained 3 months ago was 6%. His medication regimen includes metformin 1,000 mg po BID, aspirin 81 mg po daily, and lisinopril 5 mg po daily for renal protection. Stephen states that he has been having occasional headaches. Vital signs reveal a BP of 160/92, pulse of 82, and respiratory rate of 12. The physical examination is unremarkable except for mild lower extremity pedal edema and a BMI of 28.

Case Study Questions

1. What additional history should the AGNP obtain?
2. What tests should be considered?
3. What is an appropriate management plan at this time?

A 12-lead ECG reveals a normal sinus rhythm. Nonspecific T-ST wave changes are noted. Stephen denies any chest pain, shortness of breath, or fatigue. He admits to frequently eating out in restaurants with his wife and has not been monitoring his sodium intake. He does not exercise.

DYSLIPIDEMIA

Etiology

The connection between coronary artery disease (CAD) and dyslipidemia is clearly established. "Dyslipidemia" is a broad term used to define various lipid disorders, which include elevated total cholesterol, elevated low-density lipoprotein (LDL), decreased high-density lipoprotein (HDL), elevated triglycerides (TGs), or some combination of each. Dyslipidemia is the abnormal concentration of serum lipoproteins. About 50% of Americans have some form of dyslipidemia, and these people are approximately twice as likely to experience CVD compared to those with normal range levels.[8] In those with familial hypercholesterolemia, there is a substantially greater risk of CVD at an earlier age as well as premature death. Approximately 53% of adults have LDL cholesterol (LDL-C) levels that are abnormal and yet less than 50% are receiving treatment to reduce the levels. Having high LDL-C increases the person's risk for cardiovascular events, which include MI and stroke.[8]

Pathophysiology

Most cells require lipids for the manufacture and repair of plasma membranes. Cholesterol is also required for the manufacturing of substances that the body needs (e.g., bile acids, steroid hormones). Cholesterol comes from dietary intake as well as from the cells that can produce it. The cycle of lipid metabolism is very complex, so it is recommended that you review a pathophysiology book for more information. Chemical reactions in the liver result in the production of many lipoproteins that vary in density and function. There are very-low-density lipoproteins (VLDLs) that are primarily TG and protein, LDL that are mostly cholesterol and protein, and HDL that is mainly phospholipids and protein. An increased LDL is an indicator of CVD risk. Dyslipidemia is one of multiple risk factors that can raise the risk for developing CVD. The risk depends on the presence of other risk factors discussed later in this section. LDL describes several types of LDL molecules, and so measurement of some of these helps identify CVD risk. LDL-C particles are the most atherogenic and apolipoprotein B (structural protein on LDL and VLDL) are strong predictors of future coronary events. Evidence supports that for every 1% reduction on LDL-C there is a 1% reduction in coronary risk.[9] Atherosclerosis is a complicated inflammatory process where deposits of cholesterol and lipoproteins form plaque on arterial walls.

Risk Factors

Dyslipidemia can be primary or familial dyslipoproteinemias, resulting from genetic defects or caused by poor lifestyle choices or from secondary causes (Box 20.6). Race as a risk factor is not clear; however, health disparities in the Black population exist, particularly for those with diabetes.[10]

Box 20.6: Secondary Causes of Dyslipidemia

Diets high in saturated fat and cholesterol (animal products)

Metabolic syndrome

Obesity

Anorexia nervosa

Pregnancy

Type 2 diabetes mellitus

Biliary obstruction

Hypertension

Hypothyroidism

Liver disease

Chronic kidney disease

Pancreatitis

Drugs: tobacco, antivirals, antipsychotics, thiazide diuretics, beta-blockers, estrogen, alcohol, amiodarone, progestins, tamoxifen, steroids, protease inhibitors

Sedentary lifestyle

Box 20.7: Secondary Causes of Hypertension

Drugs: tobacco, alcohol, stimulants, steroids, NSAIDs, decongestants, estrogens, cyclosporine, herbal ephedra supplements, monoamine oxidase inhibitors

Metabolic disorders: Cushing syndrome, primary aldosteronism, thyroid and parathyroid disease, obesity

Pheochromocytoma

Renal parenchymal disease

Renal artery stenosis

Obstructive sleep apnea

Coarctation of the aorta

Increased intracranial pressure

Eclampsia

NSAIDs, nonsteroidal anti-inflammatory drugs.

Approach to Diagnosis

Primary prevention is the main focus of treatment, so assessing for CV risk and treating patients at higher risk is important. Dyslipidemia risk assessment and management are important. Look for signs of dyslipidemia on physical examination and search for clues that suggest the presence of atherosclerotic disease. Determine the patient's risk of atherosclerotic CV disease to help classify them into risk categories. Assess for cigarette smoking, family history of premature atherosclerosis CV (i.e., men younger than 55 years and women younger than 65 years), type 2 diabetes mellitus, hypertension, and metabolic syndrome (see Chapter 26 for more information). Xanthomas may be present on the skin and are often located around the eye. Vascular bruits may possibly be auscultated. Often, however, the patient with dyslipidemia will be asymptomatic. Newer research suggests that increased inflammatory markers, especially C-reactive protein, play an important role in the development of atherosclerosis. Measure these markers. Statins have antioxidant properties that reduce inflammation and subsequently reduce the formation of atherosclerotic plaque.

Diagnostics

The primary diagnostic approach includes obtaining a serum lipid profile and other laboratory studies to exclude secondary causes of dyslipidemia (thyroid, hepatic, kidney).

Screening Tools and Tests

The USPSTF recommends a fasting lipid profile screening in men older than 35 years of age and women older than 45 years of age every 5 years. If risk factors for atherosclerotic heart disease are present, then earlier screening is recommended. Once lipid abnormalities are identified, the NP should carefully complete a thorough review of the patient's health history, assess for other risk factors that may contribute to cardiovascular disease, review a family health history (especially for the presence of familial hyperlipidemia), and identify any possible secondary causes for the dyslipidemia.

Specific Assessment of Dyslipidemia in Adolescent and Older Adult Populations

During puberty, lipid levels fluctuate greatly. Consequently, routine lipid testing is not recommended for patients between the ages of 12 to 17 years unless the adolescent has diabetes mellitus, hypertension, a BMI greater than the 95th percentile, smokes, or has a significant family history of early-onset CAD, lipid disorder, diabetes mellitus, obesity, or chronic kidney disease. After age 17, lipid screening is recommended if risk factors are present. Lipid levels are much more stable after puberty is completed.

In adults older than 75 years of age who do not have identified ACVD, NPs must consider the individual risk versus benefit of screening and treating dyslipidemia for primary prevention. Older patients are at an increased risk of adverse effects and drug–drug interactions from statin therapy. Frank discussions with older adults should occur before screening to educate patients of plan-of-care options and patient preference for evaluation and treatment should be honored.

Management

Treatment guidelines recommended clinicians target specific LDL and HDL numbers. Guidelines released in 2013 by the American College of Cardiology and the American

Heart Association (ACC/AHA) panel shifted to identifying and treating four specific high-risk groups. The guidelines were created to prompt clinicians to develop individualized treatment plans based on calculated cardiovascular risk. Treatment of dyslipidemia is aimed at reducing the morbidity and mortality from CVD by reducing the development of atherosclerotic plaque.

Treatment of those with no known CVD should be based on estimated 10-year risk calculators that you can find online. For example, www.cvriskcalculator.com is one such calculator; http://tools/acc/org/ASCVD-Risk-Estimator-Plus is another. Adults with diabetes mellitus and/or LDL levels of at least 190 mg/dL are at high risk and should be treated regardless of estimated risk. Individuals with a 10-year risk of 12% (matches population in clinical trials) should receive treatment. Individuals with known CVD secondary prevention strategies should be put in place.

Pharmacologic

Prescribing medications is based on the patient's 10-year risk and other comorbid conditions, such as diabetes, CVD, and hypertension (see Table 20.2). The U.S. Department of Veterans Affairs and the Department of Defense have updated the guidelines for managing dyslipidemia. The following are specific to those who are 40 years or older:[11]

- In patients who have 10-year CVD risk greater than 12%, then consider moderate-dose HMG-CoA reduction inhibitor (often referred to as a statin).

- If the patient's 10-year risk is 6% to 12% and the person prefers not to take a statin, then recommend aerobic exercise and smoking cessation (if applicable) and follow-up every 2 years.

- If 10-year risk is lower than 6%, then follow up every 5 years.

Table 20.2: HMG-CoA Reductase Inhibitors (Statins)

Moderate Intensity	High Intensity
Atorvastatin (Lipitor) 10-20 mg	40–80 mg
Rosuvastatin (Crestor) 5-10 mg	20–40 mg
Simvastatin (Zocor) 20-40 mg	NA
Pravastatin (Pravachol) 40-80 mg	NA
Lovastatin (Mevacor) 40-80 mg	NA
Fluvastatin (Lescol) 80 mg (sustained release) or 40 mg twice daily	Rosuvastatin 5-10 mg
Pitavastatin (Livalo) 1-4 mg	NA

- If the patient has type 2 diabetes mellitus or an LDL equal to or greater than 190 mg/dL, recommend moderate-dose statin.

- In patients with higher CVD risk, the following are recommended stepped intensification: Maximize statin or add ezetimibe (Zetia). Consider PCSK9 inhibitor only after maximizing statin and adding ezetimibe; if myocardial infarction (MI), acute coronary syndrome (ACS), or coronary artery bypass graft/percutaneous coronary intervention (CABG/PCI) in past 6 weeks, refer for cardiac rehabilitation.

  - MI or ACS in past 12 months,

  - recurrent ACS, MI, or CVA

  - known CVD and any of the following currently, smoking, diabetes, PAD, or CABG/PCI

- In patients with HF with ejection fraction lower than 35%, ESKD, or life expectancy less than 5 years, discuss the lack of evidence demonstrating benefit and continue ongoing care and follow stepped intensification as discussed earlier.

These guidelines do not include people younger than 40 years old because they have not been studied and generally have a low risk of CVD. In addition, patients who have genetic dyslipidemia are not included in the guidelines because of limited evidence.[11] Other medications than statins for treating dyslipidemia can be seen in Table 20.3. Other guidelines focused on reducing the risk of ACVD are presented in Table 20.4.

Nonpharmacologic

The treatment for dyslipidemia should begin with lifestyle modifications. Patients should be encouraged to consume a heart-healthy diet, exercise for at least 30 minutes most days of the week, achieve and maintain an ideal weight, and avoid tobacco products. Although there is debate about what constitutes a heart-healthy diet, most authors suggest a diet low in saturated fat that contains enough total calories that allow for maintenance of desired weight. The diet should include plant sterols and stanols and aim for at least 10 g to 25 g of soluble fiber daily. This diet can be achieved with a shift away from highly processed foods to a diet rich in whole-plant foods (which are nutrient-dense but low in calorie and fat) and moderate, lean animal products. Patients should be counseled about lifestyle modifications at every visit. Unfortunately, many patients are unable to achieve risk reduction with lifestyle changes alone. Consultation with a dietitian may be helpful. Engaging in physical activity is very important, even if it is walking short distances multiple times a day.

Treatment Specific to Adolescent

Adolescents may be safely treated with statins if necessary. Because dyslipidemia is often asymptomatic until clinically significant atherosclerosis is present, adolescents with this disease process, like adults, may be nonadherent to their

Table 20.3: Examples of Other Medication Options to Treat Dyslipidemia

Drug Class	Drug Name/Dose	Lipid-Lowering Ability	Side Effects
Bile acid sequestrants	Cholestyramine 8–16 po gm daily; divided doses	12% LDL reduction	GI side effects (constipation, nausea, bloating, flatulence, vomiting)
	Colesevelam 1,875 mg po BID or 3,750 po daily	15% to 20% LDL reduction	Constipation, nausea
Fibrates	Fenofibrate Triglide 50–160 mg po daily Tricor 48–148 mg po daily	Reduces triglycerides Modest LDL reduction	Nausea, abdominal pain, increased LFTs, back pain, pancreatitis, rhabdomyolysis
	Gemfibrozil 600 mg po BID (30 minutes before meals)	Reduces triglycerides Modest LDL reduction	Nausea, abdominal pain, increased LFTs, rhabdomyolysis
Other			
Nicotinic acid (Niacin)	2 gm po TID ER 500–2gm po daily	Reduces LDL-C b10–15%	Flushing, nausea, headache, hepatotoxicity, rhabdomyolysis
Ezetimibe	10 mg po daily	Reduces LDL up to 19% Increases HDL 3%	Diarrhea, myalgia, hepatitis, rhabdomyolysis
Omega-3 acid ethyl esters	2–4 gm po daily	Reduces triglycerides by 45% but raises LDL	Indigestion, diarrhea

Table 20.4: Reducing Risk of ACVD Through Cholesterol Management

For patients with clinical ACVD, reduce LDC-C with high-intensity statin therapy or maximally tolerated statin therapy.
In very high-risk ACVD, use an LDL-C threshold of 70 mg/dL to consider the addition of nonstatin to statin therapy (statin and ezetimibe), adding PCSK9 inhibitor if appropriate.
In patients with severe primary hypercholesterolemia (LDC-C level 190 mg/dL or greater) without calculating 10-year ACVD risk, begin high-intensity statin therapy. Adding ezetimibe therapy is appropriate; if LDC-C remains over 100 mg/dL and the patient has multiple factors that increase subsequent risk of ACVD events, a PCSK9 inhibitor should be considered.
In adults 40 to 75 years without diabetes mellitus and with LDL-C 70 mg/dL or greater at a 10-year ACVD risk of 7.5% or greater, start a moderate-intensity statin if after discussing benefits versus risks the patient agrees. If statins are indicated, reduce LDL-C by 30% or greater, if 10-year risk is 20% or greater, then the goal should be to reduce the LDL-C by 50% or greater.
In patients 40 to 75 years old without diabetes mellitus and with LCL-C 70 mg/dL to 189 mg/dL at a 10-year ACVD risk of 7.5% to 19.9% and the decision about statin therapy is uncertain, consider measuring coronary artery calcium (CAC).
Adults with diabetes (40–75 years) at higher risk, especially those with multiple risk factors or those 50 to 75 years of age, it is reasonable to use a high-intensity statin to reduce the LDL-C by 50% or greater.

ACVD, atherosclerotic cardiovascular disease; LDL, low-density lipoprotein.
Source: Grundy SM, Stone NJ, Bailey AL, Blumenthal RS, Braun LT, de Ferranti S. AHA/ACC/AACVPR/AAPA/ABC/ACPM/ADA/AGS/APhA/ASPC guideline on the management of blood cholesterol: a report of the American College of Cardiology/American Heart Association task force on clinical practice guidelines. *Circulation.* 2019;25:e1082–e1143. doi:10.1161/CIR.0000000000000625

medication regimen. Detailed patient education about the risks of atherosclerosis in the presence of elevated lipids should be provided. Geriatric patients with dyslipidemia who have been previously treated and who are tolerating statin therapy may remain on moderate-intensity statin therapy for secondary prevention after age 75 years.

Patient Education

In adults evaluated for primary ACVD, a prevention risk discussion should include major risk factors (e.g., cigarette smoking, uncontrolled hypertension, elevated LDL-C, uncontrolled diabetes) and lifestyle change as appropriate. A heart-healthy lifestyle across the life course should be emphasized. In young adults (20–39 years) an assessment of lifetime risk facilitates the NP–patient discussion about the importance of reducing ACVD risk through a healthy lifestyle e.g., physical activity, heart-healthy diet). Patient education resources include the CDC, www.cdc.gov/cholesterol/materials_for_patients.htm, and the American Heart Association, www.heart.org/en/health-topics/cholesterol/prevention-and-treatment-of-high-cholesterol-hyperlipidemia.

🏠 Quality and Safety Alerts and Ethical Concerns

Before prescribing statin therapy, baseline liver function tests (LFTs) should be ordered. Routine monitoring of LFTs is no longer recommended, but care should be taken to avoid prescribing statins along with any other hepatotoxic medications. Patients should be warned to reduce or avoid the intake of alcohol with statins for this reason. If patients are unable to tolerate or refuse statin therapy, other medication classes may be used (Table 20.4). Unfortunately, evidence does **not** support their effectiveness in reducing the actual risk of cardiovascular events.

The use of moderate-intensity statin therapy for primary prevention of cardiovascular disease after age 75 is a complicated issue. Older adults are more likely to develop adverse effects or suffer drug–drug reactions from statin therapy. Subsequently, the use of statins in this instance should be carefully considered keeping risks, benefits, individual needs, and patient treatment preferences firmly in mind. Ethically, treatment of dyslipidemia in some older adults may create avoidable adverse outcomes with little cardiovascular benefit.

🕐 CLINICAL PEARLS

- Evaluate for both primary and secondary causes of dyslipidemia.
- Begin therapy with aggressive lifestyle changes.
- Determine cardiovascular risk and target high-risk groups.

EVOLVING CASE STUDY

Stephen presents for his follow-up visit 1 month later. His serum laboratory values are within normal limits except his hemoglobin A1C is 6.2% and his LDL-C level is 102. His BP is now 148/80. He reports that he has been walking 3 days per week with his wife for 30 minutes. Stephen says he has been adhering to a low-sodium diet. His pedal edema has resolved, and his physical examination is again unremarkable except for his elevated BMI.

Case Study Question

4. What plan of care should be initiated now by the AGNP?

ISCHEMIC HEART DISEASE (CHRONIC CORONARY SYNDROME)

Etiology

Ischemic heart disease (IHD), also referred to as coronary heart disease (CHD), is a cardiac disorder in which cardiac muscle perfusion (inadequate blood supply to the myocardium) is reduced due to coronary artery atherosclerosis and/or the presence of microvascular dysfunction. This preventable chronic disease is the leading cause of death for both men and women in the United States. Patients can have chronic (stable) or acute (unstable) IHD. Chronic coronary syndrome (CCS) is also referred to as stable IHD.

Pathophysiology

Chronic systemic inflammation within the vasculature leads to stenosis of the coronary arteries by plaque and alteration of the normal process of vasodilation. With time, the condition worsens as stenosis of the coronary arteries increases. Symptoms such as angina, dyspnea on exertion, fatigue, and exercise intolerance develop. The development of angina symptoms may be sudden or insidious. Some patients remain asymptomatic even with significant stenosis in the major coronary arteries because collateral circulation keeps the myocardium perfused. Rupture of coronary plaque leads to an acute coronary event.

Other patients, commonly women, suffer from cardiac syndrome X (CSX). CSX is a disease process that includes chest pain that mimics angina and ST depressions during exercise stress testing, but when cardiac catheterization occurs to better evaluate the major coronary vessels, normal or near-normal (clean) coronary vessels are found. Symptoms in patients with CSX are caused by coronary microvascular dysfunction (MVD).[12] The myocardium is fed oxygen through a network of larger coronary vessels and by countless tiny arterioles and capillaries (these are the size of a human hair). For patients with MVD, the smaller arteries fail to dilate and/or overconstrict, which leads to ischemia and symptoms. Patients with MVD are also more likely to experience vasospasms and erosion of plaque. This eroded site can lead to thrombus formation and an acute coronary event. In women, plaque erosion is more common than plaque rupture. Once thought benign, newer research reveals the syndrome leads to negative cardiac outcomes and a poor prognosis. There are three basic types of angina: typical (classic) angina, atypical angina, and nonanginal pain. Each is described in the following. IHD can be stable or unstable. "Stable angina" is defined as no significant changes in duration, frequency, or severity of symptoms in the past 2 months. Unstable angina is characterized as a worsening of ischemic symptoms.

Risk Factors

Risk factors for IHD include male gender, advancing age, a family history of IHD, hypertension, hyperlipidemia, diabetes mellitus, metabolic syndrome, smoking, and a sedentary lifestyle. Menopause and stress also increase risk. The Framingham Global predictor model assists clinicians to identify a patient's 10-year risk of developing IHD based on age, gender, cholesterol readings, SBP reading, smoking history. and current treatment of hypertension. One online risk calculator is provided on this government website at http://cvdrisk.nhlbi.nih.gov.

Approach to Diagnosis

It is important to obtain a thorough history of the patient's symptoms and risk factors. Chest pain or angina is a common presenting symptom of IHD. Inquire about specific pain location, quality, duration, frequency, and any aggravating or relieving factors. Classic angina is often described as substernal, pressure-like with radiation to the jaw, upper back, or left arm. This type of angina is often triggered by stress or exertion and is relieved by rest or nitroglycerin. Some adults present with a complaint of dyspnea on exertion as the lone complaint. This symptom is considered an angina equivalent. Other patients present with atypical chest pain described as sharp or stabbing. Atypical angina may have precipitating or alleviating factors. Nonanginal chest pain, on the other hand, is different from typical angina in quality and appears to have no discernable pattern of precipitating or alleviating factors. Regardless of presentation, all complaints of angina or angina equivalent should be carefully investigated. Other possible symptoms of IHD include fatigue, nausea, and exercise intolerance.

Although there are no consistent physical signs of IHD, the physical examination should assess for possible systemic complications of atherosclerosis. Complete a thorough evaluation of peripheral pulses and listen for vascular bruits. Identify any signs of retinopathy. Listen carefully for the presence of S3 or S4 heart sounds or murmurs. Also closely assess for any signs or symptoms of congestive HF such as lower extremity edema.

Diagnostics

Patients with suspected IHD need to be carefully evaluated. Begin with basic serum testing and consider a chest radiograph. Serum testing should include a fasting lipid panel, diabetes screen, Hs-CRP, and homocysteine levels. Also obtain a vitamin D3 level. Elevated serum lipid and glucose levels contribute to atherosclerosis development. Hs-CRP, an acute-phase inflammatory marker, is an independent risk factor for cardiovascular events. An elevated homocysteine level also confers additional cardiovascular risk. Elevated Hs-CRP and homocysteine levels are not diagnostic but do suggest underlying, chronic inflammation. A chest radiograph may be useful to identify the presence of cardiomegaly or ischemic HF.

Obtain a resting 12-lead ECG. Carefully review the ECG for ischemic changes such as ST segment elevations or depressions, peaked or inverted T waves, or the presence of a new left bundle branch block. A very important note is more than half of patients with IHD will have a normal resting ECG. Consequently, a normal ECG does not rule out the presence of IHD. A patient with acute symptoms and ECG changes should be emergently referred for inpatient admission and evaluation with a cardiologist. Serum cardiac enzymes, including troponin levels, can then identify myocardial injury. An echocardiogram can identify wall motion abnormalities (which means the myocardium is not being perfused well and so it pumps ineffectively) and measure left ventricular function/ejection fraction. Normal ejection fraction is 50% or more. A reduced ejection fraction suggests poor cardiac perfusion.

An exercise treadmill test (stress test) is a valuable diagnostic tool for IHD. The exercise testing can be done with or without myocardial perfusion studies or an echocardiogram. If abnormal, the images may reveal hypokinesia or wall motion abnormalities of the heart muscle as described previously. Additionally, a stress test offers prognostic data about BP and heart rate response to exercise, exercise tolerance, and symptomatic response to exercise.

❂ CLINICAL PEARLS

- two primary indications for patients who may benefit from undergoing coronary angiography
- angina that significantly interferes with a person's lifestyle despite maximal medical therapy that the person was able to tolerate

Another diagnostic tool to consider is a contrast-enhanced computed tomography (CT calcium scoring test) of the coronary arteries, which estimates the overall extent of coronary atherosclerosis. This test can be considered if the patient is not able to complete stress testing or with a patient who had a previous inconclusive stress test. For patients with an abnormal stress test and/or ongoing symptoms of angina, referral to a cardiologist is indicated. Cardiac catheterization is the gold standard test for evaluating the coronary vessels. Measurement of left ventricular systolic function (generally with the use of transthoracic echocardiography) can be helpful in determining the best treatment.

Special Considerations for Assessment of Adolescents and Older Adults

The risk of developing IHD increases with age. Subsequently, adolescents are generally considered to have a much lower risk of IHD than an adult over 65 years of age. Adolescents presenting with a complaint of chest pain should be evaluated for other underlying causes such as pericarditis, hypertrophic cardiomyopathy, pulmonary embolism, costochondritis, or anxiety.

There is a growing population of older adults (65 and older) with IHD; however, identifying the disease can be challenging because of the high prevalence of atypical symptoms, such as exertional dyspnea or silent myocardial ischemia. Frail, older adults may be unable to achieve the maximum targeted heart rate during stress testing or may be incapable of ambulation on a treadmill because of arthritis or orthopedic problems. Subsequently, a pharmacologic stress test is often the better diagnostic choice for older patients. Older adults also are more likely to have aortic stenosis, which is a contraindication to exercise stress testing as it can cause syncope.

Screening Tools and Tests

The USPSTF screening tests for CHD should not be routinely offered to asymptomatic, low-risk adults and should only be offered on a case-by-case basis to symptomatic patients at increased risk when the practitioner judges that the benefits to the individual outweigh the potential harms.

Management

It is important to determine the disease severity to help guide treatment and establish a prognosis. Disease severity can be assessed by performing a stress test (most common method), cardiac imaging, and angiography. Before instituting treatments, it is essential to consider benefit versus risk as you engage in shared decision-making as to what the best treatment is for the individual.

Pharmacologic

Stable, chronic IHD is managed with antianginal medications, reducing and treating risk factors, lipid-lowering therapy, and antiplatelet therapy. Antianginal therapy may include beta-blockers, calcium channel blockers, nitrates, and/or ranolazine. Many patients require treatment with a combination of medications to control symptoms. First-line therapy to decrease episodes of angina and improve or maintain physical activity is beta-blocker monotherapy. Beta-blockers should not be used in patients with vasospastic or variant (Prinzmetal) angina. In those who can't tolerate beta-blockers, alternative therapies include calcium channel blockers or long-acting nitrates. Long-acting diltiazem or verapamil or second-generation dihydropyridine (amlodipine or felodipine) are the preferred medications. Hypertension, hyperlipidemia, and diabetes mellitus should be tightly controlled.

🏠 Quality and Safety Alerts

▪ Nifedipine should be avoided as monotherapy; if used, it should be in conjunction with a beta-blocker.

  • Use of nifedipine alone increases the risk of mortality post–MI.

  • In people with hypertension, there is an increased risk of MI.

Beta-blockers reduce all-cause morbidity and mortality in patients with IHD by reducing heart rate, BP, and myocardial oxygen demand. While all beta-blockers work as described, the ACC specifically recommends the use of metoprolol succinate, bisoprolol, or carvedilol for patients with a left ventricular function of 40% or more. Long-acting calcium channel blockers also reduce all-cause morbidity and mortality in patients with IHD and are recommended for use in those unable to tolerate beta-blockers. Short-acting calcium channel blockers may cause adverse cardiac events and should be avoided.

Short- or long-acting nitrates relieve symptoms by enhancing vasodilation. Ranolazine affects the sodium channels and reduces the cardiac workload. ACEI and angiotensin II receptor blockers also reduce cardiac death and may reduce microvascular angina symptoms. Aspirin 81 mg daily or clopidogrel 75 mg daily reduces platelet aggregation and decreases the risk of coronary thrombosis.

Nonpharmacologic

Primary and secondary prevention is the cornerstone of therapy for IHD. Patients should be counseled about heart-healthy lifestyle changes such as smoking cessation, engaging in aerobic exercise for at least 30 minutes 5 days per week, and maintaining ideal weight with a lower fat diet, especially avoiding trans fats. Most studies have found that antioxidant supplements, herbs, or vitamins do not reduce cardiovascular risk, but a recent study revealed that vitamin D3 replacement dramatically reduced angina symptoms in patients with CSX.[13] Another study determined that patients eating diets high in animal protein and fat were more likely to have myocardial perfusion abnormalities.[14] Consequently, patients should be counseled to eat a whole-food, minimally processed diet rich in fruits, vegetables, greens, whole grains, and small portions of lean meats or poultry. Vitamin D3 should be replaced if the level is low.

If patients have persistent angina, enhanced external counterpulsation and spinal cord stimulation can be employed. Both relieve angina symptoms. Restorative yoga may also reduce risk factors for IHD.[15]

Treatment Specific to Adolescents and Geriatric Patients

Adolescents are unlikely to have significant IHD because of age. Risk factor management is important though in this age group. NPs should educate adolescents on the inherent risks of smoking and encourage the selection of healthy lifestyle choices to prevent the development of IHD.

Older adults often dismiss angina symptoms as "just related to aging." Educate older adults about angina symptoms and encourage them to promptly report any worsening of symptoms. Unfortunately, older adults may be sensitive to antianginal and antiplatelet medications and often develop adverse effects from treatment. Hypotension from beta-blockers, calcium channel blockers, and nitrates can occur. Bradycardia can also develop from beta-blockers and calcium channel blockers, which can cause dizziness, fatigue, syncope, and lead to falls. Ranolazine is unlikely to cause hypotension or bradycardia. Subsequently, this medication is a great choice for this age group. Antiplatelet therapy can cause significant ecchymosis. Older adults are at risk of developing gastrointestinal bleeding with antiplatelet therapy as well. If aspirin therapy is indicated, order the enteric-coated type to reduce this risk. Closely monitor heart rate and BP at each visit. Adolescents and geriatric patients with persistent angina symptoms should be referred to cardiology for further evaluation.

⚙ CLINICAL PEARLS

- Ischemic disease is rarely found in patients under 40 years of age.
- Ischemic disease can present with typical or atypical symptoms.
- The 12-lead ECG is normal in 50% of patients who do have relevant ischemic disease, so understand that this tool is not diagnostic.
- Refer symptomatic patients to a cardiac specialist.

Patient Education

Individuals should be educated about healthy lifestyle changes, such as smoking cessation, eating a heart-healthy diet, and engaging in physical activity. Patients with chronic stable angina should be seen on a regular basis (every 6–12 months). They should be informed to share with the practitioner if they are experiencing a change in physical activity (e.g., worsening of symptoms); any change in the frequency, severity, or pattern of angina; their tolerance and ability to consistently participate in the plan of care established through shared decision-making; any modification of risk factors; and new or worsened comorbid illness (e.g., CKD, diabetes).

⌂ Quality and Safety Alerts

- Avoid exercise stress tests in frail older adults or in the presence of severe aortic stenosis.
- Avoid prescribing short-acting calcium channel blockers to patients with ischemic disease.
- For postmenopausal women, hormone replacement therapy is not recommended. Several large trials have demonstrated that hormone replacement therapy increases cardiovascular risk and therefore should be avoided.
- Older adults are more likely to develop adverse effects from ischemic heart disease medical therapy. Monitor them carefully.

HEART FAILURE

Etiology

Advances in medical care for HF have led to a higher prevalence of people living with HF. Despite this, the mortality and hospitalizations of adults with HF remain high. The AHA reports that between 2013 and 2016, there about 6.2 million people in the United States with HF; worldwide there are about 23 million people worldwide with HF. The incidence and prevalence of HF in the United States over the next four decades is increasing, with an estimated increase of over 700,000 new cases by 2040[16] and 8 million by 2030.[17] Once diagnosed with HF, the mortality risk is highest at 5 years (about 50%) and substantially improves over time (about 10% after 10 years). Left ventricular dysfunction is linked to an increased risk of sudden death.[18] Acute exacerbations of HF are the leading cause of hospital admission for patients over the age of 65 years of age, which costs the United States approximately $32 billion annually. Consequently, identification and appropriate treatment of HF are imperative.

Pathophysiology

HF is a complex maladaptive, neurohormonal syndrome, which leads to impaired myocardial pumping ability. "Cardiomyopathy" is a general term that denotes a weakened myocardial muscle. Although ischemic cardiomyopathy is the most common presentation (60%–75% of all cases), the causes of HF/cardiomyopathy are numerous.

Two basic types of HF have been identified: systolic HF with impaired left ventricular function (ejection fraction below 50%) and HF with preserved left ventricular function (ejection fraction above 50%, previously called diastolic HF). In systolic HF, the left ventricle fails to pump effectively. In diastolic HF, the heart fails to relax properly, and consequently, filling is impaired. HF can be acute, chronic, or both. There are two common classifications of HF: the ACC guidelines and the New York Heart Association Functional classification (Table 20.5). The ACC's guidelines guide this section.

While the causes of myocardial dysfunction are numerous, the body's adaptive response is the same. First, the myocardium is injured or strained. The heart then compensates by remodeling the left ventricle, which means the chamber undergoes hypertrophy and reduction of its pumping ability. Over time, the body's neurohormonal response, which includes the activation of the sympathetic nervous system and the renin-angiotensin system, becomes chronic and maladaptive. Ultimately, this progresses to systolic and/or diastolic dysfunction. Cardiac output falls and filling pressures rise. Frequency, duration, and severity of HF symptoms worsen.

Risk Factors

The most common risk factors for HF include arrhythmia, hypertension, diabetes, and coronary heart disease. Patients with hypertension have a higher risk of developing HF with a preserved ejection fraction compared to those who develop HF with reduced ejection fraction.[19] Other risk factors include older age, male gender, current smoking, abnormal lipid levels, obesity, and physical inactivity.

Approach to Diagnosis

The etiology of HF must be identified for each individual. Consider the type of HF (see Table 20.6 for those with reduced LVEF). A thorough patient history is key to identifying a correctable underlying cause. Inquire about family history of coronary artery disease, congenital

Table 20.5: New York Heart Association Functional Classification

Class	Presentation/Timing of Symptoms (Fatigue, Palpitations, Dyspnea, or Angina)
I	Asymptomatic except during severe exertion
II	No symptoms at rest; symptoms begin with moderate exertion.
III	No symptoms at rest; symptoms begin with minimal exertion.
IV	Symptomatic at rest

Table 20.6: Presentation of Heart Failure With Reduced Ejection Fraction

If LVEF is less than 50 consider which findings are present:

Low-specificity/high-sensitivity findings
- Dyspnea on exertion, fatigue, weight gain, peripheral edema, age older than 60 years

Intermediate-specificity/intermediate-sensitivity findings
- Rales (crackles)
- Chest radiograph findings consistent with cardiomegaly or pleural effusion
- ECG atrial fibrillation, left atrial enlargement, LV hypertrophy, or pathologic Q waves
- Serum natriuretic peptide

    Age younger than 50: N-terminal pro B-type natriuretic peptide (NT-proBNP) 125–450 pg/mL or BNP 35–100 pg/mL

    Age 50 to 75: NT-proBNP 450–900 pg/mL or BNP 35–100 pg/mL

    Age older than 75: NT-proBNP 900–1,800 pg/mL or BNP 35–100 pg/mL

- Clinical features of CAD or moderate valvular regurgitation or stenosis
- Echocardiogram: left atrial volume index over 34 mL/m², E/A equal or greater than 0.9 and less than 2.1 or E/A equal or greater than 0.8 and E greater than 50 ncm/s

High-specificity/low-sensitivity findings
- Orthopnea, paroxysmal nocturnal dyspnea
- JVD distention, S3, pulsus alternans, or laterally displaced PMI
- Chest radiograph findings consistent with pulmonary edema
- Serum natriuretic peptide

    Age younger than 50: NT-proBNP greater than 450 pg/m: pr BNP greater than100 pg/mL

    Age 50 to 75: NT-proBNP greater than 900 pg/mL or BNO greater than 100 pg/mL

    Age older than 75: NT-proBNP greater than 1,800 pg/mL or BNP 100 pg/mL

- Clinical features of severe valvular regurgitation or stenosis
- Echocardiogram findings LVEF greater than 30%, LV end-diastolic dimension greater than 5.8 cm in men and 5.2 in women, E/e 15 or greater, E/A 2.1 or greater or inferior vena cava greater than 2.1 cm with collapse during sniff less than 50

BNP, B-type natriuretic peptide; CAD, coronary artery disease; JVD, jugular venous distention; LV, left ventricle; LVEF, left ventricular ejection fraction; PMI, point of maximal impulse.

Source: Adapted from Colucci WS. Overview of the management of heart failure with reduced ejection fraction in adults. In: Gottlieb SS, ed. *UptoDate.* UpToDate; 2021. https://www.uptodate.com/contents/overview-of-the-management-of-heart-failure-with-reduced-ejection-fraction-in-adults

cardiomyopathies, or sudden cardiac death. Identify potential risk factors for HF, such as hypertension, exposure to cardiotoxic substances (chemotherapy, heavy alcohol use, stimulant drugs, heavy metals), valvular heart disease, endocrine disorders, severe anemia, connective tissue disorders, infectious diseases, severe emotional stress, recent viral illnesses, muscular dystrophies, electrolyte disturbances, and/or recent pregnancy.

Carefully review frequency, duration, and severity of presenting symptoms. The most common symptom of HF is dyspnea, which is often worse with exertion. Other common symptoms include orthopnea, nocturnal cough, fatigue, progressive exercise intolerance, anorexia, weight gain, syncope or near syncope, palpitations, wheezing, and pedal edema. With time, patients begin to complain of insomnia and appear depressed. This is related to poor sleep quality because of nighttime symptoms. Poor cardiac output eventually leads to symptoms of peripheral hypoperfusion.

Physical examination in suspected HF should be comprehensive. Begin with general appearance. Many patients with significant HF may be well compensated and hence appear asymptomatic. Those with chronic HF often appear pale, tired, weak, and cachectic. Vital signs may reveal tachycardia with a narrow pulse pressure, pulsus alternans, and hypotension. SBP below 90 mmHg is linked to a poorer prognosis.

Jugular venous distention may be present. Auscultation of the lungs may reveal rales and/or wheezing. This suggests fluid accumulation in the interstitial lung tissue. Listen to heart sounds carefully. Auscultation of an S3 gallop heart sound strongly suggests HF. Mitral and tricuspid regurgitant murmurs or diastolic filling sounds are also common. Ascites and hepatomegaly are possible findings. Pedal edema, cool extremities, mottled skin, and poor capillary refill may be present.

When considering BNP and NT-proBNP in patients with dyspnea, a high level does not exclude other diagnoses, such as pneumonia. Consider other possible diagnoses, such as MI and pulmonary disease, such as exacerbation of COPD. Symptoms of fatigue can be due to other issues such as deconditioning, sleep apnea, and depression. In those presenting with fluid retention and complaints of leg or abdominal swelling, consider other diagnoses, such as venous thrombosis or insufficiency, kidney disease with sodium retention, drug side effects, and cirrhosis.

Diagnostics

Begin evaluation with serum testing. A comprehensive metabolic panel, complete blood count, thyroid screen, and lipid panel should be obtained. A B-type natriuretic peptide (BNP) and an N-terminal pro-B type natriuretic peptide (NT-proBNP) are natriuretic peptides that are released when the heart ventricles are dilated or under stress. Subsequently, BNP and NT-proBNP are elevated in patients with symptomatic HF.

A resting 12-lead ECG should be obtained. Examine the ECG carefully for ischemic changes. The existence of Q waves identifies previous MI, which may have damaged the myocardium, resulting in HF. Look for indications of left ventricular hypertrophy. Conduction delays such as a marked first-degree atrioventricular block are common. Atrial and ventricular arrhythmias are also quite common. If the 12-lead ECG contains ectopic beats, conduction delays, an abnormal underlying rhythm, and/or the patient complains of palpitations, a 24-hour Holter monitor should be ordered.

A chest radiograph is a helpful screening tool to identify cardiomegaly. The left ventricle is best visualized by the lateral or oblique views. The films will also help identify the presence of pleural effusions or pulmonary edema.

An echocardiogram is a very useful, cost-effective, noninvasive test to evaluate HF. The left ventricular ejection fraction can be assessed. Valvular dysfunction and wall motion abnormalities can be identified. Once HF has been identified, patients should be referred to cardiology for further testing. These tests may include exercise stress testing, cardiac magnetic resonance imaging, coronary angiography, right-sided heart catheterization, sleep studies, and myocardial biopsy.

Specific Assessment for Adolescents and Older Adults

As mentioned previously, most HF has an ischemic cause. Adolescents are unlikely to develop ischemic cardiomyopathy due to their young age. Adolescents though are susceptible to developing significant HF from genetic or acquired cardiomyopathy (such as hypertrophic cardiomyopathy), abuse of stimulants such as cocaine or amphetamines, peripartum cardiomyopathy, severe anemia, congenital valvular dysfunction, chronic arrhythmia, or as a result of inflammation or viral infection. Ask about possible illicit drug use, family history of cardiac disorders, and recent illness or pregnancy. Presenting symptoms often include exercise intolerance and unusual fatigue. Always question about the presence of palpitations or syncope, which may reveal underlying arrhythmias resulting from HF.[20]

Older adults most commonly have ischemic cardiomyopathy but should be screened for all possible causes. Carefully review the 12-lead ECG carefully for any signs of ischemia. Patients should undergo a full ischemic evaluation with a cardiologist to determine if revascularization is required. Once coronary obstructions are treated, the myocardium can recover, and left ventricular function may improve. Older patients with HF are at increased risk of developing conduction delays as well as atrial and ventricular arrhythmias. Inquire about syncopal episodes or palpitations. If present, evaluate with a 24-hour Holter monitor.

Screening Tools

HF clinical tools are available at the American Heart Association website. Get With The Guidelines®-Heart Failure is an in-hospital program for improving care by promoting consistent adherence to the latest scientific treatment guidelines and is available at www.heart.org/en/professional/quality-improvement/get-with-the-guidelines/get-with-the-guidelines-heart-failure.

The USPSTF does not recommend screening with resting exercise ECG for those at low risk, and there is not enough evidence to make screening recommendations for those at intermediate or high risk of CVD events. Screening decisions should be based on benefit versus risks; using the person's 10-year risk of CVD risk (see the earlier discussion) can help guide clinical decision-making.

Management

Management should be based on underlying cause and associated causes (see Table 20.7). The goals of care are to prevent hospitalizations, improve quality of life, and promote health and well-being. Care coordination (see Chapter 5) is an essential component of meeting these goals. Providing care that results in optimal health outcomes is complex with multiple components, which include patient self-management, appropriate and timely referral, and systems of care, with primary care providers comanaging patients with cardiology experts and other specialists as appropriate (e.g., a nephrologist for those with CKD and HF). It is very important for care coordination once a person is discharged from the hospital. Palliative care is important for patients with advanced HF to support shared decision-making about goals of care (see Chapter 8 for more information about palliative care).

Pharmacologic

Treatment for acute, inpatient HF is beyond the scope of this chapter. Patients who present with severe, symptomatic HF should be emergently referred to cardiology or the closest ED for treatment. All patients with identified or suspected HF should be referred to cardiology as soon

Table 20.7: Causes of Heart Failure

Hypertension
Ischemic heart disease
Valvular dysfunction
Aging
Volume overload
Amyloidosis
Cardiomyopathies—caused by infections or inflammation, toxin exposure (alcohol, cocaine, radiation), diabetes mellitus, idiopathic, familial, stress-induced
Connective tissue disorders

as possible. Treatment should be initiated by primary care NPs immediately while the patient awaits evaluation with the cardiologist.

Patients with Stage A HF are at risk of developing left ventricular dysfunction. Treatment for these patients is focused on managing all risk factors that can lead to HF. BP, hyperlipidemia, diabetes mellitus, obesity, metabolic syndrome, and ischemic heart disease should be aggressively managed medically and with healthy lifestyle choices.

The goal of medical therapy for chronic HF is to prolong life, lessen symptoms, and increase the quality of life and functional status of the patient. The cornerstone of therapy (Stages B–D; see Table 20.8) is the combination of an ACEI or an ARB with a beta-blocker. ACEIs can reduce remodeling and improve the ejection fraction. Start with the lowest dose and titrate to the targeted range slowly. ACEIs, even below the targeted dose range, improve left ventricular function. Carefully monitor patients for adverse effects such as hyperkalemia, renal insufficiency, hypotension, chronic dry cough, and angioedema. Patients' intolerance of ACEI inhibitors can be treated with an ARB instead. ARBs carry similar risks of ACEIs but have less incidence of angioedema and no cough. ARBs are generally more expensive than ACEIs. Sacubitril/valsartan, a combination drug that includes an ARB, has recently been approved by the Food and Drug Administration for treatment of chronic HF for both reduced and preserved EF as it reduces the risk of hospitalization and cardiovascular death.[21]

After an ACEI has been initiated and a patient is euvolemic, a beta-blocker should be initiated as well. Generally, beta-blockers are also started at a low dose and carefully titrated over several weeks to the targeted

Table 20.8: AHA/ACC Heart Failure Stages

Stage	Definition
A	Patients at risk for developing HF but who do not yet have structural heart disease or symptoms of HF
B	Patients with structural HF but who do not currently have symptoms of HF
C	Patients with structural heart disease who have prior or current symptoms of HF
D	Patients with refractory HF who require specialized interventions

ACC, American College of Cardiology; AHA, American Heart Association; HF, heart failure.

Source: Hunt et al. ACC/AHA Guidelines for the Evaluation of Chronic Heart Failure in the Adult. Circulation. 2001;104(24):2996-3007

dose. This type of medication reduces heart rate and subsequently can improve cardiac output in HF patients. There are only three beta-blockers approved for HF treatment: metoprolol succinate, bisoprolol, and carvedilol. Beta-blockers can cause symptomatic bradycardia, conduction delays, and hypotension. Heart rate and BP must be carefully monitored.

Other secondary and tertiary medications may also be added if first-line therapy fails to control symptoms. These include aldosterone receptor antagonists such as spironolactone, diuretics, combination therapy with hydralazine and isosorbide dinitrate (BiDil), and digoxin. Aldosterone inhibitors are indicated in symptomatic HF patients with a left ventricular ejection fraction of 35% or less who are already appropriately treated with an ACEI and a beta-blocker. Aldosterone is contraindicated in patients with renal insufficiency and/or hyperkalemia. Potassium and creatinine levels should be carefully monitored after starting therapy. Diuretics are used to treat volume overload but can unfortunately cause hypotension and renal insufficiency. Although diuretics do not affect morbidity or mortality in HF, they greatly reduce symptoms, which results in a better quality of life. Loop diuretics are most effective and hence are preferred. Daily weights, creatinine levels, and symptoms should guide diuretic prescribing. Digoxin can also be used to treat HF symptoms and is especially helpful for patients who also have underlying atrial fibrillation to reduce heart rate. Monitor renal status and digoxin levels closely though as digoxin is excreted largely unchanged by the kidneys. If renal status is impaired, digoxin levels can rise. BiDil provides significant benefit to African American patients with HF who remain symptomatic despite first-line treatment. It reduces preload and consequently reduces morbidity and mortality. Calcium channel blockers should be avoided in patients with systolic dysfunction as they reduce inotropy and stroke volume. Amlodipine, a long-acting dihydropyridine, is an exception and can be utilized to treat coexisting hypertension in patients with HF.

Nonpharmacologic

Patients with HF have high rates of morbidity and mortality. These patients should receive detailed education about their disease process to improve their quality of life and reduce hospitalization. Adherence to a low sodium diet (<2,000 mg daily) should be strongly encouraged. Patients should be taught to look for "hidden" sources of sodium by reading food labels carefully. Daily morning weights should be recorded. Patients should be instructed to report a weight gain of 3 lb or more in 24 hours. Diuretics can then be adjusted.

Cardiac rehabilitation and/or exercise training should be ordered. Supervised exercise is best if available as patient vital signs and heart rhythm can be closely monitored. Regular exercise improves functional capacity and overall quality of life for patients with HF.

As symptoms worsen and the left ventricular function becomes severe, HF patients should be referred to an electrophysiologist and a HF program for evaluation. These patients often benefit from device therapy called cardiac resynchronization which improves hemodynamics and lessens HF symptoms. Additionally, patients with severely reduced EF are at increased risk of sudden cardiac death due to ventricular arrhythmias. An implanted cardioverter-defibrillator greatly reduces this risk. Cardiac transplantation or insertion of a left ventricular assist device may need to be considered.

Treatment Specific to Adolescents and Older Adults With Heart Failure

Adolescents with HF have unique needs. These patients usually have non-ischemic HF, and the correct diagnosis can be overlooked or delayed as it is a less common diagnosis in this age group. Once made, the diagnosis is often frightening and overwhelming to adolescents who will require emotional support and extensive education about managing symptoms. Often, adolescents are resistant to adhering to a low sodium diet. This must be addressed in teaching. Adolescents may benefit from involvement with a HF peer support group. Include parents in teaching if appropriate.

First-line HF therapy includes treatment with an ACE inhibitor or an ARB. These medications can cause significant fetal anomalies, especially after the first trimester, and are usually contraindicated in young females for this reason. Adolescents with HF though require this medication to reverse remodeling and reduce symptoms. If the adolescent is sexually active, an effective, nonhormonal type of birth control should be used. Pregnancy is contraindicated in the presence of severe HF as this can lead to maternal death. Adolescents must be educated in detail about the risks of pregnancy in the setting of HF. Learning that you have a life-threatening illness that will prevent future pregnancies can be overwhelming for adolescents and emotional support should be offered.

Older adults with HF are often complicated and complex patients to manage. Due to age, these patients are more likely to experience adverse effects from treatment such as hypotension, bradycardia, atrioventricular block, or syncope. As such, initiate one medication at a time and start with the lowest dose and titrate slowly. Understand that many older patients will be unable to tolerate the targeted dose of ACEI or beta-blocker. A smaller dose is better than none at all. Diuretics should be used cautiously with older adults as they are more susceptible to fluid shifts and dehydration. Hypotension can often be avoided by spacing the administration time of multiple medications that may lower BP.[22] For example, give the diuretics in the morning, the ACEI in the afternoon, and the beta-blocker at bedtime.

Older adults with HF are more likely than their younger counterparts to have underlying valvular heart disease and atrial fibrillation. Identified valvular dysfunction should be closely monitored by serial echocardiograms. Significant valvular dysfunction should be referred to cardiology for workup. Complaints of palpitations, syncope, near syncope, or dizziness should be investigated with a 24-hour Holter monitor or a 10- to 30-day event monitor. If atrial fibrillation is present, the patient should be anticoagulated based on the CHASD2 score.

Some older adults may have difficulty with memory or have mild cognitive impairment, so it is essential to make sure they are able to follow through with a mutually established plan of care. Written instructions on the diet and medication regimen are very helpful. Highlight adherence with a low sodium diet and educate the patient and family about common sources of sodium concealed in processed foods. Educate the patient to keep daily logs of morning weight, heart rate, and BP. Provide the patient with specific, written instructions on when to report worsening symptoms, alterations in vital signs, or sudden changes in weight. This diagnosis is frightening to patients of all ages. Offering emotional support along with patient teaching reduces fear and increases adherence to the plan of care.

Patient Education

Taking a person/family-centered approach to care includes assuring the individual with HF has the knowledge and ability to manage HF, prevent hospitalization, and reduce the risk of comorbid conditions. The AHA has HF tools and resources that can be used for patient education and self-monitoring at home. These are available at www.heart.org/en/health-topics/heart-failure/heart-failure-tools-resources.

🏠 Quality and Safety Alerts

- Beta-blockers may worsen reactive airway disease and should be used cautiously in this patient demographic.
- Calcium channel blockers should be avoided in patients with systolic dysfunction.
- Discuss with your patients the risks associated with pregnancy in the presence of severe HF. This can, at worst, lead to maternal death. Discuss birth control with female patients of reproductive age.
- Older adults are more likely to experience adverse side effects from HF medical therapy. Start with the lowest dose of medication and titrate slowly. Monitor these patients closely.

💡 CLINICAL PEARLS

- The most common symptom of HF is dyspnea.
- The goal of medical therapy for chronic heart failure is to prolong life, lessen symptoms, and increase the quality of life and functional status of the patient.
- The cornerstone of medical therapy (Stages B-D) is the combination of an ACEI or an ARB with a beta-blocker.

📡 EMERGENCIES

Patients are at risk for acute decompensated heart failure that can result in a potentially fatal cause of acute respiratory distress. These patients need to be rapidly assessed and stabilized. In a primary care office, you may not have all the emergency equipment needed, so calling 911 is important; however, while waiting for their arrival, conduct an airway assessment and use a pulse oximetry to make sure the person has adequate oxygenation and ventilation. Use supplemental oxygen, and obtain vital signs and, if possible, an ECG. Have the patient in a seated position to facilitate respirations with less distress than if in a supine position.

EVOLVING CASE STUDY

Stephen presents to the office 3 months later. His LFTs are normal, his LDL-C has improved to 76, and his hemoglobin A1C is 5.9%. He reports he has been walking 4 to 5 days a week for 30 minutes but states that he noticed he develops mild shortness of breath when he exercises. Stephen denies having any myalgia or other side effects from the statin.

Case Study Questions

5. What important clinical questions should the AGNP ask Stephen?

6. What testing should be considered at this time?

Stephen reports that he occasionally feels "tightness" in his chest when he is active. He denies any symptoms at rest. The 12-lead ECG reveals sinus rhythm at a rate of 76 beats per minute. When compared to his previous ECG, the AGNP notes inverted T waves in his anterior leads. His BP is 140/80. Physical examination remains unremarkable.

(cont.)

Case Study Question

7. What would now be an appropriate management plan?

Two weeks later, Stephen presents to the office for his follow-up visit. His serum hs-CRP and homocysteine levels are mildly elevated. His vitamin D level is within normal limits. His exercise stress test is positive for ischemia. When questioned, Stephen reports that he continues to have dyspnea with exertion.

Case Study Question

8. What should the AGNP plan now?

Stephen is evaluated by a cardiologist, who orders a cardiac catheterization. An interventional cardiologist completes the cardiac catheterization, and Stephen is found to have nonobstructive coronary artery disease. He also has a mildly reduced systolic ejection fraction of 45%. Stephen is started on metoprolol succinate 25 mg daily. The cardiac team encouraged continued lifestyle changes and risk factor reduction to slow the progression of the disease. He is cleared to begin exercising again.

Case Study Question

9. What should the AGNP monitor with Stephen?

Stephen's serum lipid panel, CMP, CBC, and Hemoglobin A1C should be routinely monitored. The AGNP should continue to encourage healthy lifestyle choices. Stephen should be monitored for any side effects from his statin, antihypertensives, and antiplatelet therapies. A written plan of care should be provided to Stephen to ensure he understands all components of his care.

PERIPHERAL ARTERY DISEASE

Etiology

PAD is primarily caused by systemic atherosclerosis which causes stenosis of peripheral arteries. This narrowing generally begins to cause symptoms once 75% of the arterial diameter has been affected. Many patients with PAD remain asymptomatic because of the presence of collateral circulation. PAD can also be caused by arterial thrombus formation, vasospasm, collagen vascular disease, or arterial trauma. PAD occurs in 15% of people older than 55 years of age but the disease affects less than 1% of patients younger than 50 years of age. In those younger than 25 years of age, the incidence is very rare.

Pathophysiology

Atherosclerosis is a systemic disease that can affect arteries in the lower extremities. Ischemic symptoms occur when there is an imbalance between the demand for blood and the lack of supply due to atherosclerosis. There is subintimal accumulation of lipid and fibrous material that forms a plaque. This plaque can be thrombosed or rupture, causing occlusion downstream; symptoms depend on the location and severity. Middle-aged adults often experience subclinical atherosclerosis, but others have symptoms of intermittent claudication (reproduceable pain with ambulation relieved with rest). Individuals with diabetes have a risk for chronic limb-threatening ischemia (PAD along with rest pain, gangrene, or a lower limb ulceration of 2 weeks or greater). This type of ulceration can lead to tissue death and eventually require amputation. PAD can gravely affect functional capacity and quality of life.

Risk Factors

Common risk factors for the development of PAD include smoking, inactivity, obesity, diabetes, hypertension, high cholesterol, and diabetes.

Approach to Diagnosis

Begin with obtaining a thorough history. Inquire about the presence of risk factors. Ask about any previous cardiac or neurologic events, such as CAD, transient ischemic attacks, or stroke as this will alert the NP to the presence of atherosclerosis. Question the patient about the occurrence of intermittent claudication. Generally, this type of pain occurs with ambulation and is relieved with rest. In addition to pain, these patients complain of limb numbness, heaviness, and/or limb fatigue with activity. As PAD progresses, limb pain will worsen. Severe stenosis can lead to pain even at rest. Pain may also be increased at night when the patient lies flat due to decreased cardiac output and can be reduced when the limb is held dependent.[23]

Onset of pain is important for diagnosis. PAD caused by gradual stenosis of the artery from atherosclerosis is chronic and progressive in nature. On the other hand, sudden, acute ischemic pain is a medical emergency that can lead to loss of the limb. This type of pain is characterized by the "six Ps": limb pulselessness, pallor, pain, poikilothermia, paresthesias, and paralysis. The pain results from arterial occlusion caused by an arterial embolus or thrombus.

PAD leads to loss of limb hair; the presence of shiny, dry, thin skin; muscle atrophy; and trophic nail changes. Color changes are common. Extremities have significant rubor (dusky red color) or are pale. Pulses are diminished or absent. Limbs feel cool to the touch. Poor limb perfusion leads to the development of painful ulcerations which are slow to heal.

If PAD is suspected, an ABI should be ordered. This ratio is determined by dividing the systolic pressure at the ankle by the systolic pressure at the arm, which are recorded using a Doppler instrument. A normal ABI is between 1.0 and 1.4 but values between 0.9 and 1.0 are acceptable. An ABI below 0.9 is diagnostic of PAD.

Values 0.5 or less suggest severe PAD. Diabetic patients may have inaccurate ABI readings. NPs working in primary care should refer patients with abnormal ABIs to a vascular specialist for further evaluation. Angiography is considered the "gold standard" evaluation. Magnetic resonance angiography is also an accurate option for testing those with suspected PAD in the presence of renal insufficiency.

Differential diagnoses for symptoms of extremity pain or tissue loss similar to PAD include arterial thrombosis due to an aneurysm, arterial injury, arterial dissection, or thromboembolism. People with popliteal entrapment syndrome can present with intermittent claudication (IC) and should be suspected in younger patients who present with symptoms of IC but do not have risks for atherosclerotic disease. Anomalous musculoskeletal attachments or an abnormal course of the popliteal artery can cause compression of the popliteal artery with activity. Thromboangiitis obliterans (Buerger's disease) is a nonatherosclerotic disease in which there is segmental inflammatory disease that often affects the small to medium-sized arteries. Usually, patients are younger and are heavy smokers. The first presentation is usually digit ischemia, although larger vessels can be involved. Ischemic ulcers should be evaluated to determine if they are related to PAD or venous insufficiency. Neuropathic pain can cause lower limb pain as can musculoskeletal pain from osteoarthritis. Calf pain and tightness can be seen in athletes.

Specific Assessment of Adolescents and Older Adults With PAD

While PAD is quite rare in adolescents, it is possible for premature PAD to develop. Carefully review the existence of risk factors. Evaluate for the presence of hypercoagulable states, vasculitis, limb trauma, or the use of ergot migraine treatments. Patients with elevated homocysteine and C-reactive protein levels are at risk for premature PAD.

Older adults are at increased risk for developing PAD as atherosclerosis progresses with age. Twenty percent of people older than age 70 have PAD. PAD is more prevalent in those with diabetes or a history of smoking. The evaluation and treatment for PAD are the same for all age groups.

Screening Tools and Tests

Screening should be considered in those with risk factors and are asymptomatic to identify early in the presence of PAD with the goal of preventing progression and complications of PAD. Symptomatic patients should be screened as well. Patients with CAD/CVD are at increased risk of PAD so ensure they are screened appropriately with an ankle-brachial index (ABI).

Management

Most patients with PAD can be managed medically. Therapy should begin with aggressive risk factor modification in an effort to slow the progression of the disease and to reduce the incidence of death from cardiovascular events. Consultation with a vascular medicine physician should be considered for comanagement of the patient. Medical therapy includes initiating a statin, starting antiplatelet therapy, and beginning exercise rehabilitation to reduce claudication symptoms.

Pharmacologic

Initiating therapy with a statin, optimal BP, and glycemic control reduces the risks of PAD and PAD progression. Drug therapy with low-dose aspirin or clopidogrel is recommended to reduce the risk of cardiovascular events but do not directly treat the PAD. Cilostazol, a type III phosphodiesterase inhibitor, can be given to reduce symptoms of claudication. The medication has both antiplatelet and vasodilator properties.

For patients with severe disease, nonhealing wounds, or worsening symptoms despite medical therapy, the NP should refer the patient to a vascular specialist for evaluation. These patients may benefit from either surgical or endovascular revascularization with bypass grafts, angioplasty, or stents. A small percentage of patients may ultimately require amputation. Criteria to help with clinical decision-making regarding interventions is in Table 20.9.

Nonpharmacologic

Risk factor reduction includes initiating an aggressive smoking cessation program, encouraging weight loss in obese patients, and instituting tight glycemic control among diabetic patients. Patients with PAD are at increased risk of death from MI or stroke. Exercise rehabilitation that includes treadmill exercise reduces the severity of PAD symptoms and can greatly increase the walking distance before claudication symptoms occur. Patients should be encouraged to engage in aerobic exercise for at least 30 minutes 3 to 5 days each week. If

Table 20.9: Criteria for Interventions (Surgical or Percutaneous)

- The person is significantly disabled and can't engage in activities that are important to them (e.g., work, other activities); impacts quality of life.
- The patient has not had the desired response to pharmacologic and nonpharmacologic treatment.
- The characteristics of the lesion indicate that interventions are low risk and likely to lead to long-term success.
- Must take into account the history and prognosis.

they are not able to do this, encourage them to walk short distances, rest, and then repeat. Over time, they can build up to longer ambulation time.

Patient Education

Patients should be educated about what PAD is and the risk factors associated with PAD. Explaining testing procedures and treatments for PAD is also important to support shared decision-making regarding the best treatment options for the patient. The American Heart Association offers teaching aids for patients and families that are available at www.heart.org/en/health-topics/peripheral-artery-disease.

🏠 Quality and Safety Alerts

- Cilostazol should not be prescribed to patients with left ventricular dysfunction if the systolic ejection fraction is less than 40%.
- Any patient with suspected acute occlusion of a limb artery must be emergently referred to avoid loss of the limb.

💡 CLINICAL PEARLS

- The key risk factors for the development of PAD are smoking and diabetes mellitus.
- Atherosclerosis develops throughout the vascular system. If a patient is diagnosed with PAD, the NP should always evaluate the patient for the presence of ischemic heart disease as well.

CHRONIC VENOUS INSUFFICIENCY AND DEEP VEIN THROMBOSIS

Etiology

About 50% of individuals have chronic vein abnormalities; however, the rates of chronic venous insufficiency vary depending on the population studied.

Pathophysiology

Chronic venous insufficiency is essentially poor venous blood return to the heart caused by valvular incompetence, venous obstruction, varicose veins, or decreased muscular contraction around the veins (due to immobility). DVT is the development of a clot within the deep venous system. The clot usually develops from a combination of endothelial injury, venous stasis, and a hypercoagulable state commonly referred to as Virchow's triad. Once developed, the clot obstructs venous return,

which leads to venous dilation and vessel and valve damage. The clot can also embolize to the lung, causing respiratory complications and possibly death (pulmonary embolism). Symptoms include extremity pain, tenderness, and swelling. DVTs can develop on the lower and upper extremities or in the pelvis but proximal clots from the lower extremities are more likely to lead to pulmonary embolism (PE; see Chapter 19 for more information about PE).

Risk Factors

Risk factors for developing chronic venous insufficiency include age, family history, ligamentous laxity (e.g., hernia, flat feet), prolonged standing, increased BMI, smoking, lower extremity trauma, high estrogen states, pregnancy, and hereditary conditions (e.g., Klippel-Trenaunay syndrome). Risk factors for DVT are presented in Table 20.10.

Table 20.10: Risk Factors for Deep Vein Thrombosis

Stasis	Immobility related to recent travel, anesthesia, spinal cord injury, cerebrovascular accident, severe COPD, paralysis, CHF
	Older than 40 years of age
	Obesity
	Hyperviscosity
	Polycythemia
	Varicose veins
	Frailty
Hypercoagulability	Malignancy
	Increased estrogen levels
	Sepsis
	Pregnancy
	Smoking
	Nephrotic syndrome
	Chronic kidney disease
	Inflammatory bowel disease
	Inherited coagulation disorders
Endothelial injury	Surgery
	Trauma
	Intravenous catheters

CHF, congestive heart failure; COPD, chronic obstructive pulmonary disease.

Approach to Diagnosis

The diagnosis of chronic venous insufficiency is the presence of symptoms and other diagnostic testing as appropriate. Symptoms include lower extremity edema; the sensations of heaviness, fatigue, and pain in the lower extremities; dusky skin discolorations; and the development of venous stasis ulcers. Pruritus is also a common complaint. Patients can also present with telangiectasis (widened venules that cause threadlike red lines or patterns on the skin) and varicose veins. Symptoms are generally worse when the legs are dependent and lessened or relieved with elevation. Differential diagnoses can be any disease process that can cause lower extremity pain, edema, skin changes, or nonhealing wounds.

Usually, the symptoms of a DVT are unilateral but can be bilateral and in some situations the patient is asymptomatic. It is important to perform a physical examination of the legs, abdomen, and pelvis. The physical examination may reveal dilated superficial veins, unilateral edema or swelling, unilateral warmth, tenderness, erythema, pain, and tenderness along the course of the involved vein, and local or general signs of malignancy. Presentation of swelling or edema has 97% sensitivity and 33% specificity, pain 86% sensitivity and 19% specificity, and warmth 72% sensitivity and 48% specificity of the lower extremity.

Specific Assessment of Chronic Venous Insufficiency and Deep Vein Thrombosis in Adolescents and Older Adults

Assessment of these conditions is the same across all age groups. Adolescents can be at increased risk of developing a DVT if they are taking birth control pills that contain estrogen or if they sustain injury to a lower extremity. Many older adults are at greater risk of developing DVTs than younger adults due to advancing age, increased incidence of risk factors, reduced mobility, and fall-related injuries.

Diagnostics

The NP can diagnose chronic venous insufficiency by history and physical examination alone. If DVT is suspected, the probability should be assessed using a tool such as the Well's Criteria (www.mdcalc.com/wells-criteria-dvt). If the probability of DVT is low, assessment can begin with a serum D-dimer level. The D-dimer test is sensitive but lacks specificity. If the test is negative, then DVT is highly unlikely. If it is positive, DVT must still be ruled in with a venous Doppler examination. If the presence of DVT is intermediate to high, the NP should order a venous ultrasound which is considered the "gold standard" diagnostic examination. If the ultrasonography is negative for DVT, no further testing is necessary. If a pulmonary embolism is suspected, the patient should be referred for inpatient evaluation and treatment.

Management

Chronic venous insufficiency can be treated with elevation, compression, and wound care to prevent secondary infection. Weight loss, sodium restriction, and regular exercise may also reduce symptoms. Compression therapy can be achieved with compression stockings, ace wraps, or pneumatic compression boots. Patients should be advised to avoid prolonged lower extremity dependence and instructed to elevate the legs whenever possible.[24]

The goal of care when a person has a DVT is to reduce the risk of mortality and morbidity with anticoagulation therapy (unless contraindicated by the patient's current health status). Treatment of DVT is the same for all age groups. The decision to begin treatment while diagnostic testing is being done depends on your clinical evaluation and the likelihood that this is a DVT. Differential diagnoses for DVT include muscle strain or tear or twisting injury to the leg (about 40%), lymphangitis or lymph obstruction, venous insufficiency, cellulitis (only about 3% chance), and unknown (26% chance).

Pharmacological

DVT should be treated with anticoagulation therapy within 24 hours of identification. Previously this necessitated hospitalization for initial treatment with intravenous heparin therapy for 3 to 5 days while warfarin therapy was also initiated until warfarin levels were therapeutic. Patients at lower risk of developing pulmonary embolism and who do not have cancer can now be treated as an outpatient with either low-molecular-weight heparin subcutaneously first and then started on oral anticoagulation or with newer oral anticoagulants from diagnosis without the need for heparin (see Table 20.11 for details on specific regimen and dosing).

Table 20.11: Oral Anticoagulants for DVT Treatment

Coumadin	2-10 po mg daily** /+
Rivaroxaban (Xarelto)	15 mg po BID X 3 weeks, then 20 mg po daily
Apixaban (Eliquis)	10 mg po BID for 7 days, then 5 mg po BID +
Dabigatran etexilate (Pradaxa)	150 mg po BID**/+ 75 mg po BID if Crt. Clearance less than 30 mL/min
Edoxaban (Savaysa)	60 mg po daily** 30 mg po daily if Crt. Clearance less than 50 mL/min

**= Must treat DVT with 5-10 days of parenteral heparin before starting.

+ = has a reversal agent in cases of adverse, emergent bleeding.
DVT, deep vein thrombosis.

High-risk patients should be hospitalized for treatment. If the DVT is from an identifiable, modifiable cause, anticoagulant therapy is planned for 3 to 6 months. If no obvious cause is identified, the patient should be anticoagulated for 6 months. Testing for hypercoagulable states is controversial but can be considered, especially in patients with recurrent DVT. Patients with DVT should receive analgesics if necessary. Patients should be advised to elevate the affected leg and apply heat for comfort, but activity does not need to be restricted. Early activity may actually decrease the likelihood of developing chronic venous insufficiency caused by the thrombus.

When prescribing anticoagulants, you must pay attention to the risk of bleeding events. Patients who are or older than 75 years old, previous bleeding, cancer, advanced kidney disease, liver failure, thrombocytopenia, previous stroke, diabetes, anemia, and alcohol use have a higher risk for adverse bleeding.

Nonpharmacologic

Early ambulation is safe in patients with acute DVT and should be encouraged. Psychologic support may be needed in those who experience stress/anxiety regarding symptoms (e.g., pain) or if associated with chronic venous insufficiency or have concerns regarding treatment and possibility of recurrence of DVT.

Patient Education

Teaching patients about the reason for elastic graduated compression stockings and how to apply them is important. In addition, discussions about ambulation and the importance of controlling the underlying condition that put them at risk for DVT is essential.

Patient education for chronic venous insufficiency can be found at http://vasculardisease.org/flyers/chronic-venous-insufficiency-flyer.pdf and for DVT at www.cdc.gov/ncbddd/dvt/documents/dvt-factsheet_final1210.pdf.

🏠 Quality and Safety Alerts

- Older adults have a greater risk of bleeding and adverse outcomes with anticoagulants as do patients with anemia. When treating older adults though with newer oral anticoagulants, carefully consider the dose based on weight and renal function. Also be aware that these medications are quite expensive and consider cost when ordering for older adults on a limited budget.
- In older adults experiencing recurrent falls or who are at high risk for falls, be cautious about prescribing anticoagulants; the benefit must outweigh the risk.

❶ CLINICAL PEARLS

- Chronic venous insufficiency can be diagnosed clinically and does not require imaging.
- DVTs usually develop from a combination of endothelial injury, venous stasis, and a hypercoagulable state. Be aware of an individual patient's risk.
- Patients diagnosed with a DVT with low risk of developing a PE may be managed as an outpatient, which greatly reduces healthcare costs and is often more comfortable for the patient.

ARRHYTHMIAS

This last section of the chapter provides a brief introduction to arrhythmias. For more comprehensive information about arrhythmias, we recommend you consider taking a course for 12-lead ECG and/or advanced arrhythmias. NPs can face challenges evaluating and treating patients with cardiac arrhythmias in primary care, so it is important to comanage your patients with a cardiac specialist (e.g., cardiologist, cardiac NP).

Heart arrhythmias are categorized by rate, location of origin, and mechanism. The discussion that follows focuses on the basics of arrhythmias and their identification and management in a primary care setting. With the exception of premature atrial contractions (PACs), which have little clinical significance, any patient with suspected or identified arrhythmia should be referred to cardiology for evaluation.

A normal heart rate is between 60 and 100 beats per minute. A heart rate below 60 beats per minute is termed "bradycardia," and a heart rate above 100 beats per minute is called "tachycardia." Tachyarrhythmias are a result of either abnormal automaticity, triggered activity, or reentry. These rapid rhythms can originate within the ventricular tissue or above it (supraventricular). Heart blocks are conduction delays or nonconduction of electrical impulses, which can result in significant bradycardia and may lead to asystole. Arrhythmias can be caused by the presence of congenital accessory pathways, structural or ischemic heart disease, electrolyte abnormalities, defects in the sinus node, problems with the normal function of the vagal or sympathetic tone, drug toxicity, or chronic obstructive pulmonary disease.

ATRIAL ARRHYTHMIAS

Premature Atrial Contractions

PACs are a common arrhythmia. These beats are triggered from an ectopic focus within the atria. While generally benign, PACs can trigger an episode of reentrant tachyarrhythmia in some predisposed patients such as those with congenital Wolff–Parkinson–White (WPW) syndrome. PACs can be caused by stimulants, anxiety, hypokalemia, low serum magnesium levels, and ischemia. These beats are usually asymptomatic but some patients complain of "skipped beats" or palpitations.

Sinus Tachycardia

This is a sinus rhythm in which the heart rate is between 100 and 150 beats per minute. Sinus tachycardia is usually caused by the body's response to a specific metabolic state or from medications or stimulants. Common causes include fever, dehydration, anemia, pulmonary disease, and hyperthyroidism. Caffeine and nicotine use are also common causes. Withdrawal from opiates, stimulants, and alcohol may also increase heart rate.

Supraventricular Tachycardias

Supraventricular tachycardias (SVTs) are rapid heart rhythms that originate above the ventricles. SVTs include sinus tachycardia, sinus node reentry tachycardia, multifocal atrial tachycardia, paroxysmal atrial tachycardia, atrioventricular nodal reentrant tachycardia (AVNRT), atrioventricular reentrant tachycardia (AVRT), atrial fibrillation, and atrial flutter. For all but sinus tachycardia, the heart rate for each of these exceeds 150 beats per minute. The most common SVTs are AVNRT, AVRT, atrial fibrillation, and atrial flutter.

Atrioventricular Nodal Reentrant Tachycardia

This narrow complex tachycardia often presents with a ventricular rate between 150 and 250 beats per minute although it is possible to achieve even higher ventricular rates. It is generally triggered by a PAC or PVC and causes palpitations, dyspnea, and possibly syncope. Usually, AVNRT occurs in younger patients who do not have underlying structural heart disease. If it develops in an older patient with structural or ischemic heart disease, it can lead to angina or acute congestive HF. The rhythm may self-terminate, and this often results in sudden bradycardia or a brief episode of asystole resulting in syncope before normal sinus rhythm resumes.

Atrioventricular Reentrant Tachycardia

AVRT is usually a narrow complex tachycardia with a ventricular rate greater than 200 beats per minute (called orthodromic type). Antidromic AVRT presents as a wide complex QRS tachycardia. The two types can be identified by electrophysiology studies. Patients may present with palpitations, chest pain, dyspnea, or syncope.

Atrial Fibrillation

Atrial fibrillation (AF) is an irregular heart rhythm which is identified by the lack of P waves on the ECG. The ventricular rate is described as irregularly irregular. AF can occur at any rate but most commonly presents as an asymptomatic rhythm if the rate has either a very slow or very fast ventricular response. AF is categorized by cause and occurrence; it can be lone, idiopathic, new-onset, recurrent, paroxysmal, persistent, permanent, valvular, or nonvalvular. AF occurs most commonly in older individuals with valvular heart disease, coronary artery disease, HF, and/or hypertension. AF is also frequently found in obese patients, those with chronic obstructive pulmonary disease, and obstructive sleep apnea. AF can be triggered by stress, alcohol use, stimulants, PE, and metabolic abnormalities. It appears to be linked to inflammation; in addition, many patients with AF have elevated CRP levels.

Presentation of AF ranges from completely asymptomatic (often inadvertently discovered on routine physical examination) to complaints of mild palpitations, dyspnea at rest, or with fatigue. Patients in AF with a very rapid ventricular response (rates often above 170 beats per minute) may present in a hemodynamically unstable state complaining of chest pain or syncope. HF with PE in these cases is not uncommon. AF increases thromboembolic risk due to the development of thrombus, which most commonly occur in the left atrial appendage.

Ventricular Arrhythmias

Premature Ventricular Contractions

A premature ventricular contraction (PVC) is a premature beat originating from an ectopic focus in the ventricles. Like PACs, PVCs are generally benign, although they can trigger reentrant tachycardia in predisposed individuals. Patients usually complain of experiencing "skipped beats." PVCs can occur because of anxiety, electrolyte abnormalities, stimulants, and ischemia.

Ventricular Tachycardia

Three or more QRS complexes in a row originating from a ventricular focus is called ventricular tachycardia (VT). VT is either sustained (lasting more than 30 seconds) or nonsustained (NSVT), which lasts less than 30 seconds. This rhythm may be pulseless. If sustained, this requires emergent intervention.

VENTRICULAR FIBRILLATION

VF is an abnormal ventricular heart rhythm that rarely terminates spontaneously and subsequently leads to death if resuscitation and defibrillation are not initiated immediately. NPs should consider becoming certified in advanced cardiac life support (ACLS). If ACLS equipment is not available in the primary care setting, basic life support (BLS) should be initiated, and emergent care should begin immediately.

ATRIOVENTRICULAR HEART BLOCKS

These arrhythmias represent conduction disturbances between the atria and ventricles. These are classified by degrees. First-degree AV block is characterized by a PR interval greater than 200 milliseconds. Second-degree AV blocks represent the failure of conduction of one or more atrial impulses to the ventricles. There are two types of second-degree AV block: Mobitz I (also called Wenckebach) and Mobitz II. Mobitz I is a lesser block where there is a gradual prolongation of the PR interval and then a nonconducted atrial impulse occurs. Mobitz II is a higher grade block where the PR intervals remain the same, the QRS is wide, and then a nonconducted atrial impulse occurs. Mobitz II is more likely to progress to third-degree heart block. Third-degree heart block (complete heart block) is characterized by complete dissociation between atrial and ventricular electrical impulses. This generally results in a severe, symptomatic bradycardia. All patients with heart block should be referred to cardiology for evaluation. Patients with Mobitz II or complete heart block should be emergently referred for possible placement of a pacemaker. Do not allow patients in these rhythms to drive as they can progress to asystole, which is a pulseless rhythm.

General Assessment of Arrhythmias

Begin assessment with a thorough personal and family history. Pay close attention to specific cardiac symptoms. Patients with arrhythmias may be completely asymptomatic or may complain of a whole host of symptoms. Common symptoms include "skipped beats," palpitations, fatigue, dyspnea (with and without exertion), chest pain, dizziness, diaphoresis, near syncope, and syncope. Ask about the frequency and duration of symptoms. Inquire about precipitating factors.

Complete a thorough physical examination, paying close attention to any abnormal heart sounds. Determine the rate. Heart blocks are often below 40 beats per minute. Atrial fibrillation with a rapid ventricular response or other SVTs is usually too fast to count! Listen to the rhythm. Is it regular or irregular? Arrhythmias are common in the presence of valvular heart disease. Auscultate for murmurs carefully.

Obtain a 12-lead electrocardiogram (ECG). Carefully evaluate each waveform, interval, and segment on the ECG to determine if there are any abnormalities. If the ECG appears normal but the patient complains of persistent symptoms, a 24-hour Holter monitor or a 10-day event monitor can be ordered to hopefully capture the occurrence of the abnormal rhythm. If a patient experiences repeated syncopal events and abnormalities have not been identified by external monitoring, a cardiologist or electrophysiologist can implant a loop recorder in an attempt to capture and identify the problem. An echocardiogram can be considered to identify structural abnormalities. Consider serum testing to identify thyroid dysfunction, electrolyte abnormalities, and/or the presence of anemia. Also evaluate renal and liver function.

Specific Assessment of Adolescents and Older Adults With Arrhythmias

Arrhythmias can occur at any age but are more likely to occur with advancing age. This is because the aging heart often develops valvular problems, HF, ischemia, or degradation of the sinus node tissue. When evaluating each patient, keep their age in mind. An irregular heart rate in a geriatric patient is likely to be atrial fibrillation as this rhythm affects 8% to 10% of the population older than age 80. An irregular heart rate in an adolescent is more likely to be sinus arrhythmia or sinus rhythm with PACs or PVCs. In adolescents, sinus arrhythmia is a normal rhythm where the P-P interval varies related to the respiratory cycle. In adolescents presenting with symptoms suggesting arrhythmia, inquire about any specific family history of sudden cardiac death or other congenital/genetic cardiac abnormalities.

Treatment of Arrhythmias

Treatment of arrhythmias depends on the skill set of the NP and the clinical stability of the patient. In general, if a patient presents with acute symptoms and is hemodynamically unstable, the patient should be referred for emergent, inpatient treatment via ACLS guidelines. Obviously, BLS should be initiated first in an outpatient setting while the emergency medical response is activated. If, on the other hand, the patient has only intermittent symptoms and/or is hemodynamically stable, then outpatient treatment can be initiated. Many atrial and ventricular arrhythmias respond well to ablation therapies. Referral to a cardiologist to rule out structural or ischemic heart disease is wise and referral to an electrophysiologist (a cardiologist who specializes in the electrical system of the heart) should also be considered, especially if the arrhythmia is recurrent.

It is beyond the scope of this book to provide detailed treatment options for each of the many possible arrhythmias. NPs should seek certification and learn ACLS guidelines to further their education and understanding of advanced cardiac life support, especially if they plan to work within the subspecialty of cardiology. Four common arrhythmias and their treatment will be more thoroughly discussed as they occur commonly in the adolescent and geriatric populations.

TREATMENT SPECIFIC TO ADOLESCENTS AND OLDER ADULTS WITH ARRHYTHMIAS

Premature Atrial Contractions

As previously mentioned, PACs are generally considered clinically insignificant. In rare cases, they can trigger reentrant tachyarrhythmia in those with preexisting preexcitation syndromes, such as WPW syndrome. WPW can be identified on a 12-lead ECG by a PR interval less than 120 milliseconds and the presence of a slurred rise in the

QRS called a delta wave. In younger patients, PACs are most commonly caused by stimulants. Appropriate treatment therefore is to eliminate the stimulants and encourage adequate oral hydration. In older patients, they are more likely caused by HF or obstructive lung disease. ACEIs and angiotensin receptor antagonists may reduce the frequency of PACs. Educating patients that these "extra beats" are usually clinically insignificant reduces their fear. If WPW is suspected or the patient develops a symptomatic tachyarrhythmia, treatment via the ACLS guidelines should occur and referral to cardiology should be made.

Supraventricular Tachycardia

AVNRT, AVRT, AF, and atrial flutter are the most common of the SVTs. SVTs can occur in any age group, but AF and atrial flutter are more common in older adults while adolescents are more likely to develop AVNRT or AVRT.

Atrioventricular Nodal Reentrant Tachycardia

AVNRT can be slowed or terminated with vagal maneuvers. If these fail, first-line treatment is intravenous adenosine. If this fails to terminate the rhythm, beta-blockers or calcium channel blockers may be tried. If the patient becomes hemodynamically unstable, direct current cardioversion should be initiated. Long-term use of antiarrhythmic medications is not preferred for suppression of AVNRT. Catheter ablation therapy can reduce reoccurrence and, in 95% of cases, cure the patient. As such, these patients should be referred to an electrophysiologist for management.

Atrioventricular Reentrant Tachycardia

If hemodynamically unstable, direct current cardioversion should be initiated for both wide and narrow QRS complex AVRT. Narrow complex AVRT can be treated with vagal maneuvers, adenosine, or atrial pacing if the patient is medically stable. Wide complex ARVT should not be treated with adenosine, beta-blockers, or calcium channel blockers as these may actually "push" the conduction down the accessory pathways, leading to an increase in ventricular rate and the possible development of ventricular fibrillation. Antiarrhythmic medications, such as flecainide or amiodarone may be used. Synchronized cardioversion is the treatment of choice if the rhythm persists.

Once the rapid AVRT has been treated, the patient will require long-term suppression management. The treatment of choice is percutaneous catheter ablation therapy, which is effective approximately 85% to 98% of the time. Medical therapy with antiarrhythmic medications can also be considered. Again, referral to a cardiologist specializing in electrophysiology is appropriate. The primary care NP's role is to facilitate appropriate emergency care if the patient is currently in a rapid rhythm, work closely with the patient's specialists postevent, and carefully monitor the patient for recurrent symptoms. Be aware that many antiarrhythmic medications have significant adverse side effects and cause many drug–drug interactions. Monitor for these adverse effects and encourage patient compliance with the medication regimen.[25]

Atrial Fibrillation

In general, treatment of AF is focused on controlling the rate of ventricular response, anticoagulation to reduce thromboembolic risk, and, if possible, restoration to a sinus rhythm. If a patient remains in AF, despite multiple attempts to convert to sinus rhythm, then the goal of care shifts to simply controlling the ventricular rate and anticoagulation based on either a CHADS2-VASc or a CHADS2 score (see Table 20.12). The scores will indicate and guide the selection of the appropriate antithrombotic therapy. Patients with valvular AF will require therapy with IV heparin until oral Coumadin levels are therapeutic. Always carefully assess risk versus benefit of anticoagulation in patients who have had a recent history of significant bleeding, frequent falls, or who use alcohol in excess regularly. For those who cannot be anticoagulated, placement of a WATCHMAN device can be considered. This system basically occludes the left atrial appendage where most thrombi form.

In a primary care setting, all patients presenting with symptomatic AF with rapid ventricular response should be emergently referred. Treating a patient in unstable AF with a rapid ventricular response should follow ACLS guidelines and may necessitate direct current cardioversion. Stable, symptomatic patients can be treated with

Table 20.12: CHADS2/CHADVASc Scoring

CHADS2 Risk	Score
C Congestive heart failure	1
H Hypertension	1
A Age 75 years or older	2
D Diabetes mellitus	1
S2 Prior TIA or stroke	2

CHADVASc Risk	Score
C Congestive heart failure	1
H Hypertension	1
A Age 75 years or older	2
D Diabetes mellitus	1
S2 Prior TIA or stroke	2
V Vascular disease	1
A Age 65-74	1
S Sex (Female = 1 point)	1

intravenous calcium channel blockers, beta-blockers, or digoxin, and then once the rate is controlled, they should be switched to the same oral medications.

If a patient presents with nonvalvular mildly symptomatic or asymptomatic AF with a rate below 150 beats per minute, oral outpatient therapy with close daily office monitoring is preferred over admission. Patients can simply be started on an oral calcium channel blocker or a beta-blocker to reduce the heart rate. The newer oral anticoagulants are therapeutic within 1 hour of administration. These patients should be promptly referred to cardiology for evaluation. Instruct these patients that if they develop any worsening of symptoms, they should proceed to the nearest ED for evaluation.[26]

All patients with AF should be seen and evaluated by cardiology after diagnosis. If the patient fails to "chemically cardiovert" (return to a normal sinus rhythm with medications alone), direct current cardioversion should be planned once a patient has been anticoagulated for at least 1 month. Recurrent AF also may respond to catheter ablation, and so referral to an electrophysiologist should also be considered.

Atrial Flutter

Atrial flutter is the second-most common atrial tachycardia after AF. Medical therapy for atrial flutter is similar to that of AF and ACLS guidelines should be followed. Patients with atrial flutter should also be anticoagulated as discussed earlier. Referral to cardiology is appropriate.

Premature Ventricular Contractions

Occasional PVCs are usually considered benign and require no treatment as long as they are asymptomatic and do not progress to VT. For patients with symptomatic PVCs, magnesium supplementation with magnesium oxide 400 mg orally daily may reduce the incidence. Oral beta-blockers may also suppress and reduce the incidence of PVCs. Any patient with increasing frequency of PVCs or complaints of chest pain or dyspnea should undergo cardiac evaluation to rule out the presence of ischemic heart disease or HF.

🏠 Quality and Safety Alerts

- Antiarrhythmia medications are known to be proarrhythmic, which means treating one arrhythmia with a specific drug may actually cause another lethal arrhythmia to occur. Prescribe antiarrhythmic medications with great caution.
- Antiarrhythmic medications have significant adverse side effects and cause many drug-drug interactions.
- 12-lead ECGs should be repeated at least yearly if a patient is taking antiarrhythmic drugs as many can prolong the QT interval.

🅞 CLINICAL PEARLS

- Arrhythmias can be benign or malignant.
- Symptomatic patients should be fully evaluated.

FINAL PART OF EVOLVING CASE STUDY

Three months later, Stephen arrives to the primary care office complaining of worsening dyspnea and an increased heart rate when he exercises. A thorough physical examination reveals an irregular heart rate. Another 12-lead ECG is ordered by the AGNP, and this reveals atrial fibrillation, a heart rate of 100 beats per minute. The AGNP calculates the CHADS2 score to be greater than 2.

Case Study Question

10. What would now be an appropriate management plan for Stephen?

Stephen has now developed new-onset AF, but his rate is below 150 beats per minute, and he is currently only mildly symptomatic. As such, the AGNP chooses to manage the arrhythmia as an outpatient. The AGNP increase the metoprolol succinate to 50 mg po daily. His CHADS2 score indicates that he should be anticoagulated, so the AGNP initiates anticoagulation therapy. The AGNP then arranges for the patient to be seen by the cardiologist the next day. Stephen is instructed to call 911 or go to the ED if his symptoms worsen.

Stephen presents to the office 6 weeks later. Stephen converted back to normal sinus rhythm after the beta-blocker dose was increased and the cardiologist agreed with the AGNP's treatment plan. Stephen is tolerating all his medications, he has no signs or symptoms of bleeding, and his BP is 130/70. The 12-lead ECG done today reveals continued normal sinus rhythm. Stephen reports he is following his healthy lifestyle plan and eating a whole-food diet. He states that he is back to walking most days of the week with his spouse. He denies any further dyspnea or chest tightness with exercise.

CONCLUSION

This chapter has presented the most common cardiovascular conditions NPs may see in primary care. The most important aspect is taking a person-centered approach to care by individualizing cardiac risk assessment using tools provided in this chapter. Individuals should have the knowledge to be involved in shared decision-making that honors their wishes and preferences for care. The American Heart Association has evidence-based clinical guidelines to support decision-making. Decision-making regarding the diagnostics and management of CVD and potential complications involves assessing the benefit versus the risk for each patient.

REFERENCES

References for this chapter are online and available at https://connect.springerpub.com/content/book/978-0-8261-8414-6/part/part01/toc-part/ch20.

CHAPTER 21

Common Musculoskeletal Disorders Encountered in the Primary Care Setting

Damian Eker

LEARNING OBJECTIVES

At the conclusion of this chapter, the learner will be able to:

➤ Recognize the primary causes of the most frequently encountered musculoskeletal disorders in a primary care setting.

➤ Provide an overview of the anatomy and pathophysiology involved in the disease process.

➤ Discuss the signs and symptoms associated with musculoskeletal diseases.

➤ Describe the appropriate evidence-based treatment options.

INTRODUCTION

This chapter focuses on the most common musculoskeletal disorders in the adolescent and adult population encountered by nurse practitioners (NPs) in the primary care setting. Musculoskeletal disorders encompass diseases of the bones, joints, and muscles. Bones form the skeleton upon which muscles, ligaments, and tendons attach to permit movement. Musculoskeletal disorders present substantial variations in their etiology, including trauma, repetitive stress, and osteoarthritis, which are all influenced by age. Pain is one of the most common complaints related to diseases or trauma that impact musculoskeletal disorders. This chapter provides an overview, but for additional information about pain management, see Chapter 13.

OVERVIEW OF THE MUSCULOSKELETAL SYSTEM

Normal Anatomy and Physiology

The skeletal system is composed of different types of bones, but fracture risk is highest among long (e.g., femur, humerus, tibia) and irregular bones (e.g., vertebrae) due to their load-bearing function. The fracture risk is further augmented by age-related factors, such as arthritis, osteoporosis, falls, and polypharmacy.

Joints form articulations between bones and vary in complexity, structure, and degree of mobility. The joints most prone to injury are cartilaginous and synovial joints. The intervertebral discs between vertebrae are cartilaginous joints that allow slight movement to absorb shock, whereas synovial joints (e.g., elbow, knee, hip, shoulder), which allow varying degrees of mobility, are composed of a tough connective tissue capsule lined with a synovial membrane that secretes a viscous lubricating fluid. Other connective tissue elements of most synovial joints include articular cartilage found at the end of bones, ligaments that connect bones, tendons that join muscle to bone, and bursae.

There are three primary types of muscle tissue, but skeletal muscle generates the force required for movement. Skeletal muscle is made up of bundles of muscle fibers called fascicles that are covered by a layer of fascia called the epimysium. The epimysium, which is composed of connective tissue, is continuous with the muscle belly as it narrows and forms the tendon that attaches the muscle to the bone. Similarly, to the skeletal system, muscle injury is most prevalent in the high load-bearing muscles, including the lower back, quadriceps, hamstrings, calves, and biceps.

Assessment of the Musculoskeletal System

Musculoskeletal injuries are evaluated with a thorough interview and physical examination. The interview should always include questions regarding the mechanism of injury, location, and character of the pain; the presence of stiffness or swelling; and a previous history of injury.

Neurovascular Assessment

In the presence of a limb injury, the physical examination should begin with a neurovascular assessment to rule out compartment syndrome. A neurovascular assessment evaluates the five Ps: pain, pulse, pallor, paresthesia, and paralysis.[1] Pain should be assessed using a standardized scale with a high interrater reliability, such as the Numerical Pain Rating Scale, to ensure homogeneity among different examiners so that any changes in the severity of the pain can be detected.[2] It is also important to ask the patient how the pain is affecting their everyday living. The pulses distal to the site of the injury should be compared with the contralateral side. Alterations in skin color and temperature should also be assessed and compared with the opposite side. The presence of impaired sensation and paralysis should be assessed in both the unaffected and affected limbs. Hyperesthesia, hypoesthesia, and paresthesia can present in a patient suffering from compartment syndrome. Paralysis or increased pain on extension of the injured limb with passive or active range of motion (ROM) should increase suspicion for compartment syndrome as affected muscles are highly sensitive to stretch.

Compartment Syndrome

Compartment syndrome results from excessive pressure within fascial compartments of a muscle. Acute compartment syndrome due to bleeding or edema resulting from a fracture or crush injury can lead to increased pressure in a muscle compartment that compromises blood flow. A decrease in blood flow precipitates tissue ischemia and necrosis. Although uncommon, acute compartment syndrome can be life-threatening and lead to limb loss.

General Physical Examination

The neurovascular assessment is followed by inspection, palpation, and joint ROM. Inspection consists of assessing the joints for gross deformity, swelling, erythema, ecchymosis, and bilateral symmetry. Following inspection, palpation is performed to detect tenderness, warmth, deformity, and crepitus. "Crepitus" is a term used to describe a clicking, popping, or grating quality over the joint being assessed. ROM is assessed actively, with the patient responsible for moving the joint. If the patient is unable to actively move the joint, an ROM assessment is performed passively, with the examiner moving the joint. A proper assessment of ROM presupposes a firm understanding of each joint's anatomy, which is beyond the scope of this text.

Upon completion of the history and physical, imaging may be indicated based on the findings. Typically, imaging is reserved for major injuries or if conservative treatment of a suspected minor injury fails. Imaging usually begins with a plain radiograph. Plain radiography permits adequate visualization of bones, joint spaces, and alignment to aid in the diagnosis and staging of fractures, osteoarthritis, and joint injury; however, the role of plain x-ray is limited in the identification of soft tissue injuries involving tendons, ligaments, cartilage, and muscles. More complex imaging techniques, such as computed tomography (CT) or magnetic resonance imaging (MRI), may be needed in the diagnosis of soft tissue pathology. Arteriography may also be necessary if disruption of vascular supply is suspected.

Other diagnostic modalities used in musculoskeletal injury include electromyograms and nerve conduction studies. An electromyogram measures the electrical signals in skeletal muscles in the setting of weakness, spasm, or paralysis to differentiate between neurologic and muscular disorders. Nerve conduction studies are similar tests used to measure the electrical impulses in peripheral motor and sensory nerves when nerve injury is inferred based on the presenting symptoms and physical examination findings.

Musculoskeletal Injuries

The most common musculoskeletal disorders encountered in the primary care setting are related to acute injuries (e.g., sprains, strains, fractures), overuse injuries (e.g., tendonitis, bursitis), and osteoarthritis. Sports-related trauma accounts for the greatest proportion of musculoskeletal injuries in children and adolescents.[3] Among young and middle-aged adults, musculoskeletal injuries are predominantly related to trauma from recreational activities, work, and sports.[4] In adults 65 years and older, falls are the primary cause of musculoskeletal injury.[5] Osteoarthritis and osteoporosis play a key role in this pathology.

Musculoskeletal injuries involving soft tissues (e.g., muscles, ligaments, tendons), bones, and joints also occur throughout the life span. The extent of injury is contingent upon many intrinsic factors, including muscle mass, bone density, and body weight. Most injuries occur from blunt high-energy impact (e.g., falls) and repetitive strain. Acute injuries can occur in adolescents (related to sports injuries or other risky behaviors) and in older adults (falls are a common reason for injuries).

LUMBAR BACK PAIN

Etiology

Lumbar back pain is the leading cause of disability in Americans under the age of 45 and the most common presenting physical complaint in the outpatient setting.[6] Most cases of lumbar back pain occur from mechanical trauma to the muscles, ligaments, intervertebral discs, or spine. Injury to the lumbar muscles and ligaments is the leading cause of lower back pain, predominantly affecting adults aged 18 to 64.[4]

Pathophysiology

Tears in ligaments are called sprains, whereas tears in muscles or tendons are known as strains. Sprains and strains are graded from 1 to 3 based on the degree of joint instability and amount of soft tissue involved. Sprains and strains are the most common musculoskeletal injuries in adolescents and adults.[7] Symptoms of a sprain include pain, swelling, bruising, and a reduced ROM, whereas strains typically cause muscle spasms, weakness, and pain.

Lower back pain with a radiating quality that persists for more than 2 weeks may be indicative of a disc herniation. A herniated disc results from compression and rupture of the gelatinous center of the intervertebral discs between the vertebral bodies causing impingement on the spinal nerves and pain.

Risk Factors

Lower back injury tends to occur due to poor fitness level, advanced age, female gender, obesity, family history of degenerative disc disease, heavy physical activities, overstretching, and tobacco use.

Approach to Diagnosis

The differential diagnosis for acute lumbar back pain includes strains and sprains, disc herniation, osteoarthritis, and spondylolisthesis. A comprehensive medical history and physical examination are normally adequate to establish any life-threatening conditions that require immediate evaluation and treatment. Laboratory tests and radiographs are not usually indicated during the initial evaluation of lumbar back pain due to their poor diagnostic value, except in the setting of symptoms that may indicate infection or neurologic injury.

The medical history should include a review of systems that evaluates for any associated constitutional symptoms, such as chills, fever, and weight loss, as well as a thorough characterization of the pain, including onset, location, duration, quality, and aggravating and relieving factors. Bowel and bladder function should also be questioned. A detailed interview can help establish the etiology of the pain. For example, acute back pain that presents after lifting a heavy object that is described as "shooting or burning" is indicative of a herniated disc. This can be further evaluated with provocative testing, such as a straight leg raise test that can reproduce sciatica related to herniation of an intervertebral disc in the lower lumbar spine.

The physical examination of the back should include a neurologic evaluation in addition to inspection, palpation, ROM, and muscle strength testing. Any neurologic abnormalities noted during the physical examination may be stemming from spinal nerve irritation or entrapment related to osteoarthritis, spinal stenosis, disc herniation, ligamentous ossification, and spondylolisthesis.

Management

The initial treatment of strains and sprains involves avoidance of strenuous activity and cold therapy for up to 48 hours to reduce tissue inflammation and swelling. Nonsteroidal anti-inflammatory drugs (NSAIDs; see Box 21.1), muscle relaxants, and heat therapy are also used to reduce inflammation, pain, and stiffness to encourage the resumption of activity. Resuming normal activity once the swelling and pain have diminished is crucial for preventing stiffness and loss of muscle strength. Physical therapy and core strengthening exercises are encouraged during the convalescence period to preserve spinal mobility and promote proper body mechanics.

Regarding disc herniation, management is focused on reducing pain through the use of acetaminophen,

Box 21.1: Safety Issues

The NP should be cautious when prescribing NSAIDs for managing acute or chronic pain. Prescribing should be limited to short-term use. Older adults are at risk of gastrointestinal (GI) bleed due to gastritis as the result of taking NSAIDs over a longer period. In addition, NSAIDs are contraindicated in those with acute kidney injury or chronic kidney disease.

NP, nurse practitioner; NSAIDs, nonsteroidal anti-inflammatory drugs.

NSAIDs, and corticosteroids. Bedrest is no longer advocated as this contributes to muscle weakness and stiffness; rather, physical therapy with massage, electrical stimulation, and progressive muscle strengthening is beneficial in restoring activity.[8]

Patient Education

Patient education regarding lumbar back pain should be delivered in person. In-person patient education is used to complement structured education materials including pamphlets, books, and videos. Education materials provided to the client should adhere to guidelines for health literacy to promote understanding.[28]

Patient education should focus on promoting mobility and returning to regular activities when feasible. Activity should include aerobic exercise that improves cardiovascular health (such as walking or swimming), as well as specific exercises to strengthen the abdominal muscles, which are essential for supporting the lower back and preventing injury. Conservative pain management methods including the application of heat, gentle stretching, relaxation exercises, and the use of topical and oral analgesics should also be reviewed. The teach-back method should be utilized to confirm patients' understanding of their educational information.[9]

SPRAINS IN ADOLESCENTS

Ankle sprains are the most prevalent soft tissue injury in the adolescent population due to an inward rolling of the ankle.[10] Knee and wrist sprains are the next most common soft tissue injuries noted in adolescents and teenagers.[11] The majority of these injuries are a by-product of athletic involvement.

FRACTURES

Etiology

The majority of fractures in the adolescent and adult population (65 and older) are related to trauma from falls and accidents. One out of five falls in older adults results in a serious injury, such as a fracture or head injury.[29]

Pathophysiology

Fractures may be closed with intact skin or open with disruption of surrounding soft tissues, fascia, and overlying skin. In children and adults aged 18 to 64 years, fractures of the wrist, fingers, ankle, foot, and toes are the most prevalent. In contrast, hip and vertebral fractures are the most common fractures encountered in adults over the age of 64.[12] Older adults are more likely to experience pathologic fractures. Pathologic fractures occur with nominal force in a bone that has deteriorated due to the influences of disease such as osteoporosis or malignancy.

Risk Factors

The most prevalent risk factors for fractures include advancing age and a previous history of fragility fractures. Chronic corticosteroid use, low body mass index, cigarette smoking, excess alcohol ingestion, family history of fracture, and recurrent falls are other risk factors associated with fractures. There are many risk factures for falls in older adults, which are discussed in the following sections.

Approach to Diagnosis

The diagnosis of a fracture begins with an evaluation of the mechanism of injury, review of symptoms, and medical history to assess underlying risk factors. The medical history is followed by a careful physical examination to assess for tenderness around the injury, bruising, and deformity of the injured bone. If a fracture is suspected, an x-ray will be ordered to verify the diagnosis and determine treatment options.

Management

Simple fractures can be treated with closed reduction and immobilization with cast, splint, or sling and swathe. Complex fractures may require open reduction and fixation through the application of appropriate hardware, including pins, screws, plates, and rods. Internal fixation requires internal implants whereas external fixation requires the application of pins and screws into the bone introduced through the skin and secured to an external frame. In older adults, joint replacement or arthroplasty is typically required due to significant degenerative changes in the bone from osteoarthritis and osteoporosis. Similarly, with vertebral compression fractures in older adults, kyphoplasty is indicated to reduce the convalescent period.

Special Considerations for Adolescents to Young Adults

Adolescents do not have the same fracture risk as young adults. Adolescents do not have the mass or velocity to cause the same degree of injury. In addition, physiologically, adolescents' bones are softer and covered by a thicker periosteum with a richer blood supply that is less vulnerable to fracture. As a result, greenstick and buckle fractures are more common. A greenstick fracture involves a bend on one side of the bone with a partial fracture on the other side, whereas a buckle fracture causes the bone to collapse toward the damaged side. Fracture management in children also differs from other populations. Adolescents' bones heal and remodel much faster due to their dense periosteum. Recent research has demonstrated that uncomplicated fractures of the wrist, the most common fractures in young adolescents, are best managed by splinting as opposed to casting, which had been the previous standard of care.[13] However, complicated fractures, such as growth plate fractures, which affect the layer of growing tissue at the ends of long bones, must be managed more cautiously. Growth plate fractures should be managed with cast immobilization.[14]

Special Considerations for Older Adults

The link between aging and increased fracture risk as the result of osteoporosis is well established. The most common fragility fractures in older men and women are vertebral compression fractures and hip fractures. However, older women inordinately represent the highest risk population. As Burge et al.[15] noted, women account for 75% of fractures in adults older than age 64. Older females are disproportionately affected by osteoporosis, defined as a T score of −2.5 or lower on bone density testing, and have significantly higher fall rates than age-matched men.[16] Hormone-related changes can put the older women at risk of falling and should be considered when making recommendations for your patient. Furthermore, the incidence of hip fracture, which is associated with the highest rates of morbidity and mortality, is more than double in women than in men aged 65 and older.[12] Additionally, despite representing only 14% of the total number of fractures annually in the United States, hip fractures account for more than 72% of fracture-related costs.[15]

The societal cost of fractures in the geriatric population emphasizes the need for preventative care, which encompasses not only treating osteoporosis with medications (Table 21.1) but also identifying factors that increase fall risk in the most vulnerable populations. There are numerous age-related factors that contribute to fall risk, including autonomic dysfunction, loss of proprioception, sarcopenia, visual deterioration, polypharmacy, and osteoarthritis. Also important to consider is having one fall increases the risk of falls as well as fear of falling. Improving the quality of life of older adults and reducing public health expenditures on fragility fractures will require a multidisciplinary approach focused on minimizing fall risk and the early detection of osteoporosis.

The primary goal of treatment for any fracture in older adults is the rapid (as soon as possible) return to activities of daily living, baseline physical function (if possible), and pain reduction rather than restoration of perfect limb

Table 21.1: Pharmacologic Treatment of Osteoporosis

Type	Dosage	Frequency	Route
Bisphosphonates			
Alendronate (Fosamax)	70 mg	Weekly	Oral
Risedronate (Actonel)	35 mg	Weekly	Oral
Ibandronate (Boniva)	150 mg	Monthly	Oral
Zoledronic acid (Reclast)	5 mg	Annually	Intravenous
SERMs			
Raloxifene (Evista)	60 mg	Daily	Oral
Parathyroid Hormone Analog			
Teriparatide (Forteo)	20 mcg	Daily	Subcutaneously
Calcitonin salmon (Miacalcin)	200 IU (1 spray)	Daily	Intranasally
Denosumab (Prolia)	60 mcg	Q6 months	Subcutaneously

alignment or improved function. This is normally accomplished by arthroplasty or kyphoplasty as opposed to closed reduction and immobilization or bracing, which necessitates a period of reduced activity to ensure adequate bone healing. In older adults, even a moderate reduction in mobility can lead to significant deconditioning and adverse outcomes such as joint contractures, pneumonia, and depression.[17] Subsequently, despite the increased risk of complications, arthroplasty or kyphoplasty should always be considered in older adults because of the long-term improvements in functional capacity and quality of life.[18–20]

ⓘ CLINICAL PEARLS

- Older adults may not report a fall without injury, so it is important to define what a fall is and assess for fall risk at each annual visit and sooner if needed.

- Refer to an occupational therapist to perform a home safety assessment to evaluate for fall risk and provide feedback to the patient and you about possible interventions to reduce falls.

Box 21.2: Resources for Fall Prevention in Community-Residing Older Adults

- Moncada LVV, Mire LG. Preventing falls in older persons. *Am Fam Physician.* 2017;96(4):240-247. https://www.aafp.org/afp/2017/0815/afp20170815p240.pdf

- Center for Disease Control and Prevention. Older adult fall prevention: facts about falls. https://www.cdc.gov/falls/index.html

OVERUSE INJURIES IN ADULTS
Tendonitis

Etiology and Pathophysiology
Tendonitis is the disordered and progressive deterioration of collagenous fibers that make up the tendon from degenerative injury and impaired healing. Despite prevailing misconceptions, inflammation is uncommon in tendinopathies. The tendons of the rotator cuff (e.g., supraspinatus, infraspinatus, subscapularis, teres minor), patella, Achilles, and epicondyles of the elbow are the most commonly involved.

Risk Factors
Tendonitis is associated with repetitive stress from sports, recreational activities, and vocational activities (e.g., carpentry).

Approach to Diagnosis
Tendonitis is diagnosed by completion of a comprehensive history and physical. Tendonitis is a diagnosis of exclusion and should be suspected if no other source of pain can be determined. The differential diagnosis includes osteoarthritis, bursitis, and inflammatory arthritis. Imaging and laboratory analysis are normally not required. Pain related to tendonitis is aggravated by overload on the affected tendon, such as during athletic activities and vocational exposures. Pain is well localized to the affected tendon and is immediately alleviated when the offending activity is terminated. Pain can also be elicited with palpation of the tendon. Pain tends to improve during exercises as the joint is warmed up and is lessened by isometric exercises.

Management

Treatment involves rest, ice, splinting, immobilization, stretching, and progressive strengthening. NSAIDs are used for analgesia. The use of corticosteroid injections is controversial as research has not demonstrated any long-term benefits with the potential for tendon rupture.[21]

Patient Education

Education is focused on preventing overuse and excessive strain on the affected tendon. Activities should be varied, and limbs should be alternated to avoid repetitive stress. Exercise involving the affected muscle groups should be undertaken to strengthen the muscle–tendon complex. Stretching should also be incorporated before and following every activity to promote flexibility.

Bursitis

Etiology and Pathophysiology

Bursitis occurs from inflammation of a bursa sac, which serves as padding to reduce friction among the bones, tendons, and ligaments. The bursae most commonly affected by bursitis are located in the shoulder (subscapular, subacromial), elbow (olecranon), hip (trochanteric), knee (prepatellar, anserine), and ankle (retrocalcaneal).

Risk Factors

Bursitis can result from overuse injury (repetitive stressors), direct trauma, aging, and infection (septic).

Approach to Diagnosis

Bursitis is diagnosed via physical examination findings looking for tenderness overlying the location of the bursa. Cellulitis, osteoarthritis, tendonitis, fracture, and inflammatory arthritis are the differential diagnoses for bursitis. An inflamed bursa presents with erythema, warmth, swelling, and localized tenderness or stiffness. In cases of suspected septic bursitis, fluid is aspirated from the bursa and sent for analysis to confirm the infection and ensure appropriate antibiotic therapy.

Management

Management of aseptic bursitis includes PRICE (protection, rest, ice, compression, and elevation), NSAIDs, and intrabursal corticosteroid administration. In cases of suspected septic bursitis, an infectious disease specialist should be consulted as treatment will normally require intravenous antibiotics.

Patient Education

Patient education for bursitis should focus on treatment and prevention techniques. Bursitis can usually be prevented from reoccurring. Conservative home treatments including rest, cold therapy, gentle exercises, and the use of analgesics should be encouraged. Activity should be resumed for short periods of time at a slower speed following a warm-up interval. Ice therapy can be used following the resumption of activities to treat any residual pain and swelling. All joints should be cushioned from prolonged pressure, especially during occupational exposures. Bursae overlying joints and bony prominences should be cushioned during prolonged exposures.

Special Considerations for Adolescents to Young Adults

Etiology and Pathophysiology

The most prevalent overuse syndromes in adolescents are apophyseal injuries involving the medial epicondyle of the elbow (little leaguer's elbow), knee (Osgood-Schlatter disease), and heel (Sever disease). Little leaguer's elbow presents with pain at the medial epicondyle exacerbated by pitching motions. Osgood-Schlatter disease presents with anterior knee pain due to inflammation of the distal patellar tendon and tibial tuberosity from running and jumping. Similarly, severe disease occurs as a result of repetitive running and jumping, which results in inflammation of the growth plate at the posterior calcaneus. Bone growth that outpaces muscle lengthening is the common feature among apophysitis.

Risk Factors

Overtraining and specializing in a specific sport at an early age are the largest risk factors.

Approach to Diagnosis

The diagnosis of apophysitis is clinical and based primarily on the medical history and physical examination. The clinical findings consistent with apophysitis include localized swelling and pain at the apophysis exacerbated by resisted activation of the associated joint. Ultrasound imaging can be used to confirm the absence of tendon and muscle injury.[22]

Management

Apophyseal injuries normally respond to conservative treatment, including rest, icing, NSAIDs, stretching, and physical therapy.[23]

Patient Education

Patient education should focus on prevention. Parents can prevent apophysitis in adolescents by teaching them to recognize activity-related pain and early symptoms. Children who have pain with a specific physical activity should be rested until the discomfort has resolved. Proper warm-ups and stretching are essential components of all sports to promote muscle flexibility as a child grows.

Osteoarthritis

Etiology

Osteoarthritis results from the complex interplay among numerous factors that promote acute and chronic insult, including age-related wear and tear, obesity, and joint injury which triggers an imbalance between chondral matrix synthesis and matrix degradation in cartilage. The end result is progressive chondral loss that impairs cartilage repair and promotes subchondral bone injury.

Pathophysiology

Osteoarthritis is perceived as the endpoint of a dynamic series of events initiated by chondrocyte damage as a result of mechanical injury, which results in a progressive degenerative disease with activation of inflammatory chemical mediators that promote bone deterioration, osteophyte formation, and joint space narrowing. Osteoarthritis is estimated to affect 25% of the population by 2030.[24] It is the primary cause of impaired mobility in older adults.

Risk Factors

The most prominent risk factor associated with osteoarthritis is advancing age. Older adults experience altered bone remodeling, sarcopenia, reduced proprioception, and chondrocyte senescence, increasing their risk for the development of osteoarthritis. Other factors include female gender, obesity, joint trauma, metabolic bone diseases, and genetics/genomics.

Approach to Diagnosis

Diagnosis of osteoarthritis is contingent on the presence of pain as radiographic features of osteoarthritis, including joint space narrowing, osteophyte formation, subchondral bone sclerosis, and bone cysts, do not always present with symptoms.[25] The differential diagnosis includes bursitis, inflammatory arthritis, tendinopathy, septic arthritis, fibromyalgia, hypothyroidism, and neuropathy.

Management

Conservative treatments include strengthening exercises, weight loss, heat therapy, stretching, kinesiotaping, analgesics (e.g., acetaminophen, NSAIDs, tramadol), and viscoelastic joint injections (sodium hyaluronate). Total joint replacement is offered to patients with debilitating pain that no longer responds to conservative treatments. Osteoarthritis is the leading cause of elective arthroplasty in the United States.[26]

Patient Education

People with osteoarthritis often feel helpless and should be educated about useful methods to manage their symptoms and improve quality of life including the use of durable medical equipment (such as a raised toilet seat, cane, walker, grabber) to promote safety and independence, weight loss, daily low-intensity exercise (such as walking and water aerobics), and avoiding repetitive joint motions.[27]

MUSCULOSKELETAL EMERGENCIES

- Inflammation and painful swelling of a joint accompanied by constitutional symptoms of fever, chills, and general weakness may indicate septic arthritis.
- Acute respiratory distress with symptoms of hypoxemia and changes in levels of consciousness following a long bone or pelvic fracture suggest a fat embolism in the pulmonary vasculature.
- Signs and symptoms of impaired sensation, pallor, decreased ROM, and severe pain following a fracture, crush injury, or contusion should be treated with high suspicion for compartment syndrome.
- Osteomyelitis should be suspected with the sudden onset of fever, chills, and bone pain with localized swelling, erythema, and warmth within the setting of a fracture, cellulitis, or penetrating wound.

🕐 CLINICAL PEARLS

- Lumbosacral sprain is the most common cause of lower back pain.
- The initial management of lower back pain following a normal neurologic examination should include ergometric evaluation, physical therapy, and the prudent use of acetaminophen and/or NSAIDs.
- Lower back pain exacerbated by flexion of the spine is most commonly related to an injury involving the lumbar muscles and/or ligaments.
- Lower back pain provoked by extension of the spine is likely related to spinal stenosis.
- A thorough shoulder examination should include an evaluation of the cervical spine to rule out shoulder pain related to cervical spine disease.
- A frequent clinical finding in osteomyelitis is persistent pain with pronounced tenderness overlying the infected bone.

CONCLUSION

Musculoskeletal disorders are common concerns for adolescents, adults, and older adults seen in primary care settings. This chapter presented common disorders you may see in practice, but it is important to include other differential diagnoses if your assessment and treatment plan do lead to the goals of care. Refer to an orthopedic, pain, and/or rheumatology specialist as appropriate. Pain is a subjective experience, so taking a person-centered approach to pain management is essential.

CASE STUDY
PATIENT WITH KNEE PAIN

Chief Complaint: Mr. D, a 59-year-old male, presents with complaints of right knee pain.

History of Present Illness
Mr. D states that the pain is chronic and has been getting worse over the last year.

Review of Systems
Mr. D complains of right knee pain described as chronic with an aching quality and an intensity of 5 on a 10 scale that progressively becomes worse throughout the day. He also describes significant knee stiffness in the morning. He also reports steadily gaining weight over the past few years and is noted with a body mass index (BMI) of 31 kg/m². He has been taking naproxen 220 mg twice daily for the pain.

Past Medical History
Mr. D's history is noted with hypertension and hyperlipidemia.

Social History
Mr. D is employed as a warehouse supervisor with a 30 pack/year history of smoking and admits to social drinking, primarily beer over the weekend. He does not exercise regularly and admits to being sedentary when not at work.

Physical Examination
Right medial knee joint effusion with joint line tenderness and reduced extension. The joint is cool to touch. The patient is afebrile with an elevated blood pressure of 155/88.

Medications
Lisinopril 20 mg daily, naproxen 220 mg twice daily

Case Study Questions
1. What are the differential diagnoses?
2. Which diagnosis is most likely based on the physical examination and review of systems?
3. What is your treatment plan?
4. What are the modifiable risk factors, if any?

Conclusion
Based on the findings, Mr. D is likely suffering from medial compartment osteoarthritis of the right knee. The unilateral joint involvement with morning joint stiffness and progressively worsening pain is consistent with osteoarthritis. An inflammatory arthritis, such as rheumatoid arthritis (RA), will typically present with bilateral joint involvement and thickening of the synovium, with swelling and warmth of the entire joint. The joint pain in RA will normally improve with activity. RA can also affect most of the organs and manifest with systemic symptoms such as fatigue and anorexia.

In terms of the management, Mr. D is noted to be overweight and an active smoker. He should be counseled at length about smoking cessation, reducing alcohol intake, and dietary modifications to reduce his weight in order to alleviate pressure on the knees and improve joint health. He should also be educated about the importance of routine exercise to improve muscle strength and joint flexibility. The patient's education should comply with universal precautions for health literacy and utilize teach-back methods to enhance understanding.

Regarding his analgesic management, his blood pressure is noted to be elevated; under these circumstances, naproxen should be avoided as it can contribute to the hypertension. Mr. D should be encouraged to try other means of pain management, including acetaminophen, topical analgesics (e.g., diclofenac gel, transdermal lidocaine, capsaicin, menthol), cold and heat therapy, and massage.

REFERENCES
References for this chapter are online and available at https://connect.springerpub.com/content/book/978-0-8261-8414-6/part/part01/toc-part/ch21.

CHAPTER 22

Common Gastrointestinal Disorders Encountered in the Primary Care Setting

Damian Eker

LEARNING OBJECTIVES

At the conclusion of this chapter, the learner will be able to:

➤ Recognize the primary causes of the most frequently encountered gastrointestinal (GI) disorders.

➤ Describe the relevant anatomy and pathophysiology involved in the disease process.

➤ Discuss the signs and symptoms associated with GI diseases.

➤ Describe the appropriate treatment options.

INTRODUCTION

This chapter serves as an introduction to the most common GI disorders encountered in the primary care setting. The focus is on diagnosing and managing GI disorders within the framework of the most frequently presenting chief complaint.

OVERVIEW OF GASTROINTESTINAL DISORDERS

According to the National Gastrointestinal Survey, heartburn/reflux (30.9%), abdominal pain (24.8%), bloating (20.6%), diarrhea (20.2%), and constipation (19.7%) were the most commonly reported GI symptoms.[1] Numerous conditions can elicit abdominal pain, creating a diagnostic dilemma. However, a thorough understanding of physiology, along with a systematic approach to the history and physical examination, can yield valuable information and support a diagnosis.

Normal Anatomy and Physiology

Abdominal pain can be visceral, parietal, or referred. Understanding the different characteristics of each type of pain and documenting the location allows the nurse practitioner (NP) to begin to develop a logical differential diagnosis. Visceral pain is a by-product of the stimulation of pain receptors within the abdominal organs that are particularly sensitive to stretch, inflammation, and ischemia. Visceral pain is described as a dull, deep, diffuse pain perceived toward the midline. Pain resulting from bowel distention is visceral in nature. In contrast, parietal pain arises from pain receptors located in the skin and deeper tissues of the peritoneal lining. Parietal pain is described as a sharp, constant, localized pain exacerbated by movement. Acute appendicitis elicits parietal pain as the resulting inflammation irritates the parietal peritoneum. Referred pain manifests at a site distant from an affected area when nerves from both regions converge at the same level of the spinal cord. For example, right subscapular pain can result from biliary disease.

Centrally mediated abdominal pain syndrome (CAPS; formerly known as functional abdominal pain syndrome) "is characterized by continuous, nearly continuous, or frequently recurrent abdominal pain that is often severe and only rarely related to gut function. CAPS is associated with loss of function across several life domains, including work, intimacy, social/leisure, family life, and caregiving for self or others, and must be present for at least 6 months before diagnosis."[2] It can't be explained by structural or metabolic disorders and abdominal pain can be produced by or attributed to nondigestive organs (e.g., urinary or gynecologic. The patient should be evaluated for other contributing factors before a diagnosis of CAPS is made.

🄾 CLINICAL PEARLS

Approach to the patient with chronic undiagnosed abdominal pain:

▪ Perform detailed history.

▪ Determine if diffuse, nonspecific abdominal pain is present.

▪ Perform a localized pain check for Carnett's sign (test for abdominal pain involving tensing of abdominal muscles while palpating a tender spot to differentiate between local abdominal wall pain or pain of intraabdominal causes).

  ● If negative, consider functional dyspepsia or irritable bowel syndrome (IBS).

  ● If positive, consider chronic abdominal wall pain (anterior cutaneous nerve entrapment syndrome, hernia, surgical or procedure-related pain).

- Diffuse, nonspecific abdominal pain
  - CAPS
  - Narcotic bowel syndrome (patient is using opioids with increasing dose)
- Dyspareunia, dyschezia, and menstrual cycle-related diarrhea may be endometriosis (refer to gynecologist or women's health NP).

CAPS, centrally mediated abdominal pain syndrome.

Source: Pichetshote N, Pimentel M. An approach to the patient with chronic undiagnosed abdominal pain. *Am J Gastroenterol*. 2019;114:726-732. doi:10.14309/ajg.0000000000000130

General Assessment of the Abdomen

Interview and Review of Systems

During the patient interview, the NP must authentically listen and inquire about the onset, location, timing, severity, and characteristics of the pain. Within this context, all pertinent social, medical, surgical, and family history should be documented in a systematic fashion. The NP must develop a methodology to guide the interview process to ensure the inclusion of all essential medical history.

The review of systems (ROS) must be comprehensive. Documenting the absence or presence of symptoms is insufficient. A detailed ROS that delineates the distinctive characteristics of pertinent symptoms can prove invaluable in clarifying a diagnosis. For example, vomitus in the setting of recurrent nausea that contains partially digested food and lacks bile suggests a gastric outlet obstruction (GOO), whereas liquified vomitus containing bile is indicative of a small bowel obstruction. To take this one step further, vomiting associated with a small bowel obstruction will occur later and with less frequency than vomiting resulting from a gastric blockage. As depicted, all of the defining characteristics of the vomitus are crucial in differentiating the location of a GI obstruction.

If CAPS is suspected, it should distinguish from functional gastrointestinal disorders (FGID), such as functional dyspepsia and IBS (see Box 22.1). The predominant main complaint of pain with almost no other symptoms distinguishes it from these. The pain may be colicky, and after previous surgery, the pain is often described as burning.

Box 22.1: Rome IV Diagnostics Criteria

Rome IV Diagnostic Criteria* for Centrally Mediated Abdominal Pain Syndrome (CAPS)**

- Must have all of the following:
  - Continuous or nearly continuous abdominal pain
  - No or only occasional relationship of pain with physiologic events (e.g., eating, defecation, or menses) +

- Pain limits some aspect of daily functioning. ++
- The pain is not feigned.
- Pain is not explained by another GI disorder or medical condition.

*Criteria fulfilled for the last 3 months, with symptom onset at least 6 months prior to diagnosis.
**CAPS is typically associated with psychosocial comorbidity, but there is no specific psychosocial profile that can be used for the diagnosis of CAPS.
+Some degree of GI dysfunction may be present.
++Limitation of daily functioning includes impairments in work, intimacy, social/leisure, family life, and caregiving for self or others.

GENERAL PHYSICAL EXAMINATION

Physical examination of the abdomen should include observation, auscultation, percussion, and palpation. The focus should be on identifying the presence of any abnormal findings based on the patient's chief complaint, interview, and ROS. The examination should proceed in a coordinated fashion by dividing the abdomen into four main quadrants horizontally at the umbilicus and vertically from the xiphoid process of the sternum. It is a prerequisite that the examiner be familiar with the anatomy in each quadrant listed in Table 22.1 for the successful identification of pathologic findings.

Inspection

During observation, the contours and pigmentation of the abdomen should be noted. Is it flat, distended, or asymmetric? A distended abdomen may indicate constipation, excess flatus, ascites, bowel obstruction, bleeding, infection, or malignancy. Abdominal asymmetry can signal a mass or organ hypertrophy, including tumor, hernia, aortic aneurysm, diverticulitis, splenomegaly, bowel obstruction, or hepatomegaly. The presence of jaundice; engorged, superficial epigastric veins; or multiple spider

Table 22.1: GI Organs in the Four Abdominal Quadrants

RUQ	LUQ	RLQ	LLQ
Liver	Stomach	Cecum	Portions of the transverse colon
Gallbladder	Spleen	Appendix	
Duodenum	Liver (left lobe)	Ascending colon	Descending and sigmoid colon
Pancreas (head)	Pancreas (tail)	Portions of the transverse colon	
Hepatic flexure of colon	Splenic flexure of colon	Small intestine	Small intestine

GI, gastrointestinal; LLQ, left lower quadrant; LUQ, left upper quadrant; RLQ, right lower quadrant; RUQ, right upper quadrant.

angiomas may be related to liver disease. Hypertrophic, darkly pigmented scars may represent previous injury or surgical scars. A history of abdominal surgery in the setting of symptoms and physical examination findings consistent with a small bowel obstruction could indicate peritoneal adhesions.

Auscultation

Auscultation should always follow observation. All four quadrants of the abdomen should be auscultated with the diaphragm to evaluate bowel motility and the bell to listen for vascular bruits. Are bowel sounds present? The absence of bowel sounds can indicate an ileus or bowel obstruction proximal to the segment of the intestine being auscultated. The detection of a bruit over the epigastrium is suggestive of an abdominal aortic aneurysm.

Percussion

Percussion of the four abdominal quadrants elicits tympany or dullness. Tympany predominates as it corresponds with gas in the bowel, whereas dullness occurs over solid organs or fluid-filled regions. The size of the spleen and liver can be determined through percussion. The presence of a distended abdomen with dullness to percussion and hepatomegaly can imply liver disease.

Palpation

Palpation allows for localization of abdominal pain and determination of the potential etiology based on the location. Palpation may elicit guarding and rebound tenderness, which may be signs of peritoneal irritation or inflammation. For example, a positive Murphy's sign, tenderness in the right upper quadrant of the abdomen with palpation, is diagnostic of gallbladder inflammation. Completing the physical evaluation with palpation allows the NP to review any abnormal findings obtained during the previous steps of the abdominal examination.

CAUSES OF ABDOMINAL PAIN

This section will focus on the most common causes of abdominal pain encountered in the primary care setting, including gastroesophageal reflux disease (GERD), gastroenteritis, constipation, peptic ulcer disease (PUD), IBS, and cholelithiasis. FGIDs (brain-gut interaction) which includes functional dyspepsia, IBS, and chronic idiopathic constipation (CIC) are characterized by disorder motility and visceral hypersensitivity that are often worsened by psychologic distress and should be considered in your differential diagnosis. "Symptoms, including bloating and abdominal distention, are thought to result from disturbances in intestinal transit and motility, gut microflora, immune-function, gas production, visceral hypersensitivity, and central nervous systems processing."[3]

Building a trusting relationship is essential for patients to accept the biopsychosocial model of FGIDs. Before making this diagnosis, it is essential to take a structured approach to assessment and treatment as recommended in the remainder of the chapter.

🏠 Quality and Safety Alerts

Alarming symptoms suggestive of potential serious causes of gas, bloating, and belching

- Abdominal mass
- Dysphagia
- Extreme diarrhea symptoms
- Fever
- GI bleed
- Jaundice
- Lymphadenopathy
- New onset of symptoms for those 55 and older
- Odynophagia
- Symptoms of pancreatitis
- Symptoms of GI cancer
- Symptoms of ovarian cancer
- Tenesmus (rectal pain or feeling of incomplete defecation)
- Vomiting

Source: Wilkinson JM, Cozine EW, Loftus CG. Gas, bloating, and belching: approach to evaluation and management. *American Family Physician.* 2019;99(5):301–309.

GASTROESOPHAGEAL REFLUX DISEASE

Etiology and Pathophysiology

GERD is the result of excess lower esophageal sphincter relaxation causing the retrograde flow of gastric acid into the esophagus. GERD can result in erosive esophagitis, esophageal stricture, and esophageal adenocarcinoma if left untreated.

Risk Factors

Obesity, smoking, caffeine, alcohol, pregnancy, hiatal hernia, and poor diet all contribute to the development of GERD.

Approach to Diagnosis

The physical examination findings in GERD are frequently unremarkable with the exception of obesity. Therefore, a presumptive diagnosis of GERD is often based on the clinical presentation of common symptoms. Typical presenting symptoms of GERD include epigastric pain with a "burning" quality, sore throat, hoarseness, regurgitation, and globus sensation.

Management

Based on the American College of Gastroenterology updated guidelines for the treatment of GERD in 2013, empiric treatment should begin with once-daily proton pump inhibitor (PPI) therapy administered an hour before meals for a period of 8 weeks. PPI therapy can be adjusted to twice daily based on the patient's response. In addition, lifestyle modifications, such as weight loss, smoking cessation, and avoidance of alcohol and caffeine, should be encouraged. In refractory cases, endoscopy should be considered.[4]

SPECIAL CONSIDERATIONS FOR ADOLESCENTS TO YOUNG ADULTS

GERD occurs less often in adolescents, but if present typically occurs after meals. Some of the signs and symptoms may be poor weight gain or weight loss, dysphagia, chest pain, epigastric pain or nonlocalized abdominal pain, chronic cough, wheezing or hoarseness, asthma, and recurrent otitis media.[5] Diagnostic testing is not usually necessary because it has not been found to be more reliable than the history and physical. A conservative approach to treatment is the first step so adolescents should incorporate lifestyle change. If the symptoms don't improve with conservative treatment, an empiric 4-week trial using acid suppression therapy with histamine H$_2$ receptor antagonists or PPI should be considered. Prokinetic agents have been suggested to treat GERD; however, there is little evidence to support this recommendation. Antacids are not recommended for children younger than age 12 but may be a good option for adolescents experiencing dyspepsia or heartburn (will not decrease the frequency of reflux). If symptoms don't improve, referral to a gastroenterologist is recommended.[6]

SPECIAL CONSIDERATIONS FOR OLDER ADULTS

Adults older than age 50 and any individual presenting with acid reflux in setting of alarm symptoms (e.g., weight loss, anemia, hemoptysis) should be referred to gastroenterology for an upper endoscopy. Chronic acid reflux is the primary cause for the development of Barrett's esophagus, a metaplastic change in the squamous cells that line the lower esophagus, which can progress to adenocarcinoma of the esophagus.

GASTROENTERITIS

For purposes of this text, the focus is mainly on causes of acute gastroenteritis as it is more prevalent in the general population. Functional chronic dyspepsia as relates to brain–gut connection is briefly discussed.

Etiology and Pathophysiology

Gastroenteritis results from excessive inflammation of the GI tract due to viral, bacterial, and parasitic infections. Viral infections are the predominant cause of acute diarrhea in the United States. Acute diarrhea is defined as the passage of poorly formed stools at an increased frequency for a period of 2 weeks or less.[7] The most common bacterial causes of acute diarrhea in the United States are *Salmonella*, *Campylobacter*, *Shigella*, and *Escherichia coli*.[8] Gastroenteritis can cause dehydration and electrolyte imbalances, which can lead to acute kidney injury, arrhythmias, seizures, and even death.

Risk Factors

Animal exposures, consumption of undercooked and raw foods, international travel, and freshwater exposures are risk factors for gastroenteritis.

Approach to Diagnosis

During the interview, the patient should be evaluated for recent food exposures, recreational water use, travel, pet exposures, and other predisposing sources that could narrow down the potential cause (Table 22.2). The ROS should focus on symptoms of dehydration (e.g., headache, thirst, dizziness), stool characteristics (Table 22.3), the timing and onset of the symptoms in relation to potential sources, and other GI symptoms (e.g., nausea, vomiting, abdominal pain) to further refine the diagnosis.

The physical examination may reveal signs of varying degrees of dehydration (Table 22.4) consistent with a hypovolemic state. Abnormal GI examination findings are visceral abdominal pain, nonfocal abdominal distention, and hyperactive bowel sounds (borborygmi). Palpation and percussion of the abdomen are normally unremarkable in gastroenteritis. The presence of rebound tenderness or increased pain with palpation or percussion should alert the NP to a noninfectious etiology of the pain, such as cholecystitis.

Management

The priority in the treatment of gastroenteritis is to ensure rehydration, electrolyte replacement, and maintenance of ongoing fluid loss through the use of a reduced osmolarity oral rehydration solution, such as Pedialyte.[9] Sports drinks, juices, and other beverages with a high osmolarity should be avoided as they can promote diarrhea. The recommended rate of rehydration and ongoing fluid maintenance in mild to moderate dehydration in adolescents and adults is displayed in Table 22.5.[10,11] Any physical signs of severe dehydration as noted in Table 22.4 should prompt hospitalization and intravenous rehydration.

Table 22.2: Sources of Gastroenteritis

Food exposure	Food poisoning: norovirus, *Salmonella*, *E. coli*, *Campylobacter*, *Shigella*
Recreational water use	*Campylobacter*, *E. coli*, *Shigella*, *Giardia*, norovirus
Travel	Traveler's diarrhea—*E. coli*, *Campylobacter*, *Shigella*, *Salmonella*
Pet exposure	*Campylobacter* from cats and dogs, *Salmonella* from reptiles
Daycare	Rotavirus, astrovirus, norovirus, *Campylobacter*, *Shigella*, *Giardia*, and *Cryptosporidium* species
Antibiotic use	*C. difficile* infection; post-antibiotic-associated diarrhea

Table 22.3: Stool Characteristic

	Viral	**Bacterial**
Quality	Watery	Bloody or Mucoid
Quantity	Large (affects small bowel)	Small (affects large bowel)
Frequency	Fewer than 6 stools/24 hours	More than 6 stools/24 hours
Duration	1-3 days	1-14 days or longer
Vomiting	+	+/−

Table 22.4: Signs of Dehydration

	Mild to Moderate	**Severe**
Level of consciousness	Alert to irritable, listless	Lethargy, altered mental status
Blood pressure	Normal to low	Low
Pulse	Normal to tachycardic	Thready, nonpalpable
Capillary refill	Brisk to 3 seconds	Greater 3 seconds
Respirations	Normal to hyperpnea	Hyperpnea and tachypnea
Skin turgor	Normal to slow retraction	Tenting
Urine output	Normal to oliguria	Anuria

Table 22.5: Oral Rehydration Therapy in Gastroenteritis

	Rehydration	**Ongoing Fluid Loss**
Children	50-100 mL/kg over 4 hours	10 mL/kg per episode of diarrhea
Adults	2,200-4,000 mL over 4 hours	Up to 2,000 mL/day

In cases of gastroenteritis from a suspected viral etiology, supportive care with oral rehydration therapy remains the standard of care. Antimotility agents, such as loperamide, may be used in adults to reduce diarrheal episodes. Diagnostic testing is not indicated.

Diagnostic evaluation of gastroenteritis with a stool culture is recommended in the setting of severe dehydration, grossly bloody diarrhea, and in the presence of symptoms persisting for greater than 7 days.[7] Antibiotic treatment should be based on sensitivity results with the exception of Shiga toxin-producing *E. coli*. The use of antibiotics or antimotility drugs is contraindicated with Shiga toxin-producing *E. coli* as both can promote the development of hemolytic uremic syndrome. Treatment for Shiga toxin-producing *E. coli* is purely supportive at this time.[12]

Probiotics have not demonstrated any clinical evidence of efficacy in acute diarrhea due to gastroenteritis in adults. However, probiotics may be beneficial in adults with antibiotic-associated diarrhea.[7] In adolescence, studies of specific probiotics, *Lactobacillus GG* and *Saccharomyces boulardii*, have revealed statistically significant reductions in the duration and frequency of diarrhea.[13,14] Despite the ongoing debate regarding their efficacy, the use of probiotics in adolescents is generally recommended as there are no known contraindications to their use.

Despite ongoing recommendations in favor of the BRAT (bananas, rice, applesauce, toast) diet, recent research has dispelled the benefits of this diet in reducing diarrhea. To the contrary, the BRAT diet does not provide adequate nutrition when recovering from diarrhea. A diet rich in lean protein sources, complex carbohydrates, fruits, and vegetables should be resumed once a patient is rehydrated.[15]

Hand hygiene (hand washing with soap and water or use of alcohol-based hand disinfection) is the most important way to reduce transmission of microorganisms.[16] The availability of clean water and sanitary food preparation is also of importance.

More recently, the development of vaccines against pathogens that cause gastroenteritis has become a priority.

SPECIAL CONSIDERATIONS FOR ADOLESCENTS TO YOUNG ADULTS

The goals of treatment for gastroenteritis in adolescents are preventing dehydration and treating when it occurs and reducing the duration and severity of symptoms. Oral hydration solution recommendation for ages 5 to 14 is 1,200 to 2,200 mL and for ages 15 and older 2,200 to 4,000 mL given in the first 4 hours of symptoms (adolescents can have as much fluid as they want). Mild dehydration (6% or less) should be managed at home with oral hydration solution. Moderate to severe dehydration (more than 6%) should be evaluated for IV therapy. Ondansetron may need to be prescribed to treat vomiting and improve tolerance for oral hydration.

SPECIAL CONSIDERATIONS FOR OLDER ADULTS

Older adults have the highest risk of mortality and morbidity related to dehydration due to age-related physiologic differences. Older adults have a reduced water body content from increased adiposity, impaired thirst sensation, and a decreased ability to concentrate urine from age-related changes in kidney function (see Chapter 23 for more information on kidney disease).

CONSTIPATION

Etiology and Pathophysiology

Constipation, as defined by the ROME Foundation,[17] is based on the characteristics and frequency of patient complaints (Table 22.6). Constipation can be differentiated as primary or secondary. Primary constipation involves intrinsic dysfunction of the colon, anus, or rectum and is classified as normal transit, slow transit, and pelvic floor dysfunction. Secondary constipation results from extrinsic causes (e.g., metabolic, neurologic, obstructive, systemic, psychiatric, and medications). For purposes of this chapter, the focus is on the primary causes of constipation.

Normal transit constipation is the most prevalent form of constipation. It is often referred to as CIC and felt to occur along the spectrum of IBS. In normal transit constipation, stool moves through the colon at a normal physiologic rate; however, patients report symptoms of difficulty evacuating the bowel. Conversely, slow transit constipation involves delayed stool passage as a result of intrinsic colonic pathology, such as aberrant bowel innervation. Pelvic floor dysfunction, on the other hand, is a consequence of poorly coordinated relaxation of the puborectalis muscle resulting in a rectal outlet obstruction.

Risk Factors

Risk factors for constipation include advanced age, female gender, sedentary lifestyle, low socioeconomic status, low-fiber diet, inadequate fluid intake, and polypharmacy.

Table 22.6: ROME IV Criteria for Constipation

1. Two or more of the symptoms listed	• Less than three spontaneous bowel movements weekly
	• Manual maneuvers (e.g., digital extraction) to aid the passage of stool at least 25% of the time
	• Lumpy or hard stools during at least 25% of bowel movements
	• Straining during at least 25% of bowel movements
	• Sensation of incomplete bowel evacuation at least 25% of the time
	• Sensation of anorectal blockage/obstruction during at least 25% of bowel movements

Note: Criteria must be met for the previous 3 months with symptom onset at least 6 months prior to the diagnosis. Must have both of the following: loose stools rarely present without the use of laxatives and does not meet ROME IV criteria for IBS.

Source: Rome Foundation. Rome IV criteria. https://theromefoundation.org/rome-iv/rome-iv-criteria

Approach to Diagnosis

The history should include inquiries about current medications, medical history, surgical history, family history, and colorectal screening. The onset of symptoms (e.g., bloating, tenesmus, diarrhea, vomiting) should be recorded relative to any potential contributing factors (e.g., dietary changes, new medications). For instance, a patient started on an opioid could develop constipation due to a medication-induced reduction in bowel motility.

A detailed description of the patient's regular bowel pattern and any deviations from the norm, including the frequency, duration, and pattern, should be noted. Stool characteristics also need to be clearly documented (e.g., caliber, consistency, color, size) in addition to any interventions the patient may have utilized to assist the process (e.g., digital extraction, enema). During the history, the presence of any alarm symptoms, including weight loss, anemia, family history of colon cancer, recalcitrant constipation, hematochezia, and guaiac positive stool, in any patient population requires an immediate referral to a gastroenterologist.

Upon inspection, nonfocal abdominal distention or masses may indicate the presence of stool in the colon or abdominal wall hernias. This is important to note as abdominal wall hernias have the potential for impairing the intra-abdominal pressure needed for defecation. Auscultation may reveal reduced bowel sounds or borborygmi. Reduced bowel sounds can be correlated to a reduction in the haustral segmentation of the colon that propels stool. As previously discussed, borborygmi is noted proximal to an obstruction. Palpation may uncover a mass in the descending colon consistent with fecal impaction. Likewise, dullness appreciated over the left lower abdominal quadrant with percussion can also indicate stool impaction.

Management

Normal transit constipation should be suspected in patients who present with complaints of difficulty emptying their bowel in the setting of normal stool frequency. Patients may describe stool as hard, and experience generalized abdominal discomfort and bloating. Initial management should focus on dietary modifications and increased water intake as this is typically adequate to address symptoms. Dietary changes are aimed at gradually increasing fiber intake to 25 grams to 35 grams over a 2-week period to reduce unpleasant side effects, such as excess flatulence. Consulting a licensed nutritionist for more in-depth patient education can improve compliance. In terms of water intake, the goal is generally 1.5 liters to 2 liters a day. If an acceptable response is not achieved, a trial of 17 grams of polyethylene glycol once daily is indicated. The next step would be a referral to a gastroenterologist.

Slow transit constipation predominantly affects young females and is associated with fewer than one bowel movement weekly. Similarly to normal transit constipation, patients who suffer from this also complain of abdominal discomfort and bloating; however, they also commonly report the lack of an urge to defecate. The patient interview is often sufficient to differentiate between the two pathologies; however, pelvic floor dysfunction must be ruled out to confirm the diagnosis. Typically, patients with slow transit constipation do not respond to dietary changes or increased fluid intake, which have been shown to exacerbate symptoms of chronic constipation in some individuals.[18] Therefore, laxatives are normally recommended for patients with slow transit constipation. There are many types of laxatives (Table 22.7) to choose from; unfortunately, research has demonstrated pronounced variability in an individual's response.[19] As such, it is recommended that patients experiment to find the laxative or combination of laxatives that best meet their needs.[18] If laxative treatment fails, other treatment modalities may be advised through consultation with a specialist.

Pelvic floor dysfunction must be assessed with a digital rectal examination. The presence of soft stool in the rectal vault without other pathologic findings or symptoms (e.g., rectal wall mass, pain) in addition to an abnormal relaxation of the anal sphincter in response to straining is highly indicative of pelvic floor dysfunction. Pharmacologic treatment is not effective in this disorder; rather, treatment is focused on a biofeedback protocol, which has been demonstrated to be the most effective modality.[20] During biofeedback, patients are trained how to contract and relax the muscles of the pelvic floor by a licensed therapist.

SPECIAL CONSIDERATIONS FOR ADOLESCENTS TO YOUNG ADULTS

Constipation in most adolescents does not have an identifiable organic cause; rather, it is due to a learned pathologic behavioral adaptation or poor dietary intake. Constipation, common among children, often can have a negative effect on quality of life that frequently persists into adulthood. In adolescents, constipation is often functional related to painful bowel movement (BM) or other psychosocial factors (e.g., not wanting to have a BM at school) that make the person voluntarily hold the stool or poor diet. Painful defecation is the most prominent cause of constipation in adolescents.[21] In an attempt to prevent pain, the person may delay their defecation by contracting their external sphincter and gluteal muscles. If protracted,

Table 22.7: Types of Laxatives

Medications	Onset	Adverse Effects
Bulk forming Psyllium (e.g., Metamucil) Polycarbophil (e.g., FiberCon) Methylcellulose (e.g., Citrucel)	12–72 hours	Low incidence of bloating, abdominal distention
Osmotic Polyethylene glycol Lactulose Sorbitol Magnesium citrate Magnesium hydroxide	30 minutes–48 hours	Bloating, cramping, nausea. Magnesium-containing products can elevate serum magnesium, causing lethargy, hypotension, respiratory depression
Surfactants Docusate sodium	24–48 hours	None noted
Stimulants Sennosides Bisacodyl	6–12 hours	Abdominal pain, diarrhea
Chloride channel activating Lubiprostone	24 hours	Nausea
Peripheral mu-opioid antagonists Methylnaltrexone Naloxegol	30–60 minutes	Diarrhea, abdominal pain
Other Linaclotide	N/A	Diarrhea

this can lead to fecal impaction and subsequent incontinence. Additionally, stressful events can lead to negative behavioral responses that can manifest as constipation.

During the assessment, asking about recent stressors, previous and active therapies, the presence of withholding behaviors, pain or bleeding with BM, abdominal pain, fecal incontinence, and other systemic symptoms is important. Physical assessment should consider growth parameters, abdominal examination, and anorectum examination to assess for perianal sensation, anal tone, rectum size, anal wink, and amount and consistency of stool in the rectum. An adolescent who has a family history of colon cancer and has pain, weight loss, and diarrhea should have a test for occult blood. The first step to treatment for functional constipation is to provide education (www.gikids.org). Treating constipation in adolescents should focus on parent education, dietary adjustments, laxative use, and behavior modification. Dietary changes with increased fluid and increased fiber may help, as well as including probiotics.[22]

Quality and Safety Alerts

- Further evaluation is indicated for adolescents with red flags (e.g., abdominal distension, intermittent diarrhea and explosive stools, tight anal sphincter, occult blood in stool, extraintestinal symptoms like fever, vomiting) or no response to conventional treatment.
- Referral to a pediatric gastroenterologist may be needed when there are red flags for organic disease to consider further diagnostic testing and other treatments.

SPECIAL CONSIDERATIONS FOR OLDER ADULTS

Constipation is far more prevalent in the older adult population. However, it is not a normal consequence of aging and often proves more difficult to treat as the cause is commonly multifactorial. The first step in recommending a treatment protocol is taking a detailed medication and disease history. There are innumerable diseases and medications (Table 22.8) that contribute to reduced bowel motility, impaired physical function, and altered consciousness that can result in constipation. It may not always be possible to stop certain medications or adequately treat the underlying cause in many older adults. To illustrate, a patient with metastatic bone cancer and intractable pain may have to remain on chronic opioid therapy irrespective of the side effects. In this patient, the use of a peripherally acting mu-opioid antagonist, such as methylnaltrexone, may be the best treatment option.

Managing constipation in older adults should be focused on symptom improvement rather than diagnosis. As in the adult population, the initial treatment of constipation should consist of dietary modifications, increased fluid intake, and laxative use to ameliorate symptoms once all secondary causes have been investigated. Biofeedback may also be beneficial in reducing constipation in older adults with pelvic floor dysfunction with the cognitive and physical capacity to learn. Additionally, scheduled defecation following a meal can take advantage of the gastrocolic reflex. Exercise, on the other hand, has not been shown to improve constipation in older adults.[23]

Table 22.8: Medications Associated With Constipation

Class	Common Medications
NSAIDs	Ibuprofen, naproxen, meloxicam
Anticholinergics	Oxybutynin, atropine, benztropine, ipratropium, scopolamine, tolterodine
Antihistamines	Cyproheptadine, chlorphenamine, diphenhydramine, hydroxyzine, fexofenadine, loratadine, meclizine, promethazine
Antidepressants	Amitriptyline, imipramine, doxepin, mirtazapine, desipramine, fluoxetine
Iron supplements	Ferrous sulfate, ferrous gluconate
Opioids	Morphine, oxycodone, hydrocodone, codeine, Dilaudid
Antihypertensives	Clonidine, verapamil, diltiazem
Diuretics	Furosemide, bumetanide, torsemide, HCTZ
Antacids	Sucralfate, aluminum hydroxide (Maalox, Mylanta, Rolaids)
Other	Levodopa, antiepileptics

PEPTIC ULCER DISEASE

Etiology and Pathophysiology

PUD affects the stomach and proximal portion of the small intestine known as the duodenum. The primary cause of PUD is *Helicobacter pylori*. *H. pylori* disrupts the mucosal barrier protecting the gastric epithelial cells and produces cytotoxic factors including ammonia and proteases, such as vacuolating cytotoxin A. As their name suggests, cytotoxic agents cause cellular damage resulting in the ulceration that defines PUD. Other common contributing factors include nonsteroidal anti-inflammatory drugs (NSAIDs) and tobacco. NSAIDs contribute to PUD through direct cytotoxic damage and inhibition of the prostaglandin-dependent mucosal barrier. Tobacco is thought to promote PUD by potentiating the toxic effect of *H. pylori* and stimulating the production of pepsinogen, the precursor to the proteolytic enzyme pepsin.

Risk Factors

Risk factors for PUD include *H. pylori* infection, stress, consumption of spicy foods, alcohol intake, smoking, and medications (e.g., corticosteroids, NSAIDs, bisphosphanates).

🏠 Quality and Safety Alerts

- Older adults may take NSAIDs for pain and these can lead to PUD or hospitalization related to upper GI bleed.
  - The person may not have pain related to PUD until the bleed occurs.
- If NSAIDs are used, it should only be for short term.

Approach to Diagnosis

During the interview, the NP must specifically inquire about tobacco use and NSAID ingestion. Referred pain to the epigastrium is the predominant symptom and is described as having a "gnawing" and "burning" quality. Gastric ulcer pain tends to occur shortly after eating, whereas duodenal ulcer pain occurs 2 to 3 hours following a meal and may awaken the patient during sleep. Belching, bloating, nausea, anorexia, weight loss, and fatigue may also be noted in PUD. The reporting of recurrent vomiting and abdominal distention in the presence of dehydration and generalized atrophy should raise the suspicion for a GOO from an ulcer in the distal portion of the stomach, termed the pylorus.

The physical examination is often benign in PUD. Observation may reveal abdominal distention or, in rare cases, visible peristalsis in the stomach may be consistent with a GOO from a pyloric ulceration. Auscultation and percussion will be unremarkable unless GOO is present. With a GOO, there can be dullness to percussion and a succussion splash with auscultation. A succussion splash reflects fluid in the obstructed stomach. Palpation, under normal circumstances, may reveal mild epigastric tenderness.

According to Hammer et al.[24] prompt endoscopic evaluation is recommended in suspected cases of PUD in patients older than 55 and all individuals with alarm symptoms (e.g., weight loss, anemia, hemoptysis, guaiac positive stools, early satiety, dysphagia).

The presence of active *H. pylori* infection should be confirmed prior to the initiation of treatment. This can be accomplished through several methods, including urea breath tests, GI tract biopsy with rapid urease testing, and stool antigen testing. Serologic testing should be avoided as it detects antibodies to *H. pylori* and does not confirm active infection.

Management

Eradication of *H. pylori*, acid suppression, and the cessation of NSAIDs normally lead to the successful resolution of PUD. In cases of refractory PUD, an upper endoscopy should be done to confirm the diagnosis and achieve hemostasis.

First-line pharmacologic treatment of *H. pylori* consists of a PPI-based triple therapy of amoxicillin and clarithromycin or clarithromycin and metronidazole for patients allergic to penicillin for 10 to 14 days. For treatment-resistant cases, a four-drug regimen of a PPI, bismuth subsalicylate, tetracycline, and metronidazole over 10 days is recommended. Confirming *H. pylori* eradication 2 to 4 weeks following the cessation of treatment is suggested via stool antigen or UBT. Endoscopic evaluation is appropriate if confirmatory testing reveals persistent *H. pylori* infection.

🏠 Quality and Safety Alerts

- Risk of long-term use of PPI
- Acquired enteric infections such as *C. difficile*

Uncertain mechanism but postulated that related to long-term suppression of gastric acid secretion with PPT may alter colonic microbiome to decrease colonization resistance or other normal barriers to *C. difficile* proliferation

Evidence supports other risks:
- Dementia
- Pneumonia
- Acute kidney disease related to acute interstitial nephritis

- Micronutrient deficiencies (magnesium, calcium, vitamin B12)

Despite these risks, the overall quality of evidence regarding adverse effects of long-term use of PPIs is low to very low. Most of the evidence is based on observational studies. The NP must be cautious about drawing a broad conclusion based on the current evidence. PPIs have a strong positive impact on patient outcomes, so when prescribing, recommend patients have a clear indication, avoid broad off-label use, and have a prudent time-limited endpoint of prescription.

Source: Jaynes M, Kumar AB. The risks of long-term use of proton pump inhibitors: a critical review. *Ther Adv Drug Saf*. 2019;10:1-13. doi:10.1177/2042098618809927

IRRITABLE BOWEL SYNDROME

Etiology and Pathophysiology

The diagnosis of IBS (Table 22.9) is based on the presence of abdominal pain and changes in the stool characteristics without identifiable pathology.[17] IBS is twice as prevalent in females, with symptoms generally manifesting in young adults. Advanced age seems to confer a reduction in susceptibility to developing IBS. There are currently no reliable biomarkers or radiologic tests to confirm the diagnosis. IBS is a diagnosis of exclusion that occurs along a spectrum of symptoms ranging from diarrhea to constipation.

Risk Factors

Factors that increase the tendency for developing IBS include female gender, mental illness (e.g., depression, anxiety), personal history of abuse, and family history.

Approach to Diagnosis

Diagnosing IBS requires multiple invasive and noninvasive tests aimed at ruling out other intestinal conditions that have similar symptoms. Consultation with a gastroenterologist is required to confirm IBS. This is beyond the scope of this text. The focus of care for primary care providers in collaboration with GI specialists is to monitor symptoms and develop a person-centered plan of care. It is important to communicate with other providers and the patient to determine the effectiveness of treatments and evaluate for alarming symptoms that need immediate attention.

Management

General Treatment of Irritable Bowel Syndrome

IBS is categorized according to the prevailing symptoms as IBS with diarrhea (IBS-D), IBS with constipation (IBS-C), and mixed type (IBS-M).[25] Treatment is focused on managing the GI and non-GI-related symptoms of IBS

Table 22.9: ROME IV Diagnostic Criteria for Irritable Bowel Syndrome

Chronic and recurrent abdominal pain and/or altered bowel habits for at least 6 months and must have two or more of the following associated with recurrent abdominal pain 1 day/week or more in last 3 months: • related to defecation (increasing or improving pain) • associated with a change in stool frequency • associated with a change in stool form (appearance)
Patients with the following symptoms should be evaluated clinically for other diagnoses even though IBS is present: • signs or symptoms of GI bleed • unexplained iron deficiency anemia • unintentional weight loss • palpable abdominal mass or lymphadenopathy on examination • family history of colon cancer and have not had age-appropriate colon cancer screening • onset of symptoms age 50 years or more and have not had age-appropriate colon cancer screening • sudden or acute onset of new change in bowel habit

Must have the following:
• abdominal pain 4 days or more per month associated with one or more of the following:
  – related to defecation
  – a change in frequency of stool
  – a change in form (appearance of stool)
• in children with constipation, the pain does not resolve with resolution of the constipation (children in whom the pain resolves have functional constipation, not IBS)
• after appropriate evaluation, the symptoms cannot be fully explained by another medical condition

Source: Rome Foundation. Rome IV criteria. https://theromefoundation.org

to maximize quality of life. Dietary measures to gradually increase fiber intake are initially recommended despite the paucity of research to validate this.[25] Polycarbophil- and methylcellulose-containing fiber supplements are generally better tolerated than psyllium compounds because they produce less gas. Avoiding lactose, gas-producing foods (e.g., legumes, cruciferous vegetables, prunes, raisins, bananas), caffeine, and gluten may also reduce symptoms of IBS. Individuals should generally be asked to keep a detailed food diary to track the association of foods with their symptoms so that dietary plans can be customized based on tolerance. A recent review on the efficacy of probiotics with the endpoints of reducing pain or global symptoms of IBS demonstrated statistically significant outcomes; however, the most beneficial probiotics could not be determined, limiting their recommendation.[26]

Treatment of Irritable Bowel Syndrome With Constipation

Pharmacologic therapies for IBS are directed at treating the symptoms of the specific subtypes of IBS. Linaclotide (Linzess) and lubiprostone (Amitiza) are designed to treat IBS-C by attracting water into the bowel and promoting motility. Previously, tegaserod (Zelnorm) was available for managing constipation in IBS through direct stimulation of

enteric receptors. However, in 2007, the Food and Drug Administration (FDA) had the drug removed from the market over concerns regarding the risk of cardiotoxicity. Presently, tegaserod is only approved for use in refractory cases of constipation with prior authorization from the FDA.

Treatment of Irritable Bowel Syndrome With Diarrhea

Eluxadoline (Viberzi) is a mixed opioid agonist and antagonist used to reduce episodes of diarrhea in IBS without potentiating constipation. Dicyclomine and hyoscyamine are anticholinergic agents used to inhibit spasms of the viscera associated with IBS-D. Antidiarrheals, such as Lomotil and loperamide, are also used in IBS-D; however, both agents work by impairing GI motility and can promote constipation. Rifaximin (Xifaxan) is a relatively new agent in the treatment of IBS-D. Rifaximin is a derivative of the antibiotic rifampin and is believed to exert its clinical effect by degrading colonic bacteria that produce gas.

Psychotropics in the Treatment of Irritable Bowel Syndrome

Tricyclic antidepressants (TCAs) imipramine and amitriptyline are used off label to treat IBS. Both agents have shown significant efficacy in the treatment of IBS through their modulation of mood and analgesia.[25] Unfortunately, the use of TCAs in older adults is contraindicated due to their potent anticholinergic side effects, such as dizziness, confusion, and tachycardia.

CHOLELITHIASIS

Etiology and Pathophysiology

Cholelithiasis is the formation of gallstones in the gallbladder. Women have nearly double the risk of developing gallstones. The majority of gallstones diagnosed in the United States are cholesterol stones. Cholesterol stones are precipitated by excess cholesterol secretion due to obesity, estrogens, rapid weight loss, and genetic predisposition. Women in their forties also experience an increased risk for cholelithiasis due to the rapid fluctuations in estrogen levels that occur as part of the normal age-related process of menopause. Despite the relatively common prevalence of cholelithiasis, 80% of gallstones remain asymptomatic. Symptoms of cholelithiasis only occur when the normal function of the gallbladder is affected.

Risk Factors

Risk factors for cholelithiasis include obesity, female gender, age older than 40 years, pregnancy, diabetes, estrogen therapy, sedentary lifestyle, and rapid weight loss.

Approach to Diagnosis

In suspected cases of cholelithiasis, the interview should focus on the characteristics of the pain which are essential for distinguishing biliary colic from more serious conditions. Biliary colic is postprandial pain in the right upper quadrant or epigastric area of the abdomen that may radiate to the right scapula. The pain gradually intensifies over 20 minutes and then steadily declines over a 5-hour span. Biliary colic is due to a paroxysmal obstruction in the cystic duct from a gallstone. The pain is unpredictable as it only occurs when gallbladder function is interrupted. The pain is not alleviated by changes in body position, bowel movements, vomiting, or medications. Bloating, indigestion, and belching may also be reported in biliary colic. The physical examination is unremarkable in biliary colic. There are no peritoneal signs of irritation, such as rebound tenderness or guarding. Confirming cholelithiasis often requires an ultrasound of the gallbladder.

Management

The primary treatment for symptomatic cholelithiasis is a cholecystectomy, surgical removal of the gallbladder. However, in specific cases of biliary colic, such as when surgery poses a high risk, other forms of medical management may be indicated.

Other treatments for symptomatic cholelithiasis include bile salt therapy, direct solvent dissolution, and lithotripsy. Bile salt therapy involves the administration of oral ursodeoxycholic acid for a period of 6 to 18 months to dissolve gallstones. Ursodeoxycholic acid exerts its effect by reducing the cholesterol saturation of bile. However, the treatment is only effective for dissolving cholesterol stones smaller than 15 mm and carries a recurrence rate of 25% within 5 years.[27]

Direct solvent dissolution therapy involves the introduction of a solvent in the gallbladder through a percutaneously placed catheter. Despite the efficacy of the procedure, solvent dissolution therapy has fallen out of favor due to its technical complexity, elevated risk of solvent toxicity, and high rate of stone recurrence.[28] Lithotripsy, the extracorporeal transmission of ultrasound waves through the body to fragment gallstones, is also limited. As Paumgartner and Sauter[29] have indicated, this treatment modality is generally considered ineffective due to the early and high rates of stone recurrence.

SPECIAL CONSIDERATIONS FOR BARIATRICS

While dietary modifications have not been demonstrated to alter the normal progression of cholelithiasis, it is of value to note that obese patients who aggressively pursue weight loss or bariatric surgery are at an elevated risk for cholelithiasis. Therefore, it is recommended that these patients be given 600 mg of ursodeoxycholic acid daily for the prevention of gallstone formation.[30]

SPECIAL CONSIDERATIONS FOR ADOLESCENTS TO YOUNG ADULTS

Contrary to cholelithiasis in adults, gallstones in adolescents are predominantly formed from a calcium salt of unconjugated bilirubin called calcium bilirubinate. The composition of their gallstones is related to the dominant etiologies, hemolytic and hepatobiliary disorders. Hemolysis releases excess unconjugated bilirubin from the destruction of erythrocytes into the circulation, causing the supersaturation of bile with calcium bilirubinate. In many hepatobiliary disorders, the liver cannot conjugate bilirubin efficiently, which also leads to an elevation in unconjugated bilirubin levels.

The presentation and physical examination findings of cholelithiasis in adolescents are identical to those encountered in adults. In terms of treatment, laparoscopic cholecystectomy is the gold standard for treating symptomatic cholelithiasis in pediatrics.[31]

To conclude this chapter, dysphagia and colorectal cancer (CRC) screening recommendations are reviewed.

DYSPHAGIA

Etiology

Dysphagia is difficulty swallowing, irrespective of pain. Annually, dysphagia affects 1 in 25 adults in the United States.[32] During the interview, dysphagia should initially be classified as oropharyngeal or esophageal and then further categorized as neuromuscular or obstructive in etiology based on the location and nature of symptoms in addition to any associated symptoms and pertinent medical history. This classification schema allows the accurate identification of the underlying etiology of dysphagia in more than 80% of cases.[33]

Pathophysiology

The oropharyngeal phase of swallowing is composed of the voluntary movement of food from the oral cavity to the pharynx using the tongue, followed by involuntary, coordinated muscular contractions that propel food into the esophagus. Therefore, trouble initiating a swallow, coughing, choking, nasal reflux, and drooling all point to an oropharyngeal disorder. In the esophageal phase, involuntary muscular contractions of the esophagus move food toward the stomach. Symptoms of esophageal dysphagia include the sensation of food being caught in the throat or chest, odynophagia, heartburn, and chest pain.

Oropharyngeal dysphagia is the most common form of dysphagia due to strokes. Other prevalent neuromuscular causes of oropharyngeal dysphagia include Parkinson's disease, amyotrophic lateral sclerosis, multiple sclerosis, and tumors of the brainstem. Mechanical and obstructive causes of oropharyngeal dysphagia include pharyngeal diverticulum, poor dentition, tumors, pharyngeal stenosis, thyromegaly, and diseases of the cervical spine.

The most common conditions associated with esophageal dysphagia are strictures, neoplasms, webs and rings, achalasia, scleroderma, and diffuse esophageal spasms (DES).

Risk Factors

Factors associated with dysphagia include older age, GERD, and the presence of neurologic disorders (e.g., Parkinson's disease, stroke).

Approach to Diagnosis

The key to diagnosing dysphagia is the symptoms. The NP should inquire about the nature of the dysphagia. When does it occur? Do you have difficulty swallowing? Difficulty swallowing indicates an oropharyngeal cause. Do you have difficulty swallowing solids, liquids, or both? Difficulty swallowing liquids indicates a neuromuscular etiology as muscular coordination is impaired, resulting in difficulty managing the thin consistency of the liquid, while difficulty swallowing solids normally occurs with strictures or obstructive processes that narrow the lumen of the pharynx or esophagus. Impaired swallowing of liquids and solids primarily occurs in neuromuscular diseases; however, a progressive obstructive process will eventually lead to dysphagia with liquids and solids that is associated with vomiting. Is the dysphagia intermittent or progressive? Intermittent dysphagia points to a motility disturbance from a neurologic cause, whereas unremitting, progressive episodes of dysphagia point to an obstructive cause. For example, recurrent dysphagia with solids during swallowing suggests an obstructive oropharyngeal dysphagia.

In esophageal causes of dysphagia, patients will report symptoms of food getting stuck in their throat, heartburn, odynophagia (painful swallowing), and chest pain. To illustrate, DES, a neuromuscular esophageal dysphagia, is characterized by uncoordinated muscular contractions in the esophagus causing pain and dysphagia. In achalasia, the lower esophageal sphincter fails to relax, leading to the accumulation of food and liquid in the esophagus, which leads to distal esophageal enlargement and symptoms of chest pain with regurgitation. In contrast, coughing and choking are more prevalent with oropharyngeal dysphagia as the passage of food is being impaired superior to the esophagus in the pharynx, where these symptoms are normally elicited.

The physical examination in dysphagia is focused on identifying diseases that can cause dysphagia. For example, the presence of hemiparesis may indicate the history of a stroke. Tremors and bradykinesia are consistent with Parkinson's disease. Palpation of an enlarged thyroid may point to an obstructive oropharyngeal dysphagia with unremitting symptoms. Calcinosis, sclerodactyly, and telangiectasias occur in scleroderma, which is a neuromuscular cause of esophageal dysphagia.

In neuromuscular causes of dysphagia, speech therapy is consulted to perform a modified barium swallow to confirm the disorder and assess the severity. If the barium swallow is inconclusive, in suspected cases of achalasia, scleroderma, and DES, esophageal manometry can be performed to measure the pressure in the esophagus in response to swallowing. Upper endoscopy is indicated for any potential mechanical or obstructive cause of dysphagia.

Management

The treatment of dysphagia is contingent upon the cause. Dysphagia related to movement disorders, such as Parkinson's disease and myasthenia gravis, is managed with pharmacologic therapy. In other degenerative neurologic diseases, such as stroke, the risk of aspiration is assessed with a modified barium swallow study. In appropriate candidates, an oral rehabilitative treatment plan is developed by a speech therapist. Obstructive and mechanical disorders causing dysphagia are treated with resection, pneumatic dilatation, and chemotherapy based on the pathology. Achalasia and DES may also be treated with myotomy, the surgical excision of the lower esophageal sphincter. Referral to a gastroenterologist for comanagement of the patient is important.

SPECIAL CONSIDERATIONS FOR ADOLESCENTS TO YOUNG ADULTS

Age-specific causes of dysphagia in adolescents include prematurity, cerebral palsy, and congenital malformations. Management of pediatric dysphagia requires a multidisciplinary approach focused on maintaining optimal nutritional status in the context of safe feeding strategies over oral feeding.[34]

SPECIAL CONSIDERATIONS FOR OLDER ADULTS

Esophageal dysphagia with progressive, obstructive symptoms in adults older than age 65 is suspicious for malignancy and should prompt an immediate referral for an upper endoscopy. It is important to consider benefit versus risk of tube feeding in older adults with dysphagia. The risk for aspiration pneumonia may outweigh the benefit.

COLORECTAL CANCER SCREENING

The preferred method for CRC screening in average-risk non–African American individuals is a colonoscopy every 10 years starting at age 45 (Box 22.2). African Americans should begin CRC screening at the age of 45. Individuals with a first-degree relative with CRC before the age of 60 or more than one first-degree relative with CRC should undergo a screening colonoscopy every 5 years beginning at the age of 40.[35]

Box 22.2: American Cancer Society Recommendations for Colorectal Cancer Screening

- Average risk of CRC start screening at age 45
  - Personal history of CRC or certain types of polyps
  - A family history of CRC
  - A personal history of inflammatory bowel disease (ulcerative colitis or Crohn's disease diagnosed)
  - A confirmed or suspected hereditary CRC syndrome such as familial adenomatous polyposis or Lynch syndrome (hereditary nonpolyposis colon cancer)
  - A personal history of getting radiation to the abdomen or pelvis to treat prior cancer
- Adults in good health and life expectancy of more than 10 years should continue regular CRC screening through age 75.

- In adults 76 to 85, the decision to screen should be based on the person's preferences, life expectancy, overall health, and prior screening history.
- Adults over age 85 should no longer get cancer screening.

Source: American Cancer Society. American Cancer Society guideline for colorectal cancer screening. Updated November 17, 2020. https://www.cancer.org/cancer/colon-rectal-cancer/detection-diagnosis-staging/acs-recommendations.html

Patient Education

The educational strategies for GI disorders are complementary to conventional medical therapies and must utilize health literacy measures (eg, teach-back, patient-centric educational materials, information technology) to promote meaningful patient engagement. Patient education should encourage lifestyle modifications, such as the consumption of a well-balanced diet and avoidance of irritating foods including fried foods, spicy foods, acidic foods (e.g., citrus, tomatoes), garlic, onions, chocolate, and large meals. Patient education should also focus on weight loss, exercise, smoking cessation, alcohol reduction, maintaining a diet high in fiber (e.g., vegetables, beans, whole grains) and fluid intake, and developing a daily bowel routine.

GASTROINTESTINAL EMERGENCIES

- Acute onset, severe abdominal pain that is commonly associated with meals, and a benign physical examination may indicate intestinal ischemia.
- Intermittent, cramping abdominal pain accompanied by anorexia, constipation, abdominal distention, and vomiting is suspicious for bowel obstruction.
- Peritonitis should be suspected with a dull abdominal ache that rapidly progresses to severe abdominal pain that is worsened by movement and accompanied by chills, fevers, difficulty passing gas, and vomiting.

CLINICAL PEARLS

- *H. pylori* testing can be false-negative in the setting of antibiotic use and PPI therapy.
- Slow transit constipation should be treated with laxatives.
- The most common cause of acute gastroenteritis is norovirus.
- Cholelithiasis is often preceded by episodes of biliary colic.
- The abdominal pain associated with IBS improves following defecation.

CASE STUDY

Chief Complaint: Ms. A, a 63-year-old female, presents with complaints of "difficulty swallowing."

History of Present Illness: Ms. A states that her symptoms began 5 months ago and have progressively worsened with intermittent solid food dysphagia.

Review of Systems: Ms. A reports dysphagia to solids. She denies dysphagia with ingestion of liquids, nasal regurgitation, abdominal pain, weight loss, voice changes, aspiration, or choking episodes.

Past Medical History: Her medical history was notable for hypertension, type 2 diabetes mellitus, and GERD. Her current medications include metformin, amlodipine, omeprazole, glipizide, and TUMS as needed for recurrent reflux symptoms.

Social History: Ms. A is a retired secretary with a remote history of alcohol and tobacco use but has quit using both substances more than 15 years ago.

Physical Examination Findings: Neurologic examination reveals no muscle fatigability, vision issues, or cranial nerve pathologies. She is able to lift her arms above her head and rise from a seated position without difficulty. She has no difficulty swallowing water. The remainder of her examination was also unremarkable. She is afebrile with a blood pressure of 137/65 and a body mass index (BMI) of 30.5 kg/m2. Results of laboratory studies, including complete blood cell count, electrolyte panel, thyroid-stimulating hormone level, and evaluation of kidney function, was unremarkable.

Case Study Questions

1. What are the differential diagnoses?
2. Which diagnosis is most likely based on the physical examination and ROS?
3. What test is indicated to confirm the diagnosis?

Conclusion: Ms. A was referred to gastroenterology for esophagogastroduodenoscopy (EGD) and diagnosed with a benign esophageal stricture. The stricture was successfully treated with endoscopic balloon dilation. The stricture is related to long-standing GERD with recurrent esophageal inflammation and resulting scarring and narrowing over time.

In this case, patient education plays a vital role in reducing the incidence of GERD and should be developed using universal precautions for health literacy. Ms. A needs to be educated on behavioral modifications including dietary changes (e.g., avoidance of irritating foods and weight loss), exercise, and positioning following meals to reduce further sequela of GERD.

CONCLUSION

This chapter provided an overview of the most common GI disorders NPs will see in primary care. It is important to have the knowledge and skills to identify common disorders that can be managed by primary care providers and when to refer to gastroenterology. Many conditions can be managed in primary care but differentiating between urgent and nonurgent need for care is essential. This includes performing a history and physical examination on your patient and engaging in shared clinical decision-making with the patient and GI specialist; this may involve contacting the specialist to discuss the case to achieve the best outcomes for the patient.

REFERENCES

References for this chapter are online and available at https://connect.springerpub.com/content/book/978-0 -8261-8414-6/part/part01/toc-part/ch22.

CHAPTER 23

Common Kidney Disorders Encountered in the Primary Care Setting

Debra J. Hain and Dianne Sandy

LEARNING OBJECTIVES

At the conclusion of this chapter, the learner will be able to:

➤ Review screening and assessment of chronic kidney disease (CKD).

➤ Explore appropriate diagnostic testing for CKD and associated comorbidities.

➤ Discuss evidence-based treatment options.

➤ Explain alternative, holistic approaches to treatment of CKD.

➤ Summarize how culture, ethnicity, and race play a unique role on the pathophysiology and treatment of CKD.

INTRODUCTION

Chronic kidney disease (CKD) is a public health problem that affects many Americans. Nurse practitioners (NPs) will see patients in primary care who are at risk of CKD or have CKD. It is important that NPs gain knowledge and skills to identify and treat those with CKD and engage in a collaborative relationship with nephrology professionals to achieve the best patient health outcomes. This chapter provides an overview of epidemiologic data, the identification and treatment of CKD, and the most common causes of CKD, which are diabetes and hypertension. We also present a brief overview of chronic glomerulosclerosis, membranous nephropathy, and PKD. See Box 23.1 for relevant terms that may appear throughout the chapter.

OVERVIEW OF THE SYSTEM

The kidneys are vascular organs that are responsible for homeostasis of the body. The primary functions are

▪ maintenance of normal body fluid composition
  • erythropoietin
▪ excretion of waste products of metabolism and elimination of drugs and toxins
▪ regulation of blood pressure (BP)
▪ production of hormones
  • erythropoietin
  • activation of vitamin D, the final hydroxylation of vitamin D to its active form, 1,25 dihydroxy vitamin D

The renal system comprises the kidneys, ureters, bladder, and urethra (see Figure 23.1), but this chapter presents information about the kidneys only. For more information about the ureters, bladder and urethra, see Chapter 24. The kidney is a highly vascularized organ with macroscopic and microscopic anatomy.

Normal Anatomy and Physiology

The kidneys are located along the posterior abdominal wall of the retroperitoneum; each weighs about 150 g and is about 11 to 12 cm in length. The kidneys are divided into two regions: an outer cortex and an inner medulla. The cortex and medulla contain the basic functioning units of the kidney, the nephron, vasculature, nerves, and lymphatic vessels (see Figure 23.2b). Each kidney has about 1 million nephrons. The cortex has a granular appearance and the glomeruli, proximal tubule, distal tubule, cortical collecting tubules, and adjacent peritubular capillaries are located here. The medulla contains triangular wedges

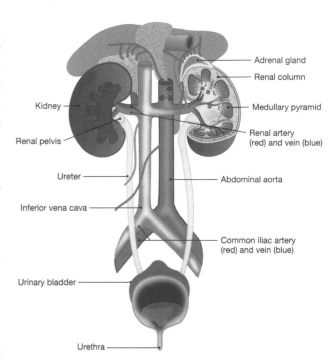

Figure 23.1: Renal (urinary) system

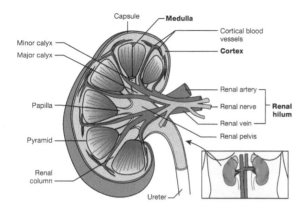

Figure 23.2a: Anatomy of the kidney

Source: Tkacs NC, Herrmann LL, Johnson RL. *Advanced Physiology and Pathophysiology: Essentials for Clinical Practice.* Springer Publishing Company; 2021.

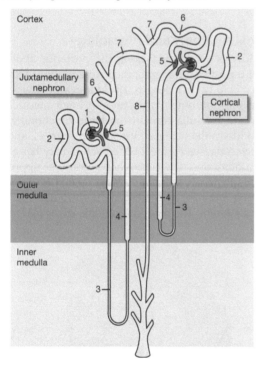

Figure 23.2b: Nephron structure

Cortical nephrons make up 85% of the nephrons of the kidney and much of the cortical volume. Juxtamedullary nephrons have long loops of Henle that descend deep within the renal medulla, making a hairpin turn before ascending back to the glomerular region: (1) Glomerulus; (2) proximal tubule; (3) loop of Henle, thin descending and ascending limbs; (4) thick ascending limb of Henle's loop; (5) macula densa of the juxtaglomerular apparatus; (6) distal tubule; (7) connecting tubule; (8) collecting duct.

Source: Tkacs NC, Herrmann LL, Johnson RL. *Advanced Physiology and Pathophysiology: Essentials for Clinical Practice.* Springer Publishing Company; 2021.

Box 23.1: Relevant Terms

Acute kidney injury (AKI): Formerly known as acute renal failure. AKI is characterized as a sudden decline in kidney function leading to uremia and disturbances in electrolytes and fluid balance. AKI may require dialysis temporarily for a time, but the patient is often expected to recover to baseline kidney function. During this time the patient is vulnerable and requires careful monitoring by the nephrology team (e.g., nephrologist, nephrology nurse practitioner) and primary care healthcare providers.

Antidiuretic hormone (ADH): Vasopressin in high plasm concentrations leads to renal vessel vasoconstriction. When present, renal blood flow and GFR decrease. ADH triggers the production of prostaglandins, and they will have their own vasoconstrictive effects, ADH is produced in hypovolemic states, and the production increases when serum osmolality and/or extracellular volume is low.

Bone and mineral metabolism disorders: Disorders involving problems with hormonal regulation of the formation and turnover of the bone. The risk of this disorder increases as kidney function declines. The disorder includes elevated phosphorus, abnormal calcium levels, vitamin D deficiency, and elevated PTH.

Excretion: Process of eliminating unnecessary substances from the body through the urine.

Glomerular filtration rate (GFR): The process by which the kidney filters the blood, removing uremic waste products and fluids. It is usually estimated using a mathematical formula. "Normal" is about 125 mL/min but declines with age even in the absence of kidney disease.

Renin-angiotensin mechanism: Critical regulator of intrarenal blood flow. The overall purpose is to maintain perfusion to vital organs when hypovolemia is present, an effect mediated by peripheral and intrarenal vasoconstriction (see Figure 23.3).

Tubular reabsorption: Movement of fluid and solutes from the tubular system into the peritubular capillaries.

Tubular secretion: Movement of solutes from the peritubular capillaries into the tubular system.

Urine protein to creatinine ratio (UPCR): Ratio of urinary protein to creatinine used to quantify the amount of excreted protein and to calculate proteinuria.

---

that have a striped appearance. The wedges are pyramids formed by the loop of Henle, medullary collecting tubules, and vasa recta. The papilla (the tapered end of the pyramid) directs urine to the major and minor calyces, which then go through the urinary system (see Chapter 24).

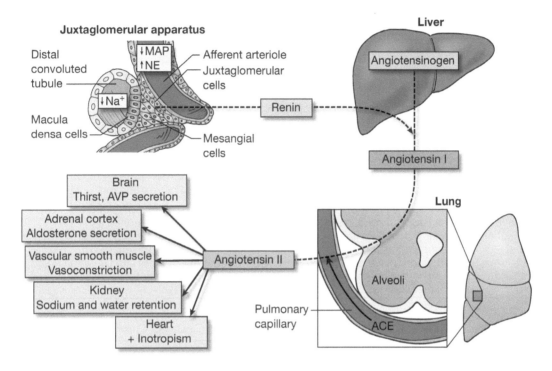

Figure 23.3: The renin-angiotensin-aldosterone system (RAAS)

Source: Tkacs NC, Herrmann LL, Johnson RL. *Advanced Physiology and Pathophysiology: Essentials for Clinical Practice.* Springer Publishing Company; 2021.

The nephron (see Figure 23.2b) is the functioning unit of the kidney, and there are two types of nephrons: cortical (85%) and juxtamedullary (15%). The glomerulus is a network of capillaries surrounded by Bowman's capsule and is responsible for selective ultrafiltration of the plasma and clearance of small molecules. The glomerulus has three layers: the endothelium, the basement membrane, and the epithelial.

The components of the tubular system, the proximal tubule, the loop of Henle, the distal tubule, and the collecting tubule each have specific structures and functions (see Table 23.1).

Glomerular filtration is the first step of the process of urine formation. For this to happen, there needs to be sufficient renal blood flow at a consistent pressure. Many things can affect this process and thus impact glomerular filtration; the kidney makes every attempt to maintain a normal glomerular filtration rate (GFR). Blood flows into the kidney via the renal artery at a rate of about 1,000 to 1,200 mL per minute (about 20% to 25% of cardiac output).

The renin–angiotensin–aldosterone system (RAAS) regulates sodium, fluid volume, and potassium homeostasis (see Figure 23.3). Angiotensin II and aldosterone have direct effects on tubular reabsorption of sodium, as well as the renal and systemic circulation to maintain or restore the effective arterial blood volume. Renin is released from the juxtaglomerular cells of the afferent arterioles in response to decreased BP, decreased sodium (occurs with hypovolemia), and increased sympathetic stimulation.

This has been an overview of the normal anatomy and physiology of the renal system; there is much more to be known about this system if the adult-gerontology nurse practitioner (AGNP) is to provide the best care for thier patient. However, it is beyond the scope of this chapter to present extensive information, so we recommend you review your advanced pathophysiology textbooks for additional anatomy and physiology information.

CHRONIC KIDNEY DISEASE

Etiology

CKD affects approximately 14% of the U.S. population, and the incidence and prevalence have been increasing. It is more common in older adults and in people of African American, Hispanic, and Native American descent. The rise in CKD has been attributed to our aging population and the increasing prevalence of lifestyle diseases, such as diabetes mellitus, hypertension, and obesity. In many cases, CKD may progress to end-stage kidney disease (ESKD), which will require treatment with kidney replacement therapy (KRT), such as hemodialysis or peritoneal dialysis or transplantation, and this can have a profound impact on morbidity, mortality, patient quality of life, and healthcare costs. The

Table 23.1: Tubular System

Proximal Tubule	Loop of Henle	Distal Tubule	Collecting Tubule
• Major site for reabsorption in nephron • 65% of filtered water and sodium reabsorbed • Other reabsorbed are filtered glucose, amino acids, water-soluble vitamins, filtered phosphate, calcium, magnesium, urea, potassium, and chloride	• Consists of thin descending limb, thin ascending limb, and thick ascending limb • Movement of solutes is by diffusion rather than active transport • Thin descending is highly permeable to water but much less permeable to urea, sodium, and most other solutes • Thin ascending is impermeable to water but transports sodium, chloride, and urea • Thick ascending is impermeable to water but sodium and chloride are major solutes that are reabsorbed. Other ions. such as potassium, bicarbonate, magnesium, and calcium are reabsorbed.	• Early DT transport sodium, chloride, bicarbonate, potassium, calcium, magnesium but is impermeable to water • Late DT site for regulation of sodium, chloride, bicarbonate, potassium, and calcium transport • Water permeability of the late DT is influenced by the antidiuretic hormone (ADH); the presence of ADH makes late DT impermeable to water.	• Water permeability is dependent on ADH. • Water absorption is minimal; dilute urine is excreted. • Dilute urine is excreted.

presence of CKD also dramatically increases a person's susceptibility to cardiovascular disease including coronary artery disease and stroke. In fact, the main cause of death in this population is related to cardiovascular disease.

CKD has been recognized as a global public health problem. In 2018, there were more than 6 million adults 18 and older who were diagnosed with CKD.[1] However, many may have not been diagnosed, particularly those in minority groups. Primary care providers (PCPs) have an important role in detecting CKD, evaluating, managing, and referring to a nephrologist and nephrology team in a timely manner. Most patients are not referred until late in the disease, which limits the ability to slow the progression, prevent complications associated with CKD, and treat comorbidities. In the United States, the most common causes of CKD are diabetes and hypertension. Both type 1 and type 2 diabetes mellitus can cause CKD, but because type 2 is more prevalent, it accounts for the majority of patients with diabetic kidney disease (DKD). Other less common but primary causes are primary glomerulonephritis (e.g., IgA nephropathy, membranous glomerulopathy), tubulointerstitial diseases, hereditary disease (e.g., autosomal polycystic kidney disease [APKD], Alport's syndrome), secondary glomerulonephritis (e.g., lupus nephritis, amyloidosis) or vasculitis, neoplasm or plasma cell dyscrasias, and other miscellaneous causes. In some situations, the cause is unknown.[2] See Table 23.2 for the most common causes of CKD.

Pathophysiology

"CKD" is defined as kidney damage or reduced estimated glomerular filtration rate (eGFR) lower than 60 mL/min/1.73 m² for 3 months or more, irrespective of the

Table 23.2: Causes of Chronic Kidney Disease

Diabetes mellitus
Hypertension
Glomerulonephritis
Chronic interstitial nephritis
Congestive cardiac failure
Liver failure
Paraproteinemia
Obstructive uropathy
Polycystic kidney disease
Nephrotoxins
Congenital renal disease
Nephrolithiasis: renal stone disease

cause. In addition, there are situations (e.g., APKD) in which the eGFR is normal, but there is still pathology. The pathology of CKD is related to the underlying cause of the disease and accelerated glomerular hypertension, systemic hypertension, inflammation, and fibrosis.[2] Markers of kidney damage (e.g., blood or protein in the urine) must be present.

Classifying CKD follows the Kidney Disease: Improving Global Outcomes (KDIGO)[3] guidelines,[3] which are abnormalities of kidney structure or function present for more than 3 months. The GFR is the rate at which plasma is filtered through the nephrons of the kidneys and is reduced in CKD. The normal GFR is greater than 90 mL/min per 1.73 m² and the stages of CKD are defined from

Stages 1 through 5 as detailed in Table 23.3. The staging of CKD is important to stratify risk, determine the likelihood of progression, and manage complications of this disease. The definition of CKD has been further refined by the assessment of albuminuria. The ratio of albumin to creatinine (ACR) is obtained in a spot urine sample and is abnormal if it is greater than 30 mg/g of creatinine. "Moderate albuminuria" is defined as an albumin-to-creatinine ratio of 30–300 mg/g of creatinine, and severely increased albuminuria is present when there is greater than 300 mg/g of creatinine. The presence of albuminuria is a marker of significant disease and may increase risk by as much as 11-fold in a patient with a GFR of 90 mL/min/1.73 m^2 (Stage 1 disease). Figure 23.4 illustrates the prevalence of the stages of CKD in the adult population in the United States and how the presence of albuminuria affects risk. The presence of albuminuria also increases cardiovascular (CV) risk.

Risk Factors

The main risk factor for CKD is having diabetes, particularly type 2 diabetes. Globally there are over 387 million people with type 2 diabetes, and with an aging population and increasing obesity, this number is expected to increase by 40% overall and more than 50% in non-White populations.[4] In the global population, about 5% have type 1 diabetes, and this is projected to increase by 30%. Hypertension is the second-most common risk factor for CKD. This chapter covers the two most common causes of CKD with a brief overview of other causes of CKD. Even though we are not discussing all of the causes of CKD, it is important that primary care AGNPs are aware of these and recognize the need for further evaluation, management, and consultation with a nephrologist.

Approach to Diagnostics

The approach to diagnosis involves identifying who is at risk (previously discussed), performing the history and

Table 23.3: Classification of CKD

Stage	Associated GFR (mL/minute/1.73 m²)
1	Greater than 90 with persistent kidney damage
2	60–89 with persistent kidney damage
3	30–59
4	15–29
5	Less than15

Source: Levey AS, Eckardt K-U, Tsukamoto Y, et al. Definition and classification of chronic kidney disease: a position statement from kidney disease: improving global outcomes (KDIGO). *Kidney Int.* 2005;67:2089-2100. doi:10.1111/j.1523-1755.2005.00365.x

Percentage of US Population by eGFR and Albuminuria Category: KDIGO 2012 and NHANES 1999-2006			Persistent albuminuria categories Description and range			
			A1	**A2**	**A3**	
			Normal to mildly increased	Moderately increased	Severely increased	
			<30 mg/g <3 mg/mmol	30-300 mg/g 3-30 mg/mmol	>300 mg/g >30mg/mmol	
GFR categories (mVmin/1.73m²) Description and range	G1	Normal or high	≥90	55.6	1.9	0.4	57.9
	G2	Mildly decreased	60-89	32.9	2.2	0.3	35.4
	G3a	Mildly to moderately decreased	45-59	3.6	0.8	0.2	4.6
	G3b	Moderately to severely decreased	30-44	1.0	0.4	0.2	1.6
	G4	Severely decreased	15-29	0.2	0.1	0.1	0.4
	G5	Kidney failure	<15	0.0	0.0	0.1	0.1
				93.3	5.4	1.3	100.0

Figure 23.4: Prevalence of CKD in the United States by GFR and albuminuria

CKD, chronic kidney disease; GFR, glomerular filtration rate.

physical examination, and implementing preventive and person-centered health promotion strategies. The next step is an evaluation of eGFR and/or the presence of albuminuria, which is presented in the diagnostics section, Box 23.3. For patients who present with an elevated serum creatinine or reduced GFR, it is important to distinguish those with relatively stable CKD from those who have acute kidney injury (AKI) or other causes for these changes. It is important to determine if there is ongoing CKD or a reversible cause of AKI (see Table 23.4). The medical history should include inquiring about exposure to potential nephrotoxins, the presence of diabetes or hypertension, family history of kidney disease or renal stones, or chronic use of nonsteroidal anti-inflammatory drugs (NSAIDs). A physical examination to identify clinical signs of CKD is necessary (see Table 23.4). Many patients may present with no clinical symptoms and have CKD detected with laboratory studies or urinalysis as part of a routine visit. Patients with more advanced disease may have weakness, anorexia, vomiting, and pruritus, and may easily fatigue. In some cases, the person may experience encephalopathy or seizures due to uremia. A review of the current BP and previous recordings of BP measurements, dietary history, and weight measurements (assess for weight loss or gain) is essential in the initial assessment of the person with CKD.

Diagnostics

Laboratory studies (Box 23.2) are important and serial testing helps the provider determine if there is a sudden change in kidney function or progression of CKD, along with evaluating for comorbidities and complications of

Table 23.4: Diagnostic Findings That Are Related to CKD

Targeted History/Physical Examination	Clinical Indication	Possible Etiology
Review of Systems	• Recent infections • Risk for STI or substance use disorder • Skin rash or arthritis • Urinary tract symptoms	• Poststreptococcal glomerulonephritis • Hepatitis B or C or HIV • Autoimmune disease (SLE) • Urinary tract infection, obstruction, or stone
Medical History	• Diabetes mellitus • Hypertension • Other potential causes of CKD • Comorbid conditions	• Moderately increased albuminuria with or without retinopathy and elevated BP • Uncontrolled BP, often with end target damage
Family History	• Equal among men and women	• Autosomal dominant polycystic disease • Sex-linked recessive disease (e.g., Alport syndrome) • Autosomal recessive polycystic kidney disease
Physical Examination	• Abdominal findings • Cardiovascular findings • Carotid bruit • Decreased peripheral pulses • Increased BP and weight gain • Peripheral edema • Musculoskeletal problems • Ophthalmoscopic findings • Skin problems	• Bruit, could indicate atherosclerotic renal artery stenosis, fibromuscular dysplasia, distended bladder, flank pain • Heart failure, ventricular hypertrophy • Carotid artery disease • Peripheral vascular disease • Hypertension, obesity • Arthritis, synovitis • Uncontrolled hypertension, diabetic retinal disease • Rash and skin changes may indicate autoimmune disease

CKD, chronic kidney disease; SLE, systemic lupus erythematosus; STI, sexually transmitted infection.
Source: Gaitonde DY, Cook DL, Rivera IM. Chronic kidney disease: detection and evaluation. *Am Fam Physician*. 2017;96:776–784. https://www.aafp.org/afp/2017/1215/p776.html; National Kidney Foundation. K/DOQI clinical practice guidelines for chronic kidney disease: evaluation, classification, and stratification.
Am J Kidney Dis. 2002;39(2 suppl 1):S1–266. https://www.sciencedirect.com/journal/american-journal-of-kidney-diseases/vol/39/issue/2/suppl/S1

Box 23.2: Laboratory Assessment

- Basic metabolic panel that includes serum creatinine for calculation of eGFR
- Complete blood count with white cell differential
- Urinalysis using reagent test strips (dipstick) and automated urine microscopy
- Quantification of urine protein and albumin by random (or "spot"), protein-to-urine creatinine ratio and albumin-to-creatinine ratio
- In some cases, may need a 24-hour urine

eGFR, estimated glomerular filtration rate.

Box 23.3: Assessment of Proteinuria

- The standard urine dipstick detects albumin but does not detect other proteins or very low levels of albumin.
- The lower limit of detection for a dipstick is 10 to 20 mg/dL so it may miss microalbuminuria.
- It is recommended that a spot urine specimen be collected and tested for albumin/creatinine ratio in patients at risk for kidney disease as this test will capture low levels of proteinuria that if present will need further evaluation.

Box 23.4: Assessment of Hematuria

- Hematuria is often detected on a urine dipstick.
- Evaluation of hematuria is based on history (e.g., prior history, upper respiratory tract infection before hematuria, travel, recent strenuous activity, previous nephrolithiasis, recent trauma, start of new medication, pelvic radiation).
- If heme-positive urine is discovered, a urine specimen should be centrifuged (if not able to do in your office, send to a laboratory).
- In the presence of white blood cells, leukocyte esterase nitrates, or symptoms of infection, it is important to rule out urinary tract infection (see Chapter 24).
- False positives can occur if there is semen, alkaline urine, oxidizing agents used to clean the perineum, or presence of bacterial peroxidase.
- Laboratory testing should be tailored to a possible etiology of hematuria.

🏠 Quality and Safety Alerts

- Contrast-induced nephropathy (CIN) is a potential risk of using iodinated CT contrast in patients with impaired kidney function, advanced age, diabetes, hypertension, heart failure, and volume depletion.
- For those receiving dialysis or who have reduced GFR, obtaining a contrast-enhanced CT or MRI should be based on the diagnostic benefits, which are beyond the scope of a primary care AGNP, so consultation with a nephrologist is important.
- If urine is very concentrated, the presence of a modest protein reaction is less likely to correspond to significant proteinuria in a 24-hour urine collection or to a spot urine albumin-to-creatinine ratio.

CKD. The urinalysis can provide information about a number of primary kidney and systemic disorders. In addition to the usual evaluation of urine (see Chapter 24), it is important to assess microalbumin. Point-of-care albumin-selective dipsticks are available for screening microalbuminuria (Box 23.3). Obtaining a urinalysis with microscopic evaluation of urine sediment is essential. The presence of hematuria, cellular casts, and crystals is suggestive of kidney disease. Sediment must be considered as a whole and interpretation should include clinical indicators based on a history and physical and laboratory findings. Assessing for hematuria is important (see Box 23.4 and Chapter 24 for more information).

Renal ultrasound can inform you about kidney size and cortical thickness, and distinguish between a solid mass and cystic kidney masses. Echogenicity (commonly attributed to CKD and has been correlated to interstitial fibrosis, tubular atrophy, and glomerulosclerosis). A computed tomography (CT) scan can provide information about the anatomy of the kidney parenchyma, vasculature, and excretory system, and evaluate a kidney mass. For a comprehensive imaging of the kidney and collecting system, an MRI may be obtained.

Referral to a nephrologist should be done if you suspect there is a need for a kidney biopsy. A kidney biopsy is usually done when there is (a) proteinuria associated with a decline in GFR, (b) proteinuria in the nephrotic range (greater than 3,500 mg/day), (c) proteinuria that may be associated with glomerular or tubular problems, and (d) persistent proteinuria greater than 500 mg/day with a patient who has systemic lupus erythematosus or other rheumatologic disorders.[5]

🔆 CLINICAL PEARLS

- Isolated proteinuria occurs when protein is greater than 300 mg per day without abnormalities in the urine sediment, GFR decline, or comorbid conditions such as diabetes, hypertension, or rheumatologic or infectious diseases.

- The gold standard for measuring proteinuria is 24-hour urine collection; however, these are rarely done because of the challenges with collection, such as transporting the specimen, and often inaccurate collections due to improper or incomplete collection techniques.

- An alternative to 24-hour urine collection is measurements of spot urine to evaluate protein or albumin-to-creatinine ratio.

- The most accurate screening occurs when a first-morning specimen is evaluated.

- Orthostatic proteinuria is seen in children and adolescents but rarely in those 30 years old or older.

- Adolescents and young adults may experience benign proteinuria or transient proteinuria; fever and vigorous exercise are often the reason. Reassessment should be done when the patient no longer has a fever or has abstained from vigorous exercise.

Screening Tools and Tests

Individuals who have diabetes or hypertension should be screened for kidney disease on an annual basis. The National Kidney Foundation (NKF) has recommended the screening of all patients with diabetes, hypertension, age older than 60 years, family history of kidney disease, or belonging to an ethnic or racial minority group. The NKF also identifies other medical risk factors, and these include exposure to known nephrotoxic agents, history of autoimmune disease, renal calculi, prior history of acute kidney injury, reduced renal mass (e.g., from prior nephrectomy), and history of low birth weight. The U.S. Preventative Services Task Force reports that there is not enough evidence to determine the potential benefits and harms of routine screening of all asymptomatic adults for CKD. This recommendation does not apply to those who have diabetes or hypertension.

Screening consists of taking a very detailed history focused on identifying the risk factors, doing a careful physical examination including BP, and then measuring serum creatinine and other laboratory studies. Individuals who are at risk for kidney disease should be screened by measuring GFR and evaluated for the presence of albuminuria (albumin/creatinine ratio in a spot urine specimen). The GFR is usually obtained by measuring a serum creatinine level and using this value in one of the approved equations to estimate GFR. The serum

creatinine level has traditionally been used to evaluate kidney function but because it is affected by a number of factors, it often either underestimates or overestimates renal function. Creatinine is a waste product of muscle and is not only filtered at the glomerulus but is also secreted by the proximal tubules. The serum creatinine level is affected by age, sex, race, and muscle mass, and therefore, patients may have similar creatinine levels but very different levels of renal function. This difference is mitigated by using GFR equations that account for these variables. The most common overall index that has been used is the Modification of Diet in Renal Disease (MDRD) equation, which is used by most laboratories to report the GFR or estimated GFR. (Box 23.5). However, the more recent Chronic Kidney Disease Epidemiology Collaboration equation (CKD-EPI) may be a better indicator of CKD (Box 23.6). Evidence supports that CKD-EPI is a better choice than MDRD because it more accurately predicts prognosis and is less biased.[6-7]

Both equations consider the patient's age, sex, and race. The coefficient of race has been controversial. The reason for this is based on the belief that Black adults have a higher mean serum creatinine value compared to non-Black (mostly White) patients for the same measured GFR. The concern at this time is inequity for Black Americans

---

Box 23.5: MDRD Equation, Variables Include Age, Race, Sex, and Serum Urea, Nitrogen, Albumin, and Creatinine Levels

MDRD GFR

GFR (mL/min/1.73 m²) = $186 \times (Pcr)^{-1.154} \times (age)^{-0.203}$ $\times$ (0.742 if female) $\times$ (1.210 if African American)

The GFR is expressed in mL/min/1.73 m²

Pcr = serum or plasma creatinine in mg/dL

GFR, glomerular filtration rate; MDRD, modification of diet in renal disease

---

Box 23.6: CKD-EPI Equation, Variables Include Age, Race, Sex, and Serum Creatinine Levels

CKD-EPI Adults

Should be used when S_{cr} is reported in mg/dL. This equation is recommended when the eGFR values above 60 mL/min/1.73 m² are desired.

GFR = $131 \times min (S_{cr}/k, 1)^{>} -1.209 \times 0.993^{age} \times 1.018$ [if female] $\times$ 1.159 [if African American]

CKD-EPI, Chronic Kidney Disease Epidemiology Collaboration; eGFR, estimated glomerular filtration rate.

for access to healthcare and timely referral to nephrology care if these equations have a coefficient of race. Cystatin C as a filtration marker may be an alternative to serum creatinine to more accurately estimate GFR and classify CKD. Cystatin C has been shown to be unaltered during inflammatory conditions, and a reduction in GFR has been correlated with reductions in serum cystatin C.[7] At this time, most laboratories report MDRD or CKD-EPI, so it is important to also consider the patient's risk factors and other indicators of CKD. Calculators for the equations can be found at www.niddk.nih.gov or www.kidney.org/professionals/kdoqi/gr_calculator.cfm.

Management

CKD cannot be generalized as one disease, but rather, it includes the primary processes causing CKD, so screening, diagnostic testing, and management should include evidence-based strategies aimed at preventing or slowing the progression and treating the underlying disease and complications of CKD. Overall goals for primary care management of CKD can be seen in Box 23.7.

It is essential that the primary care AGNP reviews medication lists in detail at every visit and inquire specifically about over-the-counter medications, as well as herbal and nutritional supplements. Many prescribed medications may have interactions that worsen kidney function, and several herbal supplements are nephrotoxic. Some patients may experience an exacerbation of their kidney disease due to underlying reversible causes that need to be identified and addressed for recovery to occur (see Table 23.5). Some medications, such as NSAIDs, which are available over the counter can be harmful to those with CKD.

Box 23.7: Goals of Primary Care Adult-Gerontology Nurse Practitioners for Managing Those With Chronic Kidney Disease

- Treatment of reversible causes of kidney disease
- Preventing or slowing the progression of CKD
- Treatment of comorbidities (complications) of CKD
- Adjusting drug doses when appropriate for the level of eGFR
- Collaborate with a nephrology expert for individuals with CKD Stage 4, 5, and ESKD to prepare for KRT
- C-management with nephrology experts when a person is receiving KRT

CKD, chronic kidney disease; eGFR, estimated glomerular filtration rate; ESKD, end-stage kidney disease; KRT, kidney replacement therapy.

Quality and Safety Alerts

- Older adults with CKD, hypertension, and/or diabetes have a high risk of cognitive impairment due to cerebrovascular disease.
- The person may have cognitive impairment that impairs their ability to manage medication safely, so when the AGNP identifies that a person may be making errors with medication management it warrants further evaluation of their cognitive status.

Box 23.8 provides recommendations of when to refer to a nephrologist. However, if the AGNP experiences challenges managing a person with CKD, consider contacting or referring to a nephrologist.

Complications Associated With Chronic Kidney Disease

Anemia

The National Kidney Foundation recommends that patients with CKD Stage 3 should be screened for anemia at least annually.[8] The World Health Organization defines "anemia" as a hemoglobin concentration of less than 13.0 g/dL in adult males and postmenopausal women, and a hemoglobin concentration of less than 12.0 g/dL for premenopausal women. Patients with CKD develop a deficiency of erythropoietin, a hormone produced by the kidney that stimulates red blood cell production in the bone marrow. As renal function deteriorates, erythropoietin production is reduced, and anemia develops. According to the

Table 23.5: Underlying Reversible Causes of Kidney Disease

Decreased Renal Perfusion	Administration of Nephrotoxic Drug
• Hypovolemia due to vomiting, diarrhea, diuretic use, bleeding, hypotension (due to myocardial dysfunction or pericardial disease)	• Aminoglycoside antibiotics (particularly unadjusted doses) • NSAIDs • Radiographic contrast material
• Infection/sepsis • Administration of drugs that lower GFR, angiotensin-converting-enzyme (ACE) inhibitors, or angiotensin receptor blockers (ARB)	Medications that interfere with either creatinine secretion or the assay used to measure the serum creatinine are • Cimetidine, • Trimethoprim, • Cefoxitin, and • Flucytosine.

GFR, glomerular filtration rate; NSAIDs, nonsteroidal anti-inflammatory drugs.

Box 23.8: Nephrology Referrals

Indications for nephrology referral:

- eGFR less than 30 mL/min/1.73^2
- Persistent UACR equal to or greater than 300 mg/g (34 mg/mmol)
- Persistent UPCR equal to or greater than 500 mg/g (56.5 mg/mmol)
- Abnormal urine microscopy (cellular casts, nonurologic hematuria, pyuria)
- History of systemic autoimmune disease
- Large cystic kidneys as seen in imaging studies or via physical examination
- Known history of multiple myeloma or monoclonal gammopathy
- Evidence of rapid decline in kidney function (reduction in eGFR greater than 5 mL/min/1.73^2 per year or decline greater than 25%)
- Single kidney eGFR less than 60 mL/min/1.73^2
- Resistant hypertension
- Recurrent or extensive nephrolithiasis
- Pregnancy
- Heredity disease such as Alport syndrome
- Difficulty in managing complications related to medications (i.e., chemotherapy)

eGFR, estimated glomerular filtration rate; UACR, urine albumin-to-creatinine ratio; UPCR, urine protein-to-creatinine ratio.

NHANES (National Health and Nutrition Examination Survey), the prevalence of anemia increases from approximately 1% in patients with a GFR of 60% to 9% at a GFR of 30% and 33% to 67% in patients with GFR 15 mL/min or less. Other factors that contribute to anemia in CKD include deficiencies of iron, vitamin B12, or folic acid and the anemia of chronic disease seen in patients with any long-standing inflammatory condition. The evaluation of anemia should include a complete blood count, absolute reticulocyte count, ferritin, serum iron, transferrin saturation levels, vitamin B12, and folate levels. (See Chapter 27 for more information about anemia.)

The availability of erythropoietin analogs has revolutionized the treatment of anemia in renal disease. Before prescribing these medications, however, all correctable causes of anemia should be addressed. Iron deficiency is very common, and correction of this often leads to an increase in hemoglobin to the target level of 10 to 11 g/dL. Adolescent females and women of childbearing age are prone to iron deficiency anemia due to menstrual losses. In the middle-aged to older adult population, iron deficiency should prompt an evaluation for occult blood loss especially from the gastrointestinal tract.

Erythropoietin-stimulating agents (ESA) are generally initiated when the Hgb is less than 10 g/dL and the iron stores are replete. In those patients who do not have ESKD and are not receiving KRT (once receiving KRT the dialysis center is responsible for providing the medication), they can be given an ESA subcutaneously at weekly, biweekly, or monthly intervals. These agents are not given to patients who have an active malignancy, who have uncontrolled hypertension, or who have had a recent stroke. Studies have shown that there is a risk of severe hypertension and stroke if they are given in doses that raise the hemoglobin to the normal range. Patients should have iron stores measured every 3 months while on erythropoietin therapy and deficiency treated as needed. Patients should be referred to a nephrologist to manage the administration of ESA and recommend or treat iron deficiencies in those with CKD. Hypoxia-inducible factor-prolyl hydroxylase domain inhibitors (HIF-PHIs) are promising new oral medications that are currently in development for treating anemia of CKD.[9]

Chronic Kidney Disease: Mineral Bone Disease

"CKD-MBD" is a term that encompasses the disorders of mineral and bone metabolism that occur with progressive deterioration in renal function. These include abnormalities of calcium, phosphorus, parathyroid hormone (PTH) and vitamin D and disorders of bone mineralization and calcification. Patients with CKD Stage 3 should have PTH and phosphorus and calcium levels measured yearly, while measurements should be made every 3 months in CKD Stages 4 and 5. Table 23.6 shows the target values for phosphorus and PTH at CKD Stages 3 to 5.[10]

As kidney function deteriorates, the excretion of phosphorus decreases, and this triggers the release of PTH from the parathyroid gland. PTH increases renal reabsorption of calcium, renal excretion of phosphorus, and the activation of vitamin D by the kidney. PTH increases the release of calcium from bone and the activated vitamin D increases the absorption of both dietary calcium and phosphorus from the gut. The increased calcium, phosphorus, and PTH levels cause increased coronary

Table 23.6: Target Phosphorus and Intact PTH Levels by Stage of CKD

Stage	Target Phosphorus (mg/dL)	Target Intact PTH (pg/mL)
3 (GFR 30–59)	2.7–4.6	35–70
4 (GFR 15–29)	2.7–4.6	70–110
5 (GFR less than 15)	3.5–5.5	150–300

CKD, chronic kidney disease; GFR, glomerular filtration rate in mL/min; PTH, parathyroid hormone.

arterial calcification and contribute to the advanced and premature coronary atherosclerosis that is typical in CKD.

As CKD progresses, serum phosphorus rises and should be treated first by restricting the intake of high phosphorus foods. These include dairy foods, nuts, meats, and commercial baked goods. Daily phosphorus intake should be limited to 800 to 1,000 mg. At CKD Stages 4 and 5, dietary restrictions may not be sufficient, and phosphate binders are given with meals to bind dietary phosphorus and decrease its absorption. There are three kinds of phosphate binders: calcium-based, such as calcium acetate; non-calcium-based, such as sevelamer carbonate and lanthanum carbonate; and the newer iron-based binders, ferric citrate and sucroferric oxyhydroxide. The calcium-based binders may cause hypercalcemia, so the total amount of elemental calcium should be limited to 1500 mg daily. The non-calcium-based binders such as sevelamer may cause gastrointestinal upset. Aluminum-based binders were used previously but are rarely prescribed now due to the potential for aluminum toxicity.

25-hydroxy vitamin D levels should be checked at least annually in patients with CKD and supplemented for levels lower than 30 ng/mL. The kidney is the site of conversion of 25-hydroxy vitamin D to 1, 25-hydroxy vitamin D, and as CKD progresses to Stage 4 and 5, this conversion is severely limited. These patients may need supplementation with the activated forms of vitamin D, such as calcitriol and paracalcitriol. Once these medications have been prescribed, serum calcium and phosphorus levels have to be monitored closely as there is a risk of the development of hypercalcemia and hyperphosphatemia. Patients who have developed elevated PTH levels, persistent hyperphosphatemia, or hyper- or hypocalcemia in the context of CKD should be referred to a nephrologist.

Metabolic Acidosis

"Metabolic acidosis" is defined as a serum bicarbonate level of less than 22 mEq/L. As kidney function declines, there is decreased excretion of ammonium and phosphate, increased acid production, and increased bicarbonate excretion. Metabolic acidosis therefore develops with worsening GFR and is present in up to 25% of patients with CKD Stage 5. Chronic metabolic acidosis is associated with significant morbidity and mortality in patients with CKD. Patients who are acidotic develop increased bone resorption, muscle catabolism, and chronic inflammation and progress to ESKD at a faster rate. In adolescents, metabolic acidosis may cause resistance to growth hormone and therefore result in stunted growth.

KDIGO recommends treating patients with oral sodium bicarbonate to maintain serum bicarbonate in the normal range (23–29 mEq/L). In patients with hypertension, the increased sodium ingestion may lead to volume retention and a mild increase in BP, but the comparative effect appears to be less for the bicarbonate salt than for the equivalent amount of sodium chloride. Randomized controlled trials have shown a slower rate of progression of kidney disease in acidotic patients prescribed bicarbonate therapy. Alkali therapy also improves the mineral bone disease of CKD and decreases PTH levels. Correcting acidosis has a positive effect on muscle metabolism, leading to a decrease in muscle breakdown and improved nutritional status.

It is important to obtain and monitor laboratory studies related to CKD-MBD, anemia, and metabolic acidosis in addition to kidney function tests (see Table 23.7) for recommended intervals.

Chronic Kidney Disease and Cardiovascular Disease

Reduced GFR and the presence of proteinuria are both associated with an increased risk of cardiovascular disease. The National Kidney Foundation, the American College of Cardiology, and the American Heart Association recommend that CKD be considered a coronary heart disease risk equivalent. Cardiovascular disease remains the leading cause of death among patients with advanced CKD, and it is important, therefore, that all modifiable risk factors be addressed. The patient should have a fasting lipid profile at the time of diagnosis and annually thereafter if the levels are within normal range. If medication is started or dosages changed, the lipid profile should be rechecked 2 to 3 months later. Per Kidney Disease Outcomes Quality Initiative (KDOQI) guidelines, the low-density lipoprotein level (LDL)[11] should be 100 mg/dL or less and in some patients with preexisting coronary artery disease, a more stringent target of 70 mg/dL is recommended.[11]

Patients with dyslipidemia should be encouraged to follow a diet that is low in cholesterol and saturated fat and high in dietary fiber. Many patients will need drug therapy to achieve the target levels and statins are the most widely used class of medications. They are generally well tolerated but there may be a slight increase in the

Table 23.7: NKF KDOQI Guidelines for Monitoring CBC, IPTH, Phosphorus, and CO_2

CKD Stage	Complete Blood Count	Intact PTH	Phosphorus/ Calcium	Total CO_2
3	12	12	12	12
4	12	3	3	3
5	12	3	1	3
Dialysis	12	3	1	1

CBC, complete blood count; CKD, chronic kidney disease; IPTH, intact parathyroid hormone; KDOQI, Kidney Disease Outcomes Quality Initiative; NKF, National Kidney Foundation; PTH, parathyroid hormone.

risk of statin-induced myopathy in patients with CKD. Hypertriglyceridemia is common in patients with CKD. Lifestyle changes including dietary changes, regular exercise, reduction of alcohol intake, weight loss, and treatment of hyperglycemia are advised for all patients.

While it is clear that patients with CKD are at heightened risk for cardiovascular disease, it is unclear whether high LDL levels are responsible for most of this increased risk. In patients with normal kidney function, higher LDL levels correlate with increased coronary risk, but the association is weaker as GFR decreases. The increased risk for coronary artery disease is likely due to nontraditional risk factors, including anemia, the chronic inflammatory state, and mineral bone disease with abnormal calcification of blood vessels.

The 2013 KDIGO guidelines also recommend screening all CKD patients with a fasting lipid profile. However, the guidelines state that all patients with CKD of 50 years or older who are predialysis age should be treated with statins or a statin/ezetimibe combination. Patients aged 18 to 49 years who are at increased cardiovascular risk should be treated with a statin. Increased risk includes known coronary disease, diabetes, prior ischemic stroke, or a greater than 10% 10-year risk of myocardial infarction or coronary death. The guidelines do not recommend following the LDL levels after the decision has been made to start therapy. This issue is somewhat controversial, and these recommendations differ significantly from the KDOQI guidelines. If indications for lipid-lowering therapy are not clear, the PCP should defer this decision to the patient's nephrologist.

Dyslipidemia in Adolescents With Chronic Kidney Disease
Adolescents with nephrotic syndrome may have grossly elevated LDL levels and will need treatment with statins. Improvement in the lipid profile usually parallels the improvement in nephrotic range proteinuria in these patients. Maintaining a diet that is low in saturated fat and cholesterol may be challenging for this population, so consultation with a renal dietitian can be beneficial.

🏠 Quality and Safety Alert

NSAIDs are over-the-counter analgesics that are commonly used and may cause progression of CKD on their own or in combination with prescribed medications. It is important that the PCP inquire specifically about the use of these agents and educate patients about their potentially harmful effects.

Special Considerations for Adolescents to Young Adults

Chapter 11 presents an overview of specific issues faced by adolescents and young adults, particularly the psychosocial aspect of becoming an adult and experiencing health problems. This population faces unique and complex psychosocial challenges when faced with CKD.[12] They constitute about 5% of the ESKD population, and their 10-year survival is from 70% to 85% with the main causes of death being cardiovascular issues and infection. Adolescent patients may present with reduced renal function due to congenital abnormalities of the kidney and urinary tract, such as reflux nephropathy, obstructive uropathy, and dysplastic kidneys. In this age group, glomerulonephritis is also an important cause. The etiology of glomerulonephritis in the adolescent includes Ig A nephropathy, post-streptococcal glomerulonephritis, lupus nephritis, and focal segmental glomerulosclerosis (FSGS).

Having CKD/ESKD interferes with growth and development. Reasons for this include metabolic acidosis, decreased caloric intake, CKD-MBD-related reduced gonadal hormone production, growth hormone resistance, and increased levels of IGF-1 binding proteins.[12] They often have a delay in puberty, which affects their psychosocial well-being. Adverse events of medications and vascular access for dialysis may lead to an altered body image. Adolescents with CKD have a higher risk of depression (see Chapters 11 and 18 for more information regarding assessment and treatment of depression). Adolescents may not focus on engaging in self-management activities because of peer pressure or wanting to be like their peers, financial issues, school/work, and future dreams.[12] Therefore, it is important to be authentically present to listen to what matters most to the adolescent and what are their future hopes and dreams as you partner with them to develop a person-centered plan of care.

Special Considerations for Older Adults

With an aging population, the AGNP needs to pay special attention to the risk for CKD in older adults. In older adults, diabetic kidney disease (DKD) and hypertensive nephrosclerosis continue to be the most common causes. Renovascular disease is uncommon but should be considered in patients who have coronary artery or peripheral vascular disease (consider vascular disease risk factors such as smoking). Membranous nephropathy may cause heavy proteinuria and CKD in older adults, and in this age group, it may be secondary to an underlying malignancy. Vasculitis can cause rapidly progressive CKD in previously healthy older adults and should always be in the differential in this population with an abrupt loss of renal function. Patients may also develop CKD secondary to hematologic conditions such as multiple myeloma, and they can present with anemia, bone pain, proteinuria, hypercalcemia, and CKD. Another important consideration is obstructive uropathy secondary to an enlarged prostate in older males.

Other causes of CKD, diabetes and hypertension, are covered later in the chapter.

Chronic Glomerulonephritis

The term "Chronic Glomerulonephritis" encompasses a broad spectrum of inflammatory conditions, both primary and secondary, that cause CKD. The condition is characterized by irreversible and progressive glomerular scarring and tubulointerstitial fibrosis, which leads to a reduction in the GFR and, in many cases, can lead to ESKD. It is the third-leading cause of ESKD, accounting for up to 10% of cases. Chronic glomerulonephritis can be a sequela of acute glomerulonephritis. Acute glomerulonephritis may result from the body's reaction to infections such as strep throat, viral hepatitis, or infectious endocarditis. The antibodies produced in response to the infection cross-react with glomerular tissues, leading to acute inflammation that manifests as proteinuria, hematuria, hypertension, and decreased renal function. This may resolve with treatment of the acute infection, but in many cases, the damage is chronic and leads to slow, progressive CKD.

Chronic glomerulonephritis can be silent clinically and may not be precipitated by an acute event. These patients may be asymptomatic but are found to have elevated creatinine and mild to moderate proteinuria or microscopic hematuria on routine examination. The prognosis of chronic glomerulonephritis depends on the cause. Rapidly progressive glomerulonephritis has an aggressive course that can lead to ESKD within weeks to months. Lupus nephritis is another important cause of chronic glomerulonephritis, and 20% of cases progress to ESKD, especially if they have certain pathologic features on biopsy. IgA nephropathy is the most common cause of glomerulonephritis worldwide with the highest incidence in people of Asian descent. The prognosis of IgA nephropathy is variable, and one-third of patients have an excellent prognosis with only intermittent proteinuria and hematuria and well-preserved renal function. One-third of patients have slowly progressive renal failure but do not develop ESRD. The remaining patients unfortunately have a relentless course of worsening kidney function, hypertension, and heavy proteinuria that leads to complete kidney failure within 10 years of diagnosis.

Membranous Nephropathy

Membranous nephropathy is characterized by heavy proteinuria which may be accompanied by progressive kidney dysfunction and usually affects patients between the ages of 30 and 50 years of age. It is an immunologically mediated disease in which immune complexes are deposited in the subepithelial space of the glomerulus. It may be idiopathic or secondary to other conditions, such as hepatitis B infection, connective tissue disease such as lupus, drugs such as NSAIDs or penicillamine, or as the presenting manifestation of a malignancy. Membranous nephropathy often requires treatment with steroids and other immunosuppressive agents and may lead to ESKD.

FSGS has emerged as the most common cause of idiopathic nephrotic syndrome in adults but may also occur secondary to a variety of conditions. These secondary causes include infections like HIV, drugs (e.g., heroin), morbid obesity, and any condition that results in nephron loss and hyperfiltration, such as chronic pyelonephritis, hypertension, or after a partial nephrectomy. FSGS usually presents with CKD and proteinuria and leads to the progression of CKD that may require dialysis. In some cases, FSGS may occur after transplantation. In some patients who do not have diabetes and have CKD with low levels of albuminuria, reducing BP does not slow the progression of CKD. The association of APOL1 and CKD in people of African ancestry indicates that this population with non-DKD and low levels of proteinuria often have an inherited disorder, which produces elevated BP after the person has CKD.[13]

Polycystic Kidney Disease

Polycystic kidney disease (PKD) is an inherited disorder in which the kidneys develop innumerable fluid-filled cysts that eventually replace the renal parenchyma, leading to markedly enlarged kidneys, hypertension, and renal failure. PKD may be of autosomal dominant inheritance or less commonly autosomal recessive inheritance. The autosomal recessive form typically presents in childhood and leads to ESKD in early childhood or adolescence. The autosomal dominant disease may present with hypertension, episodic hematuria, or abdominal pain due to the enlarged cysts in early to mid-adulthood, and then, depending on the specific mutation, patients develop gradually worsening renal failure, which may culminate in ESKD between the ages of 50 to 70 years of age. The diagnosis is often suggested by a positive family history and confirmed on imaging with renal ultrasound, CT scan, or MRI. These patients also have liver cysts and are prone to other abnormalities, such as intracranial aneurysms and mitral valve prolapse. There is a new medication, tolvaptan, that was approved in 2018 for the treatment of the rapidly progressing autosomal PKD. This medication would be prescribed by a nephrologist. Patient support can be obtained from the PKD Foundation at https://PKDcare.org

Pharmacologic

The presence of albuminuria or a GFR less than 60 mL per minute/1.73^2 increases the risk of cardiovascular disease and all-cause mortality in people with CKD. Pharmacotherapy should be aimed at slowing the progression of CKD, which includes controlling albuminuria and treating the underlying cause of CKD and complications associated with CKD (discussed later in the chapter). Increases in urine albumin excretion are a strong predictor of cardiovascular outcomes; therefore, it is important to reduce urinary albumin excretion (UAE). Medications play a key role in achieving goals of reducing urinary protein excretion and slowing the progression of CKD. Drugs of choice are angiotensin-converting-enzyme inhibitor (ACEi) or angiotensin receptor blocker (ARB); medications are discussed more in disease-specific sections. Hyperkalemia can occur in patients taking ACEi or ARB (see Box 23.9). It is recommended if possible (depending on the patient) to avoid discontinuing the ACEi or ARB; consider treating with medications for hyperkalemia and have the patient eat a low potassium diet (see Table 23.7).

Box 23.9: ACE Inhibitor, ARB, and Presence of Hyperkalemia

- Hyperkalemia (serum potassium[K+] concentration above 5.5 mEq/L) in patients prescribed an ACE-inhibitor or ARB can occur.
- The risk is highest in people with CKD and heart failure.
- Assessment of GFR and K+ should be checked before and 1 week after starting the medication.
- Attempt to manage hyperkalemia with other measures such as medications (see Table 23.8), diuretics, and low potassium diet before considering reducing or discontinuing the ACE inhibitor or ARB.
- Reduce the dose or discontinue the ACE inhibitor or ARB therapy when the patient has uncontrolled hyperkalemia despite medical management.

ACE, angiotensin-converting enzyme; ARB, angiotensin receptor blocker; CKD, chronic kidney disease; GFR, glomerular filtration rate. *Source:* Kidney Disease: Improving Global Outcomes Diabetes Work Group. KDIGO 2020 clinical practice guideline for diabetes management in chronic kidney disease. Kidney Int. 2020;98(4S):S1–S115. doi:10.1016/j.kint.2020.06.019; Momoniat T, Ilyas D, Bhandari S. ACE inhibitors and ARBs: managing potassium and renal function. *Cleve Clin J Med.* 2019;86(9):601–607. doi:10.3949/ccjm.86a.18024

🧑 CLINICAL PEARLS

Initiation of ACEi or ARB

- A reduction in GFR (about 5%-25%) can occur as the result of autoregulation, but in some cases, it may be severe (greater than 30%) in patients treated with ACEi or ARBs who have bilateral renal artery stenosis, hypertensive nephrosclerosis, heart failure, PKD, and CKD. If severe, then holding the medication until the cause is identified may be best practice.
  - Intrarenal pressure may be reduced where GFR is maintained in part by angiotensin II–induced increase in resistance at the efferent arteriole.
  - Blocking this response with these medications will relax the efferent arteriole, lower intraglomerular pressure, and reduce GFR.

- People with acute volume loss (vomiting, diarrhea) are also susceptible.
- Serum creatinine may increase a few days after starting the medication, so kidney function should be evaluated within a week of starting these medications.

🏠 Quality and Safety Alerts

- Hyperkalemia with EKG changes is a life-threatening emergency requiring emergent care.
- The patient will need stabilization of myocardium with IV calcium gluconate; shift potassium from extracellular to intracellular with IV glucose; beta-agonists (20 mg of albuterol by inhalation).
- Medications in Table 23.6 should not be given to treat acute life-threatening hyperkalemia; they can be started if needed once the patient has been stabilized.

Nonpharmacologic

Therapeutic lifestyle changes as outlined by the KDOQI guidelines are key to minimizing complications and retarding the rate of progression of CKD. Healthy lifestyle behaviors should be encouraged. Healthy People 2030 (see Box 23.11) provides goals objectives for CKD. Reducing stress is also essential; consider mindful mediation or other strategies to address stress. Educating the patient about the importance of a healthy lifestyle and things they can do to slow the progression and promote health may lead to less stress related to the unknown.

Dietary limitations can be quite complex depending on the stage of CKD and the presence of comorbidities. Many patients will need restrictions on sodium, calories, potassium, phosphorus, protein, saturated fat, and cholesterol, and this is very difficult to navigate without the expert help of a renal dietitian. Lifestyle changes include weight loss if overweight, engaging in physical activity, smoking cessation, and follow-up with PCP, nephrology, and any other subspecialists as appropriate. Dietary recommendations may change as CKD progresses; however, there are specific overall recommendations for those with CKD. Low sodium (2 grams/day) and protein (0.8–1.0 g per day) diet is important. Once individuals are receiving dialysis their protein needs change, but they will have access to a renal dietitian as part of the ESKD program. Consulting with a renal dietitian can be beneficial in developing a person-centered plan of care that considers cultural issues, other food preferences, and laboratory study results.

Regular physical activity helps to normalize BP, improve glycemic control and lipid profile, build lean body

Table 23.8: Medications to Treat Hyperkalemia (see Chapter 13 for more information about medication management)

Sodium Polystyrene Sulfonate (SPS) (Kayexalate)	Patiromer (Veltassa)	Sodium Zirconium Cyclosilicate (Lokelma)
Nonspecific organic ion-exchange resin, exchanges sodium for potassium in the colon. At this time the Food and Drug Administration (FDA) recommends avoidance of SPS prescription for patients with active gastrointestinal (GI) diseases, or history of bowl surgery. Onset variable from hours to days	Nonspecific organic ion-exchange resin; exchanges calcium for potassium in the colon Onset within 7 hours Generally tolerated by patients but the same electrolyte disorders as SPS can be seen. Monitor Mg and K+	Selective cation exchange, primarily releasing hydrogen and sodium and capturing potassium, thus increasing fecal excretion, entire GI tract, onset of action median time 2 hours
Adverse events include electrolyte disturbances: hypokalemia, hypomagnesemia, GI symptom, severe adverse events (AE) are ulceration, bleeding, ischemic colitis, perforation	Adverse events include mild GI symptoms; should be avoided in those with severe constipation, bowl obstruction, or impaction	Dose-related mild to moderate edema observed during maintenance period but resolved with diuretic therapy; dose-dependent hypokalemia Adverse events were GI disturbances and should not be used in those with constipation, impaction, or bowl obstruction.

Source: Esposito P, Conti NE, Falqui V, et al. New treatment options for hyperkalemia in patients with chronic kidney disease. J Clin Med. 2020;9:2-19. doi:10.3390/jcm9082337; Palmer BF, Carrero JJ, Clegg DJ, et al. Clinical management of hyperkalemia. Mayo Clin Proc. 2020:1-19. doi:10.1016/06j .mayocp2020.01.

mass, and reduce body fat. Patients who smoke should be strongly encouraged to stop as tobacco use increases the rate of decline of kidney function. All patients should have their health maintenance screenings performed at the recommended times and should be immunized with the pneumovax and yearly influenza vaccines. At CKD Stage 4, immunization with hepatitis B series is recommended as this will be required if the patient progresses to dialysis.

Patients with CKD need to be educated about the importance of engaging in self-management that is congruent with medical recommendations (medication regimen and diet). They should not take any over-the-counter or herbal medications without consulting their PCP/nephrologist. NSAIDs in particular can be harmful to the patient with CKD and may cause severe hyperkalemia and AKI superimposed on CKD. Commonly prescribed antibiotics, such as trimethoprim sulfamethoxazole, can also cause AKI and hyperkalemia. In the patient with CKD and coronary artery disease, if cardiac catheterization needs to be done, the patient should be made aware of the risk of contrast-induced nephropathy. This risk can be mitigated by administering IV fluids before and after the procedure and using minimal volumes of contrast.

Patients who progress to CKD Stage 4 should be prepared for the eventual need for dialysis or transplantation. Referral to a nephrologist at this time is the best way to ensure that the patient is educated about their options. If hemodialysis is chosen as the preferred modality, an AV fistula will need to be constructed and the preferred extremity should be protected from blood draws and IV access. Older

adults with CKD may have multiple comorbidities that influence decisions about pursuing dialysis, transplantation, or conservative management/palliative care (see Chapter 8). The frail older patient or the patient with significant cognitive deficits may not benefit from KRT as this therapy may not enhance either quality or quantity of life. These are often difficult choices to make, and while the ultimate decision will be made by the nephrologist, the patient, and/or their healthcare surrogate, the primary care NP who has had a long-term relationship with the patient and has guided them through their disease progression can play a valuable role. Palliative care is a viable option for frail older adults or those with advanced dementia (see Chapter 7 for more information about palliative care).

Patient Education

Patient education should include the importance of healthy living and controlling blood sugar if the person has diabetes, as well as controlling blood pressure. There are several patient educational materials that are available to assist CKD education (see Box 23.10). The following will provide key elements to think about during patient education sessions. Social determinants of health should be considered when engaging in education with a patient and developing a treatment plan (see Box 23.11). The importance of taking medications and attending medical appointments should be stressed. Nutrition is an essential aspect of care at any stage of CKD but even more so as the disease progresses to later stages. Consultation with a dietitian is something that can help individuals develop

Box 23.10: Patient Education Resources

National Kidney Foundation www.kidney.org

National Kidney Disease Education Program (NIDDK)
www.niddk.nih.gov

American Nephrology Nurses Association
www.annanurse.org

Patient Education: About Chronic Kidney Disease:
A guide for patients https://www.kidney.org

American Association of Kidney Patients https://aakp.org

Box 23.11: Social Determinants of Health-Related to CKD in the Black and Hispanic Population

■ CKD commonly seen in non-Hispanic Black (16%) and Hispanic (14%) compared to non-Hispanic White (13%) and non-Hispanic Asian (12%).

■ Lower socioeconomic status (poverty) linked to higher prevalence of lower kidney function.

■ Diabetes and hypertension (two most common reasons for CKD) are also subject to disparities due to social determinants.

■ Social determinants of poverty, race, and food insecurity worsen quality of life, particularly those with advanced CKD and can lead to the progression of the disease.

■ Limited access to quality healthcare is available.

■ Ethnic minorities, people with low socioeconomic or less than high school status, and patients with a history of environmental exposure to nephrotoxic chemicals are at risk of CKD and should be screened.

CKD, chronic kidney disease.
Source: Quinones J, Hammad Z. Social determinants of health and chronic kidney disease. *Cureus.* 2020;12(9):e10266. doi:107759/cureus.10266

a person-centered diet plan; medical nutritional therapy with a dietitian is reimbursable by Medicare. When a person is CKD Stage 4, Medicare will reimburse for kidney disease education from a nephrology expert. There are specific criteria for these benefits that involve consultation with a nephrologist.

DIABETIC KIDNEY DISEASE (DIABETIC NEPHROPATHY)

Etiology

DKD occurs in both type 1 and type 2 diabetes and is responsible for 40% to 44% of all cases of ESKD in the United States. Epidemiologic data has shown the incidence of DKD to be 25% to 40%, with about 16% developing ESKD after 30 years. Due to more intensive control of diabetes recently, the incidence of ESKD in people with type 1 diabetes is declining. People with type 2 diabetes tend to develop DKD earlier in the course of their disease. Preventing diabetes is the most effective way to reduce DKD. Factors that affect the rate of DKD onset and progression include (a) age at diagnosis; (b) family history; (c) education level; (d) male sex; (e) alcohol use; (f) uncontrolled blood sugar; (g) hypertension, not well controlled; (h) obesity; and (i) physical activity.[15]

Pathophysiology

DKD is a microvascular complication of the disease and tends to occur concurrently with retinopathy. The earliest phase of diabetic nephropathy is clinically silent and characterized by an increase in the GFR. At this stage, serum creatinine is normal and there is no proteinuria. As the pathologic damage progresses, patients develop microalbuminuria, and this eventually progresses to severely increased proteinuria and decreased GFR and may ultimately lead to ESRD. The pathologic changes of diabetic nephropathy on renal biopsy are specific and include thickening of the glomerular basement membrane and the deposition of proteinaceous nodules in the glomerulus called Kimmelstein Wilson lesions. Because the clinical course of diabetic nephropathy is well defined, renal biopsy is usually not done unless the patient

Box 23.12: Healthy People 2030 Objectives

■ Increase the proportion of adults with CKD who know they have it.

■ Reduce the proportion of adults with CKD.

■ Reduce the rate of new cases of ESKD.

■ Increase the proportion of people on Medicare who get follow-up care 3 months after acute kidney injury.

■ Reduce the proportion of adults with CKD who have elevated blood pressure.

■ Reduce the proportion of adolescents with CKD.

CKD, chronic kidney disease; ESKD, end-stage kidney disease.
Source: Office of Disease Prevention and Health Promotion. Chronic kidney disease. https://health.gov/healthypeople/objectives-and-data/browse-objectives/chronic-kidney-disease

presents with atypical features. These atypical features could include rapid deterioration of renal function, a sudden massive increase in proteinuria despite good diabetic control, heavy proteinuria or renal insufficiency at the time of diagnosis, or the absence of diabetic retinopathy. It is important for patients with diabetic nephropathy to have good diabetes control (Hgb A1c lower than 7.0%) and strict BP control with a goal of 130/80 mmHg or less. The antihypertensive classes of agents, ACEi or ARB, have been shown to reduce proteinuria in diabetic nephropathy and to retard the progression of disease (see Chapter 26 for more information on diabetes).

Risk Factors

The most important thing is identification, as management of risk factors for DKD is essential. Risk factors that are modifiable are (a) increased urinary albumin excretion, (b) elevated glucose, (c) dyslipidemia, (d) uncontrolled hypertension, (e) obesity, (f) smoking, (g) oxidative stress, and (h) inflammation. Nonmodifiable risk factors include (a) longer duration of diabetes, (b) advanced age, (c) female sex, (d) retinopathy, (e) genetic background, (f) ethnicity (African Americans), and (g) glomerular hyperfiltration.[16]

Approach to Diagnosis

Individuals with diabetes and proteinuria are more likely to progress to ESKD, so it is vital that these patients be identified and treated early. Patients should be screened for kidney disease at the time of diagnosis of type 2 diabetes and 5 years after the diagnosis of type 1 diabetes. As a PCP, the AGNP should know when it is appropriate to refer patients with CKD. Worsening proteinuria, rapid deterioration in kidney function, CKD Stage 3 or 4, or difficult-to-control hypertension are all indications for referral to a nephrologist (see Box 23.8). Poorly controlled diabetes should prompt referral to an endocrinologist as glycemic control is key to retarding the progression of the renal disease.

Diagnostics

Creatinine measurement and eGFR calculation use CKD-EPI. Diagnosis is made when the patient has evidence of kidney disease and no other primary etiology for abnormal albumin/creatinine ratio.[15] Because of the variability in urine albumin excretion, a spot-urine (mg of albumin per g of creatinine) should be obtained as described in the CKD section. If a person with diabetes has a positive test for a urinary albumin/creatinine ratio, one first needs to exclude other causes of transient proteinuria which may include fever, urinary tract infection, vigorous exercise, or congestive heart failure. Once these factors are corrected or resolved, the urine should be tested again twice in a 3- to 6-month period using a first void specimen. Albuminuria is confirmed if two of the three urine specimens are positive.

- Urine albumin (e.g., spot urine albumin-to-creatinine ratio) and eGFR should be assessed at least annually in all patients with type 2 diabetes.

Glycemic control is important to prevent macrovascular (e.g., stroke, myocardial infarction, mortality) and microvascular complications, such as retinopathy and DKD.

- Monitor HbA1c twice a year but can be measured four times per year if glycemic target is not achieved or if there is a change in antihyperglycemic medications.[14] Target HbA1C are based on the patient's tolerability and life expectancy (see Box 23.13).

Box 23.13: Target HbA1c

- Less than 6.5% of patients tolerate medications without hypoglycemia or other problems
- Less than 7% optimal for many adults
- Less than 8% in advanced kidney disease, older adult, frailty, extended duration of disease, high risk of hypoglycemia, limited life expectancy; significant medical comorbidity

Source: American Diabetes Association. Understanding A1C. https://www.diabetes.org/diabetes/a1c

- KDIGO guidelines[14] recommend individualizing HbA1c target range from less than 6.5% to less than 8.0% in patients with diabetes and CKD not treated with dialysis.

In addition to monitoring kidney function tests and other laboratory studies mentioned in the CKD section, it is important to obtain the patient's fasting lipid profile, have the patient eat a low cholesterol diet, and start a statin medication instituted as indicated.

Screening Tools and Tests

Because microalbuminuria is the earliest sign of DKD, the ADA recommends annual screening of urinary albumin (spot/urine albumin/creatinine ratio) and eGFR in people who have had type 1 diabetes for at least 5 years, those with type 2 diabetes at the time of diagnosis, and in all patients with diabetes and hypertension.

Management

Pharmacologic

All adults with diabetes and albuminuria should be started on an ACEi or ARB unless there is a contraindication. Contraindications include known allergy or intolerance to these medications, advanced renal failure, or hyperkalemia that cannot be controlled (see Boxes 23.8 and 23.13). The most common side effect of ACEi is the development of a cough, but the most serious complication is angioedema, which causes swelling of the face, lips, and pharynx and can lead to potentially fatal airway obstruction.

ACEi have been shown to reduce the risk of doubling serum creatinine and of progression to death and ESKD in people with type 1 diabetes while ARBs have been shown to be renoprotective in type 2 diabetes. Strict BP control is required with target range of 130/80 mmHg or lower in patients with diabetes with CKD. Reaching this target usually requires therapy with a diuretic as part of the antihypertensive regimen. Thiazide diuretics are used when the GFR is near normal, but in patients with impaired renal function, the more potent loop diuretics are needed.

Patients with CKD should have strict glycemic control with a target HgA1c level of 7.0%, as appropriate for the patient (see Box 23.14). This requires that individuals engage in healthy eating to achieve glycemic control and

Box 23.14: KDIGO 2020 Clinical Practice Guideline for Diabetes Management in Chronic Kidney Disease

- Recommend treatment with an ACEi or ARB be initiated in patients with diabetes, hypertension, and albuminuria and these medications should be titrated to the highest approved dose tolerated.

- Monitor changes in BP, serum creatinine, and serum potassium 2 to 4 weeks of initiate or increase in dose of ACEi or ARB.

- Continue ACEi or ARN therapy unless the serum creatinine rises by more than 30%.

- Hyperkalemia associated with the use of ACEi or ARB can often be managed to reduce serum potassium levels rather than decreasing or stopping the ACEi or ARB.

- Reduce the dose or discontinue ACEi or ARB in the setting of either symptomatic hypotension or uncontrolled hypertension despite medical treatment or to reduce uremic symptoms while treating kidney failure.

- Mineralocorticoid receptor antagonists are effective for the management of refractory hypertension but may cause hyperkalemia or a reversible decline in GFR, especially in those with a low eGFR.

KDIGO, Kidney Disease: Improving Global Outcomes.
Source: Kidney Disease: Improving Global Outcomes Diabetes Work Group. KDIGO 2020 clinical practice guideline for diabetes management in chronic kidney disease. *Kidney Int.* 2020;98(4S);S1–S115. doi:10.1016/j.kint.2020.06.019

🏠 Quality and Safety Alert

- Use only one agent at a time to block RAS. The combination of an ACEi with an ARB, or the combination of an ACEi or ARB with a direct renin inhibitor, is potentially harmful.

- Advise contraception in women who are receiving ACEi or ARB therapy and discontinue these agents in women who are considering pregnancy or who become pregnant.[14]

take medications as prescribed with the addition of insulin in type 2 diabetes if the person fails to achieve the goal with diet and oral medications. Antihyperglycemic medications for patients with type 2 diabetes mellitus (DM) and DKD should include first-line treatment with metformin (eGFR greater than 30 mL/min per 1.73²) and a sodium-glucose cotransproter-2 inhibitor (SGLT2i) and one additional medication as needed for glycemic control. When additional medication is needed, glucagon-like peptide-1 receptor agonist (GLP-1 RA) is preferred. Monitor eGFR in patients treated with metformin

and increase the frequency of monitoring in those with eGFR less than 60 mL/min/1.73.² Reduce the dose of metformin when eGFR is less than 45 mL/min per 1.73² and monitor vitamin B12 levels if a patient has been taking metformin for 4 years or more. For more information about medication management, see Chapter 13.

❶ CLINICAL PEARLS

- If the patient is at risk for hypovolemia, consider decreasing thiazide or loop diuretic before starting SGLT2i; advise patients about symptoms of volume depletion, particularly in high-risk groups such as older adults.

- Inform older adults at risk for orthostatic hypotension to slowly move from a sitting to a standing position and report episodes of possible hypotension (if they have BP readings ask them to bring to office).

- Once SGLT2i is initiated it is reasonable to continue even if the eGFR falls below 30 mL/min/1.73 m².

- GLP-1RA should not be used in combination with dipeptidyl peptidase-4 (DPP-4) inhibitors.

- The risk of hypoglycemia is low with GLP-1 RA when used alone but the risk increases when given with sulfonylureas or insulin; consider reducing the dose of sulfonylurea and/or insulin.

Source: Kidney Disease: Improving Global Outcomes Diabetes Work Group. KDIGO 2020 clinical practice guidelines for diabetes management in chronic kidney disease. *Kidney Int.* 2020;98:S1–S115. doi:10.1016/j.kint.2020.06.019

Nonpharmacologic

All patients with CKD should follow the recommendations for a healthy lifestyle as presented in the section on CKD. Patients with DKD should be encouraged to adopt a healthy lifestyle with regular exercise; KDIGO guidelines[14] recommend moderate-intensity physical activity for a cumulative duration of at least 150 minutes per week or to a level compatible with the person's cardiovascular and physical tolerance. Recommendations for physical activity should include consideration of age, ethnic background, presence of other comorbidities, and access to resources. Patients who are obese should be encouraged to lose weight and maintain an ideal body weight.

Patients should be referred to a renal dietitian for assistance with meal planning, especially if they have multiple dietary restrictions. The KDIGO[14] suggests maintaining a protein intake of 0.8 g protein/kg for those with diabetes and CKD not treated with dialysis and sodium intake of less than 2 g sodium per day. It is important to adapt dietary restrictions based on laboratory studies and patient food preferences and to consider food insecurity.

🏠 Quality and Safety Alert

- For patients at risk of falls, the AGNP should advise on the intensity of the physical activity and the type of exercises that would be safe.
- Consider physical activity that will reduce the risk of falling (e.g., Tai Chi, walking).

Patient Education

Patient education should include what was presented in the CKD section as well as a discussion of the risks of a sedentary life and obesity in those who are not engaging in physical activity. Making sure the patient understands that slowing the progression of CKD involves all the steps discussed in the previous section but that it is imperative glycemic and hypertensive control is achieved. Using positive reinforcement, discovering what matters most to the person, and avoiding negative comments (i.e., you will be on dialysis if you do not do what we recommend) are important when presenting education to the patient. The American Diabetes Association is a good resource for patient education: www.diabetes.org.

HYPERTENSION IN CHRONIC KIDNEY DISEASE

Etiology

Hypertension in those with CKD is caused by volume overload, sympathetic overactivity, sodium retention, endothelial dysfunction (impaired nitrous oxide production, oxidative stress, elevated endothelin levels), and alteration in hormonal systems that regulate BP (increased renin-angiotensin, aldosterone). Hypertension is the second most common cause of CKD and is prevalent in about 60% to 90% of patients depending on the stage of CKD.[20] In addition, "*APOL 1* renal-risk genotypes are known to be associated with a spectrum of diseases related to focal segmental glomerulosclerosis (FSGS)."[13] Many patients of African heritage who have CKD and ESKD that have been attributed to hypertensive nephrosclerosis may instead have *APOL 1*–associated disease.

Pathophysiology

Hypertensive nephrosclerosis usually occurs in patients who have had a long history of uncontrolled hypertension but may also be seen in patients whose BP has only been slightly above target. This disease results in the thickening of the walls and the narrowing of the lumens of the renal arteries and arterioles. Due to ischemic injury, the glomeruli or nephrons eventually become scarred, leading to progressive loss of function. These patients may display other evidence of hypertensive damage, such as left ventricular hypertrophy and hypertensive retinopathy. Hypertensive nephropathy is characterized by slowly progressive renal insufficiency and mild to moderate proteinuria. Hypertensive renal disease is more likely to lead to ESKD in patients of African American descent compared to Caucasians.

Renal vascular hypertension is caused by stenosis of the main renal arteries. The reduced blood supply to the kidneys leads to increased levels of the hormones renin, angiotensin, and aldosterone, which cause vasoconstriction, sodium, and water retention and thus hypertension. The stenosis may lead to a critical loss of blood supply to one or both kidneys, leading to ischemia and eventual renal failure. Atherosclerotic renal disease accounts for 75% of cases and is due to the deposition of cholesterol-filled plaques in the lumens of the main renal arteries. This occurs in older adults with multiple comorbidities and risk factors such as diabetes, preexisting essential hypertension, coronary and peripheral vascular disease, and a history of smoking. Fibromuscular renal artery disease occurs in about 25% of cases and is due to the abnormal development of fibrous tissue in the layers of the vessel wall. It is usually seen in younger females and causes the sudden onset of severe hypertension but does not cause renal failure.

Risk Factors

The prevalence of hypertension depends on the definition, but some of the risk factors include older adults, non-Hispanic Blacks, those living in rural areas, obesity, high sodium intake, physical inactivity, and heavy alcohol intake. Some medications that can increase BP are NSAIDs, sympathomimetics, diet pills, decongestants, amphetamine-like stimulants, glucocorticoids, herbal preparations, estrogen-containing contraceptives, calcineurin inhibitors, and antidepressants. The most common causes of secondary hypertension are primary aldosteronism, renal artery stenosis, and obstructive sleep apnea. Less common causes are pheochromocytoma, Cushing syndrome, and aortic coarctation.

Approach to Diagnosis

Accurate BP measurements are essential to the diagnosis of CKD and the management of hypertension is critical for slowing the progression of CKD. It is important to consider the stage of CKD, if the patient has diabetes, and proteinuria when considering the approach to diagnosis. In addition, it is essential to examine your patient before reacting to elevated BP. Remember, you do not treat numbers, but rather, you are treating a person who has come to your office for evaluation.

Diagnostics

Most BPs are obtained in an office and used to support clinical decision-making. Twenty-four-hour ambulatory BP monitoring is preferred for confirmation of hypertension; however, not every practice has access to this

Box 23.15: Definition of Normal and Abnormal BP per 2017 AHA/ACC Guideline for Patients With CKD

BP Classification	Office BP	Daytime ABPM or Home BP
Normal or elevated	Less than 130/80 mmHg	Less than 130/80 mmHg
Sustained hypertension	130/80 mmHg or greater	130/80 mmHg or greater
White coat hypertension	130/80 mmHg or greater	Less than 130/80 mmHg
Masked hypertension	Less than 130/80 mmHg	130/80 mmHg or greater

ABPM, ambulatory blood pressure monitoring; AHA/ACC, American Heart Association/American College of Cardiology; BP, blood pressure; CKD, chronic kidney disease.

diagnostic tool. This may require a referral to a nephrologist. The KDIGO 2021 Clinical Practice Guideline for the Management of Blood Pressure in CKD recommends an oscillometric BP device may be preferable to a manual BP device for standardized office BP measurement; however, standardization emphasizes adequate preparation for BP measurement and not the type of equipment. In addition, it recommends out-of-office BP measurements with ambulatory BP monitoring (ABPM) or home BP monitoring be used to complement office BP measurement. Patients can be instructed to take two readings, twice a day while sitting. The definition of hypertension based on office, ABPM, or home can be seen in Box 23.15. The AGNP should refer the patient to a nephrologist in the case of resistant hypertension (receiving three or more antihypertensive agents, one is a diuretic, without BP control) or refractory hypertension (receiving three or more antihypertensive medications, one is a thiazide-type diuretic, and the other is spironolactone without achieving BP target goal).

Other diagnostics (e.g., urinalysis, laboratory studies), as previously discussed in the CKD section, should be considered.

Screening Tools and Tests

As nephrosclerosis is the second-leading cause of CKD in the United States, the AGNP needs to be aware of the patients at high risk of nephrosclerosis in the primary care practice. African Americans have an eightfold increase in the likelihood of developing ESKD from hypertensive nephrosclerosis compared to White patients even when the BP is controlled. The link to two *APOL1* gene mutations to hypertension-related ESKD and in African Americans may explain the increased risk. Further research may also lead to guidelines for stricter targets for BP control in these patients. Other patients at risk of hypertensive nephrosclerosis are patients with a history of low birth weight or prematurity, patients who have a reduced renal mass, and patients with severely elevated BP.

Management

Most patients present with a long history of hypertension and mild proteinuria, and slowly and progressively there is a decrease in GFR. Renal biopsy is not usually done unless atypical features are present such as nephrotic range proteinuria, microscopic hematuria, and rapidly worsening renal function. Patients who have proteinuria should be treated with ACE inhibitors or ARBs. The KDIGO guidelines for treating hypertension in nondiabetic CKD patients recommend that patients without proteinuria should be treated to a goal of 140/90 mmHg. Those patients with any degree of albuminuria greater than 30 mg/24 hr should be treated to a goal of 130/80 mmHg. As with diabetic kidney disease, the importance of lifestyle changes needs to be stressed. Patients should maintain ideal body weight, exercise regularly, and adhere to a low salt diet (less than 2 g of sodium chloride daily). Despite this, many patients' hypertension and CKD Stages 3 through 5 will need multiple antihypertensive drug therapies including a diuretic to achieve their target BP.

When a patient presents to primary care with systolic BP over 180 mmHg or diastolic over 110 mmHg and is asymptomatic, a history and physical is important.

■ The evaluation should include a history of hypertension, coronary artery disease (CAD), congestive heart failure (CHF), cerebrovascular disease, CKD, peripheral vascular disease, diabetes, or sleep apnea. Ask about new medications and if taking medications that could increase BP. History should also include neurologic (orientation, any confusion, headache, vison change, seizure disorder, other neurologic deficits), cardiovascular (chest pain, shortness of breath [SOB], myocardial infarction, syncope, history of palpitations or arrhythmias), renal (urinary output, oliguria, anuria), peripheral arteries (claudication, cold extremities, weak distal pulses), and pulmonary (history of lung disease, dyspnea).

■ The physical examination should involve neurologic motor or sensory deficits, ophthalmologic changes (arteriolar narrowing, hemorrhage, papilledema), cardiovascular (arrhythmia, displace point of maximal impulse, murmur, third heart sound gallop), pulmonary (rales, hypoxia, tachypnea), and vascular (diminished or absent peripheral pulses, abdominal bruits, unequal pulses or BP, jugular vein distention). Treatment depends on your findings; for example, if the patient has signs and symptoms of target organ injury (e.g., papilledema, neurologic deficits, pulmonary edema).

■ In those that are asymptomatic and have a history of hypertension, consider adjusting the current antihypertensive medication or consider out-of-office ABPM or home monitoring and follow-up in 2 to 4 weeks. If the patient has mild symptoms, consider administering short-acting antihypertensive medication; if symptoms improve, adjust current medications or add a new medication.

- If symptoms do not improve, consider obtaining a BMP and other testing to assess target organ injury and follow-up in 1 week or consider having the patient evaluated at the emergency department.

- In the absence of acute target organ injury, the BP should be lowered to less than 160/100 mmHg but not rapidly; no more than 20% to 25% reduction of the mean arterial BP over several days to weeks. Medications can be adjusted, or another medication added, BP but it should be about 2 to 4 weeks until achieving target BP goals.[17]

Special Considerations for Adolescents to Young Adults

Hypertension is common among adolescents with CKD. The presence of hypertension and proteinuria are strong predicators of CKD progression in adolescents. BP measurements should be obtained at every office visit; however, when there is a normal BP measurement in the office, about 30% of adolescents with CKD will have masked hypertension and about 50% with elevated BP will experience white coat hypertension. Therefore, recommendations in this population are to obtain at least once a year a 24-hour ABPM.[16] The goal for treating hypertension in adolescents is to reduce the risk for target organ damage. The American Academy of Pediatrics recommends that in an adolescent with CKD, begin antihypertensive therapy when BP measures are consistently above the 90th percentile for the child's age, sex, and height or 130/80 mmHg or greater. Referral to a pediatric nephrologist is appropriate.

Special Considerations for Older Adults

An older man with hypertensive CKD and benign prostatic hypertrophy can benefit from alpha blockers. Diuretics may precipitate hyperuricemia and gout in older adults. Electrolyte imbalances are also more common in older adults. Older females in particular are prone to the development of hyponatremia with thiazide diuretics. Many patients with hypertension have isolated systolic hypertension as they get older and the diastolic pressure either stays the same or falls. This can make it difficult to achieve the stated goals for CKD, as aiming for a systolic BP goal of 130 to 140 mmHg can lead to diastolic hypotension. The risk of hypertension increases with age; the prevalence is about 27% in those younger than 60 and increases to 74% in those older than 80 years. The challenge in determining the best BP goals is related to the lack of focus on older adults (particularly those older than 80 years) in clinical trials.[18] The benefit of treating older adults is clear, but treatment decisions should include comorbidities, the presence of frailty, ability to follow instructions, the complexity of the medication regimen, supporting care (i.e., caregiver, family member), electrolytes, and renal function.[13] Thiazide diuretics (unless eGFR less than 30 mL/min/1.73 m²), ACEi, ARBs, and calcium channel blockers have demonstrated CV benefits in older adults. Beta-blockers in adults over 60 are not recommended (can worsen CV outcomes) unless they have a comorbid condition where the benefit outweighs the risk of prescribing these medications). In those with advanced CKD, loop diuretics may be prescribed but caution should be taken with older adults because of the increased risk of falls. Alpha blockers also may increase the risk of falls in this population.

Pharmacologic

(See Chapter 13 for specifics on medication management.)

Choosing medications to control BP is based on target goals of reducing CV risks and slowing the progression of CKD. The KDIGO[19] recommends that high BP and CKD be treated with a target BP (systolic BP) of less than 120 mmHg when tolerated, using standardized office BP measurements; however, for those with very limited life expectancy and symptomatic postural hypotension, less restricted BP control is warranted. The guidelines recommend starting with either an ACEi or ARB for people with high BP, CKD, with or without diabetes, and moderate or severe increased albuminuria (G1–G4, A2, A3; see Figure 23.4). The guidelines also state that it may be reasonable to treat people with high BP, CKD, and no albuminuria with or without diabetes with an ACEi or ARB.

Angiotensin-Converting-Enzyme Inhibitors

There are effective first-line agents for the treatment of hypertension in proteinuric renal disease. Because they act by reducing the GFR, patients may experience an increase in serum creatinine after starting the drugs and may also develop an increase in serum potassium. Patients should, therefore, have a metabolic panel checked 1 to 2 weeks after initiating one of these agents. An increase in serum creatinine of up to 25% may be seen. Larger increases in serum creatinine should prompt an evaluation for renal artery stenosis. The effects of ACEi and ARBs on serum creatinine and potassium often limit the use of these agents in patients with advanced CKD.

Mineralocorticoid Receptor Antagonist

Mineralocorticoid receptor antagonist (MRAs; spironolactone and eplerenone) are prescribed for resistant hypertension and to lower albuminuria in patients with diabetes and elevated urinary albumin excretion. Side effects include hyperkalemia and decline in kidney function. MRAs should be avoided in those with a high risk of hyperkalemia (e.g., hypoaldosteronism or type 4 renal tubular acidosis). Studies have shown that patients with persistent hypertension and advanced CKD (eGFR 25–45 mL/min/1.73 m²) adding patiromer compared to placebo helped keep patients on spironolactone for at least 12 weeks.[21]

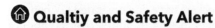 **Qualtiy and Safety Alert**

- Recommend avoiding any combination of ACEi or ARB, and direct renin inhibitor (DRI) therapy in patients with CKD, with or without diabetes.

Calcium Channel Blockers

There are two types of calcium channel blockers. The dihydropyridine calcium channel blockers (e.g., amlodipine, nifedipine) and nondihydropyridine calcium channel blockers (e.g., verapamil, diltiazem). The dihydropyridine calcium channel blockers are powerful vasodilators that do not affect cardiac contractility or conduction. The nondihydropyridine calcium channel blockers are less potent than vasodilators but have significant negative effects on cardiac contractility and conduction. These nondihydropyridine agents must therefore be cautiously used in patients with bradycardia or cardiac failure. The dihydropyridine agents are very effective antihypertensive agents, especially in patients of African descent, and are considered first-line agents in Black patients. The nondihydropyridine CCBs have been shown to be effective in reducing proteinuria and may therefore be added to ACE inhibitors or ARBs to reduce proteinuria or may be used as first-line agents for these CKD patients if ACE inhibitors or ARBs are contraindicated.

Diuretics

Most patients with hypertensive CKD will need multiple agents for control. Diuretics are first-line agents and are essential components of multidrug therapy. Thiazide diuretics are effective when the GFR is greater than 30 mL/min. Loop diuretics, such as furosemide or bumetanide, are used in CKD Stages 4 and 5. These diuretics can cause electrolyte abnormalities such as hypokalemia and hypomagnesemia. Thiazide diuretics may cause hypercalcemia. Potassium-sparing diuretics, such as aldactone and amiloride, may cause hyperkalemia in patients with a moderate to severe reduction in GFR. All the diuretics may cause or exacerbate hyperuricemia and can therefore precipitate attacks of gout.

Beta-Blockers

Beta-blockers are not first-line agents for the management of hypertensive CKD. However, there may be other indications for beta-blocker use in the CKD patient with multiple comorbidities, such as coronary artery disease or congestive heart failure. Patients with resistant hypertension and advanced renal failure may need four or more drugs for control, and beta-blockers are often part of these regimens.

Alpha Blockers

Alpha blockers, such as doxazosin or terazosin, are vasodilators but are not first-line agents for treating hypertension. They may have multiple cardiac effects, including orthostatic hypotension, palpitations, and bradycardia. They, however, can cause relaxation of smooth muscle in the prostate and lead to relief of prostate symptoms in older adult males. These agents therefore are often used for two purposes: as part of a multidrug antihypertensive regimen and for relief of nocturia, frequency, urgency, and urinary retention in the older male.

Other classes of medications used in hypertensive CKD include direct vasodilators such as hydralazine and minoxidil, and central acting agents, such as clonidine and alpha methyldopa. These are not, however, first-line agents. Hydralazine has a high incidence of side effects such as tachycardia, headache, and flushing and needs to be taken 2 to 4 times per day to be effective. Central acting agents, such as clonidine, cause drowsiness and dry mouth and, though effective, are short-acting and can lead to rebound hypertension.

Special Considerations for Adolescents to Young Adults

Engaging in recommended practices (e.g., multidrug regimen and a low sodium diet) to slow the progression of CKD can be challenging in the adolescent patient. Frequent office follow up and an interprofessional approach that uses the skills of a pharmacist and dietitian could be effective in addressing these concerns. It is also necessary to stress to sexually active adolescent females with CKD that it is important to use effective contraception because of the teratogenic effects of ACE inhibitors and ARBs and because there is a high risk of pregnancy complications and irreversible progression of CKD.[22]

Special Considerations for Older Adults

The Eighth Joint National Committee (JNC-8) recommends a higher BP target in older adults (less than 150/90 mmHg), but in adults 65 and older who reside in the community and are ambulatory, the recommendations are less than 130/80 mmHg. The CV benefits are much improved with tighter BP control. However, when considering the target BP, the AGNP should consider life expectancy and the presence of cognitive impairment.

Nonpharmacologic

The guidelines for lifestyle change are the same as those for DKD: a low sodium diet and moderate-intensity physical activity (at least 150 minutes per week), smoking cessation, and limited alcohol intake to improve CV health. It is very important that people with hypertension and kidney disease engage in self-management activities, such as taking medications as prescribed, and follow-up with healthcare providers.

Patient Education

It is important to discuss taking medications as prescribed and integrating healthy lifestyle behaviors into their everyday living. The CDC and the NKF have educational materials for patients to help gain insight into managing CKD and hypertension; these are available at www.cdc.gov/bloodpressure/index.htm and https://kidney.org. Teaching patients how to take their BP correctly before having them monitor at home is important.

CASE STUDY
PATIENT WITH HYPERTENSION, CHRONIC KIDNEY DISEASE, ANEMIA, AND ALZHEIMER'S DEMENTIA

Presented by Geriatric Care Manager (GCM): "She was found wandering in her neighborhood so they called us to get involved and we need to know what her cognitive status is before we can determine what to do next." Sally was asked how she is doing and with a big smile replied, "Very good."

History of Present Illness: Sally is an 89-year-old, community-residing female with a history of hypertension, CKD, anemia, and Alzheimer's dementia. She lived with her daughter who was her primary caregiver; however, her daughter suddenly passed away, and now she presents to your office with a GCM for an assessment of her cognitive status. She was found by a neighbor wandering outside her house, and the neighbor called the police, which is how she now has a GCM. There are no other concerns. When asked about falls or other injuries, the GCM replied, "Not that we are aware of." This is the first time you are seeing Sally. No laboratory or diagnostic tests are available. You do not have advance care planning (ACP) documents, and Sally is unable to provide this information.

Review of Systems: Sally is unable to provide the review of systems (ROS), and since she has no other family members, the NP does not have this information.

PHYSICAL EXAMINATION

Vital Signs: BP sitting 200/100 right arm and left arm 198/100, HR 82, R 18

Standing: BP 190/100, HR 100

Neuro: Alert, oriented to self and immediate surroundings, unaware of health history or that daughter has died.

Heart: Rate regular, rhythm irregular, S1, S2, no murmur

Extremities: Radial pulses 2+, pedal pulses 1+ and 1+ bilateral pedal edema

Attempted to perform cognitive assessment using valid and reliable tools but she was unable to participate due her cognitive status.

Case Study Questions

1. What are the top three differential diagnoses and rationale?

   Uncontrolled hypertension: She is not at her goal; her elevated BP is most likely related to her not taking medications as prescribed; she was living with her daughter who managed her care, and now, since her daughter died, she has been living by herself. Considering her cognitive status (consistent with moderate stage of dementia), she is unable to successfully manage her medications without assistance.

   Cognitive impairment: Her presentation of forgetfulness, repetitive statements, unawareness of current circumstances, poor insight into safety issues, and need for assistance is consistent with a moderate stage of Alzheimer's disease. Neuropsychiatric evaluation can't be completed because she would not be able to effectively participate in the completion of the tests. She may have a moderate delirium because of dehydration.

   Orthostatic hypotension due to dehydration: She most likely does not have adequate intake because she was living by herself and may not remember to drink the amount of fluid she needs.

2. What is your management plan that includes taking a person-centered approach?

   The physical examination was negative for neurofocal deficits; she is not in acute distress, so lowering her BP should include gradual titration and monitoring of response and tolerance. Unless the patient is in acute distress (neurologic, cardiovascular, respiratory), sending her to the hospital is not the best option but rather sending her home with assistance may lead to the best outcomes. Monitoring includes kidney function to detect possible increases in serum creatinine and reduced eGFR. There is the possibility of reduced eGFR related to BP-related decreased renal perfusion.

Restart the calcium channel blocker, obtain laboratory studies, and have her return in a week. Have the GCM obtain BP readings twice a day and contact you if he sees a change in her cognitive status or adverse events related to the medication.

She is not able to independently care for self. So, at this time, the NP should engage in discussions with the GCM as to the best plan for Sally (one that will honor her wishes while keeping her safe) until more permanent arrangements can be made. Educating the GCM about the importance of adequate fluid intake and assisting with medication management is essential.

Follow-Up: 1 Week Later

Sally returns to the office; her BP sitting is 170/88 left arm and 168/90 right arm and standing 166/88, HR 78, no change when standing. The GCM found the ACP documents and discovered that a nephew in another state was to be her power of attorney (POA) if something happened to her daughter. You are reviewing her laboratory studies and realize Sally has an eGFR of 18 mL/min/1.73 m^2, with albuminuria categorized as A2 (you were able to obtain previous labs and these findings were similar to labs done 6 months ago). She has been taking the prescribed calcium channel blocker since her previous visit. Her cognitive status has not changed from the previous visit, and after obtaining medical records from her previous PCP, you see that she has been diagnosed with moderate stage of Alzheimer's disease. You speak to her nephew, and he wants everything done for her, which includes dialysis if needed.

Case Study Questions

1. What are your diagnoses, including rationale? Chronic kidney disease Stage 4, moderate stage of Alzheimer's disease, hypertension not at goal
2. What category is her eGFR? G4
3. What medication should she be prescribed, including rationale? An ACEi or ARB could be beneficial to achieve control of BP, reduce albuminuria, and slow the progression of CKD.

Discuss treatment options for ESKD and how you would present this to her nephew. Recommend follow-up with her nephrologist. Palliative care may be the best option given her cognitive status. It is important to address his concerns and discover what his goals are for his aunt while remaining vigilant in honoring Sally's wishes and preferences for care (as expressed in ACP). Reviewing ACP documents and discussing possible relocation to an assisted living facility (ALF) or dementia care unit rather than remaining independently in her home should be considered, unless he is able to provide care for her in his home. It is important to take a family-centered approach and provide him with the best available evidence regarding the benefits and risks of KRT versus palliative care with no dialysis (supportive vs. curative care) as you engage in shared decision-making. The nephrology team can be extremely helpful in assisting you with this discussion, particularly if you are not comfortable discussing KRT and other options for treating advanced CKD.

CONCLUSION

The incidence and prevalence of CKD are increasing, and many adolescents and adults will first be seen by a PCP, such as an AGNP. PCPs play a key role in identifying, diagnosing, managing, and appropriate referral to a nephrologist in a timely manner. Even though it is not the focus of this chapter to provide the information regarding all causes of CKD, there is comprehensive information about the most common causes, DKD and hypertension, and a brief overview of three others. AGNPs should seek opportunities to comanage people with CKD with nephrology experts (e.g., nephrologist, NP, physician assistant). At this time, it is predicted that there will be a shortage of nephrologists, so the role of PCPs is even more critical in implementing evidence-based strategies that promote health in the complex population of adolescents, adults, and older adults with CKD.

REFERENCES

References for this chapter are online and available at https://connect.springerpub.com/content/book/978-0-8261-8414-6/part/part01/toc-part/ch23.

CHAPTER 24

Common Genitourinary Disorders Encountered in the Primary Care Setting

Humberto Reinoso and Justin M. Waryold

LEARNING OBJECTIVES

At the conclusion of this chapter, the learner will be able to:

➤ Describe the signs and symptoms of common genitourinary (GU) disease in adolescents to older adults in primary care.

➤ Review GU system assessment of adolescents to older adults in primary care.

➤ Determine a diagnosis and develop a plan of care that includes diagnostic testing and a treatment plan of common GU disease processes affecting patients from adolescence to older age in the primary care setting.

INTRODUCTION

This chapter provides an overview of the most common genitourinary (GU) system disorders that may be seen in primary care in adolescents to older adults. The GU system is composed of the kidneys, ureters, bladder, urethra, and genital organs. Large numbers of patients in primary care suffer from a variety of disease conditions that involve the GU tract, which includes the kidneys, ureters, and bladder. Refer to Chapter 25 regarding gynecology and Chapter 23 regarding nephrology for related topics regarding the kidneys and genital organs. Each disorder is presented with an overview of etiology, pathophysiology, approaches to diagnosis, risk factors, and treatment management. In addition, clinical pearls and safety issues are presented as indicated. A case study presents a clinical situation that may occur in primary care.

BENIGN PROSTATIC HYPERPLASIA

Etiology

Benign prostatic hyperplasia (BPH) is the enlargement of the prostate gland caused by an increase in the reproduction rate of the cells. The major problem with this condition is that as prostatic tissue enlarges, it compresses the urethra, where it passes through the prostate, resulting in decreased urinary flow and frequent lower urinary tract symptoms (LUTS). In a small percentage of men, untreated BPH can cause acute urinary retention, recurrent

urinary tract infections (UTIs), hydronephrosis, and even kidney disease (cause of obstructive uropathy).[1] Symptomatic patients may benefit from medical or surgical treatment. BPH is a common disorder that, with the aging U.S. population, is prevalent in primary care.

Pathophysiology

BPH involves complex pathophysiology with several endocrine and local factors and a remodeled microenvironment.[2] Its relationship to aging is well documented. The gradual growth of the prostate gland is seen through puberty with a period of rapid development following until the third decade of life. Benign hyperplasia begins around the fourth or fifth decade. Dihydrotestosterone (DHT) is necessary for normal prostatic development; however, its role in BPH is not completely clear. 5α-reductase is the most powerful of all androgen-metabolizing enzymes within the prostate. Although 5α-reductase and DHT decrease with age in the epithelium, they remain relatively constant in the stroma of the prostate gland.[2]

Risk Factors

BPH becomes increasingly common as men age. The disorder progressively increases in incidence and prevalence in men, particularly those age 50 years and older. The prevalence among U.S. men 60 years and older is about 50%, and among men 70 years or older, 90%. It is estimated that a 60-year-old man with moderate to severe symptoms would have a 13.7% chance of developing acute urinary retention in the following 10 years.[3] Age, symptoms, urinary flow rate, and prostate volume are risk factors for acute urinary retention at least in population-based studies.

Approach to Diagnosis

The clinical manifestations of BPH and LUTS include storage symptoms, such as frequency, nocturia, urgency, and urinary incontinence (UI). Male patients may experience voiding symptoms, such as a slow urinary stream, splitting or spraying of the urinary stream, hesitancy, straining to void, and/or terminal dribbling.[1] Irritative symptoms, such as frequency and urgency, are common presentations but are not specific for BPH. Differential diagnoses include UTI, prostatitis, bladder calculi, urethral stricture, or carcinoma of the prostate.[3] A digital rectal exam (DRE) should be done to assess prostate size and consistency and to detect nodules, induration, and asymmetry, all of which, if present, should raise the suspicion for malignancy. If irregularities are identified, screening for prostate cancer should be recommended on a regular basis.

Diagnostics

Diagnostic testing should include a urinalysis to assess for any infection or hematuria. There may be an elevation of the prostate-specific antigen (PSA) in either prostate cancer or BPH; therefore, the PSA value alone is not diagnostic of cancer or BPH. Acute lower urinary retention or prostatitis will also elevate the PSA.[1] Other diagnostic tests may be performed as part of the evaluation of men with BPH; however, the American Urologic Association (AUA) considers them optional. Maximal urinary flow rate, postvoid residual urine volume, and urine cystology are useful in most men with suspected BPH.

Screening Tools or Tests

The AUA has created a valid and reliable, easily reproducible index that is designed to determine BPH disease severity and evaluate response to therapy. This 35-point scale has questions about both obstructive and irritative symptoms. In addition, the International Prostate Symptom Score (IPSS) is a useful subjective assessment tool for BPH patients; it is a modification of the AUA Symptom Index. The IPSS questionnaire assesses the degree of LUTS and quality of life. Patients can fill out the IPSS form before examinations, but minimal interference from healthcare providers must be ensured. Scores of 0 to 7 are considered mild, 8 to 19 is moderate, and 20 to 35 is severe on either of these tools.

The AUA index (available at www.exchangecme.com/resourcePDF/bph/resource1.pdf) and the IPSS questionnaire (available at www.browardurologycenter.com/pdf//ipss.pdf) are sensitive and so can be used to evaluate symptoms and choose the most appropriate treatment. These should be completed at every visit if appropriate.

Management

Primary care providers and urologists have adopted a "watchful waiting" for patients with mild symptoms of BPH when other serious conditions have been ruled out. Watchful waiting refers to active surveillance by the patient and healthcare provider when BPH has little or no impact on quality of life. There are four approaches to the medical therapy of BPH when quality of life is affected: (a) alpha-adrenergic blockade relaxes the smooth muscle of the prostate, (b) antiandrogen therapy

deprives the prostate of a growth-enhancing factor, (c) combination therapy combines alpha blockades with antiandrogen therapy, and (d) anticholinergic therapy.[3] See Chapter 13 for more information about medication management.

Medications

First-line treatment for BPH includes using selective alpha-1 blockers. In clinical practice, the five selective alpha-blockers used are terazosin, tamsulosin, alfuzosin, doxazosin, and silodosin. Common side effects include orthostatic hypotension, headache, and dizziness (Table 24.1).[3] Referral to a urologist may be indicated if first-line treatment does not relieve symptoms.

Table 24.1: Common Side Effects of Alpha Blockers

Alpha-Blockers	Dosing	Safety
Terazosin	1–10 mg by mouth (PO) at bedtime (QHS) Start: 1 mg PO QHS; max 20 mg/day Clinical response may take 4 to 6 weeks	First dose might cause hypotension. *Serious reactions:* syncope, SVT, A-Fib, priapism, anaphylaxis
Tamsulosin	0.4 mg PO daily (QD) May increase to 0.8 mf PO QD after 2 to 4 weeks	*Serious reactions:* orthostatic hypotension, syncope, arrhythmia, priapism, Stevens-Johnson syndrome
Alfuzosin	10 mg PO QD Give with food; do not crush, cut, or chew	*Serious reactions:* orthostatic hypotension, syncope, hepatotoxicity, priapism, angioedema
Doxazosin	1–8 mg PO QD Start with 1 mg PO QD, then may double dose every 1 to 2 weeks. Max 8 mg/day	*Serious reactions:* orthostatic hypotension, syncope, arrhythmia, priapism, intraoperative floppy iris syndrome
Silodosin	8 mg PO QD Give with food.	*Serious reactions:* orthostatic hypotension, syncope, priapism, severe skin reaction, hypersensitivity reaction

SVT, supraventricular tachycardia.

Source: Data from Drugs.com. 2021. https://www.drugs.com

Other Treatments

Extracts of the fruit from saw palmetto (*Serenoa repens*), the American dwarf palm tree, are commonly ingested to treat benign BPH. The exact mechanisms of action of saw palmetto are unknown. Proposed mechanisms include antiandrogenic effects; inhibition of type 1 and type 2 isoenzymes of 5-alpha-reductase; inhibition of growth factors such as the insulin-like growth factor-I; relaxation of lower urinary tract smooth muscle through antagonism of muscarinic receptors; anti-inflammatory effects through inhibition of lipoxygenase, cyclooxygenase, and leukotrienes; alteration of cholesterol metabolism; antiestrogenic effects; and a decrease in available sex hormone-binding globulin. It is important that patients disclose taking these; therefore, it is important to ask specific questions about taking medications that are not prescribed.

The most common dosage of saw palmetto used in clinical trials is 160 mg twice daily of a dried lipophilic extract containing 80% to 90% fatty acids. Only mild side effects, including headache, nausea, and dizziness, have been noted with the use of saw palmetto. The 2010 AUA guidelines, based on more recent studies, do not detect a clinically meaningful effect of saw palmetto on LUTS.[3] Results from clinical trials note that saw palmetto products are generally well tolerated, with occasional reports of adverse gastrointestinal effects and headache.[4]

Patient Education

Patient education should center around symptomatology and anticipatory guidance of the disease process. Many patients with BPH have no symptoms at all. When symptoms do occur, they can include the following:

- needing to urinate often, especially at night
- having trouble starting to urinate (this means that you might have to wait or strain before urine will come out)
- having a weak urine stream
- leaking or dribbling urine
- feeling as though your bladder is not empty even after you urinate

In rare cases, BPH makes it so a man cannot urinate at all.[3] This is a serious problem. If you cannot urinate at all, call your doctor right away.

ERECTILE DYSFUNCTION

Etiology

Erectile dysfunction (ED) is defined as an inability to achieve and maintain a penile erection sufficient for satisfactory sexual intercourse. Causes of ED may stem from either physiologic, psychologic, endocrine, vascular, and/or neurologic factors. ED is part of a larger classification of male sexual dysfunction that includes diminished libido and abnormal ejaculation. Although most cases of ED have an identifiable organic cause as opposed to a psychologic cause, it is imperative for the primary care nurse practitioner (NP) to assess both the physical and mental health of the male patient presenting with sexual dysfunction symptoms. The spectrum of ED ranges from a mild form, with patients reporting two satisfactory erections out of 10 attempts, to severe, with patients reporting no satisfactory erections.[1]

Pathophysiology

The degree of contraction of cavernosal smooth muscle determines the functional state of the penis. The balance between contraction and relaxation is controlled by central and peripheral factors that involve many transmitters and transmitter systems.[2] Factors that mediate contraction in the penis include noradrenaline, endothelin-1, neuropeptide Y, prostanoids, angiotensin II, and others not yet identified. Factors that mediate relaxation include acetylcholine, nitric oxide (NO), vasoactive intestinal polypeptides, pituitary adenylyl cyclase–activating peptides, calcitonin gene-related peptides, adrenomedullin, adenosine triphosphate, and adenosine prostanoids.[5]

Risk Factors

A thorough physical examination, starting with a general appearance for any signs of depression or anxiety, should be noted. Evidence of feminization, such as gynecomastia or abnormal body hair distribution, should be assessed.[5] Perform a complete cardiovascular examination including peripheral pulses for indication of vascular etiology. A thorough genital examination to rule out any structural abnormality of the penis itself should be done. Inspect the testes and palpate for size or abnormal masses. In addition to a thorough physical examination, diagnostic tests are needed to maximize specificity in determining the cause of ED.

Approach to Diagnosis

In the United States, anywhere between 15 and 30 million men are believed to suffer from ED at some time in their lives. Aging affects sexual functioning, and more than 25% of men older than 65 years of age have ED. In 25% of the cases, medication either directly or by adverse effect may cause ED. Medications, such as antihypertensives, diuretics, or central sympatholytics, such as methyldopa, may cause loss of erection. While ED is more common in the geriatric population, men of all ages should be reminded that alcohol, tobacco, and recreational drugs increase the risk of sexual dysfunction.[5]

Diagnostics

The laboratory investigation for ED depends on information gathered during the history and physical. Laboratory testing is necessary for most patients, although not for all. On the basis of these study results, the provider should be able to determine the medical status of the patient, identify and characterize the type of dysfunction, and determine the need for additional testing (e.g., penile or pelvic blood flow studies, nocturnal penile tumescence testing, or other blood tests).[5] Laboratory tests to consider include the following:

- total, free, and bioavailable testosterone levels
- luteinizing hormone (LH)
- prolactin levels
- thyroid-stimulating hormone (TSH)
- hemoglobin A1c
- serum chemistry panel
- lipid profile
- urinalysis

Imaging studies are rarely performed, except in situations involving pelvic trauma or surgery.

Screening Tools or Tests

The evaluation of male sexual dysfunction begins with a sexual history and physical examination. During the history taking, the patient may complain of loss of desire, an inability to obtain or maintain an erection, premature ejaculation, or an absence of emission or inability to achieve orgasm.[1] Frequently, the patient has a combination of these symptoms. The International Index of Erectile Function (IIEF) is a 15-item, self-administered questionnaire (available at www.camurology.org.uk/wp-content/uploads/interpretation-of-the-iief.pdf) that can be used to assess erectile function prior to and during treatment. The history and physical examination have been reported to have 95% sensitivity but only 50% specificity in determining the cause of ED.[5]

Management

Increased physical activity and weight loss in combination with medical management of cardiovascular risk factors are effective for improving sexual function in some men. There is evidence that smoking increases the risk of ED and that stopping smoking can be beneficial.[1] As a first-line therapy for ED, the recommendation calls for phosphodiesterase-5 inhibitors (PDE-5) for its efficacy, ease of use, and favorable side effects. Sildenafil, verdenafil, tadalafil, and avanafil appear to be equally effective (Table 24.2). The rationale for the use of PDE-5 inhibitors is based on the role of NO-induced vasodilation. PDE-5 inhibitors are contraindicated in men taking nitrates and should be used cautiously in men receiving an alpha-adrenergic blocker. Other treatment options include hormone replacement, vacuum constrictive devices, penile prostheses, or penile revascularization.[5]

Medications

An increasing array of medications are available to assist in the management of ED. For any medication to be effective, the physiologic components involved in the erectile process must be functional. Serious impairments render the medication either completely or partially ineffective. In current practice, PDE-5 inhibitors are the most commonly used treatment for ED. This drug class consists of sildenafil, vardenafil, tadalafil, and avanafil.[5] Guidelines from the AUA recommend offering PDE-5 inhibitors as first-line therapy for ED unless the patient has contraindications to their use (e.g., concurrent organic nitrate therapy). Hormone replacement may benefit men with severe hypogonadism and may be useful as adjunctive therapy when other treatments are unsuccessful by themselves.[5]

Table 24.2: Phosphodiesterase-5 Inhibitors

Phosphodiesterase-5 Inhibitors (PDE-5)	Dosing	Safety
Sildenafil	25–100 mg PO once Start with 50 mg PO times; max 100 mf/dose up to 1 dose/day. Give 0.5 to 4 hours before sexual activity.	Consider starting 25 mg PO once for patient older than 65 years old *Serious reactions:* myocardial infarction (MI), stroke, ventricular arrhythmia, sudden death, anaphylaxis
Tadalafil	5–20 mg PO once Start 10 mg PO once; max 20 mg/dose up to one dose per 24 hours.	Effects last 36 hours. *Serious reactions:* hypersensitivity reaction, myocardial infarction, stroke, ventricular arrhythmia, sudden death, angina, Stevens-Johnson syndrome, syncope
Avanafil	50–200 mg PO once Start 100 mg PO once; max 200 mg/dose up to 1 dose per 24 hours	Give 15 to 30 min before sexual activity. *Serious reactions:* hypersensitivity reaction, priapism, hearing loss

Source: Data from Drugs.com. 2021. https://www.drugs.com

Replacement androgens are available in the following four forms: oral, injectable, gel, and transdermal.

An elevation of serum androgen levels has the potential to stimulate prostate growth and may increase the risk of activating a latent cancer. Periodic prostate examinations, including DREs, PSA determinations, and blood counts (i.e., complete blood count [CBC]), are recommended in all patients receiving supplemental androgens.[5] Obtaining a testosterone level during therapy is necessary for optimizing the dosage.

PROSTATITIS

Etiology

The prostate gland is subject to various inflammatory disorders that may be acute or chronic. Acute bacterial prostatitis is an infection of the prostate, usually caused by gram-negative organisms. This may result from an ascending urethral infection, reflux of infected urine, an extension of a rectal infection, or a hematogenous spread. Chronic bacterial prostatitis is a major cause of recurrent bacteriuria. A history of sexually transmitted diseases is associated with an increased risk for prostatitis symptoms.[6] Nonbacterial prostatitis has findings similar to those associated with chronic bacterial prostatitis, but no evidence of bacterial infection is present on urine culture. The clinical presentation for acute bacterial prostatitis, however, is generally well defined, and antimicrobial therapy remains the mainstay of treatment.[1] The etiology of chronic prostatitis and chronic pelvic pain syndrome (CPPS) is poorly understood but may involve an infectious or inflammatory initiator that results in neurologic injury and eventually in pelvic floor dysfunction in the form of increased pelvic tone.

Pathophysiology

Prostatitis is characterized by the presence of acute inflammatory cells in the glandular epithelium and lumens of the prostate, with chronic inflammatory cells in the periglandular tissue. However, the presence and quantity of inflammatory cells in urine or prostatic secretions do not correlate with the severity of the clinical symptoms. CPPS is diagnosed based on pain in the setting of negative cultures of urine and prostatic secretions. Neuromuscular dysfunction or congenital reflux of urine into the ejaculatory and prostatic ducts may be a precipitating factor.[6]

Approach to Diagnosis

Complaints of pelvic or perineal pain in a male patient is a common presenting symptom for acute bacterial prostatitis. Patients are typically acutely ill with fever, chills, general malaise, dysuria, and irritative urinary symptoms, such as frequency, urgency, and cloudy urine. Swelling of the inflamed prostate can cause voiding symptoms ranging from dribbling and hesitancy to acute urinary retention. The presence of typical prostatitis symptoms should prompt a DRE. On physical examination, the prostate is often warm, firm, edematous, and tender to palpation. The finding of a swollen, tender, warm, and boggy prostate on physical examination in this setting establishes the diagnosis of acute bacterial prostatitis.[1] Vigorous examination of the prostate should be avoided because of the risk of bacteremia.

Screening Tools or Tests

Although men who present with GU tract symptoms in primary care are common, acute bacterial prostatitis accounts for a small number of cases. The National Institutes of Health (NIH) has recognized and defined a classification system for prostatitis in 1999.[6] The four syndromes of prostatitis are as follows:

- **I:** Acute bacterial prostatitis
- **II:** Chronic bacterial prostatitis
- **III:** Chronic prostatitis and CPPS
  - Further classified as inflammatory or noninflammatory
- **IV:** Asymptomatic inflammatory prostatitis

Acute bacterial prostatitis occurs predominantly in sexually active men aged 30 to 50. Chronic bacterial prostatitis is more common in patients older than 50 years old with a history of a previously diagnosed UTI. Urinalysis and urine culture can confirm the presence of infection and identify pathogens. Further studies may be indicated in patients with possible complications. There is no criterion-standard diagnostic test for chronic bacterial prostatitis.[6] Most cases of chronic bacterial prostatitis can be diagnosed with history, physical examination, and urine or semen culture. If clinical evidence strongly suggests chronic prostatitis in a patient with negative cultures, a 2-week trial of antibiotics is worthwhile. If the symptoms improve, prescribe a complete course of antibiotics.[7]

The most common aerobic gram-negative bacteria involved in acute prostatitis include *Escherichia coli*, *Proteus mirabilis*, *Klebsiella*, *Pseudomonas*, and *Enterobacter*. Sexually transmitted pathogens, such as *Neisseria gonorrhoeae* and *Chlamydia trachomatis*, are possible etiologies in sexually active young men, who may have concomitant urethritis or epididymitis; however, age is not a specific risk factor for these sexually transmitted infections.

Management

Managing a patient with acute prostatitis includes antimicrobial and supportive treatment to reduce symptoms. Patients who have no major comorbidities, who have no signs or symptoms of severe sepsis, and who can reliably take and tolerate oral antibiotics can likely be managed in the outpatient setting. Hospitalization

Table 24.3: Antimicrobial Dosing and Safety

Antimicrobial	Dosing	Safety
Trimethoprim-sulfamethoxazole	1 double-strength twice daily (bid) for 4 to 6 weeks	*Serious reactions:* hypersensitivity reaction, hepatotoxicity, Stevens-Johnson syndrome, pancreatitis, renal failure, anemias, seizures, hypoglycemia, hyperkalemia
Ciprofloxacin	500 mg PO bid for 4 to 6 weeks	*Serious reactions:* hypersensitivity reaction, hepatotoxicity, QT prolongation, tendon rupture, seizures, hypoglycemia, blood dyscrasias, depression
Levofloxacin	500 mg PO QD for 4 to 6 weeks	*Serious reactions:* hypersensitivity reaction, hepatotoxicity, QT prolongation, tendon rupture, seizures, hypoglycemia, blood dyscrasias, uveitis

Source: Data from Drugs.com. 2021. https://www.drugs.com

may be necessary if the patient appears toxic or is immunocompromised. A variety of antimicrobials may be used to treat patients empirically for acute bacterial prostatitis pending culture results. Recommendations call for trimethoprim-sulfamethoxazole or a fluoroquinolone (ciprofloxacin or levofloxacin) as empiric therapy.[6] These antimicrobial agents are first-line because they achieve high levels in prostate tissue (Table 24.3).

TESTICULAR TORSION

Etiology

Normal testicular suspension ensures firm fixation of the epididymal-testicular complex posteriorly and effectively prevents twisting of the spermatic cord. An abnormal mesentery between the testis and its blood supply can predispose it to torsion if the testicle is broader than the mesentery. Contraction of the spermatic muscles shortens the spermatic cord and may initiate testicular torsion.[8] Testicular torsion may occur spontaneously, that is, during sleep,

during activity, or trauma. It is a urologic emergency that may result in infertility.

Pathophysiology

Testicular torsion is a twisting of the spermatic cord which results in compromised blood flow to the testes and acute ischemia. This occurs when the free-floating testis rotates on the spermatic cord and occludes its blood supply. The degree of torsion the testicle endures may play a role in the viability of the testicle over time. Complete torsion usually occurs when the testicle twists 360 degrees or more; incomplete or partial torsion occurs with lesser degrees of rotation.[2] The degree of torsion may extend to 720 degrees.

In addition to the extent of torsion, the duration of torsion prominently influences the rates of both immediate salvage and late testicular atrophy. Testicular salvage is most likely if the duration of torsion is less than 6 to 8 hours.[8] Generally, it is felt that the testis suffers irreversible damage after 12 hours of ischemia due to testicular torsion. If 24 hours or more elapse, testicular necrosis develops in most patients.

Risk Factors

The prevalence of testicular torsion in adult patients hospitalized with acute scrotal pain is approximately 25% to 50%.[8] Two-thirds of the cases occur between 10 and 20 years, with the peak at age 14 years. Testicular torsion is possible but rare in older men. The contributing factors of testicular torsion are usually idiopathic and spontaneous. There is a history of trauma in 20% of the cases, with one-third of patients having had prior episodes of testicular pain. Paraplegics are also at high risk for developing testicular torsion, probably as a result of constant pressure while sitting.[1]

Approach to Diagnosis

The typical presentation is a sudden onset of testicular pain that radiates to the groin. The patient may also have lower abdominal pain which may lead the clinician to consider other diagnoses such as appendicitis or gastroenteritis. There may be some associated nausea and vomiting. The cremasteric reflex should be assessed by gently stroking the skin of the upper thigh while observing the ipsilateral testis. A normal response is cremasteric contraction with elevation of the testis. The reflex is usually absent in patients with testicular torsion.[1] This helps distinguish testicular torsion from epididymitis and other causes of scrotal pain, in which the reflex is typically intact.

Diagnostics

Testicular torsion is a clinical diagnosis. If the history and physical examination suggest testicular torsion, the patient should go directly to surgery without delaying by performing imaging studies.[1] Laboratory tests are unlikely to be of consequence, as no single test has high sensitivity or specificity in diagnosing testicular torsion. Color Doppler and power Doppler ultrasonography can be used to demonstrate arterial blood flow to the testicle while providing information about scrotal anatomy and other testicular disorders.[8]

Screening Tools or Tests

The Testicular Workup for Ischemia and Suspected Torsion (TWIST) scoring system was developed for the purpose of determining the risk of testicular torsion on clinical grounds, thus decreasing the indication for ultrasound. Based on TWIST scores, patients are classified as being at low (0–2), intermediate (3–4), or high (5–6) risk.[8]

TWIST consists of the following urological history and physical examination parameters:

- testis swelling (2 points)
- hard testis (2)
- absent cremasteric reflex (1)
- nausea/vomiting (1)
- high-riding testis (1)

Management

Compression of the testicular vessels leads to ischemia of the testes within 6 hours. Failure to recognize testicular torsion and intervene immediately results in the loss of the testicle in 80% of the cases. Treatment for testicular torsion is an immediate surgical exploration with intra-operative detorsion and fixation of the testes. Manual detorsion is performed if surgical intervention is not immediately available, within 2 hours.[8] However, manual detorsion should not delay surgery.

PROSTATE CANCER

Etiology

Prostate cancer is the second-most common cancer in men worldwide. In the United States, there will be an estimated 181,000 cases of the disease and 26,100 deaths from it in 2016. More than 40% of men older than 50 years of age have been found to have prostate cancer on autopsy, and the prevalence increases with age. In U.S. men, those at highest risk for prostate cancer are African Americans, men with a family history of prostate cancer, and men with a diet high in fat, particularly animal fat.[9] Smoking has also been identified as a risk factor for prostate cancer.

Pathophysiology

The prostate is composed of acinar glands and their ducts, which are arranged in a radial fashion with the stroma containing blood vessels, lymph vessels, and nerves. Of all prostate cancers, 95% are acinar adenocarcinomas.

The epithelial cells of the prostate gland are the only source of the glycoprotein PSA. Prostate cancer is known to have propensity for the gland's posterior and apical peripheral zones; therefore, palpation through the rectal wall may help in detection. In contrast, BPH tends to affect the transition zone that surrounds the urethra.[2]

Approach to Diagnosis

Men with prostate cancer are usually asymptomatic early in the disease and may also be asymptomatic late in the disease. Presenting symptoms may include bladder-outlet symptoms or acute urinary retention with very large or locally extensive tumors. Almost 80% of men currently diagnosed with prostate cancer undergo a biopsy because of suspicious serum PSA. However, a DRE retains an important role for early detection as 20% of cases have a prostate abnormality that prompts the biopsy.[1] Rectal examination reveals a palpable hard prostate that may be localized or diffused. Asymmetric areas of induration or frank nodules are suggestive of prostate cancer.

Management

A combination of DRE and serial serum PSA determination provides the most acceptable means for excluding prostate cancer. Biopsy of the prostate is the gold standard for diagnosing and staging. Prostate tumors are classified according to the Gleason system, which is scored and scaled from 1 to 10. Gleason scoring combines two numbers and can range from 2 (*nonaggressive cancer*) to 10 (*very aggressive cancer*). Further staging of prostate cancer according to the extent of the tumor is based on additional diagnostic studies at the time of surgery.[1] The most commonly used staging system is the American Joint Committee on Cancer tumor–nodule–metastasis (TNM) system. This system grades tumors numerically within more detailed subcategories.[9] Some clinicians use a single total PSA cutoff of 4.0 for all age groups as a benchmark above which to arrange evaluations for prostate cancer. If the repeated PSA is within the normal expected values for age and is not increased more than 0.75 ng/dL compared with the prior year value, no further evaluation at that time is necessary unless there is a palpable nodule, induration, or asymmetry on DRE.[10]

Diagnostics (Common Lab and Radiology)

Patients older than age 70 years are usually offered conservative treatment as an alternative to surgery. Radiation external beam therapy or brachytherapy with implants and total androgen ablation are the general measures that are used to treat cancer in older men. In patients younger than 70 years of age, surgery is often recommended as a prostate cancer cure. The standard treatment options for prostate cancer include radical prostatectomy, radiation therapy, and watchful waiting. Treatment decisions are based often on the adverse effects, long-term risks, and financial and emotional cost of different therapies for individual patients.[1]

TESTICULAR CANCER

Etiology

Typically, the patient with testicular cancer presents with a hard lump or painless nodule on his testis that might be noted incidentally by the patient or by his sexual partner. Approximately 30% to 40% of patients complain of a dull ache or heavy sensation in the lower abdomen, perianal area, or scrotum. During physical examination, a scrotal nodule or swelling is most commonly detected in men with testicular cancer. A firm, nontender mass within the confines of the tunica albuginea is usually palpable and distinct from the spermatic cord structures.[1] As many as 10% of patients with testicular cancer will present asymptomatic, and another 10% will present with manifestations of metastasis.[11]

Pathophysiology

The testes are composed of pyramid-shaped lobules containing one to four seminiferous tubules. The seminiferous tubules empty into the rete testis located posteriorly in the hilum of the testis that then drains into the epididymis. The seminiferous tubules contain germ cells in various stages of maturation of sperm production. A primary testicular neoplasm may arise from any testicular adnexal cell component. These are divided into germinal (90%–95%) and nongerminal (sex cord-stromal) tumors.[2] The incidence of testicular cancer varies with race and socioeconomic groups.

Approach to Diagnosis

Testicular cancer is the most common solid malignancy affecting males between the ages of 15 and 35, although it accounts for about 1% of all cancers in men. Germ cell tumors (GCTs) account for 95% of testicular cancers. Testicular cancer has become one of the most curable of solid neoplasms because of remarkable treatment advances beginning in the late 1970s. Prior to that time, testicular cancer accounted for 11% of all cancer deaths in men between the ages of 25 to 34, and the 5-year survival rate was 64%. In 2014, about 380 deaths from testicular cancer were expected in the United States, with a 5-year survival rate over 95%.[11]

Management

The TNM classification of the American Joint Committee on Cancer is also used for testicular cancer. Seventy-five percent of nonseminomas can be cured with orchiectomy alone, usually with modified retroperitoneal lymph node dissection. The diagnosis of a testicular malignancy is generally established at radical orchiectomy, which also serves as the initial treatment. Subsequent therapy depends on histology and the presence or absence of more extensive disease or other risk factors. Despite this usual approach, there are men that present with advanced disease and who undergo systemic chemotherapy prior to orchiectomy.[11] Referral to a urologist is indicated with any suspected case of testicular cancer.

Diagnostics (Common Laboratory & Radiology)

The initial workup of patients with suspected testicular cancer starts with a complete history and physical examination. Laboratory tests and imaging studies include the following:

- serum alpha-fetoprotein
- serum beta subunit of human chorionic gonadotropin (beta-hCG)
- lactate dehydrogenase (LDH)
- chemistry profile
- testicular ultrasound
- high-resolution computed tomography (CT) scan of the abdomen and pelvis.[11]

MALE INFERTILITY

Etiology

Infertility is defined by the inability to achieve pregnancy after 1 year of continuous unprotective intercourse. An estimated 15% of couples are determined to be infertile; however, the cause may not be due to one partner. It has been estimated that 35% of the time infertility is due to the female partner, 30% of the time it is due to the male partner, and 20% of the time it is due to a combination of both partners, with no clear etiology 15% of the time.[12]

Pathophysiology

The pathophysiology of male infertility in more than 90% of all cases is due to low sperm counts, poor sperm quality, or both. Other common causes include hormone imbalance, chronic medical conditions such as diabetes and kidney failure, trauma or surgery to the genitals, genetic disorders, and congenital abnormalities.

Risk Factors

Common risk factors are directly associated with the male's lifestyle choices. Smoking tobacco or marijuana, excessive use of alcohol, use of anabolic steroids, psychologic stress, and excessive heat exposure are well-known factors that have been shown to reduce sperm density. Wearing tight underwear, prolonged sitting, and exposure to radiation, pesticides, or other toxins have also been reported to reduce density.

Approach to Diagnosis

The initial approach to evaluating the male for infertility starts with a comprehensive medical, surgical, and social history, inclusive of a urologic history. The urologic history should include information on the frequency and timing of sexual intercourse, the ability to achieve and maintain an erection, concerns with ejaculation, previous fertility concerns and successful pregnancies, and any problems with one's development from childhood. Following the history, the patient will undergo a traditional physical examination, including a thorough inspection of the penis and testicles, with particular attention to secondary sexual characteristics and physique. The physical examination is highly sensitive to the detection of varicocele, which is the most common correctable cause for male infertility.

Diagnostics (Common Laboratory and Radiology)

Semen Analysis

The semen analysis is the foundation of the male infertility workup. The specimen is collected by masturbation into a sterile container. The patient should have been abstinent for 2 to 3 days prior to maximize sperm number and quality. This sample is usually obtained at or close to the laboratory setting as it needs to be evaluated within 1 hour of collection. The semen is then analyzed using the reference ranges set by the World Health Organization (WHO; Table 24.4).

If the semen analysis is abnormal, further evaluation is needed, including a second specimen to be repeated in 3 months, allowing for the cycle of spermatozoa to be completed.

Table 24.4: The World Health Organization's Reference Ranges for Semen Testing

Characteristic	Normal Reference
Morphologically normal	4%
Motility (progressive)	32%
Motility (total)	40%
Sperm count	39 million per ejaculate; 15 million per mL
Vitality	58%
Volume	At least 1.5 mL

Source: Data from Department of Sexual and Reproductive Health and Research, World Health Organization. WHO Laboratory Manual for the Examination and Processing of Human Semen. 6th ed. World Health Organization; 2021. https://www.who.int/publications/i/item/9789240030787

Simultaneously, the patient should be evaluated for endocrine disorders and have noted infertility causes in up to 20% of the cases. The patient should undergo a venipuncture early for morning serum testosterone and follicle-stimulating hormone, which identify 99% of all endocrine abnormalities in men with soft testes and less than 1 million sperm per milliliter.[13]

In some cases where the examination of the scrotum is difficult, or when a varicocele is felt, an ultrasound is ordered. An ultrasound would confirm the dilatation of the testis or enlarged cysts in the epididymis or the missing vas.

Management

The management of the male with infertility starts with the treatment of the underlying cause. Patients with a varicocele may undergo surgical correction to improve sperm quality; however, there is insufficient evidence to suggest that corrective surgery will increase conception despite improved results of semen analysis.[13] Other medical treatments are limited for improving the chances of conception in men with other infertility causes. The reasons for male infertility are unknown in up to 50% of the cases. The primary care NP should seek expert consultation with a fertility specialist or reproductive endocrinologist for further evaluation and management, particularly if the initial workup is abnormal.

Patient Education

Patient education is grounded in promoting a healthy lifestyle with a focus on a heart-healthy diet and adequate exercise. Other lifestyle changes should be discussed, including cessation of tobacco, marijuana, and limiting alcohol use. Lifestyle changes may improve sperm quality in patients with no direct cause.

💡 CLINICAL PEARLS

- Male infertility accounts for 30% of the causes in couples trying to conceive, with 90% of all cases due to low sperm counts, poor sperm quality, or both.
- Obtaining a comprehensive history inclusive of an expanded urologic history and examination is imperative.
- Lifestyle changes may improve sperm quality in patients with no direct cause.

VARICOCELE

Etiology

Varicoceles commonly affect males in their late teens to the early 20s due to the fully developed testes' increased venous drainage. Studies have shown that it affects 15%

of all males and causes primary male-factor infertility in 35% of all cases.[14]

Pathophysiology

Varicocele is caused by dysfunction of the valves in the spermatic vein, most commonly occurring to the left testicle. The inadequate venous drainage leads to enlargement of the spermatic cord's pampiniform venous plexus, causing blood to pool around the scrotal structures, which results in increased heat and stress. The exact cause of this is unknown.

Risk Factors

At this time there are no known risk factors for a varicocele. Some theories suggest possible causes are elevated temperature, venous stasis and reflex, and low intratesticular testosterone.

Approach to Diagnosis

A general examination is performed, with an increased focus on the male genitalia. The penis, urethral opening, scrotum, and testicles are inspected and palpated while the patient is standing. The palpation of the testes may be uncomfortable for the patient; however, it is necessary to assess the masses. Assessment for a scrotal mass includes asking the patient to bear down (Valsalva maneuver) while standing, resulting in the dilated veins' engorgement. If a varicocele is present, a portion of the testicle will often feel like a "bag of worms."[15] Any scrotal mass should be assessed with the patient in both standing and supine positions.

Diagnostics (Common Laboratory and Radiology)

To further examine scrotal contents, the patient will undergo an ultrasound of both testicles. Color Doppler can be used to diagnose and grade varicoceles by documenting reversal of flow with or without performing a Valsalva maneuver.

Management

Surgical intervention is required to treat a varicocele for infertility reasons or if the patient is symptomatic, usually with noted reduced testicular size or a complaint of pain. Traditional surgical or percutaneous embolization may be performed as an outpatient procedure, resulting in little downtime.

🛈 CLINICAL PEARLS

- Varicoceles most often occur in males and are isolated to the left testicle.
- Varicoceles can be described as a "bag of worms" when the testicle is assessed.

- Ultrasound is necessary for further evaluation of all patients with a testicular mass.
- Surgical intervention is appropriate for the treatment of symptomatic patients and infertility.

URINARY INCONTINENCE

Etiology

The etiology of UI, also known as "leaky bladder," has been reported in women more than men. With an estimated prevalence range from 3% to 55%, the highest incidence is among pregnant women, with remission after giving birth.[16]

Pathophysiology

The pathophysiology depends on the underlying condition or cause of the UI. The most common UI types are (a) urge, (b) stress, and (c) mixed. Less common types of UI are overflow and functional. With urge UI, there is detrusor overactivity or known neurologic deficits. Stress UI involves intrinsic sphincter dysfunction and increased ureteral mobility.[17] Mixed UI is the most common type with multifactorial physiology.

Risk Factors

Common key risk factors that affect both men and women are chronic cough, obesity, prior pelvic surgeries, increasing age, overactive bladder, and cognitive and neurologic impairment. Women have a greater risk of UI with pregnancy, specifically women who have undergone vaginal deliveries and have had multiple pregnancies.[17]

Approach to Diagnosis

A comprehensive history of chronic conditions, such as diabetes and chronic cough, should be noted. An in-depth focus on the GU system should include information regarding the onset, duration, and timing of UI and associated symptoms, such as urgency, dysuria, straining, frequency, nocturia defined as more than twice nightly, and any history of UTIs. Within this focused review, the adult-gerontology nurse practitioner (AGNP) can identify other pathologies that could be causing the UI, such as multiple sclerosis, prostatitis, urinary obstruction, and vaginitis. In older adults, it is imperative to focus the history on reversible causes of UI. These factors include delirium, infection, pharmaceuticals, psychologic morbidity, excess fluid intake, restricted mobility, and stool impaction.

💡 CLINICAL PEARLS

The mnemonic **DIAPPERS** can be used to assess for UI in older adults:

- **D**elirium
- **I**nfection (UTI)
- **A**trophic urethritis and vaginitis
- **P**harmaceuticals
- **P**sychologic disorder (e.g., depression)
- **E**xcessive urine output (e.g., heart failure, diuretics, hyperglycemia)
- **R**estricted mobility
- **S**tool impaction

🏠 Quality and Safety Alert

- You must always assess if acute or chronic because an acute onset of UI and delirium may be a sign of UI in older adults (they may not have urgency, dysuria, or fever as the initial signs).

Physical examination should include an examination of the abdomen, mental status, and mobility status. A rectal examination is necessary to examine for any fecal impaction as well as rectal tone. Women may undergo a digital examination palpating the pelvic floor for muscle tone, contraction technique, and strength.

Diagnostics (Common Laboratory and Radiology)

A urinalysis is performed in all persons being evaluated for UI. This is a valuable screening tool for UTIs. If in doubt, a urine culture should be obtained. In addition to screening for infection, urinalysis detects the presence of blood, glucose, and protein and plays a role in screening for malignancy, diabetes mellitus, and renal impairment. Obtaining a urine culture is beneficial to an older adult because this population is more likely to present with nonspecific generalized symptoms that may be mistaken for another pathology.

Screening Tools and Tests

Other screening tools may be utilized, such as the cough test, voiding diaries, and pad testing, which serve as semi-objective measures for determining the UI's underlying cause.

A cough test may be performed in the office setting, whereby the patient stands with a full bladder and forcibly coughs. Any leakage is a positive test and has high sensitivity and specificity for diagnosing stress UI.

Voiding diaries is an objective measure of the average amount of urine voided, the timing and frequency of the void, and the UI frequency (a bladder diary can be found at www.urologyhealth.org/resources/bladder-diary). Additional information, such as pad usage, fluid intake, fluid type, and sensation of urgency, can provide valuable information for the NP in determining the type of UI.

Pad testing uses an absorbent perineal pad that is worn for up to 24 hours while the wearer performs normal daily life activities. The presence and volume of UI can be a useful correlate of symptoms and can determine the UI type.

Management

Treatment of UI, regardless of the etiology, starts with lifestyle changes and behavioral therapies, with the main focus placed on bladder training and pelvic floor exercises. Kegel exercises are taught to the patient to build up the pelvic floor's support through regular muscle strength training. This exercise's outcomes vary, but it has shown improvement in patients who have stress UI more than patients who have urge UI.

Pharmacologic

Medications can be used to treat urge and mixed UI when lifestyle changes and behavioral therapies are ineffective. Pharmacologic therapies should be seen as the last resort because in most studies, improvement is minimal at its best. There is no approved pharmacologic treatment for stress UI.

Anticholinergics, also known as antimuscarinics, may be used as first-line therapies in conjunction with lifestyle and behavior changes. Anticholinergics act directly on the detrusor muscle, leading to reductions in urinary urge incontinence, resulting in improvements in urinary urgency, voiding frequency, and nocturia. Starting a 4- to 8-week trial is recommended. Due to the adverse effects profile, the American Geriatrics Society recommends avoiding these medications in older adults unless no alternatives are available.[18]

The β3-adrenergic agonist is the newest class of medications used to treat urge UI (Table 24.5). Mirabegron (Myrbetriq) acts on beta-3-adrenergic receptors to relax the detrusor. A side effect of increased blood pressure (BP) can occur and should be cautiously used in patients with hypertension. Caution is needed when combining mirabegron with an anticholinergic as there is an increased risk of urinary retention.

Nonpharmacologic

- Scheduled (Timed) Voiding: Good to treat urge and functional UI in both cognitively sound and cognitively impaired older adults. The use of fixed intervals is important after evaluating common voiding patterns.
- Prompted voiding combines schedule voiding with monitoring, promoting, and verbal reinforcement.
- Pelvic Floor Muscle Exercises (Kegel): Repeated voluntary pelvic floor muscle contraction.
- Bladder Retraining: Increase interval between urge to void and voiding.

Patient Education

Patient education should be focused on lifestyle changes and behavioral therapies to achieve an age-appropriate quality of life. Patients should be made aware that

Table 24.5: Beta-3-Adrenergic Medications

Drug	Methods of Action	Adult Dosing	Prescribing Considerations
Oxybutynin	Antagonizes acetylcholine at muscarinic receptors; relaxes bladder smooth muscle, inhibits involuntary detrusor muscle contractions (anticholinergic)	Immediate Release: 5 mg PO bid-tid Extended-Release: Dose: 5–15 mg ER PO qd	Start 2.5 mg PO bid-tid in older adults Max: 5 mg PO qid Start 5–10 mg ER PO qd, may increase by 5 mg/day qwk Max: 30 mg/day ER Contraindicated for patients with urinary retention Caution in older adult patients
Tolterodine	Antagonizes acetylcholine at muscarinic receptors; relaxes bladder smooth muscle, inhibits involuntary detrusor muscle contractions (anticholinergic)	Immediate Release: Dose: 2 mg PO bid Extended-Release: 4 mg ER PO qd	May decrease dose to 1 mg PO bid May decrease dose to 2 mg ER PO qd Contraindicated for patients with urinary retention
Mirabegron	Selectively stimulates beta-3-adrenergic receptors, relaxing bladder smooth muscle	Monotherapy: 25–50 mg PO qd; Combined with an anticholinergic: 25–50 mg PO qd	Start 25 mg PO qd. Max: 50 mg/day Start 25 mg PO qd. Max: 50 mg/day Contraindicated for patients with SBP greater than 180, DBP greater than 110

DBP, diastolic blood pressure; SBP, systolic blood pressure.

pharmacotherapies have been shown not to fully resolve UI and come with side effects that can affect one's quality of life. Studies have shown that performing Kegel exercises can help control urge and stress UI to a greater extent. Women can go to www.acog.org/womens-health/faqs/urinary-incontinence, and all patients can go to www.nia.nih.gov/health/urinary-incontinence-older-adults for more information.

CLINICAL PEARLS

- Assessment for the older person with UI should include evaluation for factors, such as delirium, infection, pharmaceuticals, psychologic morbidity, excess fluid intake, restricted mobility, and stool impaction.
- Urinalysis should be performed in all persons being evaluated for UI.
- Kegel exercises have shown to be effective in the treatment of both stress and urge UI.
- Pharmacotherapy is not any more effective than lifestyle changes and behavioral therapies.

URINARY TRACT INFECTION

Etiology

The UTI is the most common bacterial infection seen in the outpatient setting, accounting for 8.6 million cases in 2007, with most of these affecting women.[19] Complications from UTIs include pyelonephritis, which may require hospitalization and result in permanent kidney damage.

Pathophysiology

The urinary tract from the kidneys to the urethral meatus is usually sterile unless it is invaded with potential urinary pathogens from the bowel entering the vagina, resulting from sexual activity. Bacteria can invade the bladder, causing cystitis, and, in some cases, invade the ureter to the kidney, causing pyelonephritis. *E. coli* is the most common microorganism, causing 75% to 95% of all uncomplicated cystitis and pyelonephritis.[19]

Risk Factors

Risk factors include sexual intercourse, the use of spermicides, and previous UTIs. There is a lack of evidence that demonstrates pre- or postcoital voiding patterns, like intake of fluids, frequent urination, wiping patterns, or type of underwear.

Approach to Diagnosis

Cystitis is usually manifested as dysuria with or without frequency, urgency, suprapubic pain, or frank hematuria. Cystitis can be challenging to diagnose because it may present itself differently in various sexes and age groups.

Careful attention to the history of the present illness will assist in the appropriate diagnosis. Therefore, these results provide little useful information when history is strongly suggestive of UTI. A urine culture is needed to provide confirmation of bacteriuria's presence and the antimicrobial susceptibility of the infecting uropathogen. This test is performed in all women with suspected pyelonephritis but is not necessary for the diagnosis of cystitis, given the reliability of the patient's history of present illness.

UTIs are the second-most common infection in the geriatric population. Typical findings, such as dysuria, polyuria, and urgency, may not always be seen in older adults. Typical manifestations of a UTI in the older adult include incontinence, decreased appetite, nausea, vomiting, abdominal pain, acute confusion, unstable gait, increased falls, and agitation. When evaluating this population, the NP must take appropriate steps to ensure no clinical evidence of a UTI when there is a high clinical suspicion.

Diagnostics (Common Laboratory and Radiology)

Initial diagnostics begin with a dipstick urinalysis in the outpatient setting. The dipstick will provide information on the presence and amount of leukocyte esterase, nitrites, and red blood cells. Dipstick urinalysis testing can be useful for rapidly screening urine for UTI possibility but may not be conclusive. The dipstick urinalysis is less specific and sensitive in older women—a population with a higher UTI rate—than in the general population.

Management

Acute uncomplicated cystitis can be treated straightforwardly with early resolution of the symptoms. Rarely does uncomplicated cystitis progress into pyelonephritis.

Due to an increase in antimicrobial resistance of uropathogenic *Escherichia coli*, treatment has become more complicated. After treatment for uncomplicated cystitis or pyelonephritis, a urine culture is not necessary if symptoms have resolved.[20] The only exceptions to this are pregnant women for whom treatment of persistent asymptomatic bacteriuria is recommended.

Pharmacologic

Empirical treatment of a 3- to 5-day course regiment is recommended for uncomplicated acute cystitis. Standard first-line therapies include nitrofurantoin monohydrate macrocrystals or double-strength trimethoprim-sulfamethoxazole. The choice of antibiotic should be individualized to the patient according to relevant factors, including, but not limited to, allergies, availability, cost, compliance, and known prevalence of resistance in the local community (Table 24.6).

Patient Education

Patient education focuses on completing a full course of antibiotics, monitoring for side effects related to the antibiotics, and resolving symptoms. A repeat culture to determine resolution is not needed unless the patient is pregnant.

🔑 CLINICAL PEARLS

- *E. coli* is the most common microorganism of all uncomplicated cystitis and pyelonephritis.
- Dipstick urinalysis is useful for rapidly screening urine for the possibility of UTI but may not be conclusive.
- Empirical treatment of a 3- to 5-day course regiment is standard for uncomplicated acute cystitis.

Table 24.6: Antibiotic Prescribing

Drug	Methods of Action	Adult Dosing	Prescribing Considerations
Nitrofurantoin	Bacteriostatic or bactericidal, depending on susceptibility and concentration; inhibits DNA, RNA, protein, and cell wall synthesis (imidazolidinedione).	*Immediate Release*: 50-100 mg PO q6h x5 days *Extended-Release*: 100 mg ER PO q12h x5 days	Give with food.
Sulfamethoxazole/ Trimethoprim	Bactericidal; sulfamethoxazole competes with para-aminobenzoic acid (PABA), inhibiting folic acid synthesis; trimethoprim selectively inhibits dihydrofolate reductase.	800 mg/160 mg 1 tab PO bid x3 days	Dosage expressed as trimethoprim Drink with plenty of fluids Caution in older adult patients

HYDROCELE

Etiology

A hydrocele is a collection of fluid, typically found in the scrotum. Hydroceles are classically found in males of all ages and are typically painless but can lead to physical and psychologic complications.

Pathophysiology

The formation of a hydrocele occurs when there is an imbalance of scrotal fluid production and absorption. This occurrence can be categorized into two types: primary and secondary hydroceles. Primary hydroceles are when the processus vaginalis of the spermatic cord fuses at term or within 1 to 2 years of birth, thus obliterating the communication between the abdomen and scrotum. Frequently, resolution occurs without intervention. Secondary hydroceles occur as a result of an underlying condition such as infection, trauma, or malignancy.[21]

Risk Factors

The risk factor associated with secondary hydroceles is directly contributed to an injury, inflammation, or infection of the testicle.

Approach to Diagnosis

The patient will usually present with an acute complaint of painless scrotal swelling in the testes. The history should ascertain any recent trauma/injury and history of inflammation or infection. Due to the scrotal swelling, the testes are often impalpable; therefore, transillumination is performed. Transillumination is one of the most common techniques used to diagnose hydroceles. This technique determines that if the light shines through the scrotum during transillumination, the mass is cystic, and if the light is blocked, the mass is solid. This technique is often used in conjunction with diagnostics to determine etiology.

Diagnostics (Common Laboratory and Radiology)

Ultrasound assessment is the recommended diagnostic tool for identifying and evaluating hydroceles. Ultrasound assists in eliminating misdiagnosis, particularly when masses accompany hydroceles.

Management

Surgical intervention is the gold standard, and it is warranted when the hydrocele becomes complicated or symptomatic. Patients who are asymptomatic or are not bothered by the hydrocele do not require intervention.[22] However, if there is a pathologic concern or if the diagnosis is in question, operative exploration is warranted.

CLINICAL PEARLS

- Transillumination is one of the most common techniques used to diagnose hydroceles.
- Ultrasound assessment is necessary to identify and evaluate assisting in eliminating misdiagnosis, mainly when masses accompany hydroceles.

CONCLUSION

GU symptoms are a common presenting complaint to primary care providers. Age-specific considerations should be applied to not only the presenting symptomology but also the treatment and prevention plan. Adolescent and elder patients, for different reasons, are at higher risk for GU disease processes. Taking a proactive approach is essential in preventing untoward events such as drug-resistant infections, urosepsis, or advanced-stage cancer.

CASE STUDY
PATIENT WITH MID- TO LOW BACK PAIN

Initial Presentation

H.B. is a 40-year-old, single, male who woke up with some mild low back pain this morning. He works for UPS and has taken extra shifts this past month. He complains of low grade fever for the last 2 days with some fatigue which he attributes to the extra workload. He denies similar episode prior.

Case Study Questions

1. List a minimum of six appropriate questions you might ask this individual.
2. What is the significance of this patient's "low-grade" fever?
3. Prioritize six possible differential diagnoses.

Medical History

- Denies any history of renal calculi or previous back pain in the past.
- Allergic to penicillin

Medications: None

Social History

- Does not smoke, drinks about two to three beers per week, denies any illicit drug use
- Sexually active, bisexual, does not use protection. Last encounter was about a week ago, described as a "hook-up" from dating site.

(cont.)

Case Study Questions

4. What additional questions do you want to ask this individual?
5. Reprioritize the list of possible differentials and provide clinical manifestations of each.

Vital Signs

- BP = 130/86; HR = 108; RR = 18
- Temp = 101 °F; Height = 5 11; Weight = 182 lb
- Review of systems (ROS): <u>Positives</u>—fever, fatigue, chills, low back pain, mild burning with urination
- All other systems negative
- Pulmonary embolism (PE): <u>Positives</u>—(+) cerebrovascular accident (CVA) tenderness right and left flank, (+) mild soft tissue tenderness to palpation lumbar spine.

Case Study Questions

6. Based on the subjective and objective data, what are the top three possible diagnoses?
7. Are there any diagnostic tests that you would like to order?

Differentials

- Low back pain, herniated disc, UTI, pyelonephritis, sexually transmitted infections (STI)
- UA:
  - Appearance: yellow and cloudy
  - SG: 1.016
  - pH: 6.5
  - Specific gravity: 1.015
  - Protein: negative

- Ketones: negative
- Glucose: negative
- Nitrites: negative
- Leukocytes: (+)
- Red blood cell (RBC): (+)

Case Study Questions

8. What is the significance of positive leukoesterase and nitrites findings with the dipstick analysis?
9. List three pathophysiologic conditions that may result in positive RBCs in the dipstick test.
10. What is your plan for this patient?

Plan

- UA and C&S
- Tylenol for fever control
- Fluoroquinolones for 14 days for mild forms of pyelonephritis. If high fever, high white blood cell (WBC), vomiting, and/or dehydration, then admit.
- Follow-up with patient in 12 to 24 hours to see if symptoms improved. Might need to be admitted for IVF and parenteral antibiotics.
- Follow-up cultures done in 2 weeks and 3 months.
- Educate patient on STIs and recommend safe sex practices.
- Order full STI panel (HIV, GC/CT, syphilis)

REFERENCES

References for this chapter are online and available at https://connect.springerpub.com/content/book/978-0-8261-8414-6/part/part01/toc-part/ch24.

CHAPTER 25

Common Gynecologic Disorders Encountered in the Primary Care Setting

Kathi Voege Harvey

LEARNING OBJECTIVES

At the conclusion of this chapter, the learner will be able to:

➤ Describe the role of the primary care adult-gerontology nurse practitioner (AGNP) in identifying and managing gynecologic disorders commonly seen in primary care practice.

➤ Differentiate normal from abnormal clinical findings in the routine gynecologic examination.

➤ Diagnose and manage common variations in the menstrual cycle.

➤ Diagnose and manage common menopausal symptoms.

➤ Diagnose and manage pelvic pain, amenorrhea, dysfunctional uterine bleeding, lichen sclerosus, and pruritus ani.

➤ Diagnose and co-manage polycystic ovary syndrome (PCOS) with the multispecialty team.

INTRODUCTION

Gynecologic disorders may at first seem like an area that should always be handled by the gynecologist, and often it is. However, the identification of a problem may be done in primary care, and when gynecologic reasons have been ruled out, patients may be asked to follow-up with their primary care provider (PCP) for further evaluation. Patients may also seek the advice and triage of their PCP first because an open and trusting relationship has previously been established, their insurance requires a referral, or the symptoms are so vague that the patient needs further guidance. It is important for the PCP to understand gynecologic disorders as they will be comanaging the patient's care over the course of treatment for many of these conditions. Some complaints of symptoms require educating the patient about normal physiologic changes that occur and what is considered pathologic. Other presentations will require active listening, a thorough history, and testing before a differential diagnosis and plan of care can be established with the patient. Because many symptoms may be cyclical, encouraging the patient to do monthly journaling may be necessary to

establish the best course of action. The age of the patient plays a key role in managing gynecologic disorders, preserving fertility during the childbearing years, and maintaining quality of life throughout the life cycle. The nurse practitioner (NP) must always consider how the disorder affects well-being and make sure to involve the patient in the plan of care.

OVERVIEW OF THE SYSTEM

Normal Anatomy and Physiology

The normal anatomy of the female genitourinary system is displayed in Figures 25.1 and 25.2. A review of these structures and their normal functions is outlined in *Advanced Health Assessment and Differential Diagnosis*.[1] As you review these structures, it is important to note the proximity of structures, as this will become critical in all aspects of the physical examination. Changes in the normal function of the colon can be misinterpreted by the patient and provider as serious gynecologic problems or overlooked as the result of constipation when further evaluation may be needed. Patients that were born with male anatomy and have undergone female reconstructive surgery will require the same gynecologic history and examination as all other patients. Evaluating symptoms requires consideration of the phase of gender transition that the patient is currently in regarding anatomic structure and hormone supplementation. As with all patients, a trusting relationship should be established through effective communication before attempting the physical examination.

There are four major hormones involved in the menstrual cycle: follicle-stimulating hormone (FSH), luteinizing hormone (LH), estrogen, and progesterone. Figure 25.3 provides a concise review of the normal menstrual cycle. Understanding the phase of the patient's menstrual cycle at the time of symptoms and evaluation plays an important part in differential diagnosis and management. Take some time to review this cycle and have a schematic available in your office as a patient teaching tool. It will be important to understand this cycle as you educate patients on normal symptoms to

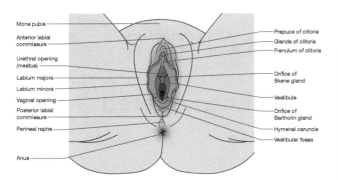

Figure 25.1: External genitourinary anatomy.

Source: Myrick KM, Karosas L, eds. *Advanced Health Assessment and Differential Diagnosis: Essentials for Clinical Practice.* Springer Publishing Company; 2021: Figure 10.1

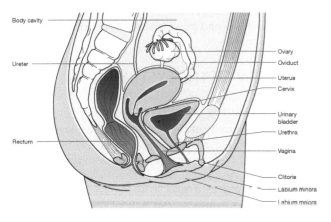

Figure 25.2: Internal genitourinary anatomy

Source: Myrick KM, Karosas L, eds. *Advanced Health Assessment and Differential Diagnosis: Essentials for Clinical Practice.* Springer Publishing Company; 2021:Figure 10.3.

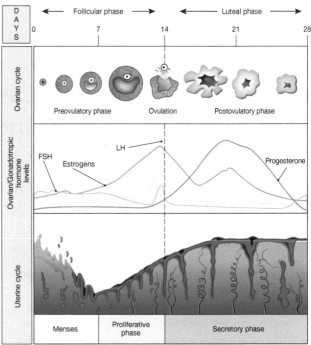

Figure 25.3: Menstrual cycle

FSH, follice-stimulating hormone; LH, luteinizing hormone.
Source: KS Gawlik, Melnyk BM, Teall AM, eds. *Evidence-Based Physical Examination: Best Practices for Health & Well-Being Assessment.* Springer Publishing Company; 2021:Figure 20.7.

expect and family planning. NPs in primary care may be called on to prescribe oral contraceptives. Other forms of contraception should be referred to a gynecologist or women's health specialist. Discuss with a pregnant patient the importance of referring to an obstetrician or a nurse-midwife. Again, it is important to have a list of trusted referrals that you have vetted. It is also important to have a clear understanding of free or low-cost obstetrical services and infant programs in your community, as many medical plans may not include coverage for pregnancy. You and your staff will also want to have a working knowledge of free and reduced-cost prescription drug plans that are available.

It is recommended that NPs co-manage any abnormal clinical findings with specialists as appropriate. Patients should always be included in any clinical discussions and their preferences as to consultants should be considered. The selection of providers that patients may be referred to should be done after careful consideration of the providers' education, training, and experience, as well as any established relationship with a provider.

CASE STUDY

MJ is a 16-year-old girl living at home with her mother and father. She has been dating her boyfriend for 2 years. MJ's mother, KJ, has been your patient for many years and reports that her daughter's moods are disrupting the family and that the pediatrician has not been able to help. KJ asks you to see her daughter as a new patient.

In your consideration of accepting MJ as a new patient:
1. What office policies would you want to discuss with her mother?
2. What privacy and patient rights does a 16-year-old girl have?
3. How would you begin a discussion to understand the mother's views on family planning?

You agree to see MJ as a new patient. When she arrives at your office with her mother, she is adamant about meeting alone with you and appears very angry. Her mother has previously agreed for you to see her alone and that she will honor her daughter's privacy. Before beginning the history, you position yourself away from your computer in a relaxed position in which you can have eye contact with MJ. You begin by introducing yourself and ask how she is doing. In taking your history, you come to understand that MJ feels irritable, has breast tenderness, and becomes emotionally sensitive 2 to 3 days before the start of her menses, and is having "terrible" abdominal pain during the first 4 days of her period. Her periods last 6 days and occur every 28 to 30 days. She is also experiencing diarrhea and sometimes bleeds through her pad and onto her clothing. She states that even between her periods, she sees a milky white odorless discharge but denies any pruritis. She shares with you that she is scared that she may have a vaginal infection and that she is not sexually active but is being pressured by her boyfriend. By the end of the interview, she appears comfortable with you and asks for your help.

Case Study Questions

1. What physical examination plan would you discuss with MJ, and how would you describe it to her before proceeding?
2. Describe the plan of care that you and MJ will develop.
3. What patient support and education do you want to convey during this first encounter?

ROUTINE GYNECOLOGIC GUIDELINES

As you have learned in previous chapters, there are guidelines for many practice areas that are based on research and expert opinion. Although it is important to consider guidelines in your clinical decision-making, it is also essential to include your expert opinion and the patient's wishes and preferences for care. The annual assessment of women is an excellent opportunity to address prevention, screening, whether the patient feels safe in their current relationship, counseling, and immunizations, based on age and risk factors. It may or may not include a pelvic and breast examination. The American College of Obstetricians and Gynecologists (ACOG) has developed an interactive tool for the annual woman's visit across the life span that can be accessed on their website.

Previously, a cervical cytology test called a Pap test to screen for cervical cancer was an annual routine part of the examination and still is in many practices. However, the need to perform this test every year has been challenged since 1984, and recently, evidence-based guidelines have been established by organizations like the United States Preventive Services Task Force (USPSTF) and evaluated by the specialty organizations like ACOG and the American Cancer Society (ACS). Many aspects of the recommendations are confusing to patients and may be of concern. Being able to make decisions is important for women who want to be able to take control of their healthcare. It is important as a healthcare provider to

read and understand these recommended changes and be able to explain them to your patients. However, it is more important to view each patient in your care as unique and apply the appropriate guidelines to their individual care.

In general, pelvic examinations with a Pap test are usually initially started at age 21 unless there are indications that the examination should be done earlier based on medical history. From age 21 to 29, a Pap alone is recommended and not human papillomavirus (HPV) screening, as this virus is very common in this age group and most of the viruses will be suppressed within 1 to 2 years without causing cancer. Performing an HPV screen at this time would lead to many false positives and unnecessary testing. However, there is currently a 9-valent HPV vaccine available for both boys and girls that should be encouraged. If the vaccine is administered before age 15, only two doses will be necessary, with the second injection 6 to 12 months after the first. The vaccine should be offered to unvaccinated women 26 years of age or younger, regardless of sexual activity, and will require a series of three injections. The vaccine was recently approved for women 26 to 45 years of age. In the first 7 years of HPV vaccination, which occurred primarily in adolescent females, clear evidence of effectiveness was demonstrated. In Australia, where the comprehensive vaccination program reached a high number of young females aged 18 to 24, a comparative study demonstrated that the prevalence of HPV genotypes in Pap smears was significantly lower in the postvaccine sample 28.7% to 6.7%, p less than 0.001.[2] Considering the efficacy of this vaccine, current vaccination rates in the United States are too low.[3] Discussion of HPV vaccination should be included as part of the routine gynecologic examination in all unvaccinated patients within the age guidelines.

Family Planning

Patients in your practice may seek your advice on safe and effective forms of birth control and/or prescriptions for oral contraceptives (OC). The most efficient way to keep current on available oral contraceptive pills is to use prescribing applications (apps) that are available on your smartphone or computer, as these are frequently changing. For other forms of contraception, the patient should be referred to a gynecologist. Chapter 11 has more information on prescribing birth control.

Emergency Contraception

If a woman of childbearing years has unprotected sex and forgets to take her birth control or may not be on any form of birth control, she may become pregnant. Emergency contraception may be indicated to prevent conception. It should also be used for women who are the victims of rape. There is an excellent patient education video available on emergency contraception on the Planned

Parenthood website (www.plannedparenthood.org/learn/morning-after-pill-emergency-contraception). The two most effective methods of emergency contraception are insertion of a copper IUD within 5 days or the oral medication Ella (Ulipristal), which must be taken within 5 days of unprotected sex. Ella requires a prescription. Plan B One Step and other pills like it are available without a prescription at most pharmacies but must be taken within 3 days to be effective.

It is important to discuss the availability, indications, and mechanism of action of emergency contraception with all patients of childbearing years. It can be included as a normal part of the gynecologic visit during the discussion on family planning so that the patient will have the information before they need it. As you delve into areas of conception, ethical issues may arise for the patient. It is just as important to listen to what the patient is not saying as well as what they are saying and to respond in a nonjudgmental way, regardless of your beliefs.

VAGINITIS

Etiology

Vaginitis is most frequently caused by infectious agents with the most common being bacterial. *Candida* vulvovaginitis and trichomoniasis account for more than 90% of infections. Between 55% and 83% of the cases are treated with over-the-counter medications for symptom relief rather than consulting providers. About 8% of White women and 18% of Black women reported vaginal symptoms in the past year.

Pathophysiology

In premenopausal women, the presence of estrogen supports the nonkeratinized stratified squamous epithelium of the vagina. The acidic vaginal environment (pH 4.0–4.5) maintains normal vaginal flora and inhibits the growth of pathogens. Disruption of this environment can lead to vaginitis.

Risk Factors

Some of the factors that can disrupt vaginal normal flora include sexually transmitted disease, antibiotics, foreign body, estrogen level, use of hygienic products, pregnancy, sexual activity, and contraceptive choice.

Approach to Diagnostics

Obtain a history to evaluate each symptom and identify the site of discomfort (Box 25.1). All women suspected of vaginitis should undergo a physical examination to assess the degree of vulvovaginal inflammation, characteristics of the vaginal discharge, and presence of lesions or foreign bodies. A pregnancy test should be performed. A speculum examination is performed to evaluate the

vagina, any vaginal discharge, and the cervix. Significant findings include signs of cervical inflammation, lesions, and pelvic or cervical motion tenderness.

Normal vaginal discharge is usually mucoid or milky white, odorless, and nonirritating. Vaginal infections are common in women during childbearing years. Postmenopausal women can have normal discharge related to atrophic vaginitis and caused by estrogen deficiency in the vaginal tissues. They often confuse this with a vaginal infection. When patients present with complaints of vaginal itching, discharge, or discomfort, it is important to rule out hypersensitivity or irritation from a source that is in contact with the vulvovaginal area, such as hygiene sprays, menstrual pads or tampons, spermicides, latex or other condoms, vaginal contraception rings, fabric softeners, laundry soaps, and diaphragms. A common source of vulvar irritation is undergarments that have been washed or dried with fabric softeners as these do not allow for the flow of air and are frequently scented.

💡 CLINICAL PEARLS

- Women can have physiologic leukorrhea during the mid-menstrual cycle close to the time of ovulation, during pregnancy, or when using estrogen-progestin contraceptives.
- Diet, sexual activity, medication, and stress can affect the volume and characteristics of vaginal discharge.

Diagnostics

Evaluate vaginal secretions with both pH and wet mount. Obtain a sample of the vaginal discharge with a cotton swab and prepare a slide to be evaluated under a microscope. If a microscope is not available, perform point-of-care testing.

Management

Women can have more than one infection at the same time. Patients should be instructed to refrain from intercourse for at least the length of the treatment. They should also be taught that when clindamycin cream is

---

Box 25.1: Common Symptoms of Vaginitis

- Women may present with one or more of the following:
  - Change in volume, color, or odor of vaginal discharge
  - Pruritus
  - Burning
  - Irritation
  - Erythema
  - Dyspareunia
  - Spotting
  - Dysuria

prescribed, as well as many other creams, it may weaken latex such as condoms and diaphragms.

Bacterial vaginosis (BV) was once thought not imperative to treat unless the patient was bothered by the discharge and odor. However, studies on BV have demonstrated an increased risk of those infected to acquire *N. gonorrhoeae*, HIV, and other sexually transmitted infections (STIs). Special consideration for treatment should be given to women with multiple sexual encounters and partners even when symptom-free. Current research supports that BV is an STI.[4]

⊙ CLINICAL PEARL

■ **Whiff Test:** Add 10% KOH to vaginal secretions. A fishy odor is positive and indicative of BV or trichomonas vaginalis.

Bacterial vaginosis, vulvovaginal candidiasis, and trichomonas vaginalis are less common in postmenopausal women. History and close attention to hormonal status are extremely important to differential diagnosis and treatment in postmenopausal women. Low-estrogen levels can cause genitourinary syndrome of menopause (vaginal atrophy). A decrease in sexual drive is normal in the perimenopause years, but the condition may be worsened by dyspareunia. Atrophic vaginitis is a common cause of dyspareunia due to the thinning and drying of vaginal tissue. It is often accompanied by vaginal pruritis without discharge, leading women to think that they have a vaginal infection and self-medicating with over-the-counter treatments that only worsen the condition.

Pharmacologic

Hormonal evaluation and possible localized estrogen treatment may increase vaginal moisture, prevent further vaginal thinning, and relieve dyspareunia and pruritis (see Box 25.2). The dose of this treatment is dependent on the response of the vaginal tissue to treatment. This treatment has been found to be safe, and there is not sufficient evidence to suggest risk in patients who are breast cancer survivors. Several natural treatments that may increase vaginal moisture are vitamin E and water-based lubrication that may be used locally at the time of intercourse.

Contamination of vaginal lubricant or STIs must also be considered in the differential diagnosis in patients presenting with vaginal discharge and itching. Postmenopausal bleeding and/or discharge are always symptoms that require further evaluation with a Pap test, pelvic ultrasonography, and possible biopsy. These symptoms may be the only indication of cancer of the cervix, endometrium, or vagina until the disease becomes more advanced.

Chemical vulvitis is a condition that has become more common with women attempting to treat incontinence

---

Box 25.2: Vaginal Estrogen Therapy

■ Low-dose vaginal estrogen is effective for moderate to severe symptoms of vaginal atrophy that are not responsive to nonhormonal interventions. Using estrogen therapy may be considered in women with symptoms of vaginal atrophy when there are low estrogen levels.

■ Estrogen therapy is associated with urinary tract benefits such as reduction of urinary tract infections and overactive bladder symptoms. Urgency and stress urinary incontinence do not improve with estrogen therapy.

■ Vaginal estradiol inserts (Yuvafem, Vagifem, Imvexxy) come in 10 mcg. Have the patient insert daily for the first 2 weeks and then twice weekly.

■ A silastic ring impregnated with estradiol (Estring) delivers estrogen locally to the vagina and releases 7.5 mcg of estradiol to the vagina daily for a period of 90 days; at this time, the ring should be replaced with a new one.

■ Vaginal estrogen cream is effective and may be more cost effective. The dose varies with the amount and type of cream used. (Premarin cream: 1 gram = 0.625 mg conjugated estrogens; Estrace and estradiol cream: 1 gram = 0.1 estradiol).

■ Low-dose vaginal estrogen therapy may be used indefinitely based on the low risk of adverse effects; the duration should be based on risks and benefits of therapy.

---

with panty liners, pads, or adult briefs. Infrequently changing these barriers causes the susceptible thinning tissue to remain in contact with urine and possible feces for long periods of time. This condition is also seen in bed-bound patients and can lead to serious local infections, as well as urinary tract or vaginal infections. The only presenting symptom may be diffuse redness of the vaginal tissue. Treatment is primarily the elimination of the causative agent. Low-dose topical steroid cream for a short period may be used to calm the area externally.

If the woman has minimal symptoms at the time of initial evaluation and you were unable to diagnose at the time of the visit, have her return to your office when she is symptomatic. If symptoms continue without a clear diagnosis, refer to a gynecologist or a women's health practitioner. Avoid empiric blind therapy because it can aggravate symptoms. Have the patient follow-up in 2 to 4 weeks after the initial intervention to evaluate response to treatment.

Patient Education

Patients should be educated about causes, treatment, and prevention of vaginitis. Patient education can be found at the ACOG: www.acog.org/womens-health/faqs/vaginitis.

SEXUALLY TRANSMITTED DISEASES OR SEXUALLY TRANSMITTED INFECTIONS

Etiology

STIs are major public health problems, regardless of sociodemographic status, that present in resource-rich and limited settings. Unfortunately, patients may be asymptomatic and not seek care until they develop complications. Identifying and treating STIs can be difficult as their presentations, available testing, and treatments vary in different settings and over time. Sexual and social history play a key part in diagnosis and treatment and must include a number of sexual partners, exposure to blood products, condom use, history of STIs in both the patient and their partners, and IV drug use. STIs may be caused by bacteria, viruses, or other organisms.

Pathophysiology

The microbes found in bodily fluids can cross into the body through mucous membranes because they are much thinner than the skin. Abrasions and cuts in the skin and mucous membranes can further increase this risk of infection. Any sexual contact has the risk of introducing microbes into the body. The usual causative agents are bacteria, fungi, protozoa, and viruses.

Risk Factors

Risks should be assessed during a routine gynecologic examination by obtaining a thorough history:

- previous STI or history of multiple sex partners
- new sex partner in past 60 days
- sex with sex partner recently treated for an STI
- no or inconsistent condom use outside a mutually monogamous sexual partnership
- trading sex for money or drugs
- sexual contact (oral, anal, penial, or vaginal) with sex workers
- meeting anonymous partners on the internet

Groups that are at risk include the following:
- young age (15 to 24 years old; see Chapter 11 for more information)
- men who have sex with men (MSM)
- history of a prior STI
- hIV positive status
- pregnant women
- admission to a correctional facility or a juvenile detention center
- illicit drug use

The risk is particularly high with sexually active adolescents and young adults. Older adults in retirement communities have a high risk because they are not fearful of pregnancy and may not consider themselves at risk of STIs. In the age of internet dating, many adults 50 and older are dating, so having the discussion with them about STI protection is very important.

Approach to Diagnosis

In evaluating, treating, and supporting patients suffering from potential STIs, it is imperative that the provider remain knowledgeable and nonjudgmental about all forms of sexual encounters. All women who undergo a gynecologic examination or during the annual visit should be asked about their sexual history and diagnostic testing for STI is based on the history (Box 25.3). It is essential to create a comfortable environment where the person trusts that what she discloses will remain confidential and handled in a nonjudgmental manner. See Box 25.4 for recommendations for screening for STI. There is a misconception among adolescents today that oral and anal sex are safe because they cannot cause pregnancy and the female will remain a "virgin." With an increased incidence in young adults of HPV-positive rectal cancer and oral cancers, dispelling this myth is imperative. Sexual contact between skin and mucous membranes of the genitals, rectum, and mouth accounts for the efficient spread of bacteria, viruses, and other organisms. Oral and anal sex can result in infections not previously considered in many differential diagnoses. Current sexual preferences, such as women who have sex with women (WSW), have provided evidence that vaginal abnormalities such as BV are actually STIs.[4] If this is an area in which a provider does not feel comfortable or capable of providing competent and compassionate care, the patient should be referred to gynecology or the county health department.

Box 25.3: Sexual History

- **Partners**
  New, multiple, or sexual partners with concomitant partners
- **Practices**
  Sexual intercourse trauma
  Anatomical sites of exposure
- **Protection**
  Condom use
- **Past History of Sexually Transmitted Infection**
  Include genital ulceration, which can increase the risk for HIV acquisition.

Box 25.4: Screening

Those at risk should be screened.

- All adolescents and women of all ages who seek counseling for an STI should be tested and receive counseling for HIV.
- All women who have sex partners with an STI should be screened.
- If younger than 25 and sexually active:

  C. trachomatis genital infection, annually

  N. gonorrhea genital infections, annually

  HIV screening, one time and consider greater frequency based on risk factors

  Cervical cancer

  Trichomonas (in settings where prevalence is high)

- Women 25 and older same as described earlier except consider hepatitis B virus infection if not vaccinated

  Hepatitis C virus based on sexual risk

  HIV if risk factors are present

- Consider chlamydia (at genital and rectal sites, according to exposure)

Review the current HPV vaccine indications and dosage schedules before ordering the vaccination as these are changing.[14]

Management

STIs are often based on a clinical assessment as testing is either limited or not available and the risk of patients not returning for follow-up care is high. With some STIs, the sexual partner may need to be treated. This often becomes a problem in primary care. If the partner is not in your practice, you cannot treat them unless you have established a chart and examined them. You can, however, refer them to their provider or the local health department. The patient's obstetrician or the local health department should be consulted before treating pregnant patients. For on-the-spot reference, an Apple or Android application named the "CDC's 2015 (most recent) STD Tx Guide" can be uploaded to your device without charge.

Pharmacologic

Bacterial STIs usually respond well to treatment. Viral STIs can be treated with antiviral drugs but persist for life. Vaccines are available for hepatitis A and B, as well as HPV infection. In the treatment of all STIs, the current Centers for Disease Control and Prenvention (CDC) guidelines should be followed and are available on its website.[17] Some STIs are reportable to the county health department in the county in which you practice. The specific diseases deemed reportable may vary from state to state at times, so it is important to follow the guidelines found on the state health department website.

Patient Education

Patient education is key to the containment and prevention of STIs. The healthcare provider should encourage an open discussion with patients about sexual behaviors and preferences. Safe sexual practice should be discussed with all patients, with special attention being given to adolescents, who may be just beginning their sexual exploration, and older adults, who may have lost their partner and are reestablishing their sexual life with a new partner.

Recently a new sexually transmitted disease was identified. Zika is a virus spread by daytime *Aedes* mosquitos. The disease itself may be symptom-free or present as a mild form of Dengue fever. Patients usually complain of a fever, headache, muscle and joint pain, and a fine macular rash that lasts approximately 7 days. The disease can be spread sexually from men and women to their partners. Women who are pregnant and become infected with the Zika virus can pass it to their fetus in utero or at the time of delivery. The virus appears to cause the birth defect microcephaly in babies born to infected mothers. With the increase of worldwide travel for business and pleasure, global dissemination of this disease can be very rapid and is tracked by the World Health Organization (WHO) and monitored within the United States by the CDC.[13]

PELVIC PAIN

Acute pelvic pain occurs in the lower abdomen or pelvis and lasts less than 3 months. When assessing a female patient, it is essential to determine if it is emergent or nonemergent by performing a rapid assessment to exclude life-threatening disorders. Checking for hemodynamic stability (vital signs, level of consciousness), determining if pregnant, and performing an abbreviated physical examination (assess for peritoneal signs, location of pain, palpable mass) will help you determine the need for emergency care.

Etiology

In the evaluation of pelvic pain in a female patient, gynecologic pathology must always be ruled out; however, gastrointestinal, urinary, musculoskeletal, and psychogenic causes must also be included in the differential diagnosis. Some causes of pelvic pain to consider that are related to the menstrual cycle are dysmenorrhea, endometriosis, and Mittelschmerz. Endometriosis may occur in adolescents; however, it is generally diagnosed in women in their late 20s. There is an increased incidence among women who have a first-degree relative with endometriosis and have shortened menstrual cycles of less than 27 days, with heavy menses lasting longer than 8 days. Dysmenorrhea beginning after years of pain-free menses is a clue to this diagnosis, as is cyclic midline pelvic pain preceding and during menses.

Approach to Diagnosis

Evaluating these conditions includes a thorough history (onset, nature of pain, date of last menstrual period, and other medical conditions, any recent surgery), a pelvic examination, urinalysis, and pregnancy test. The physical assessment should include assessing the external genitalia, speculum examination of the vagina and cervix (assess bleeding or abnormal discharge; an open cervix os suggests inevitable or incomplete abortion but does not exclude an ectopic pregnancy), bimanual examination of the uterus and bilateral adnexa, and rectal examination (thrombosed hemorrhoids, anal fissure, rectal mass).

If further information is needed, a pelvic ultrasound with or without a vaginal transducer may be helpful for structural defects, and referral to a gynecologist for further evaluation may be necessary.

Laparoscopic evaluation with biopsy may be necessary to diagnose endometriosis.

Conditions that present with pelvic pain unrelated to the menstrual cycle include the following:

■ **Pelvic Inflammatory Disease (PID)**

  ● Caused by migration of microorganisms into the upper genital tract

  ● *Chlamydia trachomatis* and *Neisseria gonorrhoeae* cause 33% to 50% of the cases[5]

  ● Risk factors include younger than age 25 and sexually active, multiple partners, unprotected sex, having a history of PID or STI, first 3 weeks following an IUD insertion

  ● Gradual onset of pelvic pain

  ● Mucopurulent cervical discharge may be present

  ● Possibly fever, dyspareunia, or dysuria

  ● Cervical motion tenderness and adnexal tenderness on bimanual examination

  ● In addition to clinical evaluation, a cervical culture should be done.

■ **Endometriosis**

  ● Presence of endometrial-like tissue outside the uterus

  ● Commonly occurs on the pelvic organs but can be found in other areas

  ● Etiology is not known.

  ● Chronic pelvic pain not associated with menstrual cycles

  ● Chronically long and heavy menses with severe pain

  ● Painful sexual activity

  ● May cause infertility

  ● Laparoscopic excision is performed for diagnosis and treatment.

  ● Hormonal treatments are used to prevent ovulation. Management can become complicated and referral to a gynecologist is appropriate.

  ● If pregnancy is the goal, refer to a gynecologist or an infertility specialist.

  ● Black women are less likely to be diagnosed with this[6] for unknown reasons.

■ **Ruptured Ectopic Pregnancy**

  ● Constant, sudden onset of pelvic pain

  ● May have vaginal bleeding which may lead to hemorrhagic shock

  ● Possible syncope

  ● Possible acute abdominal distention

  ● Immediate transportation to the ED for further evaluation is indicated. Follow-up care should be scheduled with a gynecologist.

■ **Ruptured Ovarian Cyst**

  ● Sudden onset of severe pain which gradually decreases in intensity

  ● May be associated with nausea, vomiting, or vaginal bleeding

  ● In addition to a clinical evaluation, a pelvic ultrasound is indicated.

■ **Uterine or Ovarian Cancer**

  ● Gradual onset of pain

  ● Vaginal discharge

  ● Abnormal bleeding: postmenopausal or perimenopausal recurrent menorrhagia, or frequent spotting for which no cause is apparent

  ● In the geriatric population, more definitive symptoms may include sudden loss of appetite, weight loss, dyspepsia, or change in bowel habits.

  ● In addition to a pelvic examination, pelvic ultrasound and abdominal CT are indicated.

  ● Refer to a gynecologic oncologist.

■ **Adhesions**

  ● Gradual onset of pelvic pain that progresses to chronic pain

  ● Dyspareunia

  ● Commonly seen in patients who have had previous abdominal surgery or pelvic infections

  ● Does not cause vaginal discharge or bleeding

  ● May experience nausea or vomiting

  ● This is a diagnosis of exclusion after thorough clinical evaluation and an abdominal obstruction x-ray series.

- Treatment will range from pain relievers to surgical intervention and appropriate referrals are indicated.
- **Spontaneous Abortion**
  - Delayed menses
  - Vaginal bleeding associated with cramping and lower abdominal pain that may be accompanied by the vaginal passing of tissue
  - Possible back pain
  - After clinical evaluation of these patients, referral to either the ED or an obstetrician is appropriate to ensure that no contents of the pregnancy have been retained.

A female with dysuria and pelvic pain may have a urinary tract infection, making it important to obtain a urinalysis (see Chapter 24 for more information about urinary tract infections). It is essential to note in older adults the first presentation of a UTI may be a fall or acute mental status change (e.g., confusion, delirium).

Management

Calling 911 for women with hemodynamic instability may be necessary. Vital signs demonstrating tachycardia or hypotension may indicate impending hemorrhagic shock or syncope. Postmenopausal bleeding, rebound pain, abdominal rigidity or guarding, fever, and sudden onset of pain must always be further investigated. The evaluation of pelvic pain must be thorough and timely. The treatment of pelvic pain is based on the underlying cause of the pain. Timely treatment is critical to preserve reproductive organs and functions. If a definitive diagnosis cannot be reached, referral to the ED is appropriate, as some of the causes of pelvic pain require urgent intervention.

Consider if the presentation is due to worsening of an underlying chronic disease (e.g., endometriosis, inflammatory bowel disease). Referral to a gynecologist or women's health clinician is important in situations that cannot be treated in primary care (worsening or no resolution with evidence-based treatment). If treatment of endometriosis fails and pain interferes with activities of daily life or if the patient has no desire to preserve fertility, a total abdominal hysterectomy with bilateral salpingo-oophorectomy may be recommended by the gynecologist.

🏠 Quality and Safety Alert

- Urgent evaluation in the ED is necessary whenever pelvic pain is associated with pallor, nausea, vomiting, hypotension, and tachycardia.

📶 EMERGENCIES

- Ectopic pregnancy
- Ruptured ovarian cyst (critical with significant hemorrhage; otherwise emergency)
- Ovarian torsion
- Appendicitis
- Acute inflammatory disease (PID)
- Complicated UTI (urgent)
- Urethral obstruction (urgent)

Pharmacologic

Symptomatic treatment of endometriosis includes nonsteroidal anti-inflammatory drugs (NSAIDs), combination estrogen/progestin oral contraceptives, progestins, levonorgestrel-releasing intrauterine devices, and gonadotropin-releasing hormone agonists (GnRH agonists), such as leuprolide, that temporarily suppress estrogen production. GnRH agonists should not be given for more than 6 months because they may cause long-term bone loss. If the PCP is not comfortable managing the treatment of endometriosis, referral to a gynecologist is appropriate.

Nonpharmacologic

Regardless of the patient's stated history and sexual preference, all women of childbearing years should receive a urinalysis and a pregnancy test when presenting with any pelvic symptoms and certainly before any treatments are implemented. Sexual history is important in women of all ages, as many women remain sexually active throughout their whole life. The introduction of sexual "toys" or vibrators into the vagina may cause pelvic pain related to positioning and will resolve with pelvic rest. Many patients will not share this information with their provider until a level of trust has been established.

❶ CLINICAL PEARL

- Using tampons may increase pelvic discomfort during heavy menstrual flow days by blocking the free flow of blood and causing more clots to be formed.

Patient Education

Depending on the age of the patient, describing pain in the pelvic region may be difficult. Adolescents who have recently started menstruation may not be familiar with "expected" discomforts associated with this process, and may fear something is seriously wrong. Authentic presence with these patients is extremely important during the history intake and will allow for educational opportunities that may impact the rest of these young women's lives. Helping the person understand and plan for things like heavier periods after the first day of a cycle, sudden onset of severe sharp pain at the onset of ovulation and cramping, diarrhea, or urinary frequency during menstruation may assist her in coping with these health issues. The more an adolescent knows about normal reproductive functions and possible symptoms she may experience during the menstrual cycle, the less likely the symptoms will interfere with everyday living. This can translate to less school time lost, less reporting by adolescents of "being sick," and an ability of the NP to distinguish normally expected symptoms from abnormal clinical findings. With less sexual health education being taught within the school systems, the role of the NP in this area becomes even more important.

AMENORRHEA

Etiology

Patients presenting with primary amenorrhea, or failure of menses to occur by age 15 or 2 years after the onset of puberty, should be referred to gynecology for further evaluation. Some patients present with secondary amenorrhea, which is the absence of menses for more than 3 months or three typical cycles in those who previously had regular menstrual cycles or 6 months in girls or women who had irregular menses. In the perimenopause phase, amenorrhea is expected and may occur several times before menopause (12 consecutive months of amenorrhea). Some causes of amenorrhea that the PCP should consider are pregnancy, stress-induced anovulation from excessive exercise, eating disorders, dieting, emotional stress, medications, breastfeeding, anemia, endocrine disorders, psychiatric disorders, and polycystic ovary syndrome (PCOS).

Pathophysiology

Primary amenorrhea is usually the result of a genetic or anatomical abnormality. All causes of secondary amenorrhea can also present as primary amenorrhea. The most common reasons for primary amenorrhea are gonadal dysgenesis (includes Turner syndrome), physiologic delay of puberty, Müllerian agenesis (absence of vagina and sometimes no uterus), isolated gonadotropin-releasing hormone deficiency, weight loss/anorexia nervosa, and hypopituitarism. Some causes of amenorrhea are intrauterine adhesions, pregnancy, and disorders of the hypothalamic–pituitary–-ovarian axis (hypothalamic dysfunction, pituitary dysfunction, ovarian dysfunction). PCOS can also cause amenorrhea.

Approach to Diagnosis

The first step is ruling out pregnancy with a pregnancy test. Once pregnancy is ruled out, it is important to determine if the patient has primary or secondary causes. Obtain a thorough history about changes in weight, diet, or exercise habits. Evaluate for an eating disorder or illness that may result in functional hypothalamic amenorrhea.

Ask the patient if she has had any stress that may affect her menses. Inquire about new medications, such as new initiated or discontinued oral contraceptives. Are there symptoms of estrogen deficiency (hot flashes, vaginal dryness, poor sleep, decreased libido) or hypothalamic–pituitary deficiency (headaches, visual field defects, fatigue, polyuria)? Is there galactorrhea (examine breasts) that may be hyperprolactinemia? The physical examination in women with secondary amenorrhea involves height/weight measurements (BMI greater than 30 kg/m^2 has been seen in over 50% of women with PCOS). Evaluate for hirsutism, acne, striae, acanthosis nigricans, vitiligo, and easy bruising. A vulvovaginal examination may have signs of estrogen deficiency (atrophy and dryness).

Diagnostics

After ruling out pregnancy for women with secondary amenorrhea, the laboratory testing should be done and those that may be done by the gynecologist or women's health clinician are FSH, thyroid-stimulating hormone (TSH), serum prolactin hyperprolactinemia, and estrogen to help interpret FSH values.

Management

Patients are often referred to a gynecologist or women's health clinician who will diagnose and treat her. However, it is important to co-manage your patient and have goals to treat the underlying pathology (if this can be done), help the woman with fertility (if that is what she wants), and prevent complications of the disease process (e.g., estrogen replacement). Prior to referral, a complete gynecologic history, pregnancy test, and appropriate labs or tests should be conducted and evaluated.[7] Although patients are reporting amenorrhea, which is most often anovulatory, the patient should be counseled that pregnancy may still be possible during this time.

❶ CLINICAL PEARL

- Girls who have no visible signs of puberty by age 13 should also be referred for further evaluation by an endocrinologist.

Pharmacologic

Medications are prescribed based on the cause. For example, for PCOS combined estrogen-progestin oral contraceptives are the main treatment (PCOS is discussed later in the chapter). Combination oral contraceptives (COCs) are used to manage hyperandrogenism and menstrual dysfunction. If thyroid disease is present, the women would need treatment (see Chapter 26).

Nonpharmacologic

Lifestyle changes should be discussed. Athletic women may not be consuming adequate caloric intake to match their energy expenditure. Women who are not athletic and are underweight may have nutritional deficiencies, and so nutritional counseling may be necessary. It is important to check bone density in menopausal women.

Patient Education

Discussing the reasons for absent or irregular periods and pregnancy prevention is important. PCOS is the most common cause of irregular menses so education should include the cause of PCOS and treatment. Having stress, exercising too much, burning more calories than intake, and having an eating disorder can affect the woman's body energy supply. Early menopause occurs before the age of 40. Certain types of hormonal birth control can cause issues. The ACOG has patient education material on its website: www.acog.org/womens-health/faqs/amenorrhea-absence-of-periods.

MENOPAUSE

Etiology

Menopause is a clinical diagnosis when a woman has not had a period for 12 consecutive months. In the United States, the average age for women to achieve menopause is 52. The years preceding menopause in which the woman may begin to experience change are called the perimenopausal period and vary in length and intensity of symptoms. In describing where a woman is in this process, for the sake of clarity, it is best to describe the length and timing of the menstrual cycle and attempt to place the symptoms within this timeline. Menopause before age 40 is considered abnormal and is referred to as primary ovarian insufficiency. Perimenopause occurs after the reproductive years but before menopause. The presentation may be irregular menstrual cycles, endocrine changes, and symptoms such as hot flashes. Perimenopause begins about 4 years before final menstrual period.

Approach to Diagnosis

Many women present to their PCP for vague complaints that can be difficult for them to discuss but very concerning for them. It is important to listen intently and explore these complaints with the patient while reinforcing the fact that menopause is a normal process of female progression through the life cycle. Clinical manifestations may be hot flashes, sleep disturbances, mood symptoms, and vaginal dryness. Sexual function may change because estrogen deficiency leads to decreased blood flow to the vagina and vulva. Dyspareunia (painful sexual intercourse) can also lead to reduced sexual function. Some women have memory loss and difficulty concentrating during the perimenopausal period and menopause. Menstrual migraines may worsen during the perimenopausal period. It is important to consider long-term consequences of estrogen deficiency. Bone loss can occur so obtain a bone density test. The risk of cardiovascular disease increases with menopause as does osteoarthritis. In early menopause years, women who don't take estrogen may gain fat mass and lose lean mass. The collagen of the skin and bones is reduced.

Although all women will experience menopause, each woman's experience is unique. A significant factor in the woman's ability to manage the changes that her body is going through is her understanding of the physiology. Pregnancy should also be considered in the differential diagnosis.

Management

Lifestyle modifications are always the first line of treatment for the irritating symptoms during the perimenopausal phase. The patient should always be asked what she has found to be helpful. Providers may suggest things like avoiding situations that seem to trigger or exacerbate symptoms, keeping their environment cooler than usual, using vaginal lubricants prior to sexual intercourse, and introducing sexual "toys" into their foreplay to aid in clitoral and vaginal stimulation.

Pharmacologic

For younger women experiencing perimenopausal symptoms that are disrupting their quality of life, regular cycling of the periods with oral contraceptives may be considered. This often relieves the symptoms and allows women to ease through the menopausal process. However, consideration for this treatment is on an individual basis and includes a complete evaluation of the risks associated with oral contraceptives. For older women, who have already experienced menopause, hormone replacement therapy (HRT) is a consideration, but again, only after careful consideration of each individual patient's risk has been evaluated. It is important to remember that women with a uterus must be on both estrogen and progesterone HRT, as unopposed estrogen places these women at an increased risk for endometrial cancer. If the woman is experiencing only vaginal and sexual symptoms, extremely low dose estradiol cream applied to the vagina should be considered. Although hormone therapy is the most effective method of treatment for these symptoms, it should be used with great caution and be closely monitored, with the lowest dose and shortest course of treatment being prescribed.[8]

Several clinical studies have demonstrated a moderate reduction in hot flashes with the use of selective serotonin reuptake inhibitors (SSRIs), serotonin-norepinephrine reuptake inhibitors (SNRIs), and gabapentin. Although some antidepressants improve vasomotor symptoms, they are not as effective as HRT but should be considered as an alternative.[9]

Patient Education

Some of the more common symptoms that can occur should be discussed with women in their 40s during their periodic gynecologic examinations, so they will have an understanding as their bodies begin to change. The changes in the hormonal balance preceding menopause, as well as during menopause, can lead to the following:

- hot flashes or night sweats
- increased moodiness and difficulty controlling emotional responses
- breast tenderness
- exacerbation of menstrual migraines
- vaginal dryness
- dyspareunia
- vaginal irritation and itching
- poor concentration
- memory loss
- depression
- anxiety
- insomnia
- fatigue

DYSFUNCTIONAL (ABNORMAL) UTERINE BLEEDING

Etiology

Dysfunctional uterine bleeding (DUB) presents with polymenorrhea (periods less than 21 days apart) and menorrhagia (periods greater than 7 days or 80 mL). It may cause iron deficiency anemia and infertility. DUB occurs more commonly in women older than age 45 but may be seen in approximately 20% of the adolescent population.

Pathophysiology

With 90% of DUB being anovulatory, the aim of therapeutic intervention will be to prevent endometrium proliferation caused by the lack of progesterone and an abnormal hormone cycle. This is important to decrease the patient's risk of endometrial cancer. In the remaining 10% of women with DUB, progesterone secretion may be prolonged and estrogen levels remain low, causing an irregular shedding of the endometrium and excessive bleeding during the regular menstrual cycle.

Approach to Diagnosis

DUB requires a complete history and examination with ultrasonography to rule out systemic disorders, pregnancy or complications of pregnancy, metabolic abnormalities, structural abnormalities, or medication effect, such as mismanagement by the patient of oral contraceptives.

Having the patient bring their birth control package to the visit may be helpful in teaching the proper administration. Women who are obese, especially those attempting to conceive, may present special difficulties in management and will need to be referred.

The diagnosis of DUB is made by exclusion of other potential causes. Laboratory testing includes complete blood count, pregnancy test, thyroid function testing, prolactin level, FSH, estradiol level, progesterone level during the luteal phase (after day 14 of a normal cycle), serum ferritin, coagulation tests if indicated, liver function tests, Pap test, HPV test, STI testing, and ultrasound. Test results may indicate the need for referral to a gynecologist or women's health clinician for further evaluation.

❶ CLINICAL PEARL

- Endometrial sampling is performed in patients with a thickened endometrium greater than 4 mm. It analyzes a small amount of endometrium with a sensitivity of 97.5%.

Management

If this condition persists, referral to a specialist is necessary. Referral to a gynecologist is appropriate for those with heavy bleeding, severe anemia, persistent bleeding despite treatment, or if there is suspicion of malignancy. If you think the woman may require surgery, you should refer to a gynecologist. Many PCPs are specially trained to obtain endometrial biopsies in their office, especially those working with underserved populations for whom referral to specialists is not always possible. With the development of telehealth, some organizations will provide free consultations with specialists for PCPs working with underserved and uninsured patients.

Pharmacologic

If endometrial hyperplasia is diagnosed in the premenopausal woman, medroxyprogesterone acetate 5 to 10 mg orally per day for 10 to 14 days each month may be prescribed and a repeat endometrial sampling in 3 to 6 months ordered.

After careful consideration of benefits versus risks, hormone therapy with the use of oral contraceptives and progestogens, the first line of treatment, should be discussed with the patient in shared decision-making. Hormone therapy can be very effective in suppressing endometrial development, regularizing menstruation, decreasing menstrual flow, decreasing breast tenderness, and treating dysmenorrhea. Progesterone or other progestins can be used alone if estrogen is contraindicated or COCs have been ineffective after 3 months. Treatment may include NSAIDs, which reduce bleeding and help alleviate dysmenorrhea by decreasing prostaglandin levels. Other options for the treatment of DUB are available but should be managed by a gynecologist.

Patient Education

Women should be educated about what constitutes a heavy period (having to change a pad or tampon every 1 to 2 hours because completely soaked and/or passing large blood clots, greater than 1 inch wide) as well as what is an emergency and when to contact the NP or specialist. Having a period that lasts more than 8 days and bleeding between periods are important to report. Educating women about possible diagnostic testing and treatment can help reduce their fears and support shared decision-making.

POLYCYSTIC OVARY SYNDROME

Adolescents and/or their parents may seek advice when weight becomes a problem, periods are either sporadic or absent, or acne and hirsutism are present. PCOS should be considered in the differential diagnosis in these circumstances and when there is amenorrhea. Referral to a gynecologist for further evaluation and treatment may be necessary. PCOS is an important cause for menstrual irregularity and androgen excess in women.

Etiology

PCOS is one of the most common endocrinopathies in women, affecting about 5% to 10% of women. PCOS is a systemic syndrome that is the most common reason for infertility in the United States, and the reported prevalence in women is 3% to 10%.[10] This disease process will require multispecialty team management. The exact cause is unclear, and the syndrome involves pathophysiology in several body systems.

Pathophysiology

In adolescents who present with polycystic ovarian morphology (PCOM), there seems to be an inherited autosomal dominant factor in PCOS. Evidence supports that adolescents with PCOS either had a mother with PCOM, usually without PCOS symptoms, or a parent with metabolic syndrome (see Chapter 26). More research is needed to identify specific genes that underlie the intrinsic cause of PCOS.

Risk Factors

High-risk groups include those who are obese and/or insulin resistant, who have a first-degree relative with PCOS, and who have a history of premature adrenarche. Women taking antiseizure medications have a higher frequency of PCOS. There is a high prevalence of obesity and insulin resistance in women with PCOS. They have a high risk for type 2 diabetes, dyslipidemia, and coronary heart disease. Those who have normal glucose tolerance should be rescreened at least once every 2 years unless there are indications of the need for more frequent testing. Women with impaired glucose tolerance should be screened annually to evaluate for type 2 diabetes. Obstructive sleep apnea (OSA) is common, so women should be asked about signs and symptoms of OSA (see Chapter 19 for more information). Women with PCOS have a higher prevalence of mood disorders (e.g., depression, anxiety) so screening is important (see Chapter 18 for more information about depression and anxiety).

Approach to Diagnosis

The symptoms of PCOS include early growth of axillary hair, body odor, and acne, predominantly caused by excess androgens such as DHEA being released from the adrenal cortex. Patients may complain of mild obesity and irregular periods or amenorrhea after menarche; however, some women may present with a normal weight or be underweight. After menarche, if the patient has regular menses and then develops amenorrhea, etiology other than PCOS should be considered. Hair may develop in a male or temporal balding pattern. Fatigue, inability to focus, increased blood pressure, acanthosis nigricans, and other symptoms of insulin resistance may begin to interfere with quality of life as the insulin levels rise. A pelvic examination will reveal large amounts of cervical mucus due to elevated estrogen levels. Other conditions such as Cushing syndrome or adrenal tumor should be ruled out in the workup of PCOS. The diagnosis is confirmed only when other conditions that mimic PCOS are excluded. The initial clinical evaluation is a complete history and physical, laboratory studies (FSH, prolactin, TSH, serum-free testosterone, pregnancy test, serum cortisol, serum glucose, possibly a lipid profile) depending on the age of the patient, and a pelvic ultrasound, which if positive for PCOS will often demonstrate more than 12 follicles per ovary in a pattern that is commonly referred to as a "string of pearls" by many radiologists.

In women with clinical evidence of hyperandrogenism (hirsutism, acne, male-pattern hair loss) consider obtaining serum total testosterone level (the upper limit of normal is 45 to 60 ng/Dl range). Routine measurement of serum-free testosterone is not recommended. Serum 17-hyroxyprogesterone in the early follicular phase in all women with possible PCOS should be considered to rule out non-classic congenital adrenal hyperplasia due to 21-hydroxylass deficiency. In women with oligomenorrhea/oligoovulation, consider obtaining human chorionic gonadotropin (hCG), prolactin, TSH, and FSH.

Adolescents presenting with oligomenorrhea (fewer than nine menstrual periods a year) or amenorrhea should be evaluated for PCOS. About 40% to 85% of women are overweight or obese, and insulin resistance is present regardless of weight. Women may have non-alcoholic steatohepatitis and sleep apnea. Many experts use the Rotterdam criteria to make the diagnosis: (a) oligo- and/or anovulation, (b) clinical and/or biochemical signs of hyperandrogenism, and (c) polycystic ovaries (by ultrasound).

Diagnostics

A transvaginal ultrasound (TVU) should be done in some women to look for PCOS morphology. If she meets the criteria for PCOS, an ultrasound is not generally needed. In women who are trying to conceive, a transvaginal ultrasound can identify the absence of anovulation because women with PCOS have an increased risk of anovulation and infertility. Premenopausal women with PCOS should be screened for endometrial hyperplasia or cancer via an ultrasound.

Management

The most recent evidence-based guidelines for multispecialty management of PCOS are a culmination of many guidelines over the years.[11] The PCP can begin the clinical evaluation and act as the "gatekeeper" for follow-up and co-management with all specialists involved. See Table 25.1 for more information regarding treatment.

Pharmacologic

Combined estrogen-progestin oral contraceptives are the mainstay therapy for women with PCOS. This is helpful for managing hyperandrogenism and menstrual dysfunction. Metformin has been used to treat PCOS; however, it is no longer recommended as the first-line treatment for PCOS.[16]

Nonpharmacologic

Lifestyle changes, such as diet and exercise for weight reduction, should be discussed with women who are obese or overweight.

Table 25.1: Management of Polycystic Ovary Syndrome[15]

Symptom	Treatment	Outcome	Monitor
Mild obesity	Regular exercise Healthy eating	Weight loss may induce ovulation, regularize menstrual cycles, increase insulin sensitivity	Weight, caloric intake, exercise activity
Insulin resistance	Metformin (may be used)	Increase insulin sensitivity Decrease free testosterone levels	Serum glucose levels HgbA1c levels Kidney function Liver function
Amenorrhea Ovulatory dysfunction	Oral contraception (OC) Or Intermittent progestin	Prevention of pregnancy Promote regular periods Reduce the risk of endometrial hyperplasia Reduce circulating androgens	Menstrual cycles
Hirsutism	Electrolysis Waxing Dermatology referral Spironolactone (if pregnancy is not currently desired and on OC)	Less coarse hair growth Decreased hair growth	Hair texture and growth pattern
Acne	Oral antibiotics, benzoyl peroxide, oral contraceptives, tretinoin cream, and topical antibiotics may be tried. For resistant acne, a dermatology referral is appropriate	Decreased outbreaks and eventually clear skin	Skin color, texture Monitor for adverse effects of any of the medications used
Infertility	Weight loss Referral to infertility specialist prior to implementation of PCP intervention	Increased fertility	Pregnancy tests Hormone levels

Patient Education

Treating patients with PCOS must start with a clear explanation of the disease process and plan of care with the patient and family members involved in her care. It is critical with adolescents to psychologically support them in areas of body image, peer acceptance, and real or perceived fears. Once the PCP has gained the confidence of the patient and family, the plan of care can slowly and methodically be implemented, striving to relieve symptoms and correct hormonal abnormalities. A lack of treatment places the patient at increased risk of endometrial hyperplasia, possibly leading to endometrial neoplasia, an increased risk of cardiovascular diseases, and metabolic syndrome. Sexual identity confusion and decreased sexual satisfaction can occur and need to be addressed in treatment. The U.S. Department of Health and Human Services has patient education related to PCOS on its website: www.womenshealth.gov/a-z-topics/polycystic-ovary-syndrome.

VULVAR LICHEN SCLEROSUS

Lichen sclerosus (LS) is a benign, chronic, and progressive dermatologic condition.

Etiology

Vulvar LS can occur at any age but is common in prepubertal adolescents and perimenopausal or postmenopausal women. About 1 in 30 older women to 1 in 59 women have it; the incidence seems to be increasing. The etiology is unknown but could be related to genetic factors, immunologic abnormality, and hormonal factors (low-estrogen physiologic states).

Pathophysiology

LS is a long-term skin problem that most commonly affects the anal and genital areas of postmenopausal women.

Approach to Diagnosis

The disease is not contagious, and many women may be asymptomatic. Adolescents or women may present with clinical symptoms of vulvar pruritus (hallmark of the disease) and anal discomfort (pruritus ani, painful defection, anal fissures, rectal bleeding); in adolescents, constipation may be a presenting symptom, although pain, bleeding, dyspareunia, and blisters may also occur. On physical examination, the provider may note round white atrophic papules that may coalesce into plaques. LS can also be hemorrhagic, purpuric hyperkeratotic, bullous, eroded, or ulcerated. Itching can lead to excoriations and secondary mild lichenification (thickening of the epidermis with exaggeration of the normal skin lines associated with edema) of labia minora and the prepuce).

The diagnosis is usually confirmed by biopsy. Differential diagnoses include lichen planus, lichen simplex chronicus, endogenous and exogenous dermatitis, vitiligo, candidiasis, and estrogen deficiency.

Management

Currently, the treatment for LS is topical steroids to relieve the itching and biannual pelvic examinations. Clobetasol propionate applied topically daily for 1 to 3 months has been shown to be effective in those patients that can tolerate steroids. If left untreated, the disease may progress and fuse the vagina together or cover the clitoris, disfiguring it. Surgical intervention may become necessary at this point to maintain normal bodily functions. Once LS is controlled, NPs can recommend an estrogen cream to help soften the skin around the vaginal opening.

Patient Education

LS is more common in postmenopausal women but can occur in men, adolescents, and premenopausal women. It can occur on any skin surface, but in women, most often, it is near the clitoris and on the labia. Vulvar itching is the most common symptom, but some women are asymptomatic. Early identification and treatment are important to prevent complications.

CASE STUDY
LICHEN SCLEROSUS

DP is a 75-year-old woman. She misses the days when she had a gynecologist with whom she could discuss intimate details about her healthcare. She has been experiencing itching in her vaginal and rectal area and is afraid that she has contracted a vaginal infection or STI from the toilet seat in her assisted living facility. There is no one in her facility that she can talk with about this because they will think that she has been promiscuous, and her husband died over 10 years ago.

Your clinical partner is ill, and you are covering his patients, so this is your first visit with DP. You introduce yourself to DP and state that you see that she is here for a follow-up on her high blood pressure. DP seizes the opportunity to describe her concerns with tears in her eyes. You sit beside her, establish eye contact, and listen intently as she describes her fears and concerns as well as her symptoms. You ask if you can perform a pelvic examination and explain what it will include. DP is embarrassed but anxious to have an examination. You describe your clinical findings to DP as you examine her and begin to explain your diagnosis of lichen sclerosus. You also use the opportunity to answer her misconceptions about STIs and the difference between STIs and lichen sclerosus. DP is relieved and begins to develop a plan of care with you.

Case Study Questions

1. Why do you think DP was able to discuss her concerns with you?
2. How would you describe your clinical findings?
3. In comanaging DP, and keeping in mind that you are covering for her PCP, what would the plan of care include?

PRURITUS ANI

Etiology

Pruritus ani (PA) is described as a chronic condition that can cause severe itching in the perianal area. It is a common disorder that is usually benign and affects about 1% to 5% of the general population. Approximately 75% of the cases of PA are secondary to inflammation, infection, systemic, neoplastic, and anorectal disorders. Idiopathic PA is usually from perianal fecal contamination and trauma from wiping and scratching. Although this condition is reported to have an increased prevalence in males and in persons between the ages of 30 and 50,[12] pruritis ani is probably underreported due to embarrassment or the assumption that this is a normal process of aging.

Pathophysiology

The cause of pruritis may be difficult to isolate; however, it can be caused by medication, underlying more serious systemic illnesses that may not yet have been diagnosed, sensitivity to topical exposures, fecal incontinence, poor rectal hygiene, incomplete passage of stool, or rectal prolapse. The most common anorectal diseases associated with PA are prolapsed internal hemorrhoids, abscesses, fissures, and fistulas. Inflammatory causes include contact dermatitis, inverse psoriasis, atopic dermatitis, and cutaneous squamous cell carcinoma in situ (Bowen's disease). STI and *Candida* can cause PA. Parasitic infection with *Enterobius vermicularis* (pinworm, threadworms) is associated with nocturnal PA. However, pinworms are rarely the cause of pruritis in adults.[12] In the older population, pride may prevent individuals from reporting this because of their childhood memories of pinworms, associated with "unclean people" experiencing rectal itching.

Risk Factors

Patients who have diabetes, immunocompromised people, and older adults are at risk for PA. Obesity, hyperhidrosis, and living in tropical climates are also risk factors.

Approach to Diagnosis

Those who are affected by this condition may complain of pain, irritation, and a small amount of bleeding. Interruption of sleep due to itching may also be reported. Scratching the perianal area can lead to fissures, inflammation, and infection. A thorough medical history is critical, and the PCP should be comfortable discussing the issue with the patient, but it is also important that a trusting relationship be established so the patient feels comfortable with this sensitive topic. The physical examination should include a digital examination of the anorectum area. Some patients should be referred to gastroenterology for endoscopy or sigmoidoscopy.

Important areas to cover in the medical history:

- frequency and quality of stools
- toileting accommodations (toilet, bidet, bedside commode)
- mucous leakage
- stool leakage
- sensation of incomplete evacuation
- general hygiene (products used, frequency)
- shower configuration (handheld showerhead, seat, handrails, shower chair)
- cleansing methods after bowel movements
- timing and duration of pruritis
- travel history
- current medications (prescription, herbal, over the counter and prn)
- dietary history

During routine gynecologic examinations, the rectal area should also be inspected. Further information regarding problems that the patient may be experiencing in this area can be gathered based on sharing observations with the patient and explaining that sometimes this can be an area that can cause itching. Referral to an appropriate specialist should be made for further evaluation and treatment if biopsies are indicated or the condition persists despite treatment. Examination documentation should include the Washington Hospital Center staging system to describe the severity of the condition and effectiveness of treatment (Table 25.2).

Table 25.2: Washington Hospital Center Staging Pruritus Ani

Stage 1	Normal intact skin
Stage 2	Red and inflamed skin
Stage 3	Thickened skin
Stage 4	Thickened, coarse ridges and ulcerations

Any of the following can contribute to this condition and should be considered in the differential diagnosis:

- fecal material in or around the anus
- continued moisture from saturated adult briefs, incontinence, or barrier creams
- perianal sprays or soaps used for cleansing
- scented toilet paper or wipes
- extremely acidic or sweet foods/drinks (coffee may lower the anal contraction pressure at rest and contribute to leakage of stool)

- diarrhea
- excessive and aggressive cleansing of the area
- detergents and fabric softeners
- external hemorrhoids
- rectal prolapse
- fungal or bacterial infections
- excessive skin tags
- fistula
- fissures
- anal warts

Table 25.3: Therapy Goals and Methods

Goal	Rationale	Method
Thicken stool	Minimizes leakage and allows for complete evacuation of stool	Fiber supplements: Recommended daily fiber intake is 30–40 grams
Gentle cleansing after every bowel movement	Any stool or mucus around the perianal area will set up the itching-scratching cycle	Handheld detachable showerheads and bidets. Timing of showering procedures to be completed around patient's normal bowel movement time.
Decreased irritation secondary to cleansing irritants	Many perianal products and cleansers routinely used leave a residue on the perianal area that is irritating	Unscented toilet paper and wipes Perianal cleansing with a handheld shower head or bidet after each bowel movement NO use of "spray and leave on" commercial cleansing products for perianal care.
Decreased skin damage	The perianal area must be kept dry and exposed to airflow as much as possible	Avoid tight-fitting undergarments or pants that decrease airflow to this area. Keep fingernails short to avoid increased damage when scratching. Dry area with a hairdryer on low or cool setting. Eliminate potentially irritating foods and drinks. Gradually reintroduce them into the diet as indicated by response.
Prevention of pruritis (itching)	This condition can cause the person severe discomfort, depression, and decrease their quality of life.	Attempt to isolate the cause and eliminate it, if possible. If topical antibiotics are indicated, keep in mind that ointment forms of medications are preferred as they cause less skin thinning. If antifungals are indicated: clotrimazole topical or nystatin topical. 1% hydrocortisone cream to the area bid to tid for a short period. Steroids can relieve the itching but may cause skin atrophy which would worsen this condition. Longer acting steroids such as Betamethasone dipropionate topical can be used for a short treatment cycle. Emuaid is a natural topical product that can provide instant relief. Skin barrier creams containing zinc oxide and menthol can relieve symptoms and can be combined with the steroid creams.

Management

Some older adults may have limited dexterity, infrequent bathing regimens, and may be bed-bound or rely on caregivers to help them with their perianal hygiene. Clear and detailed orders for perianal cleansing and treatment must be included in the person's plan of care. Assessing the area during bathing and after each bowel movement while thoroughly and gently cleaning the area is critical to patient care and comfort. Many of the wipes and spray solutions that are currently used for perianal care only promote or worsen the condition. In-services for the caregivers who will be caring for these patients are very important. It is an opportunity for the NP to explain why this care is critical and that it can greatly impact the patient's comfort level. Anti-itch ointment can be helpful but should not be used for more than 2 weeks. Zinc oxide skin ointment or paste can be helpful as well.

Nonpharmacologic

The goal of therapy is to have clean, dry, irritation-free, and intact skin (Table 25.3).

> ⊙ **CLINICAL PEARL**
>
> Older adults with cognitive impairment residing in memory care units or receiving care in other nursing care settings who may not be able to express themselves may act out this discomfort by constantly walking, exhibiting restlessness, tearing off or picking at adult briefs, or in other ways attempting to alleviate the discomfort and itching.

Patient Education

Good anal hygiene should be discussed. Patients should be informed about avoiding moisturizing the anal area and removing offending agents, dietary modifications, and protecting the skin. Eliminating foods that are associated with PA can help the symptoms. Foods/drinks that can irritate the anus are coffee, tea, beer, cola, chocolate, tomatoes, and citrus fruits. Tight-fitting clothing should be avoided. Hemorrhoids may be the cause, so the use of hemorrhoid creams may help and increasing fiber in the diet may help with constipation (it is important to reduce straining with bowel movement).

CONCLUSION

Many patients expect to receive all of their care from their PCP, including annual gynecologic examinations. It is important to be competent with the gynecologic examination and guidelines for care if you will include this in your practice. Possessing the skill and knowledge to provide this care will be advantageous in seeking employment. Knowing when to consult a specialist is critical and establishing a good rapport with local specialists will enhance your practice. The PCP will remain the gatekeeper for the patient and ensure that all preventative care is done even when referrals are made to specialists.

As patients come to know you, they will expect that you know them and can treat some symptoms without examining them. This is a dangerous practice. Any gynecologic complaints require a complete history, physical examination, and possible testing to establish a diagnosis and plan of care. In women of childbearing age, do not prescribe medications without first checking a pregnancy test.

REFERENCES

References for this chapter are online and available at https://connect.springerpub.com/content/book/978-0-8261-6/part/part01/toc-part/ch25.

CHAPTER 26

Common Endocrine/Metabolic Disorders Encountered in the Primary Care Setting

Sima Sitaula, Charity L. Tan, and Berit Bagley

LEARNING OBJECTIVES

At the conclusion of this chapter, the learner will be able to:

➤ Demonstrate knowledge of the etiology, pathophysiology, clinical manifestations, diagnostic tests, and medical management of endocrine disorders.

➤ Identify the components of physiologic insulin replacement for patients with diabetes.

➤ Demonstrate awareness of the American Diabetes Association's evidence-based guidelines in managing diabetes.

➤ Demonstrate the understanding of commonly encountered thyroid disorders in the primary care setting.

➤ Compare and contrast the common signs, symptoms, and physical examination findings of thyroid disorders.

➤ Understand the standard of practice for diagnosis, approach, and treatment options for thyroid conditions.

INTRODUCTION

Endocrinology is the study of the endocrine system with a focus on hormones that regulate functions in the body. The hormones produced by the organs in the body are like "messengers" that target specific organs in the body and help different parts of the body to function in metabolism, growth and development, blood sugar control, sexual development and function, mood, and blood pressure and to regulate the heart. Endocrine disorders are commonly encountered problems in clinical practice. In the primary care setting, it is important for the clinician to understand the basic clinical guidelines for type 1 diabetes, type 2 diabetes, hypothyroidism, hyperthyroidism, and thyroid nodules management. In this chapter, the adult-gerontology nurse practitioner (AGNP) will be able to identify the basic pathophysiology, interpretation of endocrine hormone tests, and general treatment options for common endocrine disorder management in primary care clinical settings. The goal of this chapter is to provide AGNPs with a practical approach to deliver safe, effective, and evidence-based care to patients with endocrine disorders.

OVERVIEW OF THE ENDOCRINE SYSTEM

The endocrine system is varied and complex with sophisticated and diverse mechanisms to regulate hormone synthesis. The primary function of the endocrine system is to maintain homeostasis through modulating tissue and organ function through the actions of blood-borne and locally acting hormones.[7] Feedback mechanisms (negative and positive) within the endocrine system regulate the amount and rate at which hormone synthesis occurs. Excess hormone production is suppressed by negative feedback whereas positive feedback prompts increased hormone reduction and release.

Normal Anatomy and Physiology

The endocrine system is composed of nine glands: the hypothalamus, the thyroid gland, the pituitary gland, the adrenals, the ovaries (female) and the testes (male), the thymus gland, the pineal gland, and the pancreas. Following is a brief description of normal anatomy and physiology; students should refer to an anatomy and physiology text for further detail.

The pancreas produces the hormone insulin with a main function of regulating glucose levels in the body. The islets of Langerhans are within the pancreas where beta cells, specialized cells within the islets, produce insulin. As with all patients, a trusting relationship should be established through effective communication before attempting the physical examination. Where there is a decreased production of insulin by the pancreas, or decreased sensitivity of the cell for reuptake of serum glucose (e.g., insulin resistance), type 2 diabetes manifests.[7]

The thyroid gland produces the thyroid hormones thyroxine (T4) and triiodothyronine (T3). Secretion of these thyroid hormones (T4 and T3) is driven by the thyroid-stimulating hormone (TSH) produced by the pituitary gland. The pituitary gland is responsible for the production of TSH, which regulates the production of thyroid hormones by the negative feedback mechanism. The hypothalamus produces thyrotropin-releasing hormone

(TRH), which stimulates the pituitary gland to produce TSH. When there are adequate circulating levels of thyroid hormone, these brain tissues will send the signal through a negative feedback loop to decrease the stimulation of the thyroid gland by downregulating the secretion of TRH and TSH. When the thyroid disorders occur within the thyroid gland itself, it is called the primary thyroid problem. When there is a disorder in the feedback process caused by the pituitary gland, it is called secondary in origin, and when the hypothalamus is involved, it is called tertiary.[1]

DIABETES

With the rising cost, prevalence, and high risk of complications and comorbidities affecting quality of life, diabetes remains a public healthcare challenge. In 2017, it was estimated that the total cost of diabetes in the United States is $327 billion, which includes $237 billion in direct medical costs and $90 billion in reduced productivity. This is an increase of 26% from the prior estimate in 2012 of $254 billion. People diagnosed with diabetes have approximately 2.3 times higher medical expenses than those without diabetes.[2] Uncontrolled diabetes has serious consequences. Per the ADA, nearly 50,000 individuals annually begin treatment for renal failure, and 44% of all new cases of renal failure are from diabetes. About 60% of all lower limb amputations (about 73,000 lower limb amputations) annually occur due to diabetes. Per the National Statistics Report of 2020, 34.2 million people (10.5% of the U S population) have diabetes, 7.3 million (21.4%) are undiagnosed, and 88 million people older than age 18 years (34.5% of the adult U.S. population) have prediabetes; in addition, 24.2 million people older than 65 years have prediabetes.[2] Immune-mediated diabetes (previously known as insulin-dependent diabetes or juvenile-onset diabetes) or type 1 diabetes accounts for 5% to 10% of all diabetes cases.

The occurrences of type 2 diabetes have increased markedly in pediatrics and adolescence due to the prevalence of obesity, particularly in minority groups, with at least a third of all new cases diagnosed in this age group.[3] There are approximately 5,000 new cases of newly diagnosed type 2 diabetes in adolescents.[4]

Etiology

Insulin is the key for moving the glucose into the cells, thus lowering the serum glucose levels. Cells in the liver, adipose tissue, and the muscle will store any excessive glucose not used as fat. Once serum glucose levels fall, the trigger for insulin release no longer exists, and the beta cells in the pancreas stop producing insulin.

Insulin resistance is the body's impaired response to serum glucose, causing the elevation of glucose levels in the blood. The sensitivity of the cells to reuptake elevated serum glucose is hindered. The pancreas then produces a larger amount of insulin. Over time, the pancreas can no longer produce enough insulin to meet the body's needs, which leads to type 2 diabetes.[5] In contrast, type 1 diabetes is the destruction of the beta cells that produce and secrete insulin, which results in absolute insulin deficiency.

Pathophysiology

In prediabetes, the pancreas produces large amounts of insulin in response to carbohydrate intake to maintain euglycemia (normal blood glucose level) until it no longer can produce enough insulin to meet the body's needs. In type 2 diabetes, there is beta-cell dysfunction causing a decrease in insulin production from the pancreas as well as insulin resistance. Hyperglycemia occurs from (a) increased caloric intake (mainly from a high-caloric consumption), (b) decreased peripheral glucose uptake (due to a lack of insulin sensitivity from cells), (c) decreased insulin secretion from the pancreas, and (d) increased gluconeogenesis from the liver.[6]

In type 1 diabetes, it is the destruction of the islet beta cell, which, in most cases, is immune-mediated; however, some cases are idiopathic. In 95% of cases, the fundamental mechanism is autoimmunity characterized by absolute insulin deficiency.[7]

Risk Factors

The presence of a family member with type 1 diabetes or the presence of other autoimmune disorders (such as celiac disease, Hashimoto thyroiditis, vitiligo, autoimmune hepatitis) is a risk factor for type 1 diabetes. Another predictive marker is the presence of islet cell antibody and or glutamic acid decarboxylase 65 (GAD 65). Islet cell antibodies are present in approximately 70% of young children at the time of diagnosis. They are typically the first marker in young children at risk of developing diabetes. GAD 65 autoantibodies are found in 80% of patients with type 1 diabetes at presentation showing autoimmunity.

The risk factors for type 2 diabetes are varied and include

- the presence of prediabetes,
- obesity (body mass index greater than or equal to 30 kg/m²),
- women who were diagnosed with gestational diabetes or birthing a baby greater than 9 pounds,
- a family member with a history of type 2 diabetes or polycystic ovary syndrome,
- presence of nonalcoholic fatty liver disease,
- a sedentary lifestyle,
- individuals older than 45 years , and
- members of certain ethnic/racial groups (African Americans, Hispanic/Latino American, Alaskan Natives, Pacific Islanders, and Asian Americans).[8]

The social determinants of health are a priority in patients with diabetes as there has been research demonstrating the effects of diabetes in low-income communities and racial and ethnic minority groups. Individuals with a high health literacy have a lower average blood glucose reading and have better knowledge of the diabetes disease process. A lower educational level is associated with a threefold higher mortality from diabetes compared to adults with a graduate degree. Having a high school education is associated with a twofold higher mortality from diabetes. Type 2 diabetes and insulin resistance are associated with food insecurity. Food insecurity is associated with lower quality food and may lead to more insulin resistance based on the accessibility of low, dense-quality food and less nutrient-dense foods that have an impact on blood glucose levels and may lead to insulin resistance. Food insecurity is always a risk factor for less than ideal diabetes management with inadequate access to quality and quantity of food. There is an increased risk of hypoglycemia with the lack of consistent availability of food. Individuals with diabetes spend two to three times more in healthcare costs compared to individuals without diabetes. At least 14% to 20% of individuals with diabetes reported reducing or delaying medications due to costs. Having access to health insurance is a strong predictor of whether quality measures of diabetes care are met. Having a good social support has been associated with a decrease in mortality and diabetes-related complications. Neighborhoods with high social cohesion are associated with a lower incidence of type 2 diabetes by at least 22%.[9]

Approach to Diagnosis

Type 1 diabetes can occur at any age, often following acute hyperglycemia/diabetes ketoacidosis (DKA). Diagnosis criteria include fasting glucose, A1C, and random glucose values, as well as auto-antibody testing. Type 1 diabetes patients typically present with an acute hyperglycemia episode with the accompanying symptoms of the 3Ps (polyuria, polyphagia, polydipsia), unintentional weight loss, and fatigue. At the time of presentation, with known risk factors, a GAD 65 antibody and hemoglobin A1c should be checked.[10] There is an association of autoimmune diseases in type 1 diabetes patients; screening for thyroid dysfunction and celiac disease should be considered. At least 17% to 30% of patients with type 1 diabetes have autoimmune thyroid disease.[3] On physical examination, individuals with type 1 diabetes are typically slim/slender or thin individuals.

Type 2 diabetes is a chronic insidious disease process and screening for diabetes in the primary setting for any individuals starting at age 45 years, on hypertension therapy or a history of cardiovascular disease, or those with risk factors is ideal. "Prediabetes" is defined as having a hemoglobin A1C of 5.7% to 6.4%, a fasting plasma glucose of 100 to 125 mg/dL, and a 2-hour plasma glucose

during a 75-g oral glucose tolerance test (OGTT) of 140 to 199 mg/dL.[10] Type 2 diabetes in adults is defined as hemoglobin A1C of 6.5% or higher, fasting plasma glucose of 126 mg/dL or higher, a 2-hour plasma glucose of 200 mg/dL or higher during OGTT, and a random plasma glucose of 200 mg/dL in individuals with signs of hyperglycemia.[6] See Table 26.1.

In type 2 diabetes patients, individuals are typically overweight or obese with a large waistline and have the presence of acanthosis nigricans (the darkening of the skin in the skin folds to the neck, upper inner thighs, under the breasts for women, or between the fingers) noticeable on physical examination.

For pediatrics or adolescence, testing for type 2 diabetes should be considered when obesity is present (body mass index at 85th percentile for age and sex or weight at 120% of ideal for height) and if any of the following two criteria are met: (a) first- or second-degree relative with type 2 diabetes, (b) minority population, or (c) presence of insulin resistance, such as acanthosis nigricans, hypertension, and dyslipidemia.[4]

Management

In type 1 diabetes, as there is insulin deficiency due to the destruction of pancreatic beta cells, exogenous insulin injections will replace indigenous insulin secretion for the duration of the patient's life span. Insulin preparations are classified by the duration of action of insulin: rapid-acting, short-acting, intermediate-acting, and basal (long-acting) insulin. A physiologic insulin regimen is ideal to include a basal/bolus (prandial) approach, which can be delivered via insulin pump, insulin pen, or syringe and vial methods (see Figure 26.1).

Basal insulin is most often considered the background insulin and short- or rapid-acting insulin is what is used to cover the carbohydrates in a meal or to correct for any hyperglycemia. Basal insulin is a 24-hour, long-lasting insulin usually taken once a day at the same time each

Table 26.1: Diagnostic Test Levels Indicating Prediabetes and Diabetes

	Prediabetes	Diabetes
HgbA1c	5.7-6.4%	6.5% or greater
Fasting glucose	100-125 mg/dL	126 mg/dL or greater
2-hour plasma glucose with a 75-gram OGTT	140-199 mg/dL	200 mg/dL or greater
Random plasma glucose		200 mg/dL with associated signs of hyperglycemia

OGTT, oral glucose tolerance test.

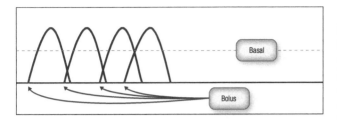

Figure 26.1: Basal and bolus insulin therapy in type 1 diabetes

day; it functions to keep blood glucose levels within a normal target range even if food is not consumed. Rapid-acting insulin is taken to cover the carbohydrates in a meal or when blood glucose levels are above target range. In individuals with type 1 diabetes, the amount of rapid-acting insulin depends on the amount of carbohydrate consumed and the level of the blood glucose level at the time. A "correction dose" of rapid-acting insulin is used to correct for blood glucose above target range. The "insulin-to-carbohydrate ratio" (ICR) is the number of units of rapid-acting insulin needed for every gram of carbohydrate consumed.[11]

Initiating Insulin Therapy in Type 1 Diabetes

When initiating insulin therapy, a baseline total daily dose (TDD) of insulin is often calculated as 0.5 × body weight in kilograms. Generally, patients with type 1 diabetes require one-half to two-thirds as basal insulin and the other one-third to one-half reserved for meals, which is calculated prior to meals depending on the number of carbohydrates.[12] For example, a 56-kg woman's calculated TDD would be 28 units (56 × 0.5) with basal insulin 14 units once a day and a set dose of rapid- or short-acting insulin of 5 units with each meal. Alternatively, premeal (or prandial insulin dose) can be calculated using the 1,700 rule to estimate the correction factor: 1,700 divided by TDD = the expected drop in glucose response to 1 unit of insulin. The 450 rule estimates the insulin-to-carbohydrate ratio: 450 divided by the TDD = the number of carbohydrates (in grams) covered by 1 unit of insulin.[13] For example, 1,700 divided by 28 = 60; 1 unit of insulin will drop the glucose by about 60 mg/dL (Note: These are estimates and clinical judgment and patient's response should determine changes). For example, 450 divided by 28 = 16; 1 unit will cover 16 grams of carbohydrates (Note: these are estimates, and clinical judgment and patient's response should determine changes).

Honeymoon Phase

Following the diagnosis of type 1 diabetes, some patients enter the "honeymoon phase." Increased endogenous insulin secretion from the working beta cells characterizes this phase. The "honeymoon phase" can last anywhere from a few weeks to months, and during this time, patients may require less insulin. Although requirements might drop to 0.2 to 0.6 units/kg/day, patients will still need insulin therapy.[12]

For individuals with prediabetes or type 2 diabetes, metformin is the first-line pharmacology therapy if renal function is adequate (glomerular filtration rate [GFR] of 45 mL/min/1.73 m² or greater). Individuals with comorbidities such as heart failure, arteriosclerotic cardiovascular (ASCVD) disease and/or kidney disease, a SGLT2 (sodium-glucose co-transporter 2) inhibitor such as empagliflozin, or a GLP-1 (glucagon-like peptide 1) such as semaglutide, is recommended barring any contraindications. Insulin is an option with individuals presenting with hemoglobin A1c of greater than 10 with symptoms, such as weight loss, hyperglycemia, polyuria, polyphagia, or polydipsia. For any concerns with hypoglycemia, the use of DDP-4 (dipeptidyl peptidase-4) agents, such as sitagliptin, can be considered. Additionally, if cost is an issue to individuals, then the pharmacology class of sulfonylureas, such as glipizide, can be considered.[14] For adolescents, only three medications are approved for use—metformin, insulin, and liraglutide.[4]

Starting insulin (long-acting or basal) on individuals with type 2 diabetes and titrating up insulin doses can be approached in this manner: 10 units of insulin a day or 0.1 to 0.2 units of insulin per kilogram per day. Increase insulin (basal or long-acting) by 5% to 15% or 1 to 4 units of insulin 1 to 2 times a week to a maximum insulin dose of 0.5 units per kilogram per day or until a fasting glucose of 80 to 130 mg/dL is achieved.[1] To add multidose insulin injection in a day or to add with a meal (also known as prandial or nutritional insulin), a TDD based on weight × 0.4 – 1 unit/kg/day = 50% basal insulin + 50% (divided into 3 = breakfast/lunch/dinner) for meals using short- or rapid-acting insulin. Therefore, with an individual with a weight of 60 kg, TDD would be as follows: 60 kg × 0.5 (can multiply anywhere from 0.4 – 1 unit/kg) =15 units of basal insulin with 5 units of rapid- or short-acting insulin for breakfast, lunch, and dinner (meals). The 50% basal insulin is to manage the glycemia in the periods of between-meal absorption and the other 50% is administered as prandial (mealtime or nutritional) insulin given to manage blood glucose after meals. Another option to basal insulin is to use intermediate-acting insulin, also known as NPH (neutral protamine hagedorn) insulin, although there is a higher risk of hypoglycemia with its variable peak and duration effect after administration. Alternatively, there is premixed insulin in which both intermediate- and rapid-acting insulin are in one vial. Examples are Novolin 70/30 or Humulin 70/30 mixtures, in which the preparation contains a mixture of 70% intermediate-acting insulin NPH and 30% regular insulin.[1] When NPH is used, typically, the TDD required would be divided into two-thirds TDD in the morning and the other third TDD dose in the evening.

Caution should be taken in managing type 2 diabetes in older adults with insulin and the use of sulfonylureas (such as glimepiride or glipizide) due to a high risk of hypoglycemia.[15]

The high cost of insulin remains a challenge and an expensive burden for individuals, especially those with type 1 diabetes, and does play a role in treatment adherence to therapy. The use of NPH and premixed insulin, as well as regular insulin, can be purchased over the counter for much less than once-a-day long-acting insulin like glargine.[11,16]

The AGNP should make referrals to the registered dietitian or certified diabetes education and care specialist (CDCES) for medical nutrition therapy (MNT) and for any further dietary modifications. Keeping physically active is also highly encouraged. In particular, with individuals with type 1 diabetes, using continuous glucose monitoring (CGM) sensors would be significantly helpful, especially in a setting of hypoglycemia unawareness. The use of an insulin pump to manage patients with type 1 diabetes is encouraged. For both adolescents and adults with obesity, metabolic surgery can also be considered.

Patient Education

Patient education is critically important in patients with diabetes of either type because of the complexity of the condition, the long-term ramifications if diabetes is poorly managed, and the high level of responsibility necessary for patients to manage their condition. The teach-back method provides for an opportunity to assess the level of understanding of the individual on what was taught. Focus on patient-centered communication by tailoring the information to the individual; for example, opportunities for individuals to return demonstrate proper insulin injection techniques or how to use a meter for glucose monitoring. Uncontrolled diabetes, over time, can have a negative effect and lead to damage to different parts of the body, both micro- (retinopathy, peripheral neuropathy) and macrovascular structures (cardiovascular, cerebrovascular).

((•)) DIABETIC EMERGENCIES

Hypoglycemia, if not treated promptly, can lead to coma and even death. Listed in Table 26.2 and Exhibits 26.1 and 26.2 are steps that the AGNP can take in teaching individuals to treat hypo- and hyperglycemia.

🏆 CLINICAL PEARL

The AGNP can manage glucose monitoring preoperatively and reduce surgical complications as well as improve mortality, improve wound healing postsurgery, and reduce the length of stay in the hospital. Table 26.3 is a chart that can help guide insulin management for perioperative care of patients with diabetes.

Table 26.2: Classification and Treatment of Hypoglycemia

Classification of Hypoglycemia

  a. Level 1: Glucose level less than 70 mg/dL and at 54 mg/dL or more

  b. Level 2: Glucose level less than 54 mg/dL

  c. Level 3: Alteration in mentation +/− assistance required for treatment of hypoglycemia event

Treatment

  a. Conscious

    1. Rule of 15: Ingest 15 grams of fast-acting glucose, repeat in 15 minutes until glucose levels reach 70 mg/dL or more

  b. Unconscious

    1. Glucagon kit

    2. Intranasal glucagon (Baqsimi)[17]

Exhibit 26.1 Hypoglycemia Overview

Hypoglycemia
LOW BLOOD SUGAR

LOW BLOOD SUGAR is blood glucose of less than 70 mg/dL.

Common causes
- Too little carbohydrate
- Too much insulin
- Extra activity or exercise

Symptoms may include
- Shaking
- Fast heartbeat
- Sweating
- Anxious
- Dizziness
- Hunger
- Impaired vision
- Weakness/fatigue
- Headache
- Irritability

continued

Treatment:

1. Test blood sugar and tell someone you feel low.
2. If below 70 mg/dL, treat by taking 15 grams of fast-acting carbohydrate.
3. Wait 15 minutes then retest blood sugar. Repeat step 2 if blood sugar is less than 80 mg/dL.

Examples of 15-gram fast-acting carbohydrates	*3-4 small glucose tablets (check label for amount of carbohydrate)*
	½ cup juice or regular soda
	Small juice box

If the person is unresponsive, glucagon (hypoglycemia rescue medication) can be given by a patient representative.

Source: Data from American Diabetes Association. Glycemic targets: standards of medical care in diabetes–2020. *Diabetes Care.* 2020;43(Suppl 1):S66–S76. doi:10.2337/dc20-s006

Exhibit 26.2: Hyperglycemia Overview

Hyperglycemia
HIGH BLOOD SUGAR

Common causes

- Too much carbohydrate
- Too little insulin
- Illness

Symptoms may include

- Extreme thirst
- Hunger
- Dry skin
- Frequent urination
- Blurred vision

Treatment:

1. Test blood sugar.
2. **If blood sugar is over 250 mg/dL or person is ill/vomiting,** test urine for ketones.
3. If urine ketones are greater than "trace," call doctor or nurse educator. High blood sugar may lead to a medical emergency if not treated.

Diabetic ketoacidosis (DKA) is a serious condition that can lead to coma or death if not treated. DKA occurs when the body is not able to use glucose for energy and begins to break down fats. When fats are used for energy versus glucose, ketones are made making the serum glucose acidic.

Symptoms of DKA may include

- Thirst
- Dry mouth
- Elevated blood sugar
- Urine ketones
- Fatigue
- Nausea, vomiting, or stomach pains
- Difficulty breathing
- Fruity odor on breath
- Confusion

Source: Tkacs NC, Herrmann L, Johnson R, eds. *Advanced Physiology and Pathophysiology: Essentials of Clinical Practice.* Springer Publishing Company; 2020:743.

Steroids are commonly used in treating patients with chronic obstructive pulmonary disease and/or asthma exacerbation. Steroids will undoubtedly affect glucose levels in individuals with diabetes, more so postprandially. The postprandial glucose levels are affected more (as opposed to the fasting glucose levels)

Table 26.3: Insulin Adjustment During Perioperative Period for Patients With Diabetes

Insulin Adjustment Guide
Oral Hypoglycemia Agents: Hold day of surgery/morning of surgery or procedure
Intermediate Insulin (NPH): Decrease usual dose by 50% the day of surgery or procedure
Long-Acting Insulin: Decrease usual dose by 20% to 40% day of surgery or procedure
Premixed Insulin (Ex: 70/30): Give one-third usual dose while NPO
Insulin Pump: Decrease usual dose (basal dose) by 20% to 40% day of surgery or procedure
Noninsulin Therapies: Hold

Sources: American Diabetes Association. Diabetes care in the hospital: standards of medical care in diabetes–2019. *Diabetes Care.* 2019;42(Suppl 1):S173-S181. doi:10.2337/dc19-S015; https://care.diabetesjournals.org/content/42/Supplement_1/S173; Duggan E, Carlson K, Umpierrez G. Perioperative hyperglycemia management an update. *Anesthesiology.* 2017;126(3):547-560. doi:10.1097/ALN.0000000000001515; Simha V, Shah P. Perioperative glucose control in patients with diabetes undergoing elective surgery. *JAMA.* 2019;321(4):399-400. doi:10.1001/jama.2018.20922

due to hepatic gluconeogenesis and impaired insulin sensitivity. Taper insulin doses with tapering of steroid use to mitigate the risk of hypoglycemia. Table 26.4 is the guide for the AGNP to use a weight base NPH dose for steroid-induced hyperglycemia.[18]

🏠 Quality and Safety Alert

Patients with diabetes may be caught in an unexpected emergency or disaster such as a fire or flood. Insulin doses may need to be adjusted or the type of insulin may need to be switched in some situations. The following is a link for the AGNP to use or refer to in the event of a disaster and when individuals are not on their typical normal routine insulin schedule or without access to their usual prescribed medications: www.diabetes.org/sites/default/files/2020-09/Switching%20Between%20Insulin%20Products%20in%20Disaster%20Response%20Situations%202020%20-%20English.pdf

Table 26.4: Guideline for Managing Steroid-Induced Hyperglycemia

Managing Steroid-Induced Hyperglycemia With NPH
• 0.4 units/kg of NPH for prednisolone doses of 40 mg/day or greater with NPH insulin dose being decreased by 0.1 unit/kg for each 10 mg/day decrease in prednisolone dose

POLYCYSTIC OVARIAN SYNDROME

PCOS is one of the most common causes of female infertility, affecting 6% to 12% (as many as 5 million) of U.S. women of reproductive age.[19] Typically, hyperandrogenemia is present, which affects ovulation and causes hirsutism and other symptoms outlined in the following text.[19] PCOS is often diagnosed with the presence of at least two out of these three criteria: dysfunction in ovulation causing irregular periods, polycystic ovaries on ultrasound, or high levels of androgens in the blood.

Etiology

The cause is unknown, but insulin resistance is present where insulin is not effectively used by the body, which increases the risk of type 2 diabetes. Genetic traits, as well as environmental factors, are thought to play a role as well.[19,20]

Pathophysiology

The altering action in luteinizing hormone (LH), insulin resistance, and hyperandrogenism are thought to contribute to the pathophysiology of PCOS. Hyperandrogenism leads to infertility due to a lack of ovulation and can cause cutaneous manifestations such as hirsutism. Insulin resistance increases hyperandrogenism, which then decreases the amount of sex hormone–binding globulin (SHBG) formation, leading to an increase of adrenal and ovarian formation of androgens.[20]

Risk Factors

The most common risk factors for this syndrome are obesity, the presence of prediabetes, or a family member with type 2 diabetes and/or PCOS.

Approach to Diagnosis

PCOS is almost a diagnosis of exclusion; however, keep in mind the following symptoms that are often present: abnormal menstrual cycles (i.e., erratic menstrual periods ranging from daily to absence), infertility due to a lack of ovulation, early (prepubertal) male pattern hair growth, acne unresponsive to treatment, history of hypertension, hyperlipidemia, or hypertriglyceridemia.

On physical examination, look for telltale signs such as acanthosis nigricans, acne, obesity, and hirsutism. Pelvic ultrasound can be ordered to look for polycystic ovaries. Blood tests, specifically the antimullerian hormone (AMH), are indicative of PCOS. Other blood work to consider are human chorionic gonadotropin (hCG), follicle-stimulating hormone (FSH), estrogen, LH, testosterone, and specifically SHBG.

Management

The first-line therapy for the presence of prediabetes or diabetes is metformin along with lifestyle changes for obesity. Electrolysis for hirsutism and topical cream for acne treatment are also recommended for patients when indicated.[20]

HYPOTHYROIDISM

The thyroid gland produces the thyroid hormones thyroxine (T4) and triiodothyronine (T3). These thyroid hormone (T4 and T3) secretions are driven by the TSH produced by the pituitary gland. The pituitary gland is responsible for the production of TSH, which regulates the production of the thyroid hormones by the negative feedback mechanism. The hypothalamus produces TRH, which stimulates the pituitary gland to produce TSH. When there are not adequate circulating levels of thyroid hormone, these brain tissues will send the signal through a negative feedback loop to increase the stimulation of the thyroid gland by increasing the secretion of TRH and TSH. Hypothyroidism is a clinical condition in which serum thyroid hormone (T3 and T4) levels are lower than the normal range or not enough to maintain normal intracellular hormone level.[21]

Etiology

The most common cause of hypothyroidism due to primary thyroid gland failure is from Hashimoto's thyroiditis. Hashimoto's thyroiditis is an autoimmune condition in which the patient has positive antithyroglobulin (anti-Tg) or anti-tissue peroxidase (anti-TPO) antibodies. These antibodies cause the autoimmune destruction of thyroid hormones and result in hypothyroidism.[1] Another common cause of hypothyroidism is from the treatment of hyperthyroidism. When a patient is treated for hyperthyroidism by thyroidectomy, postradioactive ablation, or antithyroid drugs, it can cause hypothyroidism. These treatments can decrease the thyroid hormone level to a less-than-normal range and can cause hypothyroidism. Another cause of hypothyroidism is postpartum thyroiditis, in which a woman's thyroid gland gets inflamed 4 to 6 weeks after the delivery of the baby. Initially, it can cause hyperthyroidism and later causes hypothyroidism. In some cases, acute thyroiditis caused by the viral infection may also lead to transient hypothyroidism. Other causes of hypothyroidism are congenital due to pituitary or hypothalamic disease.[21]

Pathophysiology

In primary hypothyroidism, when circulating thyroid hormones T4 and T3 are low, the pituitary gland increases the production of TSH to further stimulate the thyroid gland to increase the production of thyroid hormone. In this negative feedback mechanism, when T4 and T3 levels are low, the TSH level goes up to produce enough quantities of circulating thyroid hormone to meet the demand. Generally, the elevated level of TSH and low level of FT4 indicate hypothyroidism.[1]

Risk Factors

The following conditions increase the risk of hypothyroidism:

- Family history of hypothyroidism because hypothyroidism runs in the family
- Predominant age is older than 40
- Autoimmune disorder such as type 1 diabetes
- History of head or neck radiation as it can damage the thyroid gland and can decrease thyroid hormone production
- Treatment of hyperthyroidism with radioactive ablation, thyroidectomy, or antithyroid medications may cause hypothyroidism.
- Pituitary or hypothalamic disease can disrupt the negative feedback loop of thyroid hormone production.
- Postpartum period as women can develop postpartum thyroiditis, which can lead to hypothyroidism.

Approach to Diagnosis

It is important to know the cause of hypothyroidism as it helps to decide if treatment is indicated or not. It also helps to anticipate if treatment is needed for life or if it is temporary.

Medical history should include any family history of thyroid condition or any previous history of neck injury or radiation as these are common risk factors of hypothyroidism. A comprehensive review of the system is also very important as clinical symptoms can range from asymptomatic to myxedema coma (severe hypothyroidism). Common physical examination findings are delayed deep tendon reflexes, atrophic or enlarged thyroid gland, periorbital edema, swelling of hands and feet, dry skin, and hair loss. Common symptoms are weight gain, fatigue, cold intolerance, dry skin, constipation, depression, memory loss, and menstrual irregularities.[1] In hypothyroidism, the presenting symptoms can be vague and overlap with other conditions. Common differential diagnoses include depression, dementia, heart disease, and kidney disease as these conditions also have similar symptoms in common with hypothyroidism, such as depressed mood, memory issues, swelling of hands and feet, and fatigue.

The serum TSH is the most sensitive test to detect hypothyroidism and will be elevated in patients with hypothyroidism. If the TSH is normal, there is no need to do additional thyroid tests because 98% of the time the T4 is normal when TSH is normal. If the patient is clinically hypothyroid, TSH with free T4 should be ordered. When TSH is elevated with a low free T4, it confirms the diagnosis of hypothyroidism. When screening TSH is elevated above 5 and below 10 with a normal free T4, it is subclinical hypothyroidism, and usually, treatment is not recommended, especially in older populations. However, in some special cases, such as pregnancy, infertility, hyperlipidemia, or goiter, treatment is needed.

When hypothyroidism is originated from the hypothalamic-pituitary disease, TSH may be normal, or low even when free T4 is low (TSH does not respond proportionally to low T4). In this case, the patient should be referred to the specialist for further evaluation for a complete endocrine workup and neuroradiologic studies. If autoimmune thyroiditis is suspected, check anti-TPO antibody (preferred) or antithyroglobulin antibody. Antibodies are positive in 95% of patients with Hashimoto's thyroiditis. In hypothyroidism, lipid abnormalities and elevated CK (creatinine kinase), LDH (lactate dehydrogenase), and AST (aspartate aminotransferase) levels are common but will improve with thyroid replacement. If a nodule is suspected on the physical examination, a thyroid ultrasound should be obtained.[1]

According to the American Thyroid Association (ATA), screening with a TSH should be done for all adults beginning at age 35 years and every 5 years thereafter.[22,26]

Management

Management of hypothyroidism depends on the cause of the hypothyroidism. In most cases, treatment is indicated, but in some cases, such as subclinical hypothyroidism, treatment is not necessary. Depending on the cause, treatment may be temporary, or it may be lifelong.

The goal for thyroid replacement therapy in hypothyroidism is to normalize the TSH value. TSH in the mid- to low normal range (from 0.3–2.5 mIU/L) is desirable for most patients. In practice, TSH is usually targeted to maintain the level between 1.0 and 3.0 mIU/L (considering different labs). Overreplacement of the thyroid will cause TSH suppression (below 0.3 mIU/L) and is not appropriate for hypothyroid treatment in most patients as overreplacement is associated with an increased risk of atrial fibrillation and osteoporosis.

According to ATA guidelines, thyroid hormone replacement by levothyroxine (T4) is the standard of care for hypothyroidism.[22,26] For thyroid replacement therapy in healthy patients, the full estimated replacement dose of levothyroxine is 1.6 mcg/kg/day, and the usual starting dose is 50 to 100 mcg per day. In older patients and patients with a history of cardiac problems, the initiation of therapy should be cautioned, so begin very low (12.5 mcg–50 mcg day) and titrate more slowly. Liothyronine sodium (T3) or Cytomel is also used as an alternative medication in some cases. Low doses of 5 to 10 mcg/day in combination with levothyroxine (T4) may improve mood and neuropsychologic function. However, it is not the standard of practice to add Cytomel.

It takes about 6 to 8 weeks for the TSH level to change in the bloodstream in response to the thyroid hormone replacement. Therefore, when titrating the therapy for hypothyroidism, rechecking TSH too early could be misleading. TSH level may remain elevated for several weeks despite effective treatment. A rapid increase in the levothyroxine dose should be avoided to prevent overreplacement, which may cause thyrotoxicosis leading to excessive weight loss, irritability, and tachycardia among other symptoms. Patients with an autoimmune cause for their hypothyroidism will require lifelong thyroid hormone replacement (see Table 26.6).[1,21]

Patient Education

Patient education is focused on the proper technique of taking thyroid medication, symptoms of overreplacement or underreplacement of thyroid hormone, and frequency of lab work. Levothyroxine should be taken on an empty stomach in the morning. Patients should wait at least 30 to 45 minutes to eat breakfast. If patients are taking any iron, calcium, or multivitamins, it should be taken at least 4 hours after taking the levothyroxine to ensure proper absorption. Patients should be educated about the symptoms of an underactive thyroid, which can commonly include feeling cold, tired, and constipated; moodiness; puffy skin; and hair loss. The symptoms of an overly active thyroid can commonly include feeling hot, tired, nervous, anxious, or shaky; weight loss; hair loss; frequent bowel movements; and trouble sleeping. Female patients should be educated to notify their healthcare provider if she becomes pregnant, as the levothyroxine dose requirement increases by 25% to 50% beginning in the first trimester starting at 8 weeks. Improvement is expected 2 weeks after the treatment initiation and signs and symptoms should resolve in 3 to 6 months. In most cases, lifelong therapy is needed. The laboratory level for TSH is needed after the patient has been on levothyroxine for at least 6 weeks and should be rechecked every 6 to 8 weeks until TSH is within normal limits. After TSH normalizes, it can be checked annually, unless the patient becomes symptomatic.[21]

EMERGENCIES

Hypothyroidism emergencies are not common but severe hypothyroidism or overreplacement of hypothyroidism causing severe hyperthyroidism may lead to these thyroid-related emergencies (Table 26.5).

CLINICAL PEARL

The following are some guidelines for the AGNP in diagnosing and managing thyroid disorder and differentiating between primary, where the problem is at the thyroid gland; secondary, with the problem at the pituitary gland; or tertiary, a thyroid disorder where the problem is at the level of the hypothalamus.

Table 26.5: Treatment Guide for Hypothyroid and Hyperthyroid Emergency

Hypothyroidism Emergency
• Myxedema coma is a rare but life-threatening condition, caused by untreated, severe hypothyroidism, and may require intravenous levothyroxine and cardiopulmonary assistance. Refer the patient to the ED.

Hyperthyroidism Emergency
• Risk of thyrotoxicosis with overreplacement should be monitored
• Treatment-induced congestive heart failure (CHF) or atrial fibrillation in older patient or a patient with coronary artery disease (CAD)

Table 26.6: At a Glance: How to Manage Hypothyroidism

Hypothyroidism at a glance
• Slow and sluggish symptoms alone indicate potential low thyroid activity—obtain TSH level
• High TSH but low free T4 is hypothyroidism—treat with Levothyroxine or increase dose if already receiving medication
• High TSH greater than 5 and less than 10 and a normal T4 is subclincial hypothyroidism. Monitor the patient; treatment is usually not needed
• Normal or low TSH plus low free T4 is likely a hypothalamic-pituitary origin for hypothyroidism (refer to endocrinologist for secondary or tertiary hypothyroidism)
Hyperthyroidism at a glance
• Hyper- and overactive symptoms alone indicate potential high thyroid activity—obtain TSH level
• Low TSH, normal or high free T4 is hyperthyroidism; if being treated for hypothyroidism, decrease the dose of levothyroxine.
Other considerations during the management of hypothyroidism:
• Levothyroxine dose requirement increases during the pregnancy beginning at first trimester.
• Thyroid medication should be taken on an empty stomach without food or any other medications for optimal absorption.
Wait at least 6 to 8 weeks to recheck TSH level. TSH lags behind; even though thyroid hormone level is already normal, it takes a longer time for TSH to normalize.

TSH, thyroid-stimulating hormone.

HYPERTHYROIDISM

Hyperthyroidism is the clinical condition in which serum thyroid hormone (T3 and T4) levels are in excess and tissues are exposed to the higher level of thyroid hormones.[21]

Etiology

Graves' disease, an autoimmune condition also known as diffuse toxic goiter, is the most common cause of hyperthyroidism. It is caused by the TSI (thyroid-stimulating immunoglobulin) autoantibodies that bind to the TSH receptor (TSHR) antibodies; this increases the secretion of thyroid hormones from the thyroid gland.[1,23] The second most common cause is toxic nodular goiter in which the thyroid nodule secretes excess amounts of thyroid hormones. Postpartum thyroiditis, which is an inflammation of the thyroid gland, typically occurs 4 to 6 weeks after the delivery of the baby and can also cause hyperthyroidism. Subacute thyroiditis, possibly caused by a viral infection, also can cause hyperthyroidism. Other causes of hyperthyroidism are solitary hyperfunctioning adenoma, exposure to iodide-containing drugs (e.g., amiodarone), or administration of exogenous thyroid preparations (treatment with levothyroxine for hypothyroidism). Less common factors of hyperthyroidism are TSH-secreting pituitary tumor or human chorionic gonadotropin (hCG) from a choriocarcinoma.[21]

Pathophysiology

In hyperthyroidism, when circulating thyroid hormone levels of T4 and T3 are high, the pituitary gland decreases the production of TSH to avoid the stimulation of the thyroid gland to decrease the production of thyroid hormone. In this negative feedback mechanism, when T4 and T3 levels are high, TSH level goes down to limit the production of excessive quantities of circulating thyroid hormone to keep the balance. Generally, low or suppressed levels of TSH and high free T4 indicate hyperthyroidism.[1]

Risk Factors

Individuals with a family history of hyperthyroidism or those who have an autoimmune disease such as type 1 diabetes have an increased risk of hyperthyroidism. Those individuals undergoing treatment for hypothyroidism with thyroid hormone replacement are also at higher risk of developing hyperthyroidism due to overreplacement of the hormone.

Approach to Diagnosis

It is important to know the cause of hyperthyroidism as it helps with deciding if treatment is indicated. Also, it is helpful to anticipate if treatment is needed for life or if it is temporary.

Medical history should include any family history of a thyroid condition. A comprehensive review of the system is very important as clinical symptoms can range from mild symptoms to severe hyperthyroidism. Common physical examination findings are rapid deep tendon reflexes; enlarged thyroid with thrill or bruit; fine tremor; soft, thin hair and nails; and exophthalmos (eyelid retraction and lags). Common symptoms are unexplained weight loss, heat intolerance, nervousness, tachycardia, palpitation, anxiety, frequent bowel movement, and menstrual irregularities.[1] Common differential diagnoses of hyperthyroidism include anxiety, atrial fibrillation, psychologic problems such as panic disorder, malignancy or diabetes due to weight loss, pregnancy, and essential tremors, among others.

The serum TSH and free T4 are the most sensitive tests to detect hyperthyroidism as 95% of patients have suppressed or not detectable TSH and elevated free T4. Free T3 may be elevated too. CBC and liver function should be monitored before starting antithyroid medication. If a nodule is suspected on physical examination, thyroid ultrasound should also be obtained. Radioactive iodine uptake scanning should be considered to differentiate Graves' hyperthyroidism versus a toxic nodule.[1]

Management

The goal for the treatment of hyperthyroidism is to reduce symptoms and decrease thyroid hormone synthesis. Graves' disease can be treated by antithyroid medications, radioactive ablation, and subtotal thyroidectomy. Symptom management includes the use of beta-blockers for tremors and chest palpitation.

Antithyroid medication (methimazole or propylthiouracil [PTU]) is effective and has a rapid onset of action. In some patients, 12 to 18 months of therapy might induce lasting remission, but others require longer therapy or other treatment methods. Methimazole is more commonly used in the United States, but PTU is used during pregnancy. Antithyroid medications have a risk of low but serious complications, such as agranulocytosis. Patients on those medications who present with fever or sore throat should have leukocyte levels checked. The use of radioiodine (I-131) or radioactive iodine (RAI) ablation is the most common treatment of Graves' disease in the United States as it has fewer side effects, and in most cases, it is a permanent treatment. Hypothyroidism is the goal of the radioactive iodine ablation because it is much easier to manage hypothyroidism than hyperthyroidism. RAI is contraindicated in pregnant patients as it can lead to fetal hypothyroidism, mental retardation, and a higher risk to the baby.[1,21]

Thyroid surgery is a nonpharmacologic option. Subtotal thyroidectomy generally has a good outcome and long-term control of hyperthyroidism. It has a low risk of subsequent hypothyroidism, but it is also the most expensive approach and may trigger a perioperative exacerbation of hyperthyroidism.[23]

Patient Education

Patients should be thoroughly educated about the treatment options, outcomes, expectations, and management of hyperthyroidism. Antithyroid medication is used mostly for temporary treatment. There is a 25% to 90%

chance of permanent remission with the antithyroid drug therapy. Graves' disease has a high rate of relapse after antithyroid medication is stopped. Patients need to have labs drawn for TSH and FT4 every 4 weeks until euthyroid and then every 3 to 6 months while on antithyroid drugs. Baseline CBC before starting the antithyroid medication and repeat CBC should be checked if agranulocytosis is suspected, as antithyroid drugs may cause agranulocytosis. Also, there is a need to check liver function tests as antithyroid medication may cause hepatic abnormalities. Patients should be educated about the symptoms of underactive thyroid and overactive thyroid. Also educate patients about the symptoms of agranulocytosis (fever, chills, sore throat) and to seek medical care if that occurs.

With RAI ablation or surgery, most patients become hypothyroid and will require thyroid hormone replacement for the rest of their lives. If RAI ablation is done, the AGNP needs to monitor TSH at 6 weeks, 12 weeks, 6 months, and annually or if symptomatic. Most patients who have surgery also have an enlarged thyroid gland or compressive symptoms, such as difficulty swallowing and choking. Long-term evaluation for recurrence of hyperthyroidism or development of hypothyroidism is necessary; therefore, close follow-up is necessary.

(((•)))EMERGENCIES

Hyperthyroidism emergencies are rare, but severe hyperthyroidism may lead to these thyroid-related emergencies:

- Thyroid storm is a life-threatening, sudden, and severe hyperthyroidism. Refer to the ED for fever, severe tachycardia, and sometimes delirium. It may be precipitated by trauma, infection, or surgery. Without treatment, it is fatal.

- Refer to an endocrinologist for hyperthyroidism management during pregnancy.

⊙ CLINICAL PEARL

The following are some findings of hyperthyroidism and may help the AGNP in managing this condition. Atrial fibrillation and osteoporosis are common complications of hyperthyroidism. Older adult patients may not have any symptoms of hyperthyroidism except atrial fibrillation.

EUTHYROID GOITER AND THYROID NODULE

The enlargement of the thyroid gland with normal thyroid function is defined as "euthyroid goiter." There are three different types of euthyroid goiter: diffuse goiter, in which the thyroid gland is diffusely enlarged; multinodular goiter, in which the thyroid gland has multiple nodules; and solitary thyroid nodule, in which the thyroid gland has a single nodule.[23] Thyroid nodules can be a hot nodule/toxic nodule (thyroid-hormone-producing nodule) or cold nodule (nonfunctional nodule that does not produce any thyroid hormone) and can be benign or cancerous.

Etiology

In the United States, where iodine is sufficient, the most common cause of euthyroid goiters is chronic thyroiditis, such as Hashimoto's thyroiditis. In the other part of the world, iodine deficiency can also cause diffuse goiter.[23] However, the cause of thyroid nodule formation is unknown.[1,23]

Pathophysiology

Multinodular goiter (MNG) is caused by the hyperplasia of the thyroid follicle. MNG is most common in older adults and women and more common in iodine-deficient areas of the world, such as Southeast Asia and Africa.[23] Most patients are asymptomatic and do not require treatment. However, if compressive symptoms such as difficulty swallowing, choking, and hoarseness are present, treatment may be necessary. Subtotal thyroidectomy is the treatment of choice as it will improve the compressive symptoms caused by the enlarged thyroid gland. If the patient is a poor candidate for surgery, a high dose of radioactive iodine to shrink the thyroid gland also improves symptoms in most cases.[23]

Thyroid nodules can be classified as cold or hot depending on how they show up on a thyroid scan; hot nodules take up more radioactive iodine isotopes, so they show up easily on the thyroid scan. These hot nodules or toxic nodules can cause hyperthyroidism. Hot nodules typically do not require a fine needle aspiration (FNA) biopsy because these nodules are almost always noncancerous. If the thyroid nodule is not producing any thyroid hormones, it is called a cold nodule. If it is a cold nodule, depending on the size of the nodule, an FNA biopsy is indicated to rule out cancer.

Risk Factors

The following conditions increase the risk of thyroid nodule:

- ■ Family history exists of thyroid nodules.
- ■ Female gender, older adult, are risk factors
- ■ Iodine deficiency increases the risk of goiter.
- ■ Autoimmune disease such as Hashimoto's increases the risk of benign thyroid nodules.
- ■ Exposure to ionizing radiation to the head, neck, or chest increases the risk of thyroid cancer.

Approach to Diagnosis

It is important to know the type of thyroid nodules: functioning (toxic/hot) or nonfunctioning (cold) nodule, benign nodule, or cancerous nodule. This information will help decide if treatment is indicated or not and helps anticipate if treatment will be complex or simple.

Management

The treatment complexity of the thyroid nodule depends on the type of thyroid nodule. If it is functional and causing hyperthyroidism, the treatment goal is to normalize the thyroid hormone level. If it is a compressive nodule, the management goal is to reduce any compressive symptoms, and if it is a suspicious nodule, surgical management may be needed.

If the diffuse goiter is caused by iodine deficiency, adequate iodine intake should be ensured. However, if the patient is euthyroid and the FNA biopsy is benign, no pharmacologic therapy is needed. If the patient is hypothyroid or hyperthyroid, they should be treated according to the treatment guidelines to normalize the thyroid function. However, if the patient with diffuse goiter has compressive symptoms and is a poor candidate for surgery, a high dose of radioactive iodine to shrink the gland also improves the compressive symptoms.[1,20,23] Thyroidectomy (subtotal or total) is indicated if the FNA biopsy is positive for malignancy, or indeterminant cytology, or if compressive symptoms.[21]

Patient Education

Patient education varies depending on the type of thyroid nodule: diffuse goiter, benign thyroid nodule, or malignant thyroid nodule. Endocrinology referral can be considered after the primary screening (thyroid labs, thyroid ultrasound). Instruct patients with benign thyroid nodules and that are euthyroid that semi-annual to annual office visits are required to monitor and to determine the nodule's size and hormone levels. For those patients who have benign thyroid nodules with abnormal thyroid hormone levels and clinical manifestations, more frequent visits are required. Patients should be educated to call their provider if there are any changes in the voice, dysphasia, pain, development of lymphadenopathy, or a change in nodule size. Malignant thyroid nodule requires management from an endocrinologist and a surgeon.[21]

((•)) EMERGENCIES

Severe hyperthyroidism with toxic thyroid nodules is very rare but can be life-threatening:

- ■ Thyroid storm is a life-threatening, sudden, and severe hyperthyroidism. Refer to the ED for fever, severe tachycardia, and sometimes delirium. It may be precipitated by trauma, infection, or surgery. Without treatment, it is fatal.
- ■ Refer to an endocrinologist for hyperthyroidism management during pregnancy.

Table 26.7: Types and Presentation of Thyroid Nodules

The following show types of thyroid nodules, their presentations, and their diagnosis:

- Clinically apparent thyroid nodules occur in 6% of women and in 1% to 2% in men; 5% of these are malignant.

- Euthyroid goiter has an overall, diffusely enlarged thyroid gland. No intervention is needed unless compressive symptoms are present.

- Some thyroid nodules can be functional and produce excessive thyroid hormones. These nodules are also called hot or toxic nodules. Hot nodules are mostly benign.

- Nonfunctional nodules, known as cold nodules, have a higher risk of malignancy than hot nodules.

- Toxic/hot nodule management is either RAI ablation, antithyroid medications, or surgery.

- Cold nodule management is surveillance if FNA biopsy is benign and surgery if malignant or if compressive symptoms are present.

- Ultrasound of the thyroid gland is very helpful for monitoring the size and characteristics of nodules. TI-RADS score helps determine if FNA biopsy of the nodule is necessary or not.

- A thyroid uptake scan is preferred to evaluate hot versus cold nodules.

🕐 CLINICAL PEARL

Table 26.7 includes some guidelines for the AGNP in managing thyroid nodules, differentiating between a hot nodule and a cold nodule, and different diagnostic tools.

OTHER ENDOCRINE DISORDERS

Adrenal Insufficiency

The adrenal axis is made of a complex balance of hormones from the hypothalamus, pituitary, and adrenal glands. Any irregularity in any one of these locations can cause adrenal hypofunction or insufficiency. Primary adrenal insufficiency, also known as Addison's disease, refers to the dysfunction at the adrenal-gland level. Secondary adrenal insufficiency is caused by the loss of adrenocorticotropic hormone (ACTH) from the pituitary gland. The loss of corticotropin-releasing hormone (CHR) from the hypothalamus is referred to as tertiary adrenal insufficiency. The clinical presentation of adrenal insufficiency varies depending on the affected axis. Patients may remain undiagnosed until a significant stressor, such as surgery, illness, or infection, precipitates an adrenal crisis, which is an endocrine emergency. Some of the symptoms of adrenal insufficiency are hypotension, fatigue, nausea, vomiting, weight loss, and generalized hyperpigmentation of skin and mucosa. An early morning cortisol value drawn between 4 a.m. and 8 a.m. of less than 3 mcg/dL suggests the diagnosis of adrenal insufficiency. However, it is not a very sensitive test; therefore, the ACTH stimulation test is done to confirm the diagnosis. In this test, a baseline blood sample is drawn and then a small amount of synthetic ACTH is injected intramuscularly or intravenously. Blood samples are redrawn after the ACTH injection. Sometimes this is accompanied by a urinary 17-ketosteroid test, which is a 24-hour collection process. These patients are typically managed in an endocrinology specialty practice.

Cushing Syndrome

Cushing syndrome is a clinical condition that is caused by prolonged exposure to excessive glucocorticoids from either endogenous or exogenous sources. The most common cause of exogenous Cushing syndrome is from the long-term use of therapeutic steroids. Cushing's disease (versus Cushing syndrome) is an endogenous form and usually is caused by an ACTH-secreting pituitary adenoma. Common clinic findings include hypertension, weight gain, central obesity, facial fullness, purple striae, glucose intolerance, and infections. A 24-hour urine free cortisol test, salivary cortisol measurement, and 1-mg overnight dexamethasone suppression test are used to confirm the diagnosis. Treatment goals are to reduce the cortisol levels in the body. If the patient is on a corticosteroid, reducing the dosage over time can be helpful. If the disease is caused by a tumor, surgery may be indicated. There are medications approved for the treatment of Cushing syndrome. These patients are typically managed in an endocrinology specialty practice.

Pituitary Adenoma

The pituitary gland is responsible for producing several important signaling hormones that regulate various body functions, including ACTH, growth hormone, prolactin, and TSH, among others. Pituitary tumors can be benign or malignant but are mostly benign and slow-growing. It can be a hormone-producing functional tumor or nonfunctional tumor. Clinical presentation can be headache or vision changes due to the pressure from the tumor to the brain and nerve, along with a variety of other symptoms. Patients with functional pituitary tumors present with the symptoms caused by the excess pituitary axis hormones (such as prolactinoma, excess growth hormone, Cushing disease, TSH-secreting tumor, etc.), resulting in fatigue, growth problems, unexplained weight gain or loss, and depression, among other symptoms. The tumor is diagnosed with magnetic resonance imaging. Treatment is surgery, radiation, or medication therapy to shrink the tumor. These patients are managed in an endocrinology specialty practice.

Osteoporosis

Osteoporosis is the most common metabolic bone disorder in humans and is a growing public health concern. Osteoporosis is a condition in which new bone creation lags behind old bone removal and bones become brittle and weakened. Osteoporosis can result from either poor bone mass growth or from excessive remodeling and affects about 20% of women and about 5% of men 50 years of age and older.[24] And while the condition is more common in women, about 80,000 men are predicted to have a hip fracture and they are more likely to die than women in the first year after hip fracture.[27] Osteoporosis can cause significant morbidity and mortality, with a higher risk for a subsequent fracture and increased mortality after hospitalization.

The condition is generally asymptomatic until complications such as fractures occur, so a preventive approach using screening is important to minimize the effects of the disease. However, some people do have symptoms such as loss of 1 inch of height or more, stooping posture, bone fractures, back pain, and dyspnea due to reduced lung capacity from compressed spinal discs. Some medical conditions can increase the risk for osteoporosis such as hormone therapy for breast and prostate cancer; overactive thyroid, parathyroid, or adrenal glands; celiac or inflammatory bowel disease; and some blood disease like multiple myeloma. A sedentary lifestyle, smoking, excessive alcohol use, low calcium, and vitamin D deficiency are other risk factors.

Current screening is recommended for women 65 years and older and for younger women if there is a history of a parent having a hip fracture. The standard for diagnosis and evaluation of osteoporosis is to obtain a bone mineral density (BMD). The central and peripheral dual-energy x-ray absorptiometry (DEXA) scan is the gold standard to measure BMD. The FRAX Risk Assessment Tool can be used for screening those patients who are diagnosed with osteoporosis after the BMD is done to determine the risk of a future fracture. Patients with osteoporosis should be treated; the goal of treatment is to reduce the risk of fracture. Therefore, people with osteoporosis should consume vitamin D and calcium on a daily basis for bone health. Treatment also includes regular weight-bearing, resistance, and balance exercises.[23] There are several medications available for the treatment of osteoporosis including hormones, bisphosphonates, and biologics; the choice of which of these medications is used is dependent on the severity of disease, sex, and, to some extent, patient choice.[25]

CONCLUSION

Diabetes and thyroid disorders are very common conditions that are mostly first encountered by primary care clinicians and management is generally straightforward and cost-effective. Timely diagnosis and treatment are very beneficial for the patient. It is important for the AGNP to understand at least the most important clinical approaches for the diagnosis and treatment of diabetes and thyroid disorders. American Diabetes Association and ATA's guidelines are two of the most valuable resources to remain updated on the standard of practice. A rule of thumb regarding older adults is going low on the doses of medications and going slow in the titration of medications or therapy, which is the safe approach. Overall, the management is based on individual cases, clinical knowledge, judgment, and the patient's preferences.

There are a variety of other endocrine disorders discussed in this chapter that are often first diagnosed or at least first noticed in the primary care office, but many of these patients are referred to endocrinology for definitive diagnosis and potentially for ongoing comanagement with the primary care provider. AGNPs should be familiar with these conditions to recognize key signs and symptoms and know when to refer to the specialist.

CASE STUDY 26.1

AN ADULT FEMALE WITH UNCONTROLLED DIABETES TYPE 2

Chief Complaint

Follow-up from recent hospitalization a month ago for pyelonephritis

A 69-year-old African American female recently discharged from the hospital for pyelonephritis; noted to have hyperglycemia during hospitalization with A1c of 13.9%. Started on multidose insulin and discharged with insulin. She did not bring her SMBG as she finds it an inconvenience with her active lifestyle.

Past Medical History: Hypertension.

Family History: Mother with history of thyroid disorder. Father deceased at age 55 from MI. Maternal grandmother with history of breast cancer

Social History: Single. Lives with her daughter. Physically active—she golfs weekly, plays tennis twice a week, swims once a week. Denies ETOH use. Denies illicit drug use. (+) tobacco use—started in her late 30s, now smoking 2–4 cigarettes a week. Diet: Cooks and grocery shops for herself and daughter. Typically eats mainly two meals a day; rarely eats breakfast. Breakfast: (when she eats) oatmeal and coffee with creamer; Lunch: either soup with

(cont.)

a side of salad/sandwich with a salad and 8 oz juice; Dinner: brown rice with a protein (grilled salmon/chicken), a side of salad with 8 oz juice. Snacks on nuts/fruit throughout the day. Drinks regular Dr. Pepper 16 oz every 2 to 3 days. Admits to excessive consumption of cakes, baked goods, and ice cream in the last 3 months during the pandemic.

Medications: Atenolol; glargine 24 units SQ qHS, Aspart 8 units TID AC

Allergies: Lisinopril—angioedema

Pertinent Findings from Physical Examination

Missing some teeth. Wide gaps between teeth. Gingivitis (+) halitosis. Protuberant abdomen.

Pertinent Lab Oratory and Diagnostic Findings

Weight: 95.8 kg BMI: 37.41 kg/m^2, B/P: 163/89
HgbA1c 13.9

Assessment: 69-year-old obese (BMI 37.41 kg/m^2) female with past medical history significant for hypertension, diabetes type 2, insulin required, uncontrolled with A1c of 13.9% on multidose daily injections. She is a physically active individual with a goal of 10,000 steps 3x a week

Plan

Glycemic Targets: Premeal glucose target of 70 to 130 mg/dL

Pharmacologic Therapy[11]
Underline For Management of Diabetes:

Metformin as first-line therapy

SGLT2 or GLP1 with demonstrated CVD benefit given this patient's risk of CVD and BMI

Consider use of CGM with her active lifestyle

For Management of Hypertension:

ACE/ARBs are renal protective, but noted documented allergy to this classification of drug

Diuretics, beta-blockers, and calcium channel blockers are used as potential second or third agents

Treat to an SBP less than 140 mmHG and a diastolic blood pressure of less than 90 mmHg

For Management of Coronary Heart Disease

Aspirin, low dose, as primary preventative care for individuals with diabetes

Statin therapy—high intensity given CVD risk factor in this patient

Smoking cessation

Physical Activity

Continue with at least 150 minutes of physical activity 3 × a week

Teach-Back: Clearly states the benefits and most common side effects of metformin

Referral to medical nutrition therapy with registered dietitian and/or CDECS

Referral to ophthalmology for initial dilated examination at time of diabetes diagnosis, then every 1 to 2 years

Referral for dental care

Foot Examination Annually: with 10-g monofilament test

Urine Albumin: annually if urinary albumin is greater than 30 mg/g Cr or eGFR is lower than 60 mL/min 1.73 m^2 every 6 months

Diabetes and depression screening (PHQ9)

Vaccinations (CDC's Vaccine Information for Adults With Diabetes, 2020)

Flu vaccine annually

Pneumococcal Vaccine: once before age 65 years; two more doses after age 65 years

Hepatitis B: less than 60 years old

Tdap: once and every 10 years for a booster

Zoster (50 years old or older)

CASE STUDY 26.2

Katy, a 36-year-old female with no known past medical history, presents to clinic with symptoms of a few pounds of weight gain, feeling cold, depressed mood, dry skin, and thinning of hair. On the physical examination, Katy has delayed deep tendon reflexes, her legs appear slightly swollen but no pitting edema, her skin is dry, her nails are brittle, and her thyroid gland is slightly enlarged.

Case Study Questions

1. What is the most likely diagnosis?
2. What labs will you order?
3. What is the differential diagnosis?
4. What is the treatment option?

(cont.)

Answers

These are classic signs and symptoms of hypothyroidism. To confirm the diagnosis, two blood tests are essential.

Differential diagnosis: depression, dementia, heart disease, kidney disease

- ■ TSH (TSH will be higher than normal.)
- ■ FT4 (FT4 will be lower than normal.)

Other tests: TPO antibody may be positive indicating Hashimoto's thyroiditis as a cause for hypothyroidism. Treatment: Start levothyroxine per dose recommendation. Follow the hypothyroidism management guidelines.

CASE STUDY 26.3

Rosy is a 40-year-old healthy female who presents to the clinic with her husband with the complaints of increased anxiety, chest palpitation, unable to sleep at night, unexplained weight loss, feeling hot, and frequent bowel movements. Her husband reports that Rosy has been "very irritable and short-tempered." On the physical examination, Rosy has fine tremors of her fingers, her pulse is elevated, her thyroid gland is enlarged, and deep tendon reflexes are rapid.

Case Study Questions

1. What is the most likely diagnosis?
2. What labs will you order?
3. What is the differential diagnosis?
4. What is the treatment option?

Answers

These are classic signs and symptoms of hyperthyroidism.

Differential diagnosis: subacute hyperthyroidism, toxic multinodular goiter, thyroid adenoma, anxiety, atrial fibrillation

Do these initial blood tests.

- ■ TSH (TSH will be lower or suppressed.)
- ■ FT4 (FT4 will be higher than normal.)
- ■ FT3 (FT3 may be normal or elevated.)

Other tests: Check TSI antibody: positive means Graves' disease. Check thyroid ultrasound if a nodule is suspected on physical examination. If a nodule is present, do radioactive iodine uptake scan to rule out Graves' vs. toxic nodule

If thyroid scan uptake is isolated in the nodule area, it is the hot nodule that is producing excessive thyroid hormone, causing hyperthyroidism. If thyroid scan uptake is increased overall throughout the gland (diffuse uptake), it means it's Graves' disease.

TREATMENT

Start antithyroid medication. If symptomatic, use beta-blocker propranolol for symptoms management.

Discuss long-term treatment plan of RAI ablation or subtotal thyroidectomy and refer to an endocrinologist.

CASE STUDY 26.4

Ron, a 28-year-old male with no known past medical problem, presents to the clinic with the symptoms of sore throat, voice changes, increased anxiety, irritability, chest palpitation, weight loss, and inability to sleep at night. On the physical examination, Ron has fine tremors of his fingers, and he is experiencing tachycardia; thyroid gland is enlarged and tender.

Case Study Questions

1. What is the most likely diagnosis?
2. What labs will you order?
3. What is the differential diagnosis?
4. What is the treatment option?

Answers

Sore throat and tender thyroid gland and hyperthyroid symptoms suggest subacute hyperthyroidism. Graves' hyperthyroidism, or toxic nodular hyperthyroidism, does not cause thyroid pain.

Differential diagnosis: Graves' disease, toxic multinodular goiter, thyroid adenoma

- ■ TSH (TSH will be suppressed or low.)
- ■ FT4 (FT4 will be high.)

Other tests: TSI Antibody test will be negative.

Thyroid ultrasound: Thyroiditis but no nodule.

Thyroid uptake scan: Uptake will be low.

Treatment: Usually resolves on its own after a few weeks to months. Recommend anti-inflammatory therapy NSAID for pain and swelling. Beta-blockers are used for thyrotoxic symptoms. Patient may also need steroids. Refer to an endocrinologist for further evaluation.

(cont.)

CASE STUDY 26.5

Jane is a 40-year-old female who presents to the clinic for a routine wellness visit. On the physical examination, Jane has a slightly enlarged thyroid gland with few palpable nodules. Jane reports her mother has a history of hypothyroidism and had thyroid nodules. Patient denies any family history of thyroid cancer.

Case Study Questions

What is the most likely diagnosis?
What labs will you order?
What is the differential diagnosis?
What is the treatment option?

Answers

History of hypothyroidism and thyroid nodules in mother increases the risk of hypothyroidism in patient. On PE patient has multiple palpable thyroid nodules, which is more common in Hashimoto's thyroiditis. This information suggests that patient may have Hashimoto's thyroiditis with thyroid nodules.

Differential diagnosis: toxic multinodular goiter, thyroid adenoma, Hashimoto's thyroiditis with thyroid nodules, parathyroid adenoma

- TSH will be high or normal.
- FT4 (FT4 will be low or normal.)

Other tests: TPO Antibody test will be positive in Hashimoto's thyroiditis.

Thyroid ultrasound: May show multiple thyroid nodules.

Thyroid uptake scan: Uptake will be normal if not toxic nodule.

Treatment: Treat with levothyroxine if hypothyroid. Depending on the size and characteristics of the nodules, patient may need FNA biopsy of thyroid nodule. Refer to an endocrinologist for further evaluation.

REFERENCES

References for this chapter are online and available at https://connect.springerpub.com/content/book/978-0-8261-8414-6/part/part01/toc-part/ch26.

CHAPTER 27

Common Hematology Disorders Encountered in the Primary Care Setting

John R. Van Auker and Laura L. Van Auker

LEARNING OBJECTIVES

At the conclusion of this chapter, the learner will be able to:

➤ Review normal cellular erythropoiesis and its role in responding to conditions of anemia.

➤ Recognize the various anemias and their associated disorders and management goals.

➤ Apply a stepwise approach to determining types of anemia through signs, symptoms, and laboratory findings.

➤ Identify risk factors for acquired anemias and appropriate patient education.

➤ Recognize the various leukemias and their associated disorders and management goals.

INTRODUCTION

In this chapter, disorders of the hematologic system are discussed. This system regulates the production of the three primary cell types of the circulation, namely, red blood cells (RBCs, erythrocytes), white blood cells (WBCs, leukocytes), and platelets (thrombocytes). The primary location for this process is in the bone marrow, with multiple regulatory factors involved in the normal production of these cells (hematopoiesis). When this regulation is disrupted, disease or illness may result. When production of RBCs or erythropoiesis is diminished, decreased numbers of RBCs are produced and erythrocytopenia may result. Unregulated erythropoiesis may lead to increased RBC production with resulting polycythemia. WBC production or leukopoiesis acts similarly; when there are fewer cells produced, this results in leukocytopenia, and when WBC production is increased, leukocytosis presents. The production of platelets (thrombopoiesis) can be decreased and is called "thrombocytopenia," whereas an increase in platelet cells is termed "thrombocytosis." This chapter begins with a discussion with the normal hematopoietic process and its regulation followed by the altered processes associated with the most common disorders of hematologic origin. The impacts of aging on these disease processes will be highlighted.

OVERVIEW OF THE SYSTEM

Hematology is the study of the formed elements of the blood by way of the hematopoietic process. These formed elements develop within the bone marrow and originate from the hematopoietic stem cell (HSC) or pluripotent stem cell. The HSCs are capable of differentiating into any of the cell lineages of the blood and they are stimulated or inhibited to do so by specialized glycoproteins called hematopoietic growth factors or cytokines and colony-stimulating factors (CSF).[1] Once stimulated, the HSC will begin development down one of the two pathways in the bone marrow. One pathway is the lymphoid cell line and the other, the myeloid cell line (Figure 27.1).[2]

Along the lymphoid pathways, the cell matures into first a T-cell or B-cell precursor (lymphoblast) and eventually into a mature T-cell or B-cell lymphocyte. The B-cell lymphocyte may further progress and after migrating into tissues become a plasma cell. The myeloid pathway further differentiates into precursors of platelets (megakaryoblast), erythrocytes (pronormoblast/erythroblast), monocytes (monoblast), or granulocytes (myeloblast). Granulocytes may be neutrophils, eosinophils, or basophils. Monocytes will often migrate into the tissues where they become macrophages.

Normal Anatomy and Physiology

The formed cells of the blood—erythrocytes (RBCs), leukocytes (WBCs), and platelets—are produced through a complex array of multi-organ regulation.[3] The development of the RBC in the bone marrow is regulated by a cytokine, called erythropoietin (EPO), which is produced in the kidney. This process, known as erythropoiesis, allows for maturation of the RBC, which assembles the hemoglobin (Hgb) molecule, utilizing iron as a key element in its structure. Vitamin B12 and folate are also necessary for effective maturation. The principal function of the mature RBC is to transport oxygen, bound to Hgb, from the lungs to the tissues where oxygen is released and exchanged for carbon dioxide. The carbon dioxide attached to the Hgb molecule is then delivered back to the lungs where the Hgb releases carbon dioxide and once again binds to oxygen, thus completing the cycle.

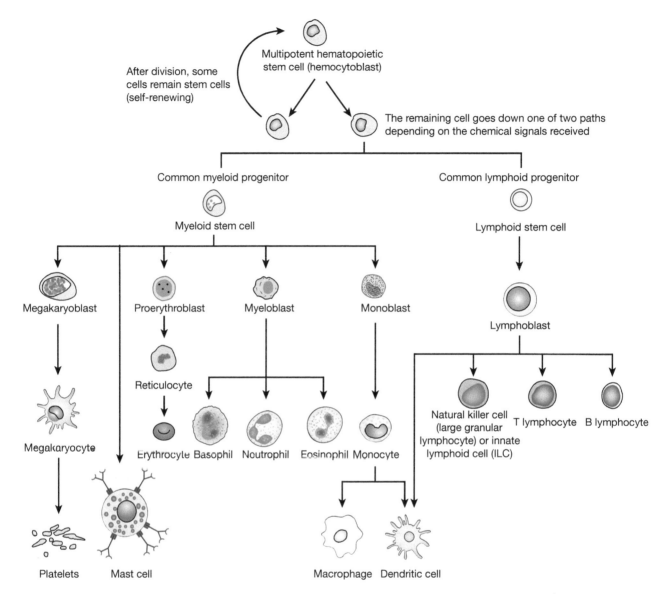

Figure 27.1: Hematopoiesis
The generation of red and white blood cells occurs in the bone marrow. A multipotent stem cell can follow a myeloid or lymphoid path before further differentiating to the final forms of the cells shown.
Source: Tkacs N, Hermann L, Johnson R, eds. *Advanced Physiology & Pathophysiology: Essentials for Clinical Practice.* Springer Publishing Company; 2021:Figure 6.5.

The respiratory by-product of carbon dioxide is expelled from the lungs during the pulmonary expiratory cycle. This cycle repeats throughout the life span of the RBC, which is approximately 120 days. At this point, RBCs are removed from circulation within the spleen by macrophages. Macrophages salvage iron from the RBC and return it to the bone marrow for continued RBC production, or iron is transported to the liver for storage for future use as ferritin.

WBCs develop into various cell lineages in the bone marrow, again under the regulation of specific cytokines or CSF. This process is called leukopoiesis. The function of the WBC is generally that of protecting the body from foreign protein whether it be organisms, cells, or particles. The WBC is also important in triggering the inflammatory process. WBCs are commonly categorized based on their staining and nuclear characteristics on the peripheral blood smear using Wright's stain. They are separated into lymphocytes, monocytes, or granulocytes. The granulocytes are further divided into neutrophils, eosinophils, or basophils based on the staining characteristics of their cytoplasm granules.

Lymphocytes are involved in the body's immune response, either producing antibodies against or by directly attacking antigens.[4] Lymphocytes serve an important function in the body's response to viral infection.

Monocytes function to identify and phagocytize foreign material. They aid lymphocytes in mounting an immune response. Monocytes can migrate to the tissues and body cavities where they become macrophages. Macrophages number more than RBCs or even skin cells in the body. Their function is varied and often dictated by the tissue or body cavity they inhabit.[5] For example, it is the macrophages within the bone marrow that are responsible for removing old RBCs to salvage iron from the Hgb molecule.

Neutrophils are one of the three granulocytes that also include eosinophils and basophils. They are the most numerous of the three and of all circulating leukocytes. Neutrophils are the first cells to respond to infection or inflammation. They function to phagocytize microorganisms and cellular debris. Neutrophils are predominantly segmented, which refers to the division of the nucleus into two to four lobes, or in more limited quantity to a band neutrophil. Band neutrophils are less mature than the segmented form and, when seen in elevated numbers, may suggest an inflammatory response.

Eosinophils are important in controlling the inflammatory response. They are capable of phagocytosis and are seen in the body's response to parasitic infection and allergic disorders such as asthma.

Basophils are involved in controlling and augmenting the inflammatory response and can release histamine, a potent vasodilator. They also assist eosinophils in controlling certain parasitic infections.

Platelets are the fragments of cytoplasm that are shed in the bone marrow from megakaryocytes. The production of megakaryocytes and subsequently platelets is regulated by the cytokine thrombopoietin (TPO). Platelets are key to initiating hemostasis by adhering to the injury site of the blood vessel (Figure 27.2). Platelets then release substances including fibrinogen that attract other platelets to aggregate at the injury site to form a plug. Fibrinogen is converted to fibrin, resulting in coagulation. The coagulation cascade involves sequential activation of clotting factors, one activating the next to achieve hemostasis. Once hemostasis is complete, a process called fibrinolysis is initiated to remove the plug after the vessel injury has been repaired.

RED BLOOD CELL DISORDERS

"Anemia" is defined as a decrease in oxygen-carrying capacity of the blood. This can be the result of an absolute decrease in the number of RBCs. It may also be combined with decreased or dysfunctional Hgb. The causes of anemia are varied, either from decreased RBC production in

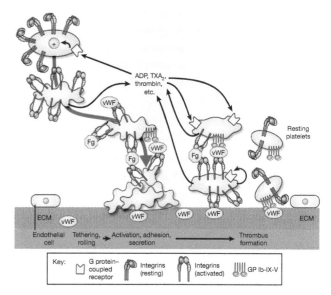

Figure 27.2: Platelet function in clot formation
Clots form at sites of vascular damage, in particular when the endothelial cell layer is disrupted and the ECM is exposed. Formation of the primary clot depends on platelet adherence to ECM, mediated by glycoprotein Ib-IX-V (GP Ib-IX-V) and vWF; platelet activation and shape change, mediated by ADP, TXA$_2$, and thrombin binding to G protein-coupled receptors; and platelets binding to fibrinogen (Fg) and to each other by activated intergrin αIIbβ$_3$ (also known as glycoprotein IIb/IIIa).

ADP, adenosine diphosphate; ECM, extracellular matrix: TXA$_2$, thromboxane A$_2$; vWF, von Willebrand factor.

Source: Tkacs N, Hermann L, Johnson R, eds. *Advanced Physiology & Pathophysiology: : Essentials for Clinical Practice.* Springer Publishing Company; 2021:Figure 8.7.

the bone marrow, an increase in RBC destruction from blood loss, both chronic and acute, or a combination of these causations.[6] Symptoms of anemia often include fatigue and dyspnea on exertion. When blood loss is minimal and prolonged, anemia may be asymptomatic as the body compensates. Laboratory studies are helpful in arriving at an accurate diagnosis so that appropriate interventions can be taken to mitigate the consequences or correct the cause of the anemia.

There are several ways of using laboratory data to classify anemias, allowing differential diagnoses to be ruled in or out. One method commonly used is to distinguish anemias starting with the size or mean corpuscular volume (MCV). The normal range for MCV is 80 fL to 100 fL and cells within this normal range are called normocytic. When the MCV is below 80 fL, the RBCs are considered microcytic. RBCs showing MCV above 100 fL are considered macrocytic. Recognizing RBC size aids in the diagnosis of various anemia types labeled microcytic, normocytic, or macrocytic anemias. Although the use of the MCV is helpful in the initial classification of anemias, it is not absolute in determining an anemia diagnosis. There are overlapping characteristics between several anemias. For example, iron deficiency anemia (IDA) is generally categorized as a microcytic, hypochromic anemia, but in earlier stages, it may present as normocytic and normochromic. Likewise, the anemia of chronic disease (ACD) and inflammation may be microcytic and hypochromic or dependent on the degree of the disease; inflammation may present as normocytic and normochromic. Additionally, it is important to recognize that concurrent conditions producing anemia of varied types may coexist. It is not uncommon that a microcytic anemia of IDA may occur in an individual also experiencing a macrocytic condition related to hypothyroidism. In this more complex circumstance, diagnosis may be hampered, and additional studies will be required to produce an accurate diagnosis.

A thorough history and physical examination are important in differentiating the cause of most anemias in conjunction with appropriate laboratory and diagnostics studies and procedures. In most anemias, patients may complain of weakness, fatigue, headaches, poor concentration, paleness, dizziness, difficulty breathing, or chest pain, as well as poor exercise tolerance. The physical examination will focus on any major medical conditions potentially contributing to anemia. Physical findings associated with anemia include pallor of the skin, mucous membranes of the conjunctiva and oral gingiva, and pale palmar creases and nailbeds. In more pronounced anemia, the patient may have tachycardia or systolic heart murmurs heard at the apex or pulmonic area. Additional physical findings of specific anemias are listed in the tables indicating physical and lab findings associated with specific anemias (Tables 27.1 and 27.2).

APPROACH TO THE ANEMIAS

There is an approach that can be utilized to facilitate diagnosing the anemias using the peripheral blood smear and the MCV; this approach can facilitate identification of the type of anemia presenting (Figure 27.3).

MICROCYTIC ANEMIA

In microcytic anemias, it is helpful to utilize the clinical manifestations and laboratory findings as an aid to arriving at the correct diagnosis.

Microcytic anemia has many causes, but the most common form in children and adults is associated with IDA. In IDA, the iron needed for RBC production is not available in adequate amounts. This can be from inadequate nutritional intake, an increase in demand, impaired

absorption, or from the most common etiology, chronic blood loss. The daily required baseline intake for iron is approximately 1 mg elemental iron. Socioeconomic factors play a role in influencing iron intake as certain iron-rich foods are expensive or not culturally recognized. Increased demand for iron occurs during rapid growth periods in childhood and adolescence, as well as during pregnancy. Impaired absorption can be the result of celiac disease, tropical sprue, and Crohn's disease. Gastrectomy and bariatric surgery inherently restrict the volume of iron-rich foods, as well as impair their absorption. Certain medications, such as proton pump inhibitors (PPIs) and H² blockers, are commonly used in the geriatric population; lower gastric acidity can affect iron absorption. Chronic blood loss is often from the gastrointestinal tract resulting from hemorrhoids, gastritis, peptic ulcers, or malignancies. The use of nonsteroidal anti-inflammatory drugs (NSAIDs) is often a cause of gastritis and ulcers, leading to chronic blood loss. Women during their reproductive years may experience heavy cyclic blood loss with abnormal menstrual bleeding or from fibroid tumors. The approach to diagnosing IDA begins with the complete blood count (CBC). The RBC count, Hgb, hematocrit (Hct), and MCV will be decreased. Additionally, iron, ferritin, and transferrin saturation will be low (Table 27.2). On physical examination, the patient may be noted to have pallor of the skin, especially of the conjunctiva and oral gingiva, and the palmar creases of the hands may be pale. Tachycardia may be noted due to increased oxygen demand from the tissues as RBCs and/or Hgb are in limited supply. The treatment of IDA is targeted at the etiology. Inadequate intake, increased iron demand, or malabsorption should focus upon dietary measures if appropriate, promoting iron-rich foods. A nutritional consult can be considered. Supplemental iron may be necessary, either taken orally or parenteral iron may be required in certain malabsorption conditions. In the case of chronic blood loss in adult males and in postmenopausal women, a gastrointestinal (GI) source is common and would warrant investigations with fecal occult blood testing, colonoscopy, and esophagogastroduodenoscopy (EGD) to evaluate the esophagus, stomach, and proximal small intestine. In menstruating women, especially during perimenopause when changes in the hormonal balance between estrogen and progesterone naturally occur, an imbalance may disrupt ovulation, resulting in abnormal uterine bleeding, causing either higher volume or extended periods of uterine shedding and blood loss. Normalizing the cycle through the use of supplemental hormones may reduce the amount and length of menstrual bleeding. Heavy bleeding caused by uterine enlargement due to fibroid tumors may eventually require surgical management. Continuous supplemental iron may be required for an extended period to maintain adequate supplies for erythropoiesis. Anemia due to medications may require alternative treatments and/or lifestyle modification.

ANEMIA OF CHRONIC DISEASE AND ANEMIA OF INFLAMMATION

The ACD and anemia of inflammation (AI) are included in the microcytic anemia category. These anemias may be seen in conditions such as chronic kidney disease (CKD), chronic obstructive pulmonary disease (COPD), or inflammatory conditions, such as inflammatory bowel disease, as well as several conditions discussed later. These anemias are collectively the second most common anemias following IDA. As with the previously discussed microcytic anemias, ACD and AI are characterized by microcytic, hypochromic RBCs. As in IDA, it is important to perform iron studies in the microcytic anemias. As previously discussed, in IDA serum iron, transferrin saturation, and ferritin levels are low. This is in contrast to the thalassemias where iron studies are normal. The anemias of chronic disease and inflammation will have low serum iron and low transferrin saturation, but "elevated" ferritin levels. It is thought that ACD and AI result from the body's defense mechanism to limit iron availability to invading organisms that would seek to utilize the host's serum iron. This may be seen in systemic infections or inflammatory disorders, such as systemic lupus erythematosus (SLE), and inflammatory bowel disorders, such as Crohn's disease. This may also occur with malignancies and chronic disorders of heart failure, COPD, and CKD. These systemic and chronic conditions are more common in older adults; therefore, ACD and AI are seen with greater frequency in the geriatric population. In the case of CKD, the essential function of producing EPO as erythropoietic glycoprotein hormone is compromised, limiting RBC production in the bone marrow. In other forms of anemia, the kidneys respond to anemia with increased circulating EPO in response to hypoxia or anemia, prompting up to a 1,000-fold increase in EPO to stimulate increased RBC production.[8] In CKD, decreased EPO production within the diseased kidneys prevents adequate circulating EPO, results in the anemia of ACD and AI, and contributes to further decline of the kidneys as well.[9] Infections, malignancies, and chronic disorders including CKD are more common in older adults, resulting in a higher incidence of ACD and AI seen in the older and geriatric populations. The management of ACD and AI is targeted at identifying the underlying condition and correcting it.[10] Evaluating ACD and AI begins with a comprehensive history and physical examination. Patient symptoms may be more related to the etiology of the anemia until the anemia is more pronounced.

Not infrequently, IDA will coexist with ACD and AI and treatment of the iron deficiency as previously discussed will be necessary. For patients with CKD, restrictive diets may put them at risk for vitamin deficiencies and may require supplementation with B12 and folic acid. Patients on dialysis are more prone to RBC destruction and at greater risk for anemia. In some instances, severe anemia will be treated with RBC transfusion in a direct effort to raise oxygen-carrying RBCs. In low EPO anemia such as CKD, a genetically engineered form of EPO may be injected or circulated during dialysis. Due to an identified increased risk to cardiovascular events of stroke and heart attack in patients with CKD, EPO is recommended only when a patient's Hgb level is below 10 g/dL.[8]

THALASSEMIAS

Thalassemias are inherited disorders causing microcytic anemia and are identified as alpha or beta thalassemia. They are inherited either as homozygous major, receiving a defective gene from each parent, or heterozygous minor, receiving a defective gene from only one parent. The minor forms of both alpha and beta thalassemias in which an individual has a single mutated gene may be referred to as an alpha or beta thalassemia gene "carrier" or thalassemia "trait." The thalassemias are an alteration of the globin chains that make up the Hgb molecule. Beta thalassemias are more common, with beta thalassemia minor being more common than the major form. Beta thalassemia minor usually results in asymptomatic anemia, but the major form of beta thalassemia typically results in severe anemia requiring regular packed red cell transfusions throughout life. Alpha thalassemia minor, much like beta thalassemia minor, usually causes mild anemia whereas alpha thalassemia major is not compatible with life and usually results in an intrauterine fetal demise. All the thalassemias are characterized by microcytic, hypochromic red cells. Unlike most anemias that typically have decreased RBCs, Hgb, and Hct, the thalassemias have a compensatory normal or elevated RBC count. Also, unlike microcytic anemias associated with low serum iron and low transferrin saturation, the thalassemias have normal iron studies. There are several reasons that identifying the thalassemias and diagnosing are important. As a microcytic anemia with low Hgb and Hct, there is a tendency to misdiagnose thalassemias as IDA. Prescribing supplemental iron replacement can lead to iron overload and resultant liver and cardiac damage. This causes a condition known as secondary hemochromatosis. Primary hemochromatosis is associated with a genetic defect causing excess iron to be absorbed from the gastrointestinal tract. This is why it is important to obtain iron studies in microcytic anemias to avoid this treatment error. Additionally, because the thalassemias are an inherited genetic disorder, it is critical that individuals who are carriers with thalassemia trait be advised of the risk for thalassemia in their offspring, especially if

Table 27.1: Physical and Lab Findings Associated With Specific Anemias

Clinical Manifestation							
Disease	Genetics	History	Symptoms	Signs	Hemolysis	Instrinsic/ Extrinsic	Hb Concentratic
Iron deficiency anemia	-	• Menorrhagia • GI loss • GI surgery • Pregnancy	• Koilonychia • Pica	• Glossitis • Cheilosis • Dysphagia	-	-	Hypochromi
Lead poisoning	-	House painted with chipped paint	• Burtonian lines • Basophilic stippling • Wrist drop • Foot drop	• Wrist drop • Foot drop • Burtonian lines	-	-	Hypochromi
Sideroblastic anemia	• Defect in ALA synthase gene • Autosomal dominant • Autosomal recessive • X-linked	• Alcohol abuse • Isoniazid use • Chloramphenicol use • Idiopathic	• Seborrheic dermatitis • Glossy tongue • Tingling	Patient presents with symptoms of vitamin B6, copper deficiency symptoms	-	-	Hypochromi
Anemia of chronic disease	-	• Rheumatoid arthritis • SLE • Neoplasm • Chronic kidney disease	• Headache • Shortness of breath		-	-	Hypochromi
Thalassemia	**α-thalassemia** • α- globin gene deletions • Cis deletions • Trans deletions **β-thalassemia** • Point mutation in splice sites and promoter sequences	Associated with parvovirus B19	**α-thalassemia** • Hydrops fetalis **β-thalassemia** • Skeletal deformities • Chipmunk facies	• Hepatomegaly • Splenomegaly	-	-	Hypochromi

| | Lab Findings | | | | | | | | | |
| | | | | | Iron Studies | | | | | |
CV	RDW	Reticulocytosis	Haptoglobin Levels	Hepicidin	Serum Iron	Serum Tfr level	Transferrin or TIBC	Ferritin	Transferrin Saturation	Specific Finding on Blood Smear
crocytic	↑	Nl or ↓	Nl	Nl	↓	↑	↑	↓	↓↓↓	• Central pallor
crocytic	Nl	Nl or ↓	Nl	Nl	Nl to ↓	Nl	Nl	Nl to ↓	-	• RBCs retain aggregates of rRNA • Basophilic stippling
crocytic	Nl	Nl or ↓	Nl	Nl	↑	Nl	Nl to ↓	↑	-	• Ringed sideroblasts
crocytic	Nl	Nl or ↓	Nl	↑	↓	Nl	↓	↑	-	NA
crocytic	Nl	• Thalassemia trait: Nl or ↓ • Thalassemia syndromes: ↑	Nl	Nl	Nl to ↑	Nl	Nl	↑	Nl to ↑	• Target cells • Anisopoikilocytosis

gastrointestinal; IBC, iron-binding capacity; MCV, mean corpuscular volume; RBC, red blood cell; RDW, red cell distribution width; SLE, temic lupus erythematosus; TIBC, transferrin and iron-binding capacity.

rce: Gibson CM. Anemia. Wikidocs; 2020, July 29. https://www.wikidoc.org/index.php/Anemia#Differentiating_Anemia_from_ er_Diseases

Table 27.2: Differentiating Anemia With Intrinsic Hemolyis From Other Diseases

Clinical Manifestation							
Disease	Genetics	History	Symptoms	Signs	Hemolysis	Intrinsic/Extrinsic	Hb Concentrat
G6PD deficiency[1]	• Defect in G6PD enzyme • X-linked recessive	• History of using • Sulfa drugs • Antimalarials • Fava Beans • Infections	• Back pain • Hemoglobinuria	Back pain	+	Intrinsic	Normochromic
Pyruvate kinase deficiency[2]	• Mutation in the *PKLR* and *PKM* gene • Autosomal recessive	Gallstones	• Hydrops fetalis • Neonatal hyperbilirubinemia • Iron overload • Perinatal complications	• Skin ulcers • Splenomegaly	+	Intrinsic	Normochromic
Sickle cell anemia[3]	Hbs point mutation causes a single amino acid replacement in β chain	• High altitude • Low oxygen • Acidosis • African American race • Parvovirus B19 infection	• Dactylitis • Priapism • Acute chest syndrome • Avascular necrosis • Stroke • Autosplenectomy • Salmonella osteomyelitis	• Dactylitis • Priapism	+	Intrinsic	Normochromic
HbC disease[4]	Glutamic acid-to-lysine mutation in β-globin	Gallstone	• Joint pains • Increased risk of infections	• Splenomegaly • Cholelithiasis • Avascular necrosis of the femoral head	+	Intrinsic	Normochromic
Paroxysmal nocturnal hemoglobinuria[5,6]	• *PIGA* gene mutations • Impaired synthesis of GPI anchor	• Associated with aplastic anemia • Thrombosis	• Fatigue • Chest pain • Dyspnea on exertion • Headache	• Chronic hemolysis • Hepatomegaly • Ascites • Papilledema • Skin nodules	+	Intrinsic	Normochromic
Hereditary spherocytosis[7]	Mutations in Ankyrin, Band 3. Protein 4.2. and spectrin	• Associated with parvovirus B19 • Cholelithiasis • Megaloblastic crisis	Aplastic crisis	• Papilledema • Skin nodules • Splenomegaly	+	Intrinsic	Normochromic

					Lab Findings					
						Iron Studies				
MCV	RDW	Reticulocytosis	Haptoglobin Levels	Hepcidin	Serum Iron	Serum Tfr Level	Transferrin or TIBC	Ferritin	Transferrin Saturation	Specific Finding on Blood Smear
Normocytic	↑	↑ but usually causes resolution within 4-7 days	↓	↓	NI to ↑	NI	↑	↑	↑	• RBC with Heinz bodies • Bite cells Blister cells
Normocytic	↑	↑	↓	NI	↑	NI	NI	↑	-	• Prickle cells • Polychromatophilic erythrocytes
Normocytic	↑	↑	1	NI or moderately ↑	NI	NI	NI or moderately ↑	1	NI	• Increased erythropoiesis • Howell-Jolly bodies • Anisocytosis
Normocytic	↑	↑	↓	NI	NI	NI	NI	↓	-	• Hemoglobin crystals inside RBCs • Target cells
Normocytic	↑	↑	↓	NI	↓	NI	↑	↓	-	NA
Normocytic	↑	↑	↓	NI	↓	NI	↑	NI	-	Small, round RBCs with less surface area and no central pallor

(continued)

Table 27.2: Differentiating Anemia With Intrinsic Hemolyis From Other Diseases (*continued*)

Clinical Manifestation							
Disease	Genetics	History	Symptoms	Signs	Hemolysis	Intrinsic/Extrinsic	Hb Concentrat
Macroangiopathic hemolytic anemia[1,2]		• DIC • TTP • HUS • SLE • HELLP syndrome • Hypertensive emergency	• Purpura • Confusion • Aphasia • Diplopia	• Numbness of an arm or hand • Jaundice • Pale conjunctiva	+	Extrinsic	Normochromic
Microangiopathic hemolytic anemia[3]	Autoimmune	Associated with • Prosthetic heart valves • Aortic stenosis	• Pallor • Fatigue	• Signs of anemia • Complications of hemolysis • Decreased vascular volume	+	Extrinsic	Normochromic
Autoimmune hemolytic anemia[4]		Associated with: • SIE • CLL • Mycoplasma pneumonia	• Painful blue fingers and toes on exposure to cold temperature • Chest pain • Chills • Dizziness • Tachycardia • Headache • Fatigue	• Painful, blue fingers and toes with cold weather	+	Extrinsic	Normochromic
Infection[5]		Associated with • Malaria • Babesia	Fever	• Fever • Signs of shock • Headache	+	Extrinsic	Normochromic

					Iron Studies					
Lab Findings										
MCV	RDW	Reticulocytosis	Haptoglobin Levels	Hepcidin	Serum Iron	Serum Tfr Level	Transferrin or TIBC	Ferritin	Transferrin Saturation	Specific Finding on Blood Smear
Normocytic	↑	↑	↓	Nl	↓	Nl	-	↑	-	Helmet cells
Normocytic	↑	↑	↓	Nl	↓	Nl	-	-	-	Spherocytes or schistocytes
Normocytic	↑	↑	↓	Nl	↓	Nl	-	-	-	RBC agglutination
Normocytic	↑	↑	↓	Nl	Nl	Nl	-	-	-	• Trophozoite • Maltese crosses

Differentiating Microcytic Anemia From Other Diseases
To review the differential diagnosis of anemia, see external links below.

External links
Emedicine on chronic anemia (http://www.emedicine.com/EMERG/topic734.htm)
FP Notebook (http://www.fpnotebook.com/HEM7.htm)
American Family Physician (http://www.findarticles.com/p/articles/mi_m3225/is_n7_v55/ai_19463577)
Overview (vet) (http://www.vet.uga.edu/vpp/clerk/mwoods/)

CLL, chronic lymphocytic leukemia; DIC, disseminated intravascular coagulation; GI, gastrointestinal; HEELP, hemolysis, elevated liver enzymes and low platelets; HUS, hemolytic uremic syndrome; IBC, iron binding capacity; MCV, mean corpuscular volume; RBC, red blood cell; RDW, red blood cell distribution width; SLE, systemic lupus erythematosus; TIBC, transferrin and iron-binding capacity; TTP, thrombotic thrombocytopenic purpura.

Source: Gibson CM. Anemia. Wikidocs; 2020, July 29. https://www.wikidoc.org/index.php/Anemia#Differentiating_Anemia_from_Other_Diseases

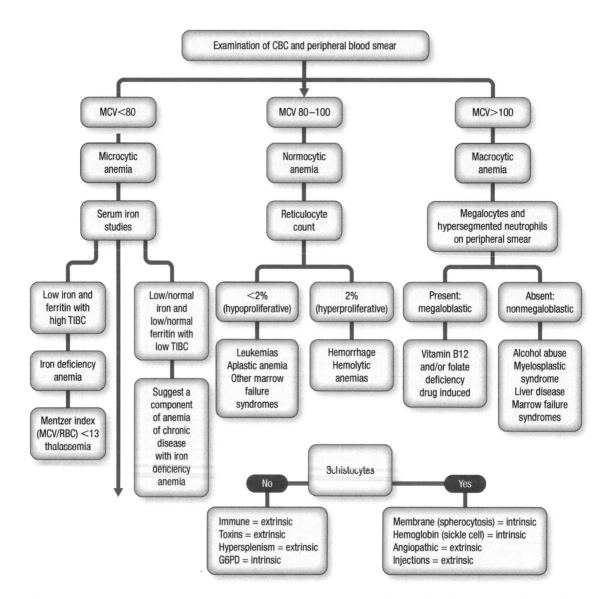

Figure 27.3: Recommended approach to determining anemia type based upon the CBC and peripheral blood smear

Begin by using the CBC and peripheral blood smear to note the presence of anemia.
- **MCV is less than 80 fL = Microcytic anemia**

Serum iron studies (iron, ferritin, and TIBC): Low iron and ferritin with high TIBC = Iron deficiency anemia (IDA), Low/normal iron and low/normal ferritin with low TIBC = Anemia of chronic disease with IDA
  - Determine Mentzer Index less than 13= Thalassemia

- **MCV is greater than 100 fL = Macrocytic anemia**

Megalocytes and hypersegmented neutrophils: present = Megaloblastic anemia–vitamin B12 or folate deficiency or drug-induced; Absent = Nonmegaloblastic anemia–alcohol abuse, myelodysplastic syndrome, liver disease, congenital bone marrow failure syndromes

- **MCV is normal 80-100 fL = Normocytic anemia**

Reticulocyte count: Less than 2% = Hyperproliferative–leukemias, aplastic anemia, other marrow failure syndromes; Greater than 2%= Hyperproliferative–hemorrhage or hemolytic anemias. Check peripheral smear for schistocytes: Present = Intrinsic defect–membrane = Hereditary spherocytosis–hemoglobin = Sickle cell; Present = Extrinsic-angiopathic–infections; Absent = Intrinsic defect–G6PD; Absent = Extrinsic defect–immune–toxins–hypersplenism

MCV, mean corpuscular volume; RBC, red blood cell; TIBC, transferrin and iron-binding capacity.

both parents carry alpha thalassemia trait, which could produce a homozygous thalassemia resulting in fetal demise. Genetic counseling referral is strongly advised. Beta thalassemia may be diagnosed through Hgb electrophoresis. Alpha thalassemia is diagnosed using DNA analysis. Beta thalassemia is associated with ethnic heritage from the Mediterranean geographic regions. Alpha thalassemia is more common in those with family heritage from Asia and Africa. The thalassemias, while less common than IDA, are an important differential to consider in all cases of identified microcytic anemia.

MACROCYTIC ANEMIAS

The macrocytic anemias are characterized as having an MCV greater than 100 fL. They are also associated with a low reticulocyte (retic) count, indicating an underproductive bone marrow. Macrocytic anemias are further distinguished as being either megaloblastic or nonmegaloblastic. In the megaloblastic anemias, DNA synthesis is abnormal whereas DNA synthesis appears normal in the nonmegaloblastic anemias. Normal DNA synthesis is necessary for normal development of RBCs in the bone marrow. If not present, normal divisions of RBC precursors are inhibited. This results in RBCs that are larger than normal (megaloblastic) with MCVs as high as 120 fL. Essential nutrients for DNA synthesis include folate and vitamin B12. Deficiencies of either folate or B12 are the predominant causation of the macrocytic anemias. Low levels of vitamin B12 may occur due to inadequate dietary intake and are more commonly seen in strict vegetarian and vegan diets, which lack the cobalamin found in meats and dairy products, which often necessitates B12 supplementation. Poor absorption of B12 may occur in the small intestine where absorption is aided by the presence of intrinsic factor. Absorption is reduced in a number of conditions such as gastritis, including alcoholic gastritis, *Helicobacter pylori* (*H. pylori*) infection, celiac disease, and inflammatory bowel conditions, such as Crohn's disease. Individuals with a history of total or partial gastrectomy such as with bariatric weight loss surgery have a reduction of surface area for absorption to occur. Additionally, medications that affect gastric acidity, especially PPIs, hamper the release of vitamin B12 from its food source, limiting absorption. The geriatric population is more prone to gastroesophageal reflux disease (GERD) as the lower esophageal sphincter becomes less compliant with age, increasing the associated use of PPIs and H2 acid blockers. This population is also more likely to experience musculoskeletal conditions, such as arthritis, with increasing use of NSAIDs leading to increased risk of gastritis.

In B12 deficiency anemia, the peripheral blood smear will show macrocytes that are oval and hypochromic. It is also thought that the associated defective DNA synthesis

seen in B12 anemia affects neutrophils and results in hypersegmentation of the neutrophils beyond the two to four nuclear lobes seen in normal neutrophilic cells. This hypersegmentation is common to all the megaloblastic anemias with five to seven or more lobes seen. The reporting of hypersegmented neutrophils is nearly pathognomonic for megaloblastic anemias and the diagnosis is further supported by a CBC with low RBCs, and low Hgb and Hct. Measurement of the serum vitamin B12 will be reduced below 200 pg/mL.[10] Further laboratory testing for B12 deficiency may be confirmed through the measurement of serum methylmalonic acid (MMA), which will be inversely elevated due to the absence of sufficient vitamin B12.

A lack of intrinsic factor necessary to absorb vitamin B12 may rarely occur as an inherited autosomal recessive autoimmune disorder. Most commonly, an autoimmune process develops in adulthood that attacks and destroys parietal cells in the stomach lining and inhibits the production of intrinsic factor, leading to cobalamin deficiency required for B12 absorption predominantly in the ileum. This autoimmune process is called pernicious anemia and manifests as low serum B12 levels. While pernicious anemia can occur at any age with an incidence of 0.1% in the general population, in the United States, it is most common among those older than 60 years. The median age for onset is 70 to 80 years, with an incidence of 1.9% in those over age 60, with slightly more women than men being affected. It has a lower incidence in those of Asian descent and somewhat higher in those of Scandinavian, European, and North American heritage.

Symptoms of vitamin B12 anemia are similar to all the anemias where patients may experience fatigue, pallor, dizziness, shortness of breath, lightheadedness, decreased cognition, and tachycardia. However, vitamin B12 is necessary for myelin formation in the nervous system and demyelination of nerves can accompany B12 deficiency. Neurologic findings may include peripheral neuropathy, paresthesia, weakness, and alterations in balance causing ataxia. Neuropsychiatric changes may include personality changes and psychosis. These symptoms may be insidious in onset resulting in delayed diagnosis. In the most severe cases of untreated neurologic pernicious anemia, death from anemia may occur. The approach to the patient requires a careful and complete past medical and family history. There is increasing recognition of the association with other autoimmune disorders such as type 1 diabetes, vitiligo, and autoimmune thyroid disorder.[10] Therefore, autoimmune risk factors in family and personal history are elicited as well as evaluation of dietary habits and medication use. A complete physical examination should focus on neurologic, hematologic, and gastrointestinal risk factors and findings. Laboratory studies will include a CBC, serum B12, and a peripheral smear. When B12 deficiency is confirmed, further testing may provide the diagnosis of pernicious anemia by evaluation for intrinsic factor deficiency and other autoimmune indicators. Folic acid deficiency, as discussed later, will further differentiate the diagnosis.

Treatment in the early stages may include improved dietary B12 consumption or supplementation with high-dose oral B12 tablets. Sublingual and intranasal forms are also available. When lack of intrinsic factor is the primary causation or neurologic symptoms are present, intramuscular B12 must be initiated. Prompt treatment is essential as common anemia symptoms are reversible by replacing B12 stores, but neurologic symptoms may be permanent.[2]

FOLATE DEFICIENCY ANEMIA

Folate deficiency anemia is another megaloblastic anemia associated with elevated MCV. Similar to vitamin B12 anemia, folate (vitamin B9) deficiency anemia can be caused by a number of factors, with insufficient dietary intake as the primary etiology. Folate deficiency is relatively uncommon in the United States as a result of an action by the U.S. Food and Drug Administration in 1998 requiring food manufacturers to add folate as a food additive to common breads and cereals. This was in response to research demonstrating an association in the incidence of births with neural tube defects that were the result of maternal folate insufficiency during pregnancy. They also recommended pregnant women supplement with folic acid 400 mcg/day in addition to a varied diet with folate fortified foods.[11] As this impact occurs early in pregnancy, women of childbearing age are also recommended to take supplemental folic acid. Populations that remain vulnerable to folate deficiency due to malabsorption or dietary malnutrition include those with alcohol abuse disorder, malabsorption syndromes, lower socioeconomic status, and older adults. Folate is absorbed in the small intestine and autoimmune conditions such as tropical sprue and celiac disease (gluten-sensitive enteropathy) can affect folate levels.

Like vitamin B12 anemia, the peripheral smear in folate deficiency anemia exhibits a macrocytic, hyperchromic RBC, and hypersegmented neutrophils. The CBC will reveal anemia in association with decreased serum folate levels. Symptoms of folate deficiency are not unlike those of B12 megaloblastic anemia with fatigue, weakness, poor concentration, shortness of breath, heart palpitations, irritability, and headache as common symptoms. Folate deficiency may present with additional symptoms such as skin, fingernail pigmentation, hair, and oral mucosal changes. Stomatitis and angular cheilosis may be seen as well as gastrointestinal complaints. Unlike B12 anemia, folate deficiency is not associated with the peripheral neuropathies. Dietary adjustments or supplementation with folic acid will promptly replenish folate stores in the liver. Elevated levels of homocysteine have been associated with folate deficiency, and current research is focusing upon conditions, such as cardiovascular disease, in which homocysteine reduction with folate supplementation may prove beneficial.[11]

Although macrocytic anemias are predominantly megaloblastic as a result of vitamin B12 or folate deficiency, the nonmegaloblastic anemias are worthy of mention for inclusion on the list of anemia differentials. Alcohol abuse disorder can cause macrocytosis, and in some individuals, anemia is also present. Alcohol is a toxin to the bone marrow and abuse is linked to altered maturation in RBC precursors. WBC and platelet precursors are also often affected.[11] Nonalcoholic liver disease can lead to macrocytic anemias resulting from viral and medication-induced forms of hepatitis. Myelodysplastic syndromes (MDS), disorders affecting the bone marrow, may be a source of megaloblastic anemia when dysfunction occurs in the HSC lines that produce normal RBCs, WBCs, and platelets. Symptoms of MDS are similar to all the anemias, but MDS may manifest other conditions and symptomology associated with reduced WBCs (i.e., infections) or decreased platelets (easy bruising or bleeding). There are myriad causes of MDS, such as cancer radiation and chemotherapies, tobacco abuse, and pesticide or heavy metal exposures. Older adults are especially at risk for a form of MDS lacking a clear etiology. During one's lifetime, HSCs replicate many times and random chromosomal mutations are possible. The risk of random abnormal replication increases with age, resulting in age-related random cell replication errors. The true cause is unknown. It is recognized that those that do experience MDS anemia have a higher risk of developing acute myelocytic leukemia.[5] Treatment of MDS may include chemotherapy or even bone marrow transplant.

HEMOLYTIC ANEMIA

Hemolytic anemias can be the result of intrinsic or extrinsic causes. Clinical manifestations and laboratory studies can help distinguish between the causes and further lead to a definitive diagnosis.

The life span of the typical RBC is approximately 120 days. The senescent expired cells are normally removed in the spleen and liver by macrophages where the RBC undergoes hemolysis or cell rupture. Premature hemolysis will signal an increase in EPO in order to stimulate RBC production. This is reflected in an increase of reticulocytes entering the circulation as evidenced by elevated retic counts on blood hematology lab studies ordered following identification of anemia. In abnormal hemolysis, this destruction can occur in the spleen or liver and is termed "extravascular hemolysis." When the hemolysis occurs within the blood vessels themselves, it is termed "intravascular hemolysis." If hemolysis outpaces RBC production, anemia will result. Hemolytic anemia can further be categorized as being the result of intrinsic defects within the RBC or extrinsic disorders occurring outside of the RBC.

Intrinsic hemolytic anemias are typically inherited disorders and can be the result of cell membrane abnormalities such as spherocytosis in which the normal bi-concave appearance of the RBC is lost. Sickle cell disease or trait, one form of morphologic change that occurs during membrane oxidative stress, causes the RBCs to deform into a sickle shape. Enzyme abnormalities, such as G6PD deficiency, alters the Hgb and the cell membrane. Disorders that cause these cell morphologic changes render the RBC defective and result in premature hemolysis. When hemolysis occurs, the contents of the RBC are exposed. If the hemolysis is intravascular, contents in the plasma cause an increase in iron and bilirubin. RBCs are also rich in potassium and lactate dehydrogenase (LDH), which will become elevated. Haptoglobin, the glycoprotein that binds free Hgb, will engage to salvage the iron supplies. In intravascular hemolysis, haptoglobin levels are low relative to the degree of the hemolytic event. The Hgb in the plasma is filtered by the kidneys and the urine may be positive for Hgb. The peripheral blood smear will show RBC fragmentation called schistocytes. In hereditary spherocytosis, spherocytes will be seen, and in sickle cell anemia, sickled cells will be seen.

The symptoms and physical examination of patients with the hemolytic anemias may manifest systemically as in sickle cell anemia, in which the abnormal cells and intravascular hemolytic process clog the capillary beds. Splenomegaly and hepatomegaly with jaundice may present. In sickle cell anemia, the sickle cell shape is rigid and prone to sticking and clumping along vessel walls resulting in vascular blockage and vessel ischemia. The patient experiences severe pain at the site of the microvascular blockage, which may manifest as stroke-like symptoms and headache, joint and bone pain, abdominal pain, and swelling of the hands and feet. As there is no cure for sickle cell anemia, individuals experience sickle cell crises into adulthood. Management focuses on avoiding oxidative stress through avoiding low oxygen exposure such as during airplane travel, tobacco use, pollutants, and emphasis on the promotion of a healthy lifestyle. If sickle cell crises are frequent or severe, the individual may require transfusions or a splenectomy. Medical care of all hemolytic anemias should involve comprehensive involvement with appropriate specialists. End-organ damage is a common risk leading to chronic health conditions in multiple systems, such as hypertension and risk to infection. Preventing inherited hemolytic anemias should be addressed through genetic counseling as a primary goal in preconceptual counseling.

Extrinsic hemolysis is an acquired disorder through autoimmune activation which may occur in transfusion reactions, in certain infections and toxin exposure, or in autoimmune conditions such as SLE. This immune activation occurs when antibodies attach to antigens on the RBC surface. The antigen–antibody complex is recognized by the macrophages that remove the targeted RBCs. Hypersplenism (overactive spleen) can also cause hemolysis. Angiopathic disorders can be microangiopathic such as in disseminated intravascular coagulation (DIC), thrombotic thrombocytopenia purpura (TTP), hemolytic uremic syndrome (HUS), or macroangiopathic as a response to prosthetic heart valves or aortic stenosis. In microangiopathic hemolysis, there is an atypical coagulation process that forms fibrin strands in the vessels. These strands trap RBCs that create increased sheer forces leading to cell hemolysis. In macroangiopathic hemolysis, artificial or atypical surfaces, such as prosthetic valves or aortic stenosis, create an increased force on the RBCs, leading to cell destruction and hemolysis. Lab findings in extravascular hemolysis show an elevated retic count and bilirubin with decreased haptoglobin and iron. The Coombs test, which detects anti-RBC antibodies, will be positive in immune-mediated hemolysis. Symptoms will vary from mild to severe depending on the cause of hemolysis. Patients may describe fever or confusion in addition to the typical symptoms of anemia discussed previously. On physical examination, jaundice, tachycardia, heart murmur, hepatosplenomegaly, and dark urine may be noted. Treatment is targeted at the etiology of the hemolytic events and may require an immediate response as in transfusion reaction hemolysis or require a chronic strategy to negate effects of mechanical hemolysis with prosthetic valve devices including RBC replacement through transfusion.

POLYCYTHEMIA

An increase in RBCs (polycythemia) can be the result of a primary or secondary etiology. Primary polycythemia is usually the result of a malignancy, such as in polycythemia vera (PV), a myeloproliferative disorder. Secondary polycythemia is more common and is the result of an increase in RBC cell mass as a compensatory response to sensed low oxygen levels. This may be seen in COPD, smoking, high altitude habitation, renal artery stenosis, or in EPO-producing tumors. Except in EPO-producing tumors, the driving force behind the polycythemia is hypoxia. Hypoxia stimulates increased EPO secretion and increased RBC production in the bone marrow. Blood viscosity is elevated, which can lead to intravascular thrombosis. Lab findings show an increased RBC count and elevated Hgb and Hct. The peripheral smear is normal. EPO levels are elevated. Symptoms of polycythemia may include vertigo, tinnitus, headache, and visual disturbances. Physical examination may reveal plethora, a condition of reddening of the skin and mucous membranes. Individuals are described as having a ruddy complexion. In dark-skinned individuals, the skin may appear pale.

Splenomegaly is more suggestive of primary PV.[12] Treatment is targeted at addressing the causative source such as optimizing COPD therapies, smoking cessation, renal stenting, and consideration of tumor etiologies. If the cause cannot be mitigated, routine phlebotomy may be required to prevent the potential risks from thrombosis in severe polycythemia.[5]

WHITE BLOOD CELL DISORDERS

Recall that leukocytes are produced in the bone marrow and the production or inhibition is under the control of specific CSF. Disorders of the WBCs that relate to increases or decreases in a particular WBC lineage will involve these CSFs (Table 27.3).

Disorders of WBCs can be separated into nonmalignant and malignant conditions. In the nonmalignant disorders, elevated neutrophils, or neutrophilia, are often seen as a response to acute infection, most typically bacterial. Inflammatory reactions seen in conditions of rheumatoid arthritis, pancreatitis, burns, or acute myocardial infarction can also stimulate neutrophilia. Neutrophilia may also be seen in conditions of uremia, diabetic acidosis, poisoning, or insect envenomation. Acute hemorrhage and hemolytic anemia may be seen to stimulate neutrophilia as well as steroid use. The bone marrow contains a large reserve of neutrophils that can be quickly mobilized as needed to respond to acute events. Young neutrophils, also called bands, can be seen in large numbers when the demand for neutrophils is increased.

Neutropenia, which is a decrease in neutrophils, is seen when a significant infection is overwhelming, during radiation or chemotherapy, with splenic sequestration or in some autoimmune disorders and viral infections.[9] Significant neutropenia puts the body at increased risk for opportunistic infection, which can quickly progress to sepsis. A useful measurement to help stratify the risk is provided by most automated hematology analyzers and is termed the absolute neutrophil count (ANC). This measurement is calculated by multiplying the WBC count by the percent neutrophils including bands, from a manual or automated differential. When the ANC is low fewer than 1,000 cells/μL), the risk for infection is significant.

Eosinophils are a type of WBC that participate in allergic reactions and destroy certain agents that are foreign to the body such as parasites. It is common to see eosinophilia, elevated level of eosinophils in allergic reactions to drugs, and in allergen-stimulated conditions such as allergic rhinitis, allergic asthma, and atopic dermatoses. Certain infections such as scarlet fever and autoimmune disorders such as SLE may have increased eosinophil counts. Hypereosinophilic syndromes (HES) are rare but may cause organ damage and require targeted evaluation and management by specialists. Patient symptoms of eosinophilia may include urticaric rash, fatigue, fever,

sweats, and unexplained weight loss. Eosinopenia, low eosinophil count, can be seen during stress reactions where the adrenal glands produce endogenous glucocorticoids, as well as from exogenous steroid use. There are no adverse effects of eosinopenia.[5]

Basophilia, a condition of elevated basophilic white cells, is quite uncommon but can be seen in hypothyroidism, ulcerative colitis, and with certain infections including influenza. When basophilia is identified it is most commonly associated with the malignancy of chronic myelogenous leukemia (CML), which will be discussed later under leukemias. Basopenia, low basophil count, is difficult to evaluate due to the small percentage of leukocytes (0%–2%) that basophils represent. There are reports of decreased numbers associated with some cases of hyperthyroidism.[9]

Elevated monocytes or monocytosis is most commonly seen with bacterial infections, such as tuberculosis (TB), subacute bacterial endocarditis (SBE), and in cases of syphilis. Malaria and Rocky Mountain spotted fever may also present with elevated monocytes. Monocytopenia, low monocyte count, is seen with steroid use and in HIV and Epstein–Barr virus.

Lymphocytosis, an elevated lymphocyte count, is frequently associated with infectious mononucleosis infections, with hepatitis, cytomegalovirus, and influenza. Each of these infections is also associated with reactive changes in the lymphocyte nucleus and/or cytoplasm. This will be present in qualitative WBC disorders. Increased numbers of lymphocytes are seen in certain bacterial infections such as TB, brucellosis, and pertussis. Lymphocytopenia, depressed lymphocyte counts, can be seen with steroid therapy, radiation, and chemotherapies. Congenital forms of lymphocytopenia are extremely rare but acquired lymphocytopenia is more common in autoimmune conditions, such as SLE, myasthenia gravis, or rheumatoid arthritis, all of which may have a genetic predisposition. The viral conditions of HIV/AIDS are associated with a decreased lymphocyte count when not controlled by therapeutics.

QUALITATIVE DESCRIPTIVE DISORDERS OF WHITE BLOOD CELLS

There are additional nonmalignant WBC disorders that are qualitative abnormalities based on cellular morphology as opposed to quantitative cell counts. The cellular descriptions report WBC findings involving the cytoplasm and/or the cellular nucleus. The most common qualitative abnormalities are associated with neutrophilic WBCs. Identifying these abnormalities requires microscopic evaluation of the CBC using Wright's staining of the peripheral blood smear. "Toxic granulation" involves the cytoplasm of some neutrophils and is seen with infections or inflammatory conditions. "Döhle bodies" are found in the cytoplasm of neutrophils

Table 27.3: Conditions Associated With White Blood Cell Abnormalities

Condition	Cause	Example
Neutrophil		
Neutrophilia	Inflammation or tissue necrosis	Surgery, burns, MI, pneumonitis, rheumatic fever, RA
	Infection	Gram-positive (staphylococci, streptococci, pneumococci), gram-negative (*Escherichia coli*, *Pseudomonas* species)
	Physiologic	Exercise, extreme heat or cold, third-trimester pregnancy, emotional distress
	Hematologic	Acute hemorrhage, hemolysis, myeloproliferative disorder, CGI.
	Drugs or chemicals	Epinephrine, steroids, heparin, histamine, endotoxin
	Metabolic	Diabetes (acidosis), eclampsia, gout, thyroid storm
	Neoplasms	Liver, GI tract, bone marrow
Neutropenia	Decreased marrow production	Radiation, chemotherapy, leukemia, aplastic anemia, abnormal granulopoiesis (megaloblastic anemia)
	Increased destruction	Splenomegaly, hemodialysis, immune reaction
	Infection	Gram-negative (typhoid), viral (influenza, hepatitis B, measles, mumps, rubella), severe infection, protozoal infections (malaria)
Eosinophil		
Eosinophilia	Allergy (type I)	Asthma, hay fever, drug sensitivity
	Infection	Parasites (trichinosis, hookworm), chronic (fungal, leprosy, TB)
	Malignancies	CMI, lung, stomach, ovary, Hodgkin lymphoma
	Dermatoses	Pemphigus, exfoliative dermatitis (drug-induced)
	Drugs	Digitalis, heparin, streptomycin, tryptophan (eosinophilia myalgia syndrome), penicillins, propranolol
Eosinopenia	Stress response	Trauma, shock, burns, surgery, mental distress
	Drugs	Steroids (Cushing syndrome)
Basophil		
Basophilia	Inflammation	Infection (measles, chickenpox), hypersensitivity reaction (immediate)
	Hematologic	Myeloproliferative disorders (CGI, polycythemia vera, Hodgkin lymphoma, hemolytic anemia)
	Endocrine	Myxedema, antithyroid therapy
Basopenia	Physiologic	Pregnancy, ovulation, stress
	Endocrine	Graves' disease

(continued)

Table 27.3: Conditions Associated With White Blood Cell Abnormalities (*continued*)

Condition	Cause	Example
Monocyte		
Monocytosis	Infection	Bacterial: SBE, TB, recovery phase of infection
		Rickettsiae: Rocky Mountain spotted fever, typhoid fever
		Protozoa; malaria
	Hematologic	Monocytic leukemia, myeloproliferative disorders, Hodgkin lymphoma agranulocytosis
	Physiologic	Normal newborn
Monocytopenia	Rare	Chronic diseases: ulcerative colitis, Crohn disease, RA, SLE
Lymphocyte		
Lymphocytosis	Physiologic	4 months to 4 years
	Acute infections	Infectious mononucleosis, CMV infection, pertussis, hepatitis, mycoplasma pneumonia, typhoid
	Chronic infections	Congenital syphilis, tertiary syphilis
	Endocrine	Thyrotoxicosis, adrenal insufficiency
	Malignancies	ALL, CLL, lymphosarcoma cell leukemia
Lymphocytopenia	Immune deficiency syndromes	AIDS, agammaglobulinemia
	Lymphocyte destruction	Steroids (Cushing syndrome), radiation, chemotherapy
	Malignancies	Hodgkin lymphoma
	Debilitating illness	CHF, renal failure, TB, SLF, aplastic anemia

Source: Reproduced with permission from McCance K, Huether S. *Pathophysiology: The Biologic Basis for Disease in Adults and Children*. 8th ed. Mosby; 2018.
AIDS, acquired immunodeficiency syndrome;ALL, acute lymphocytic leukemia; CGL, chronic granulocytic leukemia; CHF, congestive heart failure; CLL, chronic lymphocytic leukemia; CML, chronic myelocytic leukemia; CMV, cytomegalovirus; GL, gastrointestinal; MI, Myocardial infarction; RA, rheumatoid arthritis; SBE, subacute bacterial endocarditis; SLE, systemic lupus erythematosus; TB, tuberculosis; WBC, white blood cell.

and bands, may represent infection or sepsis, and may be seen normally in pregnancy. "Toxic vacuolation" involves the cytoplasm and is evidence of phagocytosis of bacterial and fungal organisms by neutrophils during sepsis. "Hypersegmented neutrophils" mentioned previously are noted when six or more lobes are noted in the nucleus. These cells are seen in megaloblastic anemias such as B12 and folate deficiency anemias. "Reactive or atypical lymphocytes" are noted for dark blue cytoplasm or nucleoli noted within the nucleus. "Atypical lymphs" are usually associated with lymphocytosis and therefore will be associated with the previously discussed conditions of lymphocytosis. "Smudge cells" are lymphocytes that are seen on the peripheral smear. They are seen in greater numbers in chronic lymphocytic leukemia (CLL), in which lymphocytes tend to be more fragile. "Auer rods" are seen in the cytoplasm of myeloblasts and promyelocytes and are indicative of acute myelogenous leukemia.

MALIGNANT WHITE BLOOD CELL DISORDERS

Malignant WBC disorders include multiple conditions, such as the leukemias and lymphomas, including both Hodgkin and non-Hodgkin, myeloma, and multiple myeloma. This also includes myeloproliferative disorders such as PV, essential thrombocythemia (ET), and MDS. The leukemias are summarized in Table 27.4, including clinical manifestations, laboratory findings, and demographics. There is variability in the leukemias as to whether the disease presents aggressively or as more indolent. Acute leukemias tend to be aggressive and will require close, acute management and treatment involving specialists such as a hematologist/oncologist. The more indolent leukemias, such as CLL and CML, may be managed in consultation with the specialist, much like a chronic disease such as diabetes or hypertension. Best practice dictates that hematologic findings, symptoms, and physical examination findings support a timely and accurate diagnosis with prompt specialty referral as appropriate. The primary care clinician will remain an important coordinating member of the healthcare team. Preventive health measures such as recommended laboratory screening, immunizations, and screening procedures such as mammograms or colonoscopy, remain essential to optimal health outcomes even in the face of malignant WBC disorders.

The WBC disorders and malignancies share similar symptoms, and often a clear picture of the underlying disease process may be challenging. Nonspecific symptoms of fatigue, weakness, dizziness, headache, and decreased appetite are common, but their persistence and progression warrant concern. Bleeding, bruising, weight loss, and night sweats are more ominous for malignancy. In the early stages of WBC disorders and malignancies, there may be nonspecific, limited, or normal physical findings. In the older adults, this may be further compounded by chronic disease conditions. The presence of pallor, unusual bruising, and mild lymphadenopathy rarely will provide a singular diagnosis. However, when widespread LAD is present with hepatomegaly or splenomegaly and associated abdominal tenderness, a deeper evaluation should be pursued. Targeted laboratory and imaging studies coupled with patient risk factors will elicit a narrower list of differentials for diagnosis and management. More advanced studies ordered by the primary care clinician at the direction of a consulting hematologist/oncologist may proceed while awaiting the consult visit. The initial laboratory studies with the previously mentioned symptoms should include CBC with peripheral smear and differential, metabolic panel, TSH, LDH, uric acid, and PT/PTT (prothrombin time/partial thromboplastin time). In the presence of bone pain, radiology may be appropriate, and ultrasonography of the abdomen if abdominal pain is present.

Only brief mention is made of the lymphomas and myelomas as these disorders will be managed primarily by a specialist in hematology or oncology. The reader is encouraged to access further resources in oncology references.

PLATELET DISORDERS

Platelets are an essential component in providing homeostasis and control of bleeding. Disorders of platelets are defined as qualitative or quantitative causes. Quantitative disorders involve either too few platelets, thrombocytopenia, or excessive platelets in thrombocythemia. Thrombocytopenia may occur from a variety of etiologies including decreased production in the bone marrow. TPO is the cytokine produced in the kidney and liver to regulate the production of platelets by the bone marrow. When renal or hepatic dysfunction occurs, platelet production may be affected, resulting in lower levels. Disorders within the

bone marrow such as hematologic malignancies seen in leukemia or, more commonly, deficiencies of iron, B12, and folate may also affect platelet production. Certain medications such as thiazide diuretics, estrogen, or chemotherapy agents may cause decreased platelet survival and may lead to diminished platelet levels. A condition of hypersplenism may enhance the sequestering of platelets as well as viral infections which may reduce platelet survival. Certain immune disorders such as immune thrombocytopenia purpura (ITP) will result in cell destruction when platelets are coated with an autoantibody that is recognized by macrophages within the spleen where the platelets will be removed. ITP is often a chronic condition in adults ages 20 to 50 years, while in children, it presents as an acute self-limiting event in response to viral illness. Symptoms of ITP are petechiae and purpura that may progress to life-threatening hemorrhage. Treatment consists of the use of steroids and intravenous immunoglobulins may be necessary. Refractory cases may necessitate splenectomy. TPP is a less common cause for low platelets. It is a coagulopathy that results in platelet aggregation called microthrombi. Forming in the arterioles and capillary beds, it precipitates thrombotic ischemia, affecting the kidneys, heart, and brain. The coagulation defect involves the von Willebrand clotting factor (VWF) and is predominant in women in their third decade of life. The microthrombi cause decreased platelets and an associated hemolytic anemia and schistocytes may be seen on the peripheral smear. Bilirubin and LDH levels may be notably elevated. Treatment may include the use of fresh frozen plasma (FFP), plasmapheresis, and steroids. Splenectomy may be considered in refractory cases.

Thrombocythemia is the elevation of platelet levels and can be a secondary response to infection or inflammation. Primary thrombocythemia or ET is a chronic myeloproliferative disorder, which includes other conditions such as PV or CML noted previously. ET is an alteration of the HSC in the bone marrow. The thrombi form more commonly in arteries of the heart or kidneys rather than in the venous system where deep vein thrombus and pulmonary emboli may form. Microvascular thrombi cause symptoms of headache, paresthesias, transischemic attack (TIA), and visual disturbances. This disorder typically presents initially between ages 50 and 60, with equal gender distribution. Lab findings show platelets elevated (600,000 or higher), with normal coagulation studies (PT/PTT). Splenomegaly is often a key finding. Treatment is not curative but targeted at preventing thrombosis and hemorrhage.

Qualitative, also referred to as functional, platelet disorders result in increased bleeding in the presence of normal platelet levels. The disorders may be congenital or acquired. Congenital disorders are uncommon and are the result of defects in platelet adhesion, aggregation, or secretory function. Adhesion dysfunction is caused by a defect in platelet binding to the von

Table 27.4: Leukemias

Clinical Manifestation				
Disease	Etiology	Demography	History	Symptoms
Acute myelogenous leukemia[2,3]	• Clonal proliferation of malignant myeloid blast cells in the bone marrow • Genetic abnormalities t(8;21), inv(16), and t(15;17)	• The most common leukemia in adults • Median age of 63 years old	Smoking, previous chemotherapy or radiation therapy, myelodysplastic syndrome, and exposure to the chemical benzene	• Fatigue • Bleeding
Acute lymphoblastic leukemia[4,5]	• Arrest of lymphoblasts • Chromosomal translocations: t(9;22), t(12;21), t(5;14), t(1;19)	• The most common cancer in children • Peak 2-5 years of age • Boys > girls	• History of cancer • History of drug exposure	• Generalized weakness • Fatigue • Bleeding
Chronic myelogenous leukemia[6,7]	• Dysregulated production and uncontrolled proliferation of mature and maturing granulocytes • *BCR-ABL1* fusion gene • Autosomal dominant mutation	Median age 50 years old		• Generalized weakness • Fatigue • Early satiety • Abdominal fullness • Bleeding
Chronic lymphocytic leukemia[8]	Progressive accumulation of monoclonal B lymphocytes	• The most common leukemia in adults in western countries • M > F • Median age 70 years old	• Positive family history • Exposure to herbicides or insecticides	• Bleeding • Abdominal pain • Generalized weakness • Anorexia

Laboratory Findings				
gns	Laboratory	Histopathology	Gold Standard Diagnosis	Associated Findings
Bone tenderness Dyspnea Leukemia cutis Swelling of the gums Chloroma Rare LAP	• Anemia • Thrombocytopenia • Leukocytosis or leukopenia	• Leukemic blasts • Positive Auer rods	Flow cytometry greater than 20% blasts of myeloid lineage	• Persistent or frequent infections • Fatal within weeks or months if left untreated • Down syndrome or Bloom syndrome
Hepatosplenomegaly LAP Dyspnea Pallor Papilledema Nuchal rigidity Cranial nerve palsy Testicular enlargement Mediastinal mass	• Anemia • Thrombocytopenia • Normal or slightly increased WBC counts	• Lymphoblasts • Atypical cells	Bone marrow biopsy	CNS involvement
Asymptomatic Blast crisis Excessive sweating Papilledema Tenderness over the lower sternum Hepatosplenomegaly	• Anemia • WBC greater than 100,000/microL • Absolute basophilia and eosinophilia • Plt greater than 600,000 to 700,000/microL • Low leukocyte alkaline phosphatase • High uric acid	• All cells of the neutrophilic series, from myeloblasts to mature neutrophils • Myelocyte bulge	Bone marrow biopsy	• Acute gouty arthritis • Venous obstruction
LAP (most common sign) Hepatosplenomegaly Skin lesions (leukemia cutis) Night sweats Muscle wasting	• Anemia • Thrombocytopenia • Absolute lymphocytosis greater than 5,000 cells/μl • Neutropenia • Positive direct Coombs test • Hypogammaglobulinemia • Elevated lactate dehydrogenase and beta-2 microglobulin	• Presence of smudge cells • Monoclonality of kappa- and lambda-producing B cells • Express CD19, CD20, CD23, and CD5 on the cell surface	Flow cytometry of the peripheral blood	• Extranodal involvement of skin, kidney, lung, and spine • Membranoproliferative glomerulonephritis • Autoimmune hemolytic anemia

(continued)

Table 27.4: Leukemias (*continued*)

Clinical Manifestation				
Disease	Etiology	Demography	History	Symptoms
Hairy cell leukemia[9,10]	• Accumulation of small mature B cell lymphoid cells with abundant cytoplasm and "hairy" projections • BRAF mutation	• Uncommon • Median age 50 to 55 years old • M >> F • More common in Caucasians than Blacks	Exposures to ionizing radiation, pesticides, and farming	• Generalized weakness • Fatigue • Early satiety • Abdominal fullness • Bleeding
Large granular lymphocytic leukemia[11,12]	Clonal proliferation of cytotoxic T cells Dysregulation of apoptosis through abnormalities in the Fas/Fas ligand pathway	• Rare • Median age 60 years • M = F	• Autoimmune diseases • Lymphoproliferative disorders	• Generalized weakness • Fatigue
Chronic neutrophilic leukemia[9]	• Mature granulocytic proliferation in the blood and bone marrow • Point mutations in the *CSF3R* gene	• Very rare • M = F	Multiple myeloma	• Generalized weakness • Fatigue
Chronic eosinophilic leukemia	• There is no known cause for chronic eosinophilic leukemia. • It hasn't been linked to a specific chromosome or genetic abnormality.	Unknown	Unknown	• Constitutional symptoms • Rash • Rhinitis • Gastritis • Thromboembolism-related
Myelodysplastic syndrome				• Constitutional symptoms • Bleeding

		Laboratory Findings		
gns	Laboratory	Histopathology	Gold Standard Diagnosis	Associated Findings
Asymptomatic Splenomegaly Spontaneous splenic rupture Skin rash Ascites Pleural effusion	• Cytopenia • Leukocytosis in 10% to 20% • Azotemia • Abnormal liver function tests • Hypergammaglobulinemia	• Pancytopenia with monocytopenia and circulating tumor cells characteristic of HCL • Dry bone marrow	Analysis of peripheral blood + immunophenotyping by flow cytometry	Vasculitis
ostly asymptomatic	• Modest lymphocytosis • Neutropenia • Anemia • Thrombocytopenia	• Large lymphocytes with a condensed round or oval nucleus, abundant pale basophilic cytoplasm, and small azurophilic granules	Biopsy and flow cytometry + T-cell receptor gene rearrangement studies	Recurrent bacterial infection
Hepatosplenomegaly Pruritus Gout	• Peripheral blood neutrophilia greater than 25 × 109/L with myeloid precursors (promyelocytes, myelocytes, metamyelocytes) • Elevated leukocyte alkaline phosphatase	• Toxic granulation in the neutrophils • Nuclear hypersegmentation • Increased myeloid: erythroid ratio greater than 20:1	• WHO diagnostic criteria include leukocytosis of 25 or more × 109/L • More than 80% neutrophils, • Less than 10% circulating neutrophil precursors with blasts	• Poor prognosis • Absence of the Philadelphia chromosome or a *BCR/ABL* fusion gene
Hypertension Eczema, mucosal ulcers, erythema Angioedema Ataxia Anemia Lymphadenopathy Hepatosplenomegaly	• Leukocytosis with left shift • Eosinophilia • Basophilia • Monocytosis • Anemia • Thrombocytopenia • ↑ B12 levels • ↑ LDH	Hypercelluar with ↑ eosinophilic precursors, ↑ eosinophils, and atypical mononuclear cells		• Heart failure • Lung fibrosis • Encephalopathy • Erythema annulare centrifugam
Pallor Petechiae Organomegaly	• Pancytopenia	• Hypercellular/normocellular bone marrow with dysplastic changes • Macro-ovalocytes • Basophilic stippling • Howell-Jolly body		• Leukemia transformation • Acquired pseudo-Pelger-Huët anomaly • Infection

(continued)

Table 27.4: Leukemias (*continued*)

Clinical Manifestation				
Disease	Etiology	Demography	History	Symptoms
Adult T-cell leukemia/ lymphoma (ATLL)[13-18]	• Adult T-cell leukemia is caused by an infection with HTLV. • Common genetic mutations involved in the development of adult T-cell leukemia can be found here.	• The incidence of adult T-cell leukemia increases with age, and the median age at diagnosis is 57 years. • Males are more commonly affected with adult T-cell leukemia than females. • The male to female ratio is approximately 1.4 to 1.	• Abdominal pain • Constipation • Nausea and vomiting • Fatigue • Generalized weakness • Cough • Recurrent infections	• Fever • Weight loss • Recurrent bleeding • Anorexia • Night sweats • Bone pain • Hypercalcemia
Sezary syndrome[20-27]	• The cause of Sezary syndrome has not been identified. • Sezary syndrome might have one or more of the chromosomal abnormalities, such as the loss or gain of genetic material.	• The prevalence of Sezary syndrome is not unknown. • The median age at diagnosis of Sézary syndrome is 60 years of age. • Sezary syndrome is more commonly observed among older adult patients. • Males are more commonly affected with Sezary syndrome than females (2:1).	• The majority of Sezary syndrome patients present with developing lymphadenopathy and erythroderma for weeks to months. • Early clinical features of Sezary syndrome include: • Mimic psoriasis • Chronic eczema • Atopic dermatitis • Leprosy • Lichenoid pityriasis • In Sezary syndrome, single or multiple lesions (thin erythematous plaques or flat patch) is a typical skin involvement in the gluteal region or thighs.[28] • Patients with Sezary syndrome often have a history of several years of eczematous *or* dermatitis skin lesions before the diagnosis is finally established.	• Widespread erythema • In Sezary syndrome, widespread erythema can be finely scaly, indurated, or even resemble livedo reticularis • Indurated • Resemble livedo reticularis • Erythema (not seen in some patients) • The severity of erythema body surface area (BSA) involved may wax and wane (>80% of BSA) • Patches and plaques to erythroderma • Keratosis pilaris • Alopecia (hair loss) • Ectropion • Keratoderma • Hypertrophic nails • Erosions • Lichenification • Trouble regulating body temperature • Abnormalities of fingernails and toenails • Lymphadenopathy • Viscer
Differentiating Leukemia From Other Diseases Leukemia must be differentiated from various diseases that cause weight loss, night sweats, hepatosplenomegaly, and palpable lymph nodes, such as hairy cell leukemia, prolymphocytic leukemia, follicular lymphoma, and mantle cell lymphoma. Based on the expression of cell surface markers, the table differentiates different types of leukemia from other diseases that cause similar clinical presentations.[1]				

CNS, central nervous system; HTLV, human T-lymphotropic virus; WBC, white blood cell; WHO, World Health Organization.

Source: Fischbach F, Fischbach M. *Fischbach's A Manual of Laboratory and Diagnostic Tests.* 10th ed. Wolters Kluwer; 2017; Gibson CM. *Leukemia.* Wikidocs; 2020, July 29. https://www.wikidoc.org/index.php/Leukemia

Willebrand *factor* of the endothelium membrane of the blood vessels. This leads to impaired hemostasis and is termed von Willebrand *disease*. Dysfunction of platelet aggregation is caused by a deficiency in a protein needed to form fibrinogen bridges between platelets to create a plug. Acquired qualitative disorders are more common and often belong to two principal etiologies: drug-related and systemic conditions. Systemic disorders that affect platelet function include myeloproliferative neoplasms (i.e., PV, CML), liver disease (reduction in clotting factors), chronic renal disease (uremia), and leukemia. Certain drugs may induce platelet function defects including ASA, NSAIDs, most calcium channel blockers, and some beta-blocker hypertensive medication, cephalosporin and beta-lactam antibiotics, alcohol, and some herbs such as cumin and turmeric. Qualitative platelet disorders can lead to a range of symptoms from petechiae and purpura to hemorrhage. Treatment should be directed at the cause such as liver and renal disease, lifestyle changes to limit alcohol use, and avoidance of impacting herbal and prescription medications.

CONCLUSION

The study of hematology involves a wide range of essential functions within the human body.[14] Blood cells nourish and protect at both cellular and major organ levels. Dysfunction within RBCs, WBCs, and platelets may significantly impact homeostasis in both acute and chronic ways. The astute clinician will integrate patient history, symptomology, and physical signs to appropriately select laboratory and imaging studies to arrive at timely and accurate diagnoses. A strong knowledge of hematology will provide essential skills for developing differentials in hematologic conditions and provide for a strong evidence-based practice.

CASE STUDY
MALABSORPTION-ASSOCIATED B12 DEFICIENCY

PATIENT COMPLAINT

"I have been feeling really tired over the past 6 months and there are times when I feel dizzy and lightheaded, almost like I might fall. I get plenty of sleep and I usually walk but I worry about falling now. I know I am getting older, but it seems like it is getting harder to even think anymore. My brain is full of fog and I'm worried something might be wrong, so I scheduled my annual examination."

HISTORY OF PRESENT ILLNESS/REVIEW OF SYSTEMS

Ms. H. is a 70-year-old female being seen today for her Medicare wellness visit that she does each year. She has been generally healthy until her current complaints. She now complains of fatigue, lightheadedness, and dizziness, sometimes associated with change of position. She reports she has new numbness and tingling in her toes. She has a fear of falling, occasions of feeling "foggy-brained," and less alert when doing her crossword puzzles. In the past, she has had a good appetite and stable weight, but 9 months ago, she was diagnosed with celiac gluten intolerance and has struggled to find foods to meet her new dietary restrictions. Her "gut" has always caused her problems with periods of intermittent nausea and diarrhea after certain foods. She currently denies fever, chills, nausea, vomiting, diarrhea, melena, hematuria, or abdominal pain. She denies changes in hearing or vision, sleep, or exercise patterns. No headaches or other neurologic symptoms other than the mental changes, imbalance, and tingling in her feet. She denies recent illness or injuries. She denies depression.

PAST MEDICAL/FAMILY HISTORY

Ms. H. has been a patient at the clinic for over 20 years, and has been generally healthy until her celiac diagnosis 9 months ago. She was widowed 15 years ago and lives alone. She reports difficulty in managing the low-gluten diet. She has a history of hypertension and is well controlled on an angiotensin-converting-enzyme (ACE) inhibitor. She has mild osteoarthritis in both knees and uses occasional ibuprofen or Tylenol to treat her symptoms about twice weekly. Family is remarkable for type 2 diabetes in her mother and one of her two sisters. She is not aware of any family history of dementia or Alzheimer's.

PHYSICAL EXAMINATION

VS: Normal, T 98.8 °F, BP 138/78, pulse 80, respirations 20, weight 146 lb with BMI of 24. A 70-year-old female who appears her stated age and is well nourished and well developed in no acute distress. Conjunctiva and gingiva are slightly pale, as are her palmar creases. Lungs, heart, and abdominal examination are normal. Neurological examination reveals lack of sensation to filament testing in both feet but sparing the heels and ankles. Vibratory sense is diminished and correlates to filament test.

LABORATORY FINDINGS

RBC (3.74×10^6 per/mcL), Hgb (10.1 g/dL), Hct. (30.6%), all low with a low retic count (0.2%). MCV is elevated (105 fL), differential shows normal platelets, but macrocytic, hypochromic RBCs, and there are reported hypersegmented neutrophils. Ferritin and iron studies are normal. Vitamin B12 (106 pg/mL) is low, MMA (505 nmol/L) is elevated. Thyroid, vitamin D, and chemistry panel are normal.

Case Study Questions

1. Explain the patient's fatigue and lightheadedness.
2. How is her past medical history involved?
3. What explains her balance, numbness/tingling, and cognitive complaints?
4. What treatment and by what route of administration would you recommend?

REFERENCES

References for this chapter are online and available at https://connect.springerpub.com/content/book/978-0-8261-8414-6/part/part01/toc-part/ch27.

CHAPTER 28

Aging, Immunity, and Infection

Sumathi Sankaran-Walters and Elise Buser

LEARNING OBJECTIVES

At the conclusion of this chapter, the learner will be able to:

➤ Review the basic concepts of immunology, including the innate immune system, adaptive immune system, and cellular mediators of the immune response.

➤ Identify the effects of aging on the innate immune system.

➤ Define "inflammaging."

➤ List the effects of aging on the regenerative capacity of the innate immune system.

➤ Discuss the interactions of age and the adaptive immune response.

➤ Describe the changes in the gut mucosal immune function and the microbiome in aging.

➤ List five infections that are common in older adults and discuss the pathophysiology of these infections.

➤ Review the vaccines that are recommended in older adults.

INTRODUCTION

From birth to death, the body's immune system ebbs and flows. These changes have a great impact on a person's response to infection, injury, and vaccinations. Additionally, gender and hormones also play a role in the immune response and can impact outcomes. In this chapter, we review the basic concepts in immunology, changes that occur with aging, and common infections in older adults. We also discuss the immune response to vaccination and special considerations in infection control in older adults.

DEFENSE MECHANISMS AND THE IMMUNE SYSTEM

The Innate Immune System

Present at birth, the innate immune system is the first line of defense. It includes the skin, mucosa, and the microbiome present on both skin and mucosa. Antibacterial peptides such as defensins and lysozymes are found in mucous secretions, perspiration, saliva, and tears. Thus, in addition to the mechanical barrier, this chemical barrier aids in the prevention of infection. All the surfaces of the body are colonized by resident microbes known as the microbiome. The distribution and diversity of these organisms are specific to a person as well as to the surface they inhabit. They prevent infection by two mechanisms. First, they occupy space and prevent the growth of pathogenic organisms. Second, they secrete compounds that inhibit the growth of other organisms.[1] In addition, they help with digestion in the gut through the production of essential vitamins such as B12. When this first line of defense is disrupted, infections such as *Clostridium difficile* diarrhea can occur. For example, when patients in the hospital are given antibiotics, the good bacteria in the gut that contribute to this first line of defense are destroyed. This allows harmful bacteria such as *C. difficile* to colonize, resulting in the diarrhea and other nosocomial infections.

Once these skin or mucosal surfaces are breached and a pathogen enters the body, inflammation is the second line of defense. Inflammation is also nonspecific and occurs in response to both an infection as well as to tissue damage. Inflammation takes seconds to minutes to occur and is associated with the classic features of swelling, redness, and the flooding of inflammatory cells to the area of damage. Part of this process includes the extravasation of white blood cells such as neutrophils from the local blood vessels into the tissue. To initiate the process of inflammation, antigen–antibody complexes, as well as lipopolysaccharide (LPS) and other antigens, activate the complement system. Through a cascade of responses, C3b (opsonin), C3a (anaphylatoxin), and C5a (anaphylatoxin, chemotactic factor) are produced that then activate mast cells, macrophages, and other innate immune cells. Additionally, the kinin system is activated, which produces bradykinin. Bradykinin in turn increases vascular permeability and thereby allows for the influx of neutrophils to the area of damage. In addition, bradykinin causes pain—a key element of inflammation. The last contributor to inflammation is the clotting system that, when activated, produces a clot to stop the bleeding and a fibrin meshwork to promote healing (Figure 28.1).

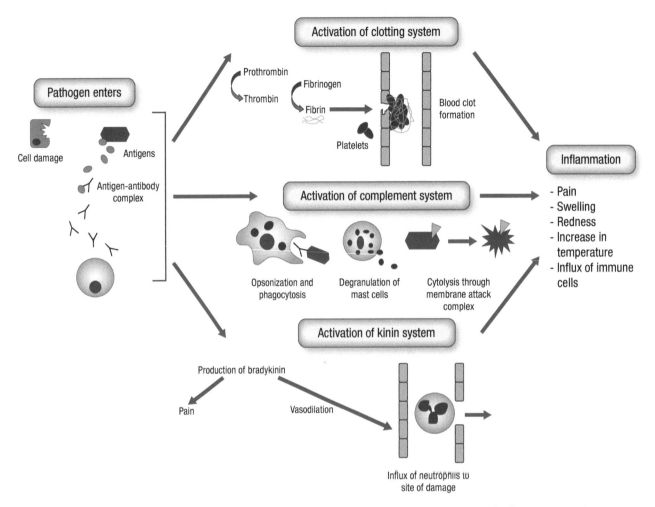

Figure 28.1: Activation of inflammation. Several pathways contribute to the activation of inflammation. These innate pathways include the clotting system, the complement system, and the kinin system. In response to tissue injury, the three systems complement each other, resulting in inflammation.

Cells of the Innate Immune System

The cells of the innate immune system include mast cells, macrophages, and granulocytes (Table 28.1). Together, mast cells and macrophages initiate inflammation by recognition of pathogens expressing pathogen-associated molecular patterns (PAMPs) and damage-associated molecular patterns (DAMPs; Figure 28.2). Pattern recognition receptors are present in both the membrane and the cytoplasm of these cells and include Toll-like receptors (TLR), nucleotide-binding-like receptors (NLR-like), and nucleotide oligomerization domain–like receptors (NOD-like). PAMPs are common to many organisms and both mast cells and macrophages express pattern recognition receptors that recognize PAMPs. TLRs present on these cells span the cell membrane and recognize PAMPs. NLR-like and nucleotide NOD-like receptors are cytoplasmic receptors that also recognize PAMPs and

DAMPs and, when activated, signal the cell to increase the production of cytokines and chemokines.[2]

Mast cells are present near surfaces and when active release histamine that, in turn, increases the inflammation by inducing vasodilation. Macrophages are members of the innate immune system and are derived from blood monocytes, which are white blood cells that can go on to differentiate into various immune cells (Table 28.1). These monocytes will leave the general circulation and migrate to specific tissues in the body where they can go on to differentiate into macrophages. The macrophage population is therefore highly diversified as macrophages will specialize based on the tissues in which they are found. A few types of common macrophages found in tissues throughout the body include alveolar macrophages found in lung alveoli, Kupffer cells found in the liver, and microglia found in the central nervous system. The main roles of

Table 28.1: Cell Functions

Type	Functions	Key
Basophils	• Migrate from blood to site of infection through chemotaxis • Mediate immune cell responses, prevent clotting and cause vasodilation • Involved in allergic response	
B cells	• Develop in bone marrow and mature in secondary lymphoid organs through antigen contact • Secrete antibodies against specific antigens • Maintain "memory" of a pathogen	
CD4+ T cells	• Recognize antigens presented by APC on MHC class 2 molecules • Release cytokines that mediate the response of other immune cells • Activate B cells and allow for antibody generation	
CD8+ T cells	• Recognize antigens presented on MHC class 1 molecules • Destroy cancerous cells and infected cells • Kill infected cells through cytokine release, cytotoxic granule release, and Fas/FasL interactions	

Cell Type	Functions	Key
Monocytes	• Circulate in peripheral blood until migration into surrounding tissues • Differentiate into macrophages and dendritic cells • Once differentiated, perform phagocytosis, release cytokines, and present antigens to other immune cells	
Dendritic cells	• Sample surrounding environment for pathogens • Process antigen material and present peptides on cell surface for other immune cells to recognize • Migrate to lymph nodes to activate other immune cells	
Natural killer cells	• Recognize receptors expressed by infected cells and cancerous cells • Kill infected cells and tumor cells • Secrete cytokines that enhance immune response of macrophages and dendritic cells	
Neutrophils	• Most abundant leukocyte • Migrate from blood to site of infection through chemotaxis • Fight invading microbes through phagocytosis and degranulation	
Eosinophils	• Migrate from blood to site of infection through chemotaxis • Release effector molecules to defend against viral and parasitic infections • Involved in allergic response and autoimmune disorders	

APC, antigen-presenting cells; MHC, major histocompatibility complex.

macrophages are to detect invading pathogens, phagocytose them, and destroy them by producing reactive oxygen species such as nitric oxide. Macrophages release tumor necrosis factor α (TNF-α), interleukins (ILs), interferons, and other cytokines that promote inflammation. The neutrophil PMN, also known as the polymorphonuclear neutrophil, is the predominant phagocytic cell early inflammation.[3] It exits the circulation through retracted endothelial junctions by a process called diapedesis and moves to the inflammatory site by chemotaxis.

Mediators of the Innate Immune System

Cytokines (which translates to "cell movement") are a group of small proteins used in cell signaling and are produced primarily by lymphocytes and macrophages, as well as by fibroblasts and vascular endothelial and epithelial cells. They activate the growth and differentiation of leukocytes and contribute to systemic inflammatory changes, such as fever. There are many types of cytokines, and they are classified loosely into chemokines, interferons, interleukins, lymphokines, and TNFs. The most important interleukins that initiate and promote inflammation are IL-1 and IL-6. IL-2, IL-8, and IL-12 and they are important for the activation of neutrophils and natural killer (NK) cells. Interferons, such as interferon gamma, are produced by cells that are infected by viruses. Once released from infected cells, interferons can stimulate neighboring healthy cells

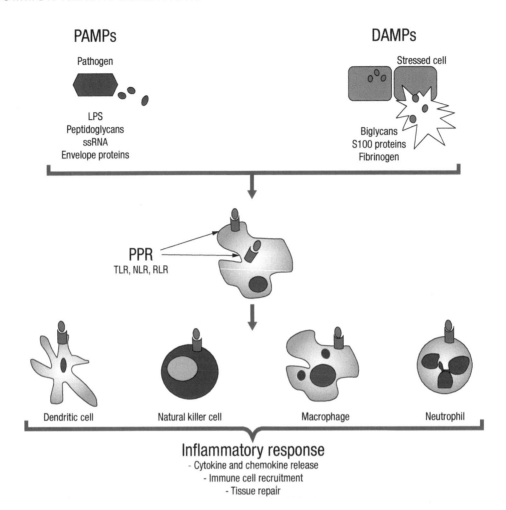

PAMPs

Pathogen

LPS
Peptidoglycans
ssRNA
Envelope proteins

DAMPs

Stressed cell

Biglycans
S100 proteins
Fibrinogen

PPR
TLR, NLR, RLR

Dendritic cell   Natural killer cell   Macrophage   Neutrophil

Inflammatory response
- Cytokine and chemokine release
- Immune cell recruitment
- Tissue repair

Figure 28.2: PAMPs (pathogen-associated molecular patterns) and DAMPS (damage-associated molecular patterns) are small molecular motifs that trigger an inflammatory response. Both these molecular signatures are conserved and recognized by Toll-like receptors on immune cells. This recognition results in the immediate immune activation and inflammation associated with infection and tissue injury.

to produce substances that prevent viral infection. TNF-α is produced when pattern recognition receptors (PRR) binding on the macrophages sends intracellular messengers to the nucleus that activate NF-κB, a transcription factor that, in turn, promotes the expression of other cytokines and chemokines. TNF-α has multiple proinflammatory effects and immune functions, such as promotion of apoptosis, chemotaxis, cellular proliferation, and inflammation.[4]

Control of the Innate Immune System

Controlling inflammation is as important as the initiation of inflammation. This involves regulating inflammatory cells and enzymes and containing the inflammatory response to the area of injury or infection. Anti-inflammatory cytokines, such as transforming growth factor–β (TGF–β) and IL–10, downregulate the inflammatory response. The TGF–β superfamily signaling plays a critical

role in the regulation of cell growth, differentiation, and development. TGF-β is produced predominantly by macrophages while IL-10 is produced by macrophages and T-helper (Th) 2 cells.

Mechanisms of Pathogen Elimination by the Innate Immune System

One of the main early mechanisms by which pathogens are eliminated is through the process of phagocytosis. In this multistep process, a phagocytic cell such as a macrophage surrounds a pathogen and uses its plasma membrane to engulf the pathogen or foreign debris, resulting in the destruction of the pathogens and foreign debris. The steps of phagocytosis include recognition and attachment, engulfment, the formation of a phagosome, the formation of a phagolysosome, and the eventual destruction of the pathogen or foreign debris. Phagocytic cells engulf microorganisms, enclosing them within phagocytic vacuoles

Antigen uptake
or synthesis

Antigen presentation

T-cell dependent
effector functions

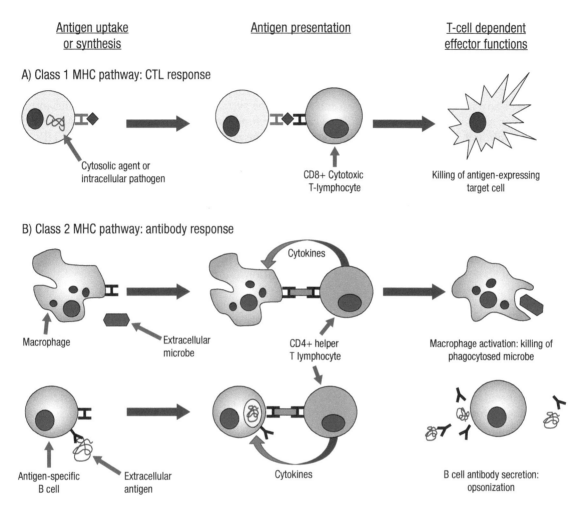

A) Class 1 MHC pathway: CTL response

Cytosolic agent or
intracellular pathogen

CD8+ Cytotoxic
T-lymphocyte

Killing of antigen-expressing
target cell

B) Class 2 MHC pathway: antibody response

Cytokines

Macrophage

Extracellular
microbe

CD4+ helper
T lymphocyte

Macrophage activation: killing of
phagocytosed microbe

Antigen-specific
B cell

Extracellular
antigen

Cytokines

B cell antibody secretion:
opsonization

Figure 28.3: Overview of the adaptive immune response: Antigen is presented to the immune system in context with MCH molecules. The two arms of the adaptive immune system, while not mutually exclusive, activate the killing of infected or damaged cells via the cytotoxic T-lymphocytic response or activate extracellular targeting of pathogens via the antibody response mediated by CD4+ T lymphocyte and B lymphocyte.

CTL, cytotoxic T-lymphocytic; MHC, major histocompatibility complex.

(phagolysosomes). The vacuoles contain toxins (especially metabolites of oxygen) and/or enzymes that kill and digest the microorganisms. Opsonization is the process by which pathogens are coated by complement C3b and antibodies and targeted for phagocytosis. This process, in addition to creating a target for the phagocytes, improves the binding and the process of phagocytosis.[5]

The innate response to parasites involves the eosinophils which release products that control the inflammatory response (Table 28.1). IL-5 plays a central role in inducing activation and recruitment of eosinophils to sites of infection, while eotaxin also promotes eosinophilia. Eosinophils are able to phagocytose parasites and destroy them. Other cells of innate immunity include dendritic cells which function as messengers between the innate and acquired (adaptive) immune systems, and NK cells that detect certain invaders and cancer cells.

The Adaptive Immune System

Adaptive (acquired) immunity is the third line of defense (Figure 28.3). It differs from inflammation and the innate response because it is slower to develop, more specific, and has a memory that makes it much longer lived. Following phagocytosis, portions of the pathogens are presented to the lymphocytes in the lymphoid tissue.

The Cells of the Adaptive Immune System

Lymphocytes are the primary cells of the adaptive immune system. There are two arms of the adaptive immune system, each with its own activation cascade. The two main types of lymphocytes—B lymphocytes and T lymphocytes—have distinct functions. B lymphocytes or B cells are responsible for humoral immunity that is mediated by circulating antibodies and targets extracellular pathogens in general (Figure 28.3). T cells are responsible for cell-mediated immunity, in which they kill targets directly or stimulate the activity of other leukocytes to kill cells harboring intracellular pathogens or abnormal cells. When there is a break in the innate immune system, which includes skin and mucosa, pathogens can enter the body. Many individuals carry *Neisseria meningitidis* in their nares. Some of these organisms can enter the body resulting in meningitis. Following the innate response, the adaptive immune response takes over and often results in control of the bacteria. This can be amplified and can happen sooner when the person has received the meningococcus vaccine, which trains the adaptive immune response to respond appropriately to the pathogen. In the case of HIV infection there is a failure of the adaptive immune response which results in acquired immunodeficiency.

The induction of an immune response, or clonal selection, begins when antigen enters the individual's body and interacts with antigen-presenting cells (APCs; e.g., dendritic cells, macrophages, B cells). To induce an optimal cellular or humoral immune response, APCs must present antigens to Th cells. The antigen is processed in the APCs and presented on the cell surface by molecules of the major histocompatibility complex (MHC). The specific MHC molecule (class I or class II) that presents antigen determines which cell will respond to that antigen. "Th" cells require that the antigen be presented in a complex with MHC class II molecules. MHC class II molecules are found only on APCs. "Tc" cells require that the antigen be presented by MHC class I molecules.

The T Lymphocytes

T lymphocytes or T cells are derived from multipotent hematopoietic stem cells present in the bone marrow, and they will ultimately go on to mature in the thymus (Table 28.1). A mature T cell will express T-cell receptors as well as their associated co-receptor—either CD4 or CD8. However, there are T cells that have been identified to have both the CD4 and CD8 receptors, termed "double-positive T cells."[6] As T cells are maturing in the thymus, the genes encoding the T-cell receptor will undergo rearrangement and this leads to the formation of different T cells, each expressing a unique T-cell receptor whose structure depends on the arrangement of receptor-encoding genes. Once rearrangement is completed and the T-cell receptors are expressed, maturing T cells will need to undergo both positive and negative selection before they can finish maturation. Undergoing positive and negative selection will ultimately decrease the likelihood of T cells attacking the body's own cells. At the end of maturation, the goal is to have produced T cells that express a variety of T-cell receptors that only bind to foreign antigens that are combined with self–major histocompatibility complexes I and II (MHC I and MHC II) on the surface of other immune cells such as dendritic

cells, macrophages, and B cells. If these T cells pass both positive and negative selection, they will then be able to complete maturation and become the various subsets of T cells, which include helper T cells, cytotoxic T cells, and regulatory T cells.[6] This component of the adaptive immune system, although slower, is specific and has memory function. The importance of the adaptive immune system is exemplified by two pathogens: HIV and *Staphylococcus*. In the case of HIV infection, the virus infects and kills CD4+ T cells. These cells are the gatekeepers of the immune system, and their destruction puts the entire system in disarray, resulting in immunodeficiency syndrome. In toxic shock syndrome, the toxins of *Staphylococcus aureus* can bypass the elegant signaling system characterizing adaptive immunity and can directly stimulate the immune response resulting in massive inflammation and tissue injury.

Helper T cells serve several purposes. They are needed to help activate B cells and macrophages as well as to help activate cytotoxic T cells so they can attack and eliminate infected host cells. To activate these various other immune system cells, helper T cells are activated by dendritic cells that have ingested a pathogen, broken up the antigen that was presented by the pathogen, and are now presenting a part of this antigen on the dendritic cell's own cell surface along with an associated MHC II molecule (Figure 28.3). An activated helper T cell will begin to divide rapidly and differentiate into memory T cells and effector T cells. Memory T cells will express the same T-cell receptors as the helper T cell they are derived from and will allow the body to mount a faster immune response should it become infected again with the same pathogen. Effector T cells, on the other hand, can release cytokines that can activate macrophages and cytotoxic T cells to begin fighting off an infection. These cytokines can also stimulate B cells to secrete specific types of antibodies. One of the most important roles of effector T cells is to activate B cells that are already bound to an antigen.

Cytotoxic T cells are a special type of T cell that can recognize and mount an immune response toward host cells that have been infected by a virus or bacteria (Table 28.1). These pathogens are protected from antibodies once they make their way into cells and therefore the cells themselves must be eliminated to rid the body of the invading pathogen. This action will be carried out by cytotoxic T cells. An activated cytotoxic T cell will proliferate and differentiate into another type of memory T cell, the effector T cell. These effector T cells also can induce apoptosis in the infected host cell after binding at the cell surface (Figure 28.3). Cytotoxic T cells can also recognize and mount a response to cancer cells. Regulatory T cells work to modify and control the body's overall immune response as well as to maintain the immune system's tolerance to self-antigens that are presented on cells throughout the body.[6]

Proteins called CD4 and CD8 are expressed on developing T cells. As the cell matures, it retains either the CD4 molecule or the CD8 molecule, but not both. Eventually CD4 cells develop into Th cells and CD8 cells become T-cytotoxic cells (Tc cells). Other mature T cells include T-regulatory cells (Treg cells) and memory cells. The generation of clonal diversity concludes when immunocompetent T and B cells migrate from the primary lymphoid organs into the circulation and secondary lymphoid organs to await antigen.

The B Lymphocytes

The B cell is the second of the two important lymphocytes that make up the adaptive immune system. Like T cells, B cells are formed from multipotent hematopoietic stem cells present in the bone marrow. After formation in the bone marrow, B cells move into the lymphatic system where they will go on to circulate throughout the body and continue to mature. A mature B cell that has not yet been bound to an antigen will express thousands of one specific type of antibody on its cell surface. These are commonly known as membrane-bound antibodies, and all antibodies on the surface of an individual B cell will have the same unique antigen-binding site. Other types of antibodies found on other B-cell surfaces will have different antigen-binding sites. During development, a rearrangement of the genes that encode the antibodies produced by the B cell will determine which type of antibody, and therefore which type of antigen-binding site, will be presented on the cell's surface. Rearrangement allows for a wide array of antibodies and antigen-binding sites to be produced, ultimately allowing the immune system to respond to a variety of invading pathogens.

A mature B cell must be activated by the binding of the antigen that the specific type of antibodies on the B-cell surface can recognize. Once the B cell is bound to the antigen, the cell can phagocytose the pathogen, break it down, and present a piece of the antigen on its cell surface attached to an MHC II molecule. At this point, helper T cell-derived effector T cells that can recognize and bind this same antigen will bind to the antigen on the B cell's surface. This interaction completes the activation of the B cell by allowing it to begin to proliferate and differentiate (Figure 28.1). Thus, after binding an antigen, engulfing the associated pathogen, and presenting a part of the antigen on its cell surface for an effector T cell to bind to, the B cell can now officially begin to divide and differentiate into effector B cells and memory B cells. Each of these types of cells plays a unique and crucial role in mounting an immune response toward an invading pathogen. Along with producing many memory B cells, an activated B cell will also produce effector B cells. Effector B cells will essentially become antibody-producing factories. An effector B cell will produce the same antibodies as the B

cell it is derived from, but instead of inserting these antibodies in the membrane, it will instead secrete these antibodies so that they can enter circulation and mark the associated pathogen for elimination by other immune cells.

AGING AND IMMUNE FUNCTION

Innate immunity is the first aspect of the immune response to develop and the last to be lost as organisms age. However, even innate immunity decreases with aging, and this is due to the process of immunosenescence. Cellular senescence is considered to be a pre-encoded cancer suppressor mechanism characterized by cell cycle arrest, loss of proliferation capacity, global cell enlargement, characteristic misshaped nuclei, presence of chromatin foci with persistent DNA damage response, increased nuclear factor-κB (NF-κB) signaling, and resistance to apoptosis, which occurs in immune cells as well[7,8] (Figure 28.2). There are many theories on the cause of this process and one such theory involves the hematopoietic stem cells (HSC).[9] As HSCs age they give rise to immune cells that exhibit reduced homing, as well as altered processes of differentiation. This weakened innate immune response increases the risk of infection in the older adult. Specifically, the decreased activity of HSCs causes several cellular components of innate immunity to be deficient in number (e.g., tissue macrophages) or to have diminished activity (e.g., neutrophil chemotaxis, degranulation, and phagocytosis). Another theory involves an age-related decrease in the expression and function of several TLRs, which reduces the ability of the innate immune system to recognize pathogens and present antigens in the context of MHC. The function of the transcription factor NF-κB is also altered with decreased expression of adhesion molecules on immune cells and reduces the ability of cells to attach and destroy pathogens. Immune cell senescence, as with generalized cellular senescence, can be triggered by many stimuli[10,11] (Figure 28.2). These include critical telomere shortening, persistent DNA damage, oncogene activation or inactivation, epigenetic alterations, mitochondrial dysfunction, and exposure to DAMPs that are released by stressed cells. There exists some evidence that the phenotypic manifestations induced by different triggers are heterogeneous. In addition, other factors such as a history of cancer, chemotherapy, HIV infection, and therapies for chronic illnesses also accelerate the aging of the immune system.[12]

Inflammaging

Over the course of life, the immune system reacts to some pathogens more often than others. In addition, the immune system loses some of its regulatory capacity, which results in unregulated tissue inflammation known as inflammaging (Figure 28.4).[13,14] "Inflammaging" is defined as a chronic, sterile, low-grade

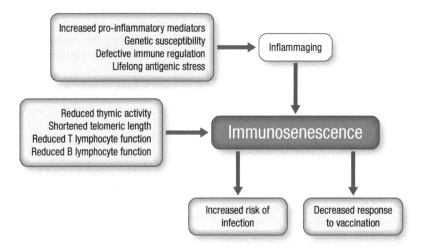

Figure 28.4: Factors influencing the development of immunosenescence and inflammaging. A host of factors contribute to inflammaging and immunosenescence, most of which are currently nonmodifiable factors. More research is needed into identifying means to slow the process and improve health in older adults.

inflammation that occurs with aging. This is usually accompanied by increased levels of several cytokines such as IL-1, IL-1 receptor antagonist protein (IL-1RN), IL-6, IL-8, IL-13, IL-18, C-reactive protein (CRP), IFNα and IFNβ, transforming growth factor-β (TGF-β), TNF and its soluble receptors (TNF receptor superfamily members 1A and 1B), and serum amyloid A, as well as reactive oxygen species.[15] Because these molecules are in circulation, they have a systemic effect on the body and an increased risk for chronic inflammatory diseases (e.g., heart disease, metabolic syndrome, diabetes) that occur with aging. There are many likely causes for the acceleration of this process that have been studied extensively in recent years. These include genetic susceptibility, central obesity, increased gut permeability, changes to microbiota composition, cellular senescence, NLRP3 inflammasome activation, oxidative stress caused by dysfunctional mitochondria, immune cell dysregulation, and chronic infections. In addition, part of inflammaging is caused by chronic infections (e.g., human immunodeficiency virus [HIV] or human cytomegalovirus CMV] infection) and intrinsic defective mechanisms in immune cells that might involve metabolic stress, as well as age-related changes in microRNA transcription.[16]

Regenerative Capacity

Other factors affect innate immunity and wound healing in older adults. Older adults often sustain injuries due to decreased mobility and sensation, as well as changes in skin integrity. Aging also alters the tissue microenvironment and macrophage function through changes in

wound healing angiogenesis and fibrosis. Collagen fibers become thicker, and a certain percentage of elastin is lost, further contributing to a loss of protection. The regenerative capability of the skin is maintained with aging, but the epidermis undergoes age-associated changes that include atrophy of the underlying capillaries and a loss of subcutaneous fat. In addition, older adults often suffer from venous stasis and arterial insufficiency. The decrease of perfusion makes older adults more susceptible than younger people to the adverse effects of hypoxia in the wound bed, as well as reduction in chemotaxis of neutrophils to the site of injury. Fibroblasts also have a slower rate of proliferation over the course of aging, and therefore, wound healing is attenuated as fibroblasts are important in scar formation.[17] Taken together, the process of healing is delayed.

Aging and the Adaptive Immune Response

Adaptive immune function also decreases with age as a result of changes in both lymphocyte function and relative lymphocyte populations due to decreased function of HSCs. At the cellular level, the most prominent features of immunosenescence include a decrease in the number of naïve lymphocytes, which are cells that have not yet encountered an antigen.[7] This is a result both of a reduction in thymic output of T cells and of fewer bone marrow early progenitor B cells.[18,19] Additionally, there is an increase in oligoclonally expanded and functionally incompetent memory lymphocytes due to repeated exposure to common antigens such as those of CMV and other chronic viral infections. Because of these changes, the diversity of the antigen-recognition repertoire is markedly decreased with age, recusing the ability of these cells to detect and recognize a wide variety of antigens. Studies have shown TCR Vβ chain usage in human peripheral T cells and the antigen-recognition repertoire of T cells decreases from approximately 108 in young adults to 106 in the older adults.[20] The causes of age-associated decline in the generation of naïve cells are likely to be multifactorial and to involve changes in growth factors and/or hormones, hematopoietic progenitor cells, and their surrounding microenvironment as well as other comorbid conditions.

The accumulation of memory cells with age may reflect an adaptive response to the decline of production of naïve lymphocytes through homeostatic expansion as well as the cumulative effect of past and persistent viral infections.[21] These changes make the older individual more susceptible to infectious disease and cancer and less able to respond to vaccination, as discussed at the end of this chapter.

While many of these changes are age-related, one must recognize that chronic illnesses have the same effects as aging and can, in fact, accelerate the aging process. The ability to respond to new antigens diminishes as the number of peripheral naïve T and B cells declines due to the decrease in the diversity of the TCR and BCR repertoire. The thymus atrophies from infancy, resulting in an exponential decline in T-cell production with a half-life of about 16 years.[22] This is accompanied by decreased production of thymic hormones and a subsequently decreased capacity to mediate T-cell differentiation. The capacity of Th cells to produce IL-2 declines, which is needed for proliferation. Thus, there is a shift in the populations of T-cell subtypes with Tc cells significantly outnumbering Th cells. Some subsets of memory T cells are lost, thus reducing the repertoire of antigens that the T cells are able to recognize. However, age-related changes in the composition of memory CD4+ T-cell subsets such as central and effector memory cells have also been implicated for the impaired immune response to both viral infections such as the influenza virus and to vaccines. Clonal expansion of CD8+ T cells, especially those CD28− CD8+ T cells, presents another prominent age-associated change. These are differentiated CD8 T cells that lack a second receptor. As a result, there is a reduction of naïve CD8+ T-cell output, and some degree of oligoclonal expansion of CD8+ T cells with age is commonly observed in healthy older adults. Such changes may reflect a compensatory mechanism to control latent viral infections or to fill available T-cell space in the lymphoid organs. When clonal expansion reaches a critical level, the diversity of the T-cell repertoire is reduced, and the ability of immune protection to new infection is compromised. In fact, clonal expansion of CD28− CD8+ T cells appears to be directly responsible for increased infections and a failed response to vaccines in the older adults.

B-cell function is also altered with age as shown by decreases in specific antibody production in response to antigenic challenge. This is a direct result of loss of BCR repertoire, but a decrease in the number of circulating memory B cells is also observed. In older people, there is an increase in a subset of B cells called age-associated B cells (ABCs). ABCs are paradoxically associated with an increased presentation of antigen, a release of cytokines, and secretion of antibodies; however, a significant proportion of these antibodies are autoantibodies and contribute to autoimmune disease.[23] This excess of antibodies also adds to inflammaging, which then augments the nonspecific inflammation associated with aging.

GUT MUCOSAL IMMUNE FUNCTION IN AGING

The gastrointestinal (GI) tract carries out the functions of food processing and digestion, nutrient absorption, and expulsion of waste in addition to harboring about 90% of the body's lymphocytes within the gut-associated lymphoid tissue (GALT).[24] The intestinal structure is composed of simple columnar epithelium, mucosa, submucosa, smooth muscle, and serosa. Glandular epithelium is present along the entire length of the gut in the form of goblet cells, which secrete mucus that lubricates the passage of food and protects the tissue from digestive enzymes. This mucous layer is also home to the millions of microbes that inhabit the gut. As one ages, many changes occur in the microenvironment of the small intestine. These include alterations in the composition, pH, and thickness of the mucous layer as well as changes in the composition of the microbiome. Inflammaging occurs in the gut and mucosal surfaces as well and determines how we age at the epithelial level.[25] In general, the cytokine expression in older adults at the mucosal level is increased. It may be the result of reduced epithelial barrier integrity resulting in increased bacterial translocation, especially in the context of other comorbidities.[26] This, in turn, may result in increased exposure to LPS and the resulting immune activation.[27] Additionally, a dysregulated Th17-type effector function of immune cells is associated with leaky gut and inflammatory phenotype of aging.[27,28] A range of environmental factors including smoking, infections such as CMV, and obesity may contribute to systemic low-grade inflammatory activity in older individuals.[21,29] The physiologic conditions caused by other viruses such as HIV, Epstein–Barr virus, and herpes zoster, among others, also play a role in inflammation. In the context of chronic infection and other comorbid conditions, the cytotoxic T-lymphocytic (CTL) response to CMV accelerates immunosenescence and reduces the immune responses originating from the mucosa.

While absorption abnormalities in the aged are common, the effects of aging on gut function and reconstitution following injury are not fully understood and have yet to be significantly investigated. Disorders of the GI tract in older adults include diarrhea and constipation, adverse reaction to drugs, esophageal and swallowing disorders, gastric and peptic ulcer disease, gastroparesis, and increased intestinal permeability.[30] A study utilizing the baboon model has shown that gastrointestinal permeability was higher in colonic biopsies in aging monkeys. Compared to younger animals, the GI epithelium of older animals showed decreased expression of tight junction proteins including Zonula Occludens-1, OCLN, and junctional adhesion molecule-A (JAM-A). Furthermore, CLDN-2, a pore-forming tight-junction protein, showed increased expression. Inflammatory cytokines interferon gamma (IFN-γ), IL-6, and IL-1β were also found to be increased in colonic biopsies from old baboons compared to young baboons and have previously been shown to directly hinder tight junction complex formation.[30] These studies indicate that increased colonic permeability via age-associated remodeling of intestinal epithelial tight junction proteins may be an important component of gastrointestinal dysfunction.

Role of Gut Microbiome

The effects of aging on the gut microbiome are also an important component of immunosenescence. The extensive colonization of the gut has been associated with many disorders and health outcomes, including healthy aging. In the colon alone there are more than 1 trillion microbes that exert an effect on the mucosa and are affected by the secretions of the mucosa. Studies have demonstrated major shifts in bacterial species in the aged as compared to younger controls.[31] Aging is associated with an increase in facultative anaerobes and a reduction in beneficial bacteria, such as bacteroides and bifidobacteria.[31,32] Aging is also associated with decreased stability and increased diversity of the gut microbiota. The shift in the diversity of the intestinal microbiota toward conditionally pathogenic and primarily pathogenic microorganisms changes the local intestinal chemical and immunologic parameters and induces the translocation of the gut bacteria into local lymphoid tissue, thus increasing the systemic microbial load.[27] These factors contribute to an increase in permeability of the intestinal and blood-brain barriers and the penetration of pathologic microflora and their metabolites into the brain. These inflammatory changes may contribute to diseases such as Alzheimer's disease.[33] Bacteria such as *Lactobacillus plantarum* have shown promise in animal studies to improve barrier function by reducing IL-1β associated inflammation. This highlights the role of probiotics, prebiotics, and other supplements that may be needed to improve health in older adults at the mucosal interphase.

THE EFFECTS OF SEX HORMONES ON IMMUNOSENESCENCE AND INFLAMMAGING

Gender influences the immune system through sex hormones and the endocrine system. Women have an increased risk of developing autoimmune conditions which may be influenced by sex hormones. Following menopause, the levels of estrogen in a woman decrease drastically and this has been shown to mitigate immune responses and predispose older women to infections and disease. During menopause, there is also an increase in pro-inflammatory serum markers (IL-1, IL-6, TNF-α), an increased response of the body's cells to these cytokines, a decrease in CD4 T and B lymphocytes, and a decrease in the cytotoxic activity of NK cells.[34,35] These inflammatory changes are nonspecific and often occur in the absence of a pathogen, thus contributing to inflammaging.

The aging process affects sexual dimorphism regarding immunocompetence and disease susceptibility. As women age and lose the positive effects of estradiol, aging women lose their immunological advantage. Under some conditions, women have increased susceptibility and mortality, especially in infections such as hepatitis, meningococcus, and pneumococcus. Protective effects of estrogen are thought to enable premenopausal women to clear the hepatitis C virus, and women progress slower through the disease than age-matched men. After menopause, these sex-dependent advantages are lost and treatment efficacy was severely decreased.[36] In addition, the secretion of IL-10, an anti-inflammatory cytokine, was increased in older women but not in age-matched men. Alternatively, in infections, such as influenza and COVID-19, in which the immune response is the primary cause for morbidity and mortality, postmenopausal women may have a slight advantage over their male counterparts.[37]

AGING AND INFECTIOUS DISEASES

The most common infections that occur in seniors include bacterial pneumonia, influenza, skin infections, gastrointestinal infections, and urinary tract infection. Of these, bacterial pneumonia is most common. Taken together, these infections are some of the leading causes of morbidity and mortality in older adults. A decade ago, infectious diseases were the leading cause of death in individuals older than age 65. With the advent of vaccinations and antibiotics, cardiovascular disease, cancer, and stroke now are the leading causes of death. However, immunosenescence, comorbid chronic diseases like diabetes, and alterations in normal physiologic organ functions may still modify the frequency and severity of infections in older patients. Mechanisms such as increased body temperature and pain may be less obvious in older adults and severe infections of the respiratory and urinary tracts may be missed, resulting in severe sepsis at the time of diagnosis. Due to various comorbid conditions, surgery, and other factors, hospitalized older adult patients are more susceptible to catheter-associated infections and *C. difficile* infections as discussed in this section.

Respiratory Infections

Respiratory infection (most commonly pneumonia) is the most common infection in older adults. *Streptococcus pneumoniae* is the most common pathogen associated with pneumonia. The rates of hospitalization are also higher in older adults with pneumonia compared to younger patients, and these rates rise exponentially for patients in nursing homes.[38] This has been especially true with severe acute respiratory syndrome coronavirus 2 (SARS-CoV-2) infections. In this age group, the symptoms are not clearly indicative of any one diagnosis and may include fatigue, anorexia, falls, delirium, and confusion as opposed to the standard symptoms such as fever, chills, productive cough, and shortness of breath.[39] These symptoms in an older patient with suspected pneumonia need to be investigated by chest x-rays and a computed tomography (CT) scan to rule out other causes. Additional diagnostics may be needed if pneumonia is accompanied by sepsis or if sepsis is suspected. The systemic inflammatory response (SIRS) criteria and the CURB-65 (confusion, urea, respiratory rate, blood pressure, 65 years) also help in the determination of severity and decisions on hospitalization. Repeated episodes of pneumonia may be the result of underlying conditions such as lung cancer or chronic obstructive pulmonary disease. These underlying conditions also predispose the patient to other less common pathogens such as *Haemophilus influenzae*, *Moraxella catarrhalis*, and *Legionella pneumophila*, as well as antibiotic-resistant bacteria. Viral pneumonia may be caused by pathogens like influenza, SARS-CoV-2 and rhinovirus, and often include a component of bacterial pneumonia as well, especially in hospitalized patients. Infections like influenza have a much higher mortality rate in older adults compared to younger patients. In the 2018 to 2019 flu season, people older than 65 years had an influenza-related mortality rate of over 48% compared to 9% in patients between the ages of 50 and 64.

Recently, infection with SARS-CoV-2 has resulted in significant morbidity and mortality in older adults.[40] The COVID-19 pandemic has been especially devastating to older adults and those living in nursing homes and care facilities. There is an increased risk of hospitalization or death as the age increases. As age advances, the disruption of both innate and adaptive arms of the immune system, the continual production of inflammatory mediators and cytokines, and aberrant ciliary function and ciliary ultrastructural anomalies together contribute to the increased susceptibility to SARS-CoV-2 in older adults. In addition to a higher susceptibility due to aging, epidemiologic studies revealed sex-specific differences in the incidence and mortality in humans after SARS-CoV-2 infection, with males experiencing higher mortality compared to females. Interestingly, this sex-dependent increase in disease severity after pathogenic SARS-CoV-2 infection is more pronounced with advancing age. As with all the other infections discussed here, the symptoms of COVID-19 in older adults are not limited to the classic fever, insistent cough, and shortness of breath but also include confusion, loss of orientation, excessive sleep, loss of appetite, loss of balance, and falls. On admission, dyspnea, lymphocytopenia, comorbidities including cardiovascular disease and chronic obstructive pulmonary disease, and acute respiratory distress syndrome were predictive of a poor outcome. The long-term effects of COVID-19 on the health of older patients are not known. In the aged, immune responses to vaccination are also often weak or defective whereas autoimmunity increases. Therefore, in designing vaccines against SARS-CoV-2, it will be important to consider that older people may not respond as well to vaccines as younger individuals.

Urinary Tract Infections

Urinary tract infections (UTIs) are the second-most common type of infection in the older population. In the absence of typical clinical symptoms of an infection, it is important to differentiate asymptomatic bacteriuria from symptomatic bacteriuria. The development of UTIs in older adults is so insidious that it is the cause of sepsis in about 30% of cases.[41] In hospitalized patients, an indwelling catheter is often associated with UTI and the most common organisms include *Escherichia coli*, *Candida spp.*, *Enterococcus spp.*, and *Pseudomonas aeruginosa*. As with pneumonia, in these groups of patients, with fever and/or other signs compatible with infection, urine and blood cultures should always be obtained. These labs should be obtained even in the absence of classic symptoms. A UTI that is refractory to antibiotics should be tested for antibiotic-resistant strains of bacteria. Multidrug resistance occurs particularly in the gram-negative bacteria and includes extended-spectrum beta-lactamase production and/or carbapenem-resistant *Enterobacteriaceae* and recently emerging colistin-resistant gram-negative bacilli. If a fungal infection such as candida is suspected, an indwelling catheter is usually the origin, and management involves replacing or removing the catheter. Minimizing the duration of catheter use is often useful in preventing or managing UTIs in older persons.

Systemic Infections

Bacteremia is often associated with central lines in older patients while sepsis is associated with respiratory tract infection or UTIs. About 65% of sepsis cases occur in older adults over the age of 65 with a fatality rate of 27.7%, which is higher than the general population. Methicillin-resistant *S. aureus* (MRSA) is the most common pathogen in bacteremia. In this case as well, the symptoms are subtle, vague, and include cognitive impairment and functional disability. In some studies, this physical and cognitive decline persisted for up to 8 years following the sepsis diagnosis and treatment.[42] Sepsis not only affects the patient but also family members or caregivers. It has been reported that especially wives of older sepsis survivors were at greater risk of developing depression, which demonstrates the importance of recognizing stress in family caregivers.

Gastrointestinal Infections

GI infections trail UTIs in older adults in terms of incidence. However, they are associated with significantly higher mortality. Older adults are more prone to dehydration and electrolyte disturbances that are associated with GI infections. The increased incidence of infections with pathogens, such as *C. difficile,* is due to the increased rates of hospitalization in older adults in addition to antibiotic use and immunosuppression.[43] A recent analysis indicated that overall health status, including infections; healthcare utilization; acute conditions in the past year; and frailty indicators are the most important determinants of *C. difficile* infection (CDI) risk in an older population. Thus, an older person in critical condition will be more likely to have a severe CDI than will a person of similar age or older without any comorbidity or previous hospitalization.

Risk Factors

Other chronic diseases that predispose older adults include chronic kidney disease, heart failure, and lung failure, along with physiologic changes caused by aging, frailty, and nutritional problems; these which lead to an increased frequency and severity of infections in geriatric patients. The incidence of chronic and end-stage renal disease and the need for dialysis increases with age. It remains controversial whether older patients with peritoneal dialysis have an increased risk of peritonitis than their younger counterparts. There is consensus that the risk of recurrence of peritonitis and short-term mortality is high in this group of older adults due to the presence of atypical organisms associated with peritonitis such as fungi, atypical mycobacterium, *Listeria monocytogenes*, and others. Heart failure is another chronic disease whose incidence increases with age. Older patients who are hospitalized for the management of heart failure are more prone to infection due to multiple organ system disorders. Pneumonia, intra-abdominal acid-related peritonitis, and dermatitis due to lower extremity edema are among the most common infections in these patients.

Infections such as tuberculosis and infective endocarditis are also common in older persons. Tuberculosis tends to be extrapulmonary in older patients.

Additional factors play a role in the increased susceptibility to infections. Venous stasis predisposes patients to stasis ulcers that are chronic nonhealing ulcers. Conditions such as diabetes predispose patients to ulcers in the feet that may go unnoticed for extended periods of time and provide a focus for infection. These can progress to osteomyelitis as well. Arterial insufficiency also allows for chronic nonhealing ulcers as well as pressure ulcers in nonmobile patients. Taken together, all infections account for about 30% of mortality seen in older adults prior to the COVID-19 epidemic.

VACCINATION AND AGING

While age-related changes of the immune system contribute to increased incidence and severity of infections in older adults this is accentuated by the suboptimal ability of older adult individuals to respond to vaccines.[44,45] Vaccination is the most effective measure to prevent infections, and vaccination recommendations in most countries include specific guidelines for older adults. For example, vaccination against influenza and *Streptococcus pneumoniae* is usually recommended for persons with underlying diseases and for older adults (Table 28.2). Vaccination against herpes zoster is also recommended. Additionally, several vaccines are recommended for all adults, which include regular booster shots against tetanus/diphtheria/pertussis/polio, and some vaccines are recommended for specific groups, for example, vaccination against tick-borne encephalitis in endemic areas or travel vaccines.[46] Decisions on these vaccinations are made after serious consideration of the risk of exposure to these illnesses.[47]

Much of the reduced response to vaccination can be attributed to immunosenescence characterized by a decrease in T-cell numbers and TCR diversity. This reduced ability of T cells to recognize pathogens results in increased susceptibility to novel and new pathogens such as West Nile virus or SARS-CoV-2 and to any potential vaccine toward a novel pathogen. A muted immune response to known and recurrent pathogens such as influenza is due to the decrease in naïve T cells, as well as memory T-cell dysfunction. One proposed mechanism includes the Th17 response that has a central role in the production of T cells and the maintenance of their functionality at mucosal surfaces. The declines in efficiency with age are due to the combination of the limited life span of naïve cells, reduced thymic function, and decrease in recruitment of naïve cells into activated and memory T-cell pools. Despite these change, vaccination is strongly recommended in older adults. The commonly recommended vaccines in the United States are outlined in Table 28.2.

Table 28.2: Vaccinations Recommended in Older Adults

Vaccine	Pathogen	Age Group and Frequency
Influenza inactivated (IIV) or Influenza recombinant (RIV)	Influenza A and Influenza B	Annual for all age groups
Tetanus, diphtheria, pertussis (Tdap or Td)	*Clostridium tetani, Corynebacterium diphtheriae, Bordetella pertussis*	Every 10 years for all ages
Zoster recombinant (RZV) (preferred) or Zoster live (ZVL)	Varicella zoster	2 doses greater than 50 yrs Or 1 dose greater than 65 yrs
Pneumococcal polysaccharide (PPSV23)	*Streptococcus pneumoniae*	I dose greater than 65 yrs
COVID vaccine	SARS CoV2	For all age groups greater than 12 years

Most currently used vaccines are less effective in older individuals due to their decreased immunogenicity. There are many ways to improve the response to vaccination that include higher doses and using adjuvants and alternate delivery routes. These have been shown to be partially effective, but the final response is still lower than that in younger adults. These potential strategies to improve their immunogenicity were all implemented for influenza vaccines, where they induced moderately higher antibody concentrations.

SPECIAL CONSIDERATIONS IN INFECTION CONTROL IN OLDER ADULTS

Because the geriatric population is a heterogeneous group of patients ranging from healthy active adults to patients with chronic illnesses, care and infection control in this group is of utmost importance. The first and most important measure is to limit surgical/invasive interventions to the most essential and for the shortest possible duration. These interventions may include central lines and urinary catheterizations. This effectively reduces the risk of nosocomial infections. In addition, early mobilization and feeding of patients also improves outcomes. Because people do not always present with the common signs and symptoms of infection, early detection of infections is also important. Aphasia, hearing loss, and cognitive impairment may further complicate our ability to diagnose and treat older adults.

Clinical trials have indicated that in the in-patient setting the following infection control policies are effective. First, vaccines against influenza, pneumococcus, and diphtheria/tetanus have effectively reduced rates of hospitalization.[48] Second, hand hygiene plays an important role in reducing MRSA and VRE infections. For example, *C. difficile* infection has been shown to be successfully controlled through the use of a restrictive antibiotic policy.

Finally, team-based care of older adults, including in the setting of infectious diseases, is effective in the successful management of care. Well-implemented team-based care has the potential to improve the comprehensiveness, coordination, efficiency, effectiveness, and value of care, as well as the satisfaction of patients and providers. Research also links patient-centered care to positive outcomes, including improved physician–patient communication and relationships, higher patient satisfaction, better recall of information and treatment adherence, better recovery, and improved health outcomes. Thus, using evidence-based care in geriatrics and involving a team that includes family caregivers is essential for improving outcomes. In summary, there are many aspects of medicine that are unique to geriatrics, and they can be used to optimize care for this population.

CONCLUSION

The effects of aging on immune function are not completely understood. The main mechanism for immune dysfunction is immunosenescence, which is accentuated by the process of inflammaging. This results in an increased risk of respiratory infections, including COVID-19. Although the effectiveness of vaccines is less than optimal, vaccination is still one of the key means of prevention of infections and is a means to improve quality of life in older adults.

REFERENCES

References for this chapter are online and available at https://connect.springerpub.com/content/book/978-0-8261-8414-6/part/part01/toc-part/ch28.

Index